# Aging: Clinical Perspectives on Spatial Memory and Emotional Perception

# Aging: Clinical Perspectives on Spatial Memory and Emotional Perception

Editor: Robyn Parker

MURPHY & MOORE
www.murphy-moorepublishing.com

www.murphy-moorepublishing.com

MURPHY & MOORE

**Cataloging-in-Publication Data**

Aging : clinical perspectives on spatial memory and emotional perception / edited by Robyn Parker.
p. cm.
Includes bibliographical references and index.
ISBN 978-1-63987-030-1
1. Older people--Diseases--Treatment. 2. Older people--Health and hygiene. 3. Cognitive neuroscience.
4. Clinical neuropsychology. 5. Aging--Psychological aspects. I. Parker, Robyn.
RC953.5 .A35 2022
615.547--dc23



Murphy & Moore Publishing,
1 Rockefeller Plaza,
New York City, NY 10020, USA

ISBN 978-1-63987-030-1 (Hardback)

# Contents

# Preface

The gradual process due to which people become older is termed as aging. It is associated with a plethora of biological, psychological, physiological, environmental and behavioral changes. Emotions are considered to be vital to the healthy functioning of the human body. There have been various studies on the impact of aging upon emotions as well as its effect on perception, experience and memory. Some theories state that there is a deterioration of emotional function among the elderly population. On the other hand, there are theories and researches which suggest that the ability of solving emotional problems increases with age. Spatial memory refers to the cognitive process which helps a person to remember different locations along with the spatial relations between them. It deteriorates in most adults after the age of 60. This book includes some of the vital pieces of work being conducted across the world, on various topics related to aging and emotional perception. The readers would gain knowledge that would broaden their perspective about this area of research. This book will prove to be immensely beneficial to students and researchers in this field.

This book is the end result of constructive efforts and intensive research done by experts in this field. The aim of this book is to enlighten the readers with recent information in this area of research. The information provided in this profound book would serve as a valuable reference to students and researchers in this field.

At the end, I would like to thank all the authors for devoting their precious time and providing their valuable contribution to this book. I would also like to express my gratitude to my fellow colleagues who encouraged me throughout the process.

**Editor**

# 1

# Age-related differences in neural recruitment during the use of cognitive reappraisal and selective attention as emotion regulation strategies

***Eric S. Allard* and Elizabeth A. Kensinger***

*Cognitive and Affective Neuroscience Laboratory, Department of Psychology, Boston College, Chestnut Hill, MA, USA*

**Edited by:**
*Natalie Ebner, University of Florida, USA*

**Reviewed by:**
*Natalie Ebner, University of Florida, USA*
*Nichole Lighthall, Duke University, USA*
*Brittany Shane Cassidy, Brandeis University, USA*

***Correspondence:**
*Eric S. Allard, Cognitive and Affective Neuroscience Laboratory, Department of Psychology, Boston College, 140 Commonwealth Avenue, Chestnut Hill, MA 02467, USA*
*e-mail: eric.allard@bc.edu*

The present study examined age differences in the timing and neural recruitment within lateral and medial PFC while younger and older adults hedonically regulated their responses to unpleasant film clips. When analyses focused on activity during the emotional peak of the film clip (the most emotionally salient portion of the film), several age differences emerged. When comparing regulation to passive viewing (combined effects of selective attention and reappraisal) younger adults showed greater regulation related activity in lateral PFC (DLPFC, VLPFC, OFC) and medial PFC (ACC) while older adults showed greater activation within a region DLPFC. When assessing distinct effects of the regulation conditions, an ANOVA revealed a significant Age × Regulation Condition interaction within bilateral DLPFC and ACC; older adults but not young adults showed greater recruitment within these regions for reappraisal than selective attention. When examining activity at the onset of the film clip and at its emotional peak, the timing of reappraisal-related activity within VLPFC differed between age groups: younger adults showed greater activity at film onset while older adults showed heightened activity during the peak. Our results suggest that older adults rely more heavily on PFC recruitment when engaging cognitively demanding reappraisal strategies while PFC-mediated regulation might not be as task-specific for younger adults. Older adults' greater reliance on cognitive control processing during emotion regulation may also be reflected in the time needed to implement these strategies.

**Keywords: aging, emotion regulation, fMRI, selective attention, reappraisal**

## INTRODUCTION

Despite normative declines in several areas of functioning (e.g., cognition and health) older adults report relatively high levels of emotional well-being (Carstensen and Mikels, 2005). One prevailing theory in the psychology of human aging suggests that older adults are motivated to maximize emotional well-being due to limits in future time perspective (Carstensen et al., 1999). Self-report studies have shown that older adults are more motivated to regulate emotion as compared to their younger counterparts (Kennedy et al., 2004; Kliegel et al., 2007). Furthermore, this enhanced motivation can be shown in reported attempts to actively enhance well-being through the use of particular emotion regulation strategies (Gross et al., 1997).

One of the most studied regulatory strategies is cognitive reappraisal. Cognitive reappraisal is a strategy that involves the reinterpretation of a stimulus/situation in order to change its meaning and emotional impact. Reappraisal draws upon processes associated with cognitive control and executive functioning (Ochsner and Gross, 2005). Several neuroimaging studies have identified a series of brain systems involved in active attempts to reappraise affect including dorsolateral, ventrolateral, and dorsomedial prefrontal cortex (PFC) and posterior parietal cortex (Ochsner et al., 2004; Kalisch, 2009; Winecoff et al., 2011; Silvers et al., 2013). These aforementioned regions have been shown to correspond with specific cognitive control processes likely to support emotion regulation (Ochsner and Gross, 2008). In a recent meta-analysis, Buhle et al. (2013) observed activity in regions of dorsolateral (DLPFC), ventrolateral (VLPFC), and dorsomedial (DMPFC) prefrontal cortex during reappraisal tasks. Their results supported predictions that DLPFC activation may support the manipulation of affective appraisals in working memory, VLPFC may aid the selection and inhibition of appraisals (e.g., selecting a non-affective appraisal or positive reappraisal while trying to inhibit a negative appraisal), and DMPFC may reflect processes related to updating the success of chosen appraisals (e.g., was the desired affective state obtained?). Older age is associated with declines in volumetric gray matter in several PFC regions (Raz et al., 2004; Grieve et al., 2005; Fjell et al., 2009), raising questions regarding whether older adults are able to use reappraisal strategies as successfully as younger adults (see Gross et al., 1997; John and Gross, 2004; Urry and Gross, 2010 for this debate).

Very few studies have directly assessed age differences in neural recruitment when performing specific emotion regulation strategies. Current evidence suggests that older adults activate PFC regions to a lesser extent than younger adults during hedonic regulation (e.g., diminishing negative affect) and that this limited activation might relate to older adults' reduced success at deploying reappraisal-type strategies. For instance, Opitz et al.

(2012) had a group of younger and older adults perform hedonic and non-hedonic reappraisal (decrease and increase emotional reactions) in response to negative images in a series of fMRI tasks. In this study, older adults showed reduced DMPFC and VLPFC activation when reappraising negative images as compared to younger adults. Furthermore, diminished activation in VLPFC among older adults was accompanied by difficulty in decreasing negative responses to those images. Similar results were observed in another recent study in which older adults reported more negative affect in response to negative images when attempting to downreglate negative reactions as compared to younger adults (Winecoff et al., 2011). Furthermore, in this study, older adults showed reduced activation in a region of VLPFC when reappraising negative images as compared to younger adults. Taken together, these results suggest that older adults may be less effective than their younger adult counterparts in using reappraisal strategies to decrease negative affect (see also Tucker et al., 2012), perhaps because reappraisal relies on cognitive processes within lateral PFC that diminish with age (e.g., diminished VLPFC recruitment corresponding to a difficulty with inhibiting prepotent negative responses; Silvers et al., 2013).

Although past research has examined the effect of aging on neural mechanisms supporting cognitive reappraisal, less work has assessed the effects of aging on other antecedent strategies that may be less cognitively demanding. In their SOC-ER (selective optimization with compensation in emotion regulation) model, Urry and Gross (2010) proposed that older adults use less cognitively demanding regulatory strategies, such as situation selection/modification or attention deployment, rather than strategies such as reappraisal or suppression that rely heavily on cognitive control processing. This model fits well with evidence that older adults show a "positivity effect" (either positive engagement or negative avoidance) in visual attention in response to emotional stimuli (Isaacowitz et al., 2006), perhaps reflecting older adults' attempts to use selective attention as a regulatory strategy (Isaacowitz et al., 2008, 2009b) because it does not heavily impinge on cognitive resources (Allard et al., 2010). In cases where cognitive resources are constrained (e.g., in divided attention tasks), there is research suggesting that older adults will not/cannot preferentially engage with information in line with presumed emotion regulation goals (see Mather and Knight, 2005; Knight et al., 2007). Thus, emotion regulation processes might proceed more efficiently for older adults in situations where a full complement of cognitive control resources is available.

For the current study, we compared younger and older adults' neural recruitment while implementing two different types of antecedent emotion regulation strategies. We asked participants to regulate their emotions using selective attention or cognitive reappraisal. Given past research demonstrating older adults' diminished recruitment of lateral and medial PFC regions for certain forms of reappraisal as compared to younger adults, and their difficulty in using reappraisal to successfully regulate in real time (Opitz et al., 2012), we expected older adults in our sample to display reductions in the speed or level of recruitment of lateral and medial PFC during emotion regulation. However, it was less clear how the type of emotion regulation strategy would affect younger and older adults' recruitment of PFC regions. We used relatively long (40 s) film clips so we could examine a more protracted time course of emotion regulation. By using stimuli with a long duration, we could adjudicate between three plausible alternative outcomes regarding age-related changes in PFC recruitment. First, there may be a main effect of age, such that regardless of the strategy used, older adults may chronically under-recruit PFC when regulating their emotions, even when given time to implement the strategy. Second, there may be an interaction between age and time course for strategy implementation, such that older adults may require more time to recruit PFC processes, but when given sufficient time, they may recruit them in the same manner as younger adults. This prediction is based on previous evidence suggesting that the implementation of processes assumed to be in the service of emotion regulation (e.g., cognitive disengagement from negative stimuli) might take some time to execute for older adults (Isaacowitz et al., 2009a). Third, older adults' implementation of PFC processes may be affected by the task demands (i.e., type of regulatory strategy), yielding different effects of age and time course for cognitive reappraisal and selective attention.

To examine these alternatives, we recruited a group of younger (18–34) and older (55–85) adults to complete selective attention and cognitive reappraisal tasks during an fMRI scan session. We presented participants with a series of positive, negative, and neutral film clips within three scanning conditions: passive viewing, selective attention, and reappraisal. Emotional film clips were used in order to provide a dynamic, emotionally evocative stimulus set for examining age differences in neural recruitment in response to specific emotion regulation strategies. We focus our main analyses on the downregulation of negative affect in response to negative videos, consistent with the focus of the majority of studies that have compared younger (see meta-analysis by Diekhof et al., 2011) and older adults' neural responsivity to emotional inputs (particularly in the context of reappraisal: Urry et al., 2006, 2009; van Reekum et al., 2007; Opitz et al., 2012).

## MATERIALS AND METHODS

### PARTICIPANTS

Forty-five younger (25 female, *range* = 18–35 years; $M = 23.40$, $SD = 4.39$) and 42 older adults (25 females, *range* = 55–85; $M = 69.21$, $SD = 8.62$) participated in this study. Eleven younger adults and 12 older adults were excluded from subsequent analyses due to poor data quality (i.e., excessive motion artifacts: greater than $\pm 5$ mm of head motion; $<20$ motion outliers within each scan run as determined by an artifact correction procedure) or a failure to complete all three functional scans. The final sample included 34 younger (16 females, $M = 23.79$, $SD = 4.33$) and 30 older adults (20 females, $M = 68.47$, $SD = 8.14$) who had no history of psychiatric, neurological, or learning disorders nor any history or current use of psychiatric medication. Younger and older adults performed somewhat similarly on a variety of cognitive ability measures (younger adults outperformed older adults on only 2 out of 5 tasks assessing frontal lobe functioning derived from

**Table 1 | Additional demographic and cognitive variables.**

| Variable/Test | Young adults | | Older adults | | F |
|---|---|---|---|---|---|
| | M | SD | M | SD | |
| Education | 16.27 | 1.96 | 16.37 | 2.44 | 0.031 |
| Shipley | 33.54 | 3.01 | 35.37 | 3.17 | 5.07* |
| Digit back[a] | 8.39 | 2.36 | 7.87 | 2.33 | 0.729 |
| FAS[b] | 48.07 | 10.82 | 48.03 | 12.59 | 0.00 |
| WISC[c] | 5.89 | 0.42 | 5.23 | 1.43 | 5.51* |
| Arithmetic[d] | 15.68 | 3.39 | 15.03 | 2.75 | 0.638 |
| Mental control[e] | 30.69 | 4.15 | 26.10 | 5.49 | 7.24* |

[a–e]*Glisky frontal lobe tasks (Glisky et al., 1995).*

*$^*p < 0.05$.*

Glisky et al. (1995); see **Table 1**). Informed consent was obtained from all participants in accordance with the Boston College Institutional Review Board. All participants received $25/h. for their participation.

## STIMULI

We used a series of emotional and neutral film clips as stimuli for the fMRI scan sessions. We focused our analysis for the present study on the neural activity to the negative stimuli. The clips were obtained from television programs, feature films, and documentaries. Positive and negative clips included a variety of emotional scenarios. For instance, positive videos included amusing situations (e.g., standup comedy routine) or more tender/heartwarming scenarios (e.g., a married couple talking about how they first met). Negative videos included fear/sad/disgust scenarios (e.g., a woman being threatened on the phone; a man comforting his dying dog; a man digging through a messy toilet). A separate group of 14 younger and 14 older adults rated each clip on dimensions of valence and arousal. Ratings were made on a scale from 1 (*highly unpleasant, non-arousing*) to 9 (*highly pleasant, highly arousing*). Based on these ratings, a total of 45 clips (18 positive, 18 negative, 9 neutral) were selected for inclusion in the study. Positive and negative videos were matched on ratings of valence and arousal between younger and older adults: Positive-Valence ($M_{young} = 7.31$, $SD = 0.63$; $M_{old} = 7.46$, $SD = 0.81$; $p = 0.45$); Positive-Arousal ($M_{young} = 6.19$, $SD = 0.46$; $M_{old} = 6.60$, $SD = 0.82$; $p = 0.10$); Negative-Valence ($M_{young} = 2.19$, $SD = 0.79$; $M_{old} = 2.12$, $SD = 1.14$; $p = 0.76$); Negative-Arousal ($M_{young} = 7.05$, $SD = 0.79$; $M_{old} = 7.19$, $SD = 0.69$; $p = 0.46$); Neutral-Valence ($M_{young} = 5.28$, $SD = 0.26$; $M_{old} = 5.47$, $SD = 0.39$; $p = 0.20$). For each scan session, the order in which a particular clip was presented (whether it appeared in the passive viewing, selective attention, or reappraisal condition) was randomized across participants. Presentation of the clips was also pseudorandomized within each condition with the caveat that no more than three clips of the same valence were presented consecutively. Stimulus presentation was accomplished using SR Research EyeLink 1000 software (Kanata, Ontario, CA) during the scan session; although this presentation program acquired eye tracking data from participants, the eye tracking data are not reported here.

## PROCEDURE

Before entering the MRI scanner, participants were instructed that they would view a series of emotional and neutral film clips during three functional scan runs. Within each run, six positive, six negative, and three neutral clips were presented. Participants were told that they would be given specific instructions on how to view the film clips with a series of instructions presented to them while in the scanner. Each regulation task (passive viewing, selective attention, and reappraisal) was performed within separate scan runs. For the "passive viewing" task, participants were instructed that they would view a series of 15 film clips; they should "view the clips naturally, as if at home watching television." For the selective attention condition, participants were instructed to "focus on areas of the screen that would help increase positive and decrease any negatives feelings/reactions in response to the clips." For the reappraisal condition, participants were provided with hedonic regulation instructions. When presented with negative clips, participants were instructed to utilize their choice of two strategies: detached reappraisal ("Try to distance yourself from the events being portrayed by reminding yourself that what you are viewing is a fictional event; these are just actors portraying a role.") and positive reappraisal ("Try to put a positive spin on the outcome of the event being portrayed. For example, if you see a clip of a car accident, try to imagine that no one was seriously injured/killed, and everyone walked away from the accident relatively unharmed."). We provided these strategies as options for participants given that certain clips might lend themselves to be more easily reinterpreted with one strategy or the other (or perhaps even both).

## TRIAL STRUCTURE

A black fixation cross was shown on the center of a gray screen for 10, 12, 14, 16, or 18 s. Each video was presented for 40 s[1]. During the passive viewing condition, the instruction "view" was presented on the bottom of the screen 4-s post-stimulus onset and remained on the screen for 3 s. This timing for the instruction phase has been used in previous research (see Opitz et al., 2012). Using the same timing and screen placement, for the selective attention condition, the instruction "avoid negative" was presented along with the negative videos and for the reappraisal condition, "decrease negative" was presented. In all three conditions, each video was followed by an inter-trial interval consisting of a black fixation cross for an average of 14 s (jittered between 10 and 18 s). The presentation order of the three conditions was varied across participants.

## DATA ACQUISITIONAND ANALYSIS

Images were acquired on a 3 Tesla Siemens Tim Trio MRI scanner using a 12-channel head coil. Stimuli were projected onto a screen located at the back of the magnet bore, and

[1]The instructions were embedded within videos for 14 younger and 13 older adults participants across all three conditions, while reappraisal instructions were embedded within videos for all participants. When assessing results from the remaining 20 younger and 17 older adult participants who did not have visual prompts within the selective attention and passive viewing videos, our main results remained relatively unchanged.

participants viewed stimuli using a mirror attached to the head coil. T1-weighted localizer images and a T1-weighted inversion recovery echo planar image required for auto-alignment were collected. Anatomical data were collected with a multiplanar rapidly acquired gradient-echo (MEMPRAGE) sequence ($TR = 2200$ ms; $TEs = 1.64, 3.5, 5.36, 7.22$; flip angle $= 7°$; FOV $= 256 \times 256$ mm; slice thickness $= 1$ mm, no gap; $1 \times 1 \times 1$ mm resolution). Functional images were collected using a T2*-weighted echo-planar imaging (EPI) sequence with the following parameters: $TR = 2000$ ms, $TE = 30$ ms, FOV $= 216$ mm, flip angle $= 85°$. Thirty interleaved near axial slices were collected in a $3 \times 3 \times 3.6$ mm matrix (slice thickness $= 3$ mm with a 20% skip).

Preprocessing and data analysis were conducted in SPM8 (Welcome Department of Cognitive Neurology, London). Preprocessing steps were as follows: slice timing correction; motion correction using a six parameter, rigid body transformation algorithm; normalization to the Montreal Neurological Institute (MNI) template (resampling at 2 mm isotropic voxels); and spatial smoothing using a 8 mm full-width half maximum isotropic Gaussian kernel.

We first incorporated a slow event-related design anchored to the onset of the most emotionally salient portion of each film clip, what we will refer to as the "emotional peak" portion. This peak (assessed in seconds) was determined by the researchers and corroborated by two younger and two older adult naïve raters. An interclass correlation analysis was conducted to assess inter-rater reliability. There was adequate agreement amongst raters for determining the emotional peak ($\alpha = 0.79$). Final peak ratings were determined by the majority consensus among raters (e.g., 3/5 or 4/5 raters) agreeing on a peaks falling within a range of 1–3 s, whereby the average of that range was used as the peak value (in whole seconds). For this first set of analysis, we used a general linear model incorporating task effects for the negative films in the three viewing conditions (passive, selective attention, reappraisal), along with three linear regressors to account for the three runs, at the single subject level. These models were used to create contrasts between conditions of interest. All contrasts utilized an explicit mask that encompassed all of the PFC, anterior cingulate gyrus, and the amygdala (created using MARINA; Walter et al., 2003) in order to focus our analyses on apriori regions of interest.

We contrasted the combined effects of the two regulation conditions relative to passive viewing (selective attention + reappraisal > passive viewing and passive viewing > selective attention + reappraisal), conducting these contrasts both collapsing across the age groups and also separately for each age group. We also conducted an Age × Condition [regulation (selective attention + reappraisal) vs. passive viewing] ANOVA. These first analyses determined potential age similarities and/or differences in neural recruitment when asked to regulate vs. passively view the clips. These initial analyses also addressed our general prediction that older adults would show diminished activation in response to the regulation conditions relative to younger adults.

Next, we assessed distinct effects of the two regulation conditions for younger and older adults. These analyses specifically addressed whether younger and older adults differed in their activity profile as a function of the specific regulatory strategy used. We first examined activation for each age group in contrasts comparing the two regulatory conditions (selective attention > reappraisal and reappraisal > selective attention). To reveal regions that showed an Age (young vs. old) × Regulation Condition (selective attention vs. reappraisal) interaction, we conducted a separate ANOVA.

Although these prior analyses were based on activity at the peak emotional moment of the film clip, a final analytical approach was used to assess whether age differences in the timing of neural activation might contribute to the observed effects. This analytic approach modeled both the instruction-related activity (modeled as an event starting 4-s post-stimulus onset; see Opitz et al., 2012) and peak-emotion activity (modeled as an event occurring at the most emotionally salient portion of the film clip) for the film clips in the selective attention and reappraisal conditions. An ANOVA was used to reveal regions within the amygdala-PFC mask that showed an Age (young vs. old) × Condition (selective attention vs. reappraisal) × Phase (instruction-onset vs. peak-emotion).

For all analyses, differences in activation are reported for regions consisting of at least 10 voxels, active at $p < 0.005$, unless otherwise specified. This combination of threshold and voxel extent has recently been justified as appropriate in studies equally concerned with Type I and Type II error (see Lieberman and Cunningham, 2009), and in the present study represents a more conservative combination because we limited our search space to the amygdala-PFC mask. AlphaSim (B.D. Ward) revealed a slightly higher voxel extent threshold, of 17 voxels, each active at $p < 0.005$, was required to correct for multiple comparisons across this search space at $p < 0.05$. Notations are provided throughout the results tables to indicate clusters that did not reach this voxel extent. For regions that emerged from a Two or Three-Way interaction in any of our ANOVA analyses, we extracted parameter estimates and plotted the activity within a *post-hoc* region of interest (ROI), defining ROIs within Marsbar (Brett et al., 2002) and plotting the activity using REX (downloaded from http://web.mit.edu/swg/rex/) to reveal the basis for the interaction.

## RESULTS

### IMAGING RESULTS

#### *Effects of passive viewing and emotion regulation separately for younger and older adults at the emotional peak*

Again, all analyses focused on negative film clip presentation. We first examined the passive viewing > emotion regulation and emotion regulation > passive viewing contrasts separately for each age group (See **Tables 2A,B** for results when collapsing across age groups). Older adults showed greater activity in left DLPFC, left VLPFC, and OFC for passive viewing relative to emotion regulation (See **Table 2C**). Only one cluster within DLPFC was revealed in the emotion regulation > passive viewing contrast for older adults (See **Table 2D**). For younger adults, the contrast resulting in greater PFC activity was reversed. Only one region of right precentral gyrus was more active in the passive viewing > selective attention contrast (See **Table 2E**). However, several regions emerged in the emotion regulation > passive viewing contrast for younger adults (See **Table 2F**). These included left ACC, left VLPFC, bilateral DLPFC, and bilateral OFC.

**Table 2 | Activation across emotion regulation conditions relative to passive viewing.**

| Brain region | BA | X | Y | Z | K extent | t-score | $p_{uncorrected}$ |
|---|---|---|---|---|---|---|---|
| **A. REGIONS OBSERVED IN THE PASSIVE VIEWING > EMOTION REGULATION CONTRAST (COLLAPSED ACROSS AGE)** | | | | | | | |
| Left post-central gyrus | 2 | −42 | −20 | 19 | 40 | 3.23 | 0.001 |
| Left precentral gyrus | 6+ | −40 | 2 | 12 | 11 | 3.24 | 0.001 |
| Left superior frontal gyrus (DLPFC) | 8+ | −16 | 31 | 37 | 14 | 2.89 | 0.003 |
| | 8/9+ | −16 | 45 | 36 | 14 | 2.96 | 0.002 |
| **B. REGIONS OBSERVED IN THE EMOTION REGULATION > PASSIVE VIEWING CONTRAST (COLLAPSED ACROSS AGE)** | | | | | | | |
| Left superior frontal gyrus* | 6 | −20 | −3 | 50 | 30 | 3.75 | 0.000 |
| Right middle frontal gyrus | 6+ | 24 | −1 | 48 | 12 | 3.12 | 0.001 |
| Right precentral gyrus* | 6 | 34 | 2 | 31 | 101 | 3.66 | 0.000 |
| **C. REGIONS OBSERVED IN THE PASSIVE VIEWING > EMOTION REGULATION CONTRAST FOR OLDER ADULTS** | | | | | | | |
| Left inferior frontal gyrus (VLPFC) | 45 | −51 | 20 | 10 | 33 | 3.22 | 0.002 |
| Left superior frontal gyrus (DLPFC) | 9 | −10 | 50 | 36 | 212 | 4.03 | 0.000 |
| Left medial frontal gyrus (DLPFC) | 9+ | −8 | 51 | 18 | 12 | 3.12 | 0.002 |
| Orbitofrontal cortex | 10 | 0 | 56 | 3 | 224 | 3.89 | 0.000 |
| **D. REGIONS OBSERVED IN THE EMOTION REGULATION > PASSIVE VIEWING CONTRAST FOR OLDER ADULTS** | | | | | | | |
| Middle frontal gyrus (DLPFC) | 9 | 32 | 15 | 31 | 28 | 3.74 | 0.000 |
| **E. REGIONS OBSERVED IN THE PASSIVE VIEWING > EMOTION REGULATION CONTRAST FOR YOUNGER ADULTS** | | | | | | | |
| Right precentral gyrus | 4+ | 42 | −6 | 18 | 11 | 3.30 | 0.001 |
| **F. REGIONS OBSERVED IN THE EMOTION REGULATION > PASSIVE VIEWING CONTRAST FOR YOUNGER ADULTS** | | | | | | | |
| Left anterior cingulate cortex (ACC) | 32 | −10 | 21 | 38 | 192 | 4.10 | 0.000 |
| Left inferior frontal gyrus (VLPFC) | 11/47 | −34 | 25 | −6 | 53 | 3.50 | 0.001 |
| Left middle frontal gyrus (DLPFC) | 46 | −44 | 29 | 34 | 44 | 3.41 | 0.001 |
| Right middle frontal gyrus (DLPFC) | 9/46 | 42 | 33 | 37 | 252 | 3.69 | 0.000 |
| Left orbitofrontal cortex (OFC) | 10 | −48 | 48 | −9 | 32 | 3.48 | 0.001 |
| Right orbitofrontal cortex (OFC) | 10 | 8 | 67 | 10 | 28 | 4.19 | 0.000 |
| **G. REGIONS SHOWING AN AGE × CONDITION INTERACTION (COMBINED EMOTION REGULATION VS. PASSIVE VIEWING)** | | | | | | | |
| Left middle frontal gyrus (DLPFC) | 9/46 | −46 | 31 | 42 | 35 | *F*-score 11.89 | 0.001 |
| Right superior frontal gyrus (DLPFC) | 9/46+ | 44 | 35 | 33 | 11 | 9.70 | 0.002 |
| | 9/46 | 28 | 52 | 29 | 152 | 15.42 | 0.000 |

*Stereotaxic coordinates based on the Talairach atlas (Talairach and Tournoux, 1988). All coordinates correspond to clusters that met a voxel extent threshold = 17, $p < 0.005$.*

**Nearby cluster observed within a separate conjunction analysis (reappraisal > passive viewing masked with selective attention > passive viewing).*

*+Cluster did not reach 17-voxel extent threshold to correct for multiple comparisons at $p < 0.005$.*

### Regions showing an Age × Condition (combined regulation vs. passive viewing) interaction at the emotional peak

An ANOVA confirmed a different activity profile for younger and older adults within three regions of DLPFC (**Table 2G**; **Figure 1A**). When the parameter estimates from these regions were examined, within two regions of right DLPFC (BA 9/46, peak at Talairach coordinates: 28 52 29; BA 9/46, peak at Talairach coordinates: 44 35 33), older adults showed greater activity than younger adults during passive viewing but less activity than younger adults during emotion regulation. Within the region of left DLPFC (BA 9/46, peak at Talairach coordinates: −46 31 32), younger adults but not older adults showed greater activity for emotion regulation relative to passive viewing[2].

### Comparing effects of reappraisal and selective attention for younger and older adults at the emotional peak

The previous analysis suggested greater PFC activity for emotion regulation in younger as compared to older adults. However, this could reflect less overlapping activity within the two regulation conditions for older adults. Thus, we next examined activation patterns between the selective attention and reappraisal condition for younger and older adults. Significant activation patterns occurred for different contrast analyses for each age group: reappraisal > selective attention for older adults and selective

[2]It was possible that results of the Age × Condition interactions (both collapsing across regulation condition and separately for selective attention and reappraisal) were primarily driven by age differences in activation within the passive viewing condition. We examined older adult > younger adult and younger adult > older adult contrasts for just the passive viewing condition. Only one significant cluster emerged in these analyses (DLPFC, BA 45/46; Talairach coordinates: 36 26 24), and was observed in the older adult > younger adult contrast. When we used this result as an exclusive mask and reran our interaction analyses, our previous results remained unchanged. This suggests that the observed Age × Condition interactions were not primarily the result of age differences in activation within the passive viewing condition.

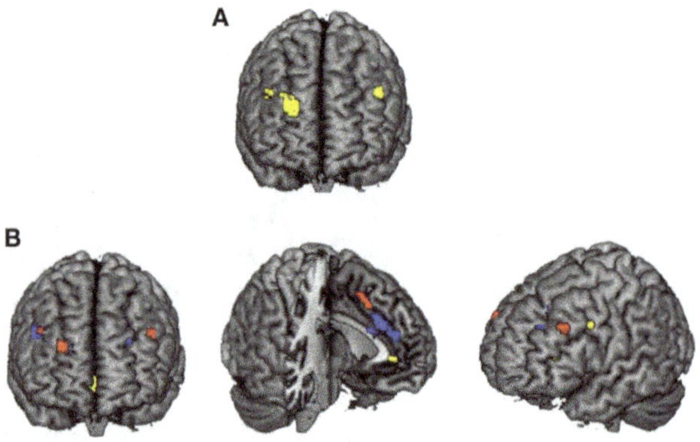


**FIGURE 1 | PFC engagement during emotion regulation.** DLPFC activation observed for the Age × Combined Regulation interaction analyses **(A)** and overlays of activity for selective attention > reappraisal for younger adults in blue, reappraisal > selective attention for older adults in yellow, and the Age × Regulation Condition interaction in red **(B)**.

attention > reappraisal for younger adults (no significant clusters were observed in the respective opposite contrast for both age groups; **Figure 1B**). For older adults, activation was greater for reappraisal relative to selective attention in posterior cingulate, ACC, bilateral VLPFC, and OFC (See **Table 3A**). For younger adults, activity was greater for selective attention relative to reappraisal in bilateral DLPFC, VLPFC, and DMPFC (See **Table 3B, Figure 1B**).

#### *Regions showing an Age × Regulation Condition interaction*

A significant Age × Regulation Condition interaction (**Table 3C, Figure 1B**) was observed within a region of ACC (BA 32; peak at Talairach coordinate: −4 12 45), right DLPFC (BA 46; peak at Talairach coordinate: 46 31 33), and left DLPFC (BA 9/46; peak at Talairach coordinate: −44 33 32).Although these regions were similar to those revealed in the younger adults' contrast of selective attention > reappraisal, the regions were not overlapping (compare red and blue regions in **Figure 1B**). In each of the regions identified by this ANOVA, younger adults showed similar activation for the two regulation conditions while older adults showed greater activity for reappraisal as compared to selective attention, particularly within the right DLPFC region. Thus, this ANOVA revealed that older adults showed greater differentiation in PFC recruitment for the two regulatory strategies than did younger adults.

#### *Phase analysis: activity at film-onset and emotional-peak*

To clarify whether differences noted above might be due to age differences in the timing of regulatory processes, the next analysis examined age differences in activity at instruction-onset and at the emotional peak of the negative videos across the two regulation conditions. An Age × Condition × Phase ANOVA was assessed. Focusing on the three-way interaction, activation was revealed within two regions of VLPFC, although the voxel extent in neither region reached the 10-voxel cutoff ($K = 5$ voxels and 8 voxels); thus, this activity must be interpreted tentatively. Parameter estimates extracted from each VLPFC region(BA 47, peak at Talairach coordinates: 24 25 −13, $p_{uncorrected} = 0.003$, 8 voxels; −22 31 −8, $p_{uncorrected} = 0.008$, 5 voxels) revealed that activity was greater for reappraisal than for selective attention during the onset of the video relative to the emotional peak for younger adults (activity at the peak was greater for selective attention than for reappraisal). For older adults, activity within right VLPFC was greater at the emotional peak during reappraisal than selective attention, while activity was greater at the onset for selective attention than reappraisal. Within left VLPFC, onset and peak activity was slightly greater for reappraisal compared to selective attention for older adults (**Figure 2**). These results suggest that, particularly within right VLPFC, compared to younger adults, older adults may have delayed engagement of regulatory processes during reappraisal.

## DISCUSSION

The current study investigated the neural mechanisms underlying the hedonic regulation of negative affect in a sample of younger and older adults, examining the effect of regulation strategy (reappraisal vs. selective attention) and the time course of strategy implementation on activity within PFC. We first examined potential overlap across the two age groups in activity that was stronger for emotion regulation relative to passive viewing. These results revealed little overlap in PFC regions supporting regulation relative to passive viewing when collapsing our results across age. More age differences than similarities emerged when we examined the age groups separately. The combined effects of the two regulation strategies relative to passive viewing were more robust for younger adults, with activation observed within lateral and medial PFC. This suggests that younger adults may have more common activation within regions implicated in cognitive emotion regulation networks for both strategies than older adults. Thus, older adults might be showing more differentiation with selective attention and reappraisal.

Indeed, when examining distinct effects for each regulation strategy, further age differences emerged. In some PFC regions, there was a complete age-related reversal in the strategy that utilized the most activity: older adults recruited lateral and medial PFC regions more for reappraisal relative to selective attention while younger adults recruited lateral and medial PFC regions more for selective attention relative to reappraisal. Older adults' greater reliance on lateral and medial PFC activation for reappraisal than selective attention could relate to the heightened cognitive demand that older adults must meet in order to engage these challenging reappraisal strategies. If older adults' implementation of reappraisal processes is less efficient, they may require greater neural engagement than younger adults in order to achieve the same successful regulatory outcome.

Partial support for the interpretation that older adults' reappraisal processes may be engaged less efficiently than younger adults' comes from our phasic analysis of the time course of strategy implementation. This analysis revealed that within two regions of VLPFC, activity was greater for reappraisal than for selective attention during the instruction onset of negative videos for younger adults but not until the emotional-peak of the videos for older adults.

**Table 3 | Activation within the reappraisal and selective attention conditions for younger and older adults.**

| Brain region | BA | X | Y | Z | K extent | t-score | $p_{uncorrected}$ |
|---|---|---|---|---|---|---|---|
| **A. REGIONS OBSERVED IN THE REAPPRAISAL > SELECTIVE ATTENTION CONTRAST FOR OLDER ADULTS** | | | | | | | |
| Left posterior cingulate cortex | 31 | −16 | −33 | 40 | 28 | 4.34 | 0.000 |
| Left inferior frontal gyrus (VLPFC) | 44+ | −50 | 9 | 35 | 15 | 3.21 | 0.002 |
| | 45 | −38 | 34 | 11 | 55 | 3.81 | 0.000 |
| Left orbitofrontal cortex (OFC) | 11 | −20 | 40 | −12 | 41 | 3.92 | 0.000 |
| Right inferior frontal gyrus (VLPFC) | 47 | 32 | 42 | −12 | 25 | 3.60 | 0.001 |
| Anterior cingulate cortex (ACC) | 32 | 6 | 43 | −2 | 302 | 4.35 | 0.000 |
| **B. REGIONS OBSERVED IN THE SELECTIVE ATTENTION > REAPPRAISAL CONTRAST FOR YOUNGER ADULTS** | | | | | | | |
| Left middle frontal gyrus (DLPFC) | 6 | −22 | 10 | 47 | 68 | 3.57 | 0.001 |
| | 9/46 | −24 | 40 | 27 | 25 | 3.13 | 0.002 |
| Anterior cingulate cortex (ACC)* | 32 | −10 | 21 | 30 | 282 | 4.06 | 0.000 |
| Left inferior frontal gyrus (VLPFC)* | 47 | −36 | 25 | −5 | 119 | 3.53 | 0.001 |
| Right middle frontal gyrus (DLPFC)* | 9/46 | 48 | 29 | 30 | 45 | 3.37 | 0.001 |
| Left superior frontal gyrus (DMPFC) | 8 | −12 | 31 | 43 | 62 | 3.79 | 0.000 |
| **C. REGIONS SHOWING AN AGE × REGULATION CONDITION INTERACTION (REAPPRAISAL VS. SELECTIVE ATTENTION)** | | | | | | | |
| Left middle frontal gyrus (DLPFC) | 9/46 | −44 | 33 | 32 | 19 | *F*-score 7.00 | 0.001 |
| Right middle frontal gyrus (DLPFC) | 46+ | 46 | 31 | 33 | 11 | 6.13 | 0.003 |
| Anterior cingulate gyrus (ACC) | 32 | −4 | 12 | 45 | 77 | 6.47 | 0.002 |

*Stereotaxic coordinates based on the Talairach atlas (Talairach and Tournoux, 1988). All coordinates correspond to clusters that met a voxel extent threshold = 17, $p < 0.005$ (no significant clusters revealed in the opposite contrast for each age group).*

**Nearby cluster observed within a separate conjunction analysis (selective attention > reappraisal masked with selective attention > passive viewing).*

*+Cluster did not reach 17-voxel extent threshold to correct for multiple comparisons at $p < 0.005$.*

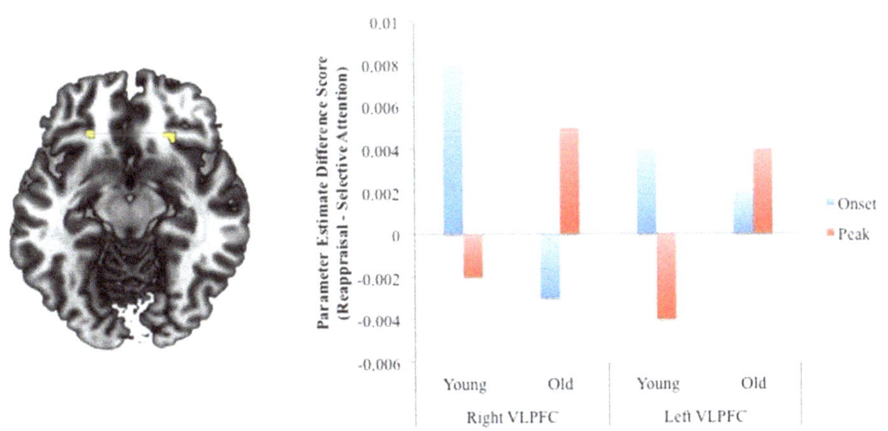


**FIGURE 2 | Regions revealed in the Age × Regulation × Phase interaction analysis.** For ease of presentation, we created difference scores for activity at the onset and emotional peak for the selective attention and regulation conditions separately for younger and older adults. Scores greater than 0 indicate greater reappraisal-related activity and scores less than zero indicate greater selective attention-related activity.

This time course shift might reflect different possibilities for older adults' reappraisal deployment. For one, it is possible that delayed reappraisal-related recruitment in PFC reflects neural decrements related to cognitive slowing (Salthouse, 1995). Such neural decrements would suggest that reappraisal processes require significant effort for older adults to deploy, consistent with behavioral evidence arguing that older adults need sufficient time to recruit cognitive resources for preferentially avoiding negative stimuli (Isaacowitz et al., 2009a). It is plausible that older adults needed more time to select out their preferred reappraisal tactic once they made the initial appraisal (Wager et al., 2008), or they might have had difficulty inhibiting prepotent negative affective responses when attempting to reappraise (Winecoff et al., 2011). Because reappraisal is often most effective when processes are deployed before the emotional response has reached its peak (Goldin et al., 2008), older adults may need to recruit more processes than younger adults because they are attempting to regulate a more intense or mature emotional response. In contrast, by engaging processes earlier, younger adults may successfully curtail the development of a strong emotional response and thereby minimize the cognitive resources required for reappraisal. This latter explanation may also relate to why, for younger adults, selective attention may recruit more activity within PFC regions at the emotional peak than reappraisal: early-acting reappraisal may negate the need for subsequent reappraisal during a film clip, whereas attentional selection of hedonic information at an early time point within a film is unlikely to meaningfully impact the need to select hedonic information at a later time point.

In contrast to a neural-limitation account for the timing effects among older adults, it is possible that the time course of PFC recruitment reflects intentional discretion in terms of strategy deployment. While it is possible that reappraisal is more effective before an emotional response reaches its peak, older adults might be sophisticated enough to wait for the necessary moment when a reappraisal strategy needs to be deployed (i.e., when the most emotionally salient portion of an event/stimulus has emerged). Previous studies assessing reappraisal strategies have not done so over a protracted time course (typically only 2–8 s for stimulus presentation; Winecoff et al., 2011; Opitz et al., 2012) or with more dynamic stimuli (static images as opposed to video stimuli). Thus, older adults might be more motivated to engage in proficient reappraisal strategies with stimuli that are particularly engaging and over a time course suited for full reappraisal deployment. Overall, while these timing effects should be interpreted with caution given the small cluster extents revealed in the analysis, the results are suggestive of the importance of considering age differences not only in the magnitude of recruited PFC processes but also in the time course over which the processes are recruited. Future research should attempt to adjudicate how potential age-related differences in the timing of regulation deployment reflects aspects of ability vs. motivation in the successful use of particular emotion regulation strategies.

In addition to revealing that there are some PFC regions that show age reversals in strategy recruitment, the results also demonstrated that there are PFC regions (namely DLPFC and ACC) in which older adults show more differentiation in the strategy (i.e., reappraisal) that elicits the most activity. Younger adults recruited these to downregulate negative affect by both reappraisal and selective attention. Although prior research has not compared reappraisal and selective attention, this general recruitment in younger adults is consistent with studies that have observed heightened lateral PFC, particularly DLPFC, both when reappraising negative stimuli (Ochsner et al., 2002; Phan et al., 2005; McRae et al., 2010) and when examining attentional deployment strategies (including selective attention; see Silvers et al., 2013, and see Corebetta and Shulman, 2002, for a review of the role of DLPFC in attentional control). Conversely, older adults did not show much in the way of overlapping effects of the two regulation strategies within PFC regions. At first glance, these results seem to be in line with recent work suggesting that older adults do not activate lateral PFC regions to the same extent as younger adults when instructed to regulate negative affective responses (Winecoff et al., 2011; Opitz et al., 2012). However, the lack of PFC recruitment when examining common activation of the two regulation conditions as compared to passive viewing appears instead to relate to discrepant activation patterns across the two strategies when compared to passive viewing for older adults and may suggest that the method of hedonic regulation has a greater impact on the neural processes recruited by older adults than by younger adults.

To our knowledge, only two studies (Winecoff et al., 2011; Opitz et al., 2012) have compared samples of younger and older adults during fMRI investigations of cognitive emotion regulation, and both of these studies employed conditions examining age differences in neural activation when hedonically regulating via reappraisal. Results from these two studies revealed greater lateral and medial PFC activation during reappraisal of negative stimuli in younger as compared to older adults. Conversely, our results suggest that older adults show greater reappraisal related activity within lateral and medial PFC. Although our findings could be consistent with work suggesting that emotion regulation is particularly taxing to cognitive control resources for older adults (see Kryla-Lighthall and Mather, 2009; Urry and Gross, 2010), thus requiring more PFC processes, and more time, for older adults to achieve regulation, the question remains as to why our results seem at odds with those of Opitz et al. and Winecoff et al. One possibility, as mentioned earlier, could be the timing of neural recruitment observed. Whether older adults seem to under-recruit or over-recruit PFC regions during reappraisal may depend on whether activity is measured early in a trial or late in a trial. There are also other design and methodological differences that could lead older adults in our study to implement PFC processes in the service of reappraisal. Most notably, we employed dynamic, emotional film clips, as opposed to static IAPS images. Not only were these films temporally extended, allowing older adults time to implement the regulatory strategies, they might have been particularly engaging. This might have enhanced older adults' ability or motivation to utilize a reappraisal strategy that they report using effectively in their daily lives (see Gross et al., 1997; John and Gross, 2004). Support for this possibility, that older adults successfully use reappraisal when motivated to do so, comes from behavioral evidence revealing that older adults might actually be more successful than younger adults at down-regulating affective responses to negative videos (Scheibe and Blanchard-Fields, 2009). It will be interesting for future research to compare older adults' regulatory processes across different time courses and with stimuli that elicit varying motivations for regulation.

## LIMITATIONS AND FUTURE DIRECTIONS

Some limitations should be noted. For one, we did not control the type of reappraisal tactic used by younger and older adults. This provides potential confounds in determining differences in activation patterns across age groups for reappraisal. It is possible that the different age groups were utilizing different strategies (see Shiota and Levenson, 2009, for a discussion), but we have no way of knowing which strategy was most preferred or if more than one strategy was engaged during any specific trial. Whether older adults recruit regulatory control regions within the PFC when utilizing more of a positive reframing rather than a distancing/detached reappraisal tactic needs to be addressed further in the future.

We were also limited by our assessment of regulatory outcomes. We did not examine regulation success on a trial-by-trial basis, which would help determine how well individuals engaged a particular strategy when the efficacy of that strategy was likely to still be in mind. We did assess self-reported affect at the end of each scan run, whereby both younger and older adults showed a modest increase in mood after the regulation runs as compared to passive viewing. However, no effects of age or interactions with age and regulation condition emerged. Furthermore, when we assessed stimulus ratings for the video clips after the fMRI session, there was no effect of regulation condition on the ratings. Although it could be susceptible to demand characteristics, assessing affect (i.e., self-reported mood and stimulus ratings) at the end of each trial might have provided a more accurate portrayal as to how well individuals actually performed the strategy and whether the strategy was effective in eliciting the desired regulatory response/outcome.

Finally, while positive videos were also presented to participants, they were not included in the present paper. This was mainly for logistical reasons and to keep our focus on testing hypotheses relevant to the limited literature in this area that has focused on the regulation of negative affect. However, future analyses will include an assessment of age effects on hedonic regulation of positive stimuli to more fully assess how individuals regulate toward positive affective states (by either increasing positive and/or decreasing negative affect).

In spite of the aforementioned limitations, the present study emphasizes that older adults do recruit lateral and medial PFC regions in response to regulatory instructions. They recruit PFC regions more for reappraisal than for selective attention, perhaps reflecting their need to compensate for less efficient or effective cognitive control processing in order to engage challenging regulation strategies. Consistent with this interpretation that older adults' PFC recruitment during reappraisal may be less efficient than younger adults', the timing of reappraisal-related activity in VLPFC was delayed for older adults compared to younger adults. While older adults implemented VLPFC processes the moment reappraisal instructions were given, older adults did not deploy them until the experienced emotion was likely at its peak. The present findings suggest a need for future research to disentangle age differences in the neural underpinnings involved in executing a variety of cognitive emotion regulation strategies and to examine the implementation of these processes over extended time intervals. This line of research may help to explain which strategies are going to be more or less effective for younger and older adults in achieving regulatory success and enhanced emotional well-being.

## ACKNOWLEDGMENTS

This research was supported in part by NIMH Grant MH080833, the Dana Foundation, and a Searle Scholar Program Grant awarded to Elizabeth A. Kensinger. We would like to thank Halle Zucker, Jenny Wong, John Morris, Kelly Durham, Meghan Horn, Sarah Scott, John Ksander, and Nadia Haddara for their assistance with participant recruitment and data collection. The authors have no competing interests to disclose.

## REFERENCES

Allard, E. S., Wadlinger, H. A., and Isaacowitz, D. M. (2010). Positive gaze preferences in older adults: assessing the role of cognitive effort with pupil dilation. *Aging Neuropsychol. C* 17, 296–311. doi: 10.1080/13825580903265681

Brett, M., Anton, J. L., Valbregue, R., and Poline, J. B. (2002). "Region of interest analysis using an SPM toolbox [abstract]," in *8th International Conference on Functional Mapping of the Human Brain* (Sendai), CD-ROM in *Neuroimage* 16.

Buhle, J. T., Silvers, J. A., Wager, T. D., Lopez, R., Onyemekwu, C., Kober, H., et al. (2013). Cognitive reappraisal of emotion: a meta-analysis of human neuroimaging studies. *Cereb. Cortex.* doi: 10.1093/cercor/bht154. [Epub ahead of print].

Carstensen, L. L., Isaacowitz, D. M., and Charles, S. T. (1999). Taking time seriously: a theory of socioemotional selectivity. *Am. Psychol.* 54, 165–181. doi: 10.1037/0003-066X.54.3.165

Carstensen, L. L., and Mikels, J. A. (2005). At the intersection of emotion and cognition. *Curr. Dir. Psychol. Sci.* 14, 117–121. doi: 10.1111/j.0963-7214.2005.00348.x

Corebetta, M., and Shulman, G. L. (2002). Control of goal-directed and stimulus-driven attention in the brain. *Nat. Rev. Neurosci.* 3, 201–215. doi: 10.1038/nrn755

Diekhof, E. K., Geier, K., Falkai, P., and Gruber, O. (2011). Fear is only as deep as the mind allows: a coordinate-based meta-analysis of neuroimaging studies on the regulation of negative affect. *Neuroimage* 58, 275–285. doi: 10.1016/j.neuroimage.2011.05.073

Fjell, A. M., Walhovd, K. B., Fennema-Notestine, C., McEvoy, L. K., Hagler, D. J., Holland, D., et al. (2009). One-year brain atrophy evident in healthy aging. *J. Neurosci.* 29, 15223–15231. doi: 10.1523/JNEUROSCI.3252-09.2009

Glisky, E. L., Polster, M. R., and Routhieaux, B. C. (1995). Double dissociation between item and source memory. *Neuropsychology* 9, 229–235. doi: 10.1037//0894-4105.9.2.229

Goldin, P. R., McRae, K., Ramel, W., and Gross, J. J. (2008). The neural bases of emotion regulation: reappraisal and suppression of negative emotion. *Biol. Psychiatry* 63, 577–586. doi: 10.1016/j.biopsych.2007.05.031

Grieve, S. M., Clark, C. R., Williams, L. M., Peduto, A. J., and Gordon, E. (2005). Preservation of limbic and paralimbic structures in aging. *Hum. Brain Mapp.* 25, 391–401. doi: 10.1002/hbm.20115

Gross, J. J., Carstensen, L. L., Pasupathi, M., Tsai, J., Gottestam, K., and Hsu, A. Y. C. (1997). Emotion and aging: experience, expression, and control. *Psychol. Aging* 12, 590–599. doi: 10.1037/0882-7974.12.4.590

Isaacowitz, D. M., Allard, E. S., Murphy, N. A., and Schlangel, M. (2009a). The time course of age related preferences toward positive and negative stimuli. *J. Gerontol. B Psychol. Sci. Soc. Sci.* 64B, 188–192. doi: 10.1093/geronb/gbn036

Isaacowitz, D. M., Toner, K., Goren, D., and Wilson, H. R. (2008). Looking while unhappy: mood congruent gaze in young adults, positive gaze in older adults. *Psychol. Sci.* 19, 848–853. doi: 10.1111/j.1467-9280.2008.02167.x

Isaacowitz, D. M., Toner, K., and Neupert, S. D. (2009b). Use of gaze for real-time mood regulation: effects of age and attentional functioning. *Psychol. Aging* 24, 989–994. doi: 10.1037/a0017706

Isaacowitz, D. M., Wadlinger, H. A., Goren, D., and Wilson, H. R. (2006). Selective preference in visual fixation away from negative images in old age? an eye tracking study. *Psychol. Aging* 21, 40–48. doi: 10.1037/0882-7974.21.1.40

John, O. P., and Gross, J. J. (2004). Healthy and unhealthy emotion regulation: personality processes, individual differences, and lifespan development. *J. Pers.* 72, 1301–1334. doi: 10.1111/j.1467-6494.2004.00298.x

Kalisch. R. (2009). The functional neuroanatomy of reappraisal: time matters. *Neurosci. Biobehav. Rev.* 33, 1215–1226. doi: 10.1016/j.neubiorev.2009.06.003

Kennedy, Q., Mather, M., and Carstensen, L. L. (2004). Aging and emotional memory: the forgettable nature of negative images for older adults. *Psychol. Sci.* 15, 208–214. doi: 10.1111/j.0956-7976.2004.01503011.x

Kliegel, M., Jäger, T., and Phillips, L. H. (2007). Emotional development across adulthood: differential age-related emotional reactivity and emotion regulation in a negative mood induction procedure. *Int. J. Aging Hum. Dev.* 64, 217–244. doi: 10.2190/U48Q-0063-3318-1175

Knight, M., Seymour, T. L., Gaunt, J. T., Baker, C., Nesmith, K., and Mather, M. (2007). Aging and goal-directed emotional attention: distraction reverses emotional biases. *Emotion* 7, 705–714. doi: 10.1037/1528-3542.7.4.705

Kryla-Lighthall, N., and Mather, M. (2009). "The role of cognitive control in older adults' emotional well-being," in *Handbook of Theories of Aging, 2nd Edn,* eds V. Berngtson, D. Gans, N. Putney, and M. Silverstein (New York, NY: Springer Publishing), 323–344.

Lieberman, M. D., and Cunningham, W. A. (2009). Type I and Type II error concerns in fMRI research: re-balancing the scale. *Soc. Cogn. Affect. Neuroscie.* 4, 423–428. doi: 10.1093/scan/nsp052

Mather, M., and Knight, M. (2005). Goal-directed memory: the role of cognitive control in older adults' emotional memory. *Psychol. Aging* 20, 554–570. doi: 10.1037/0882-7974.20.4.554

McRae, K., Hughes, B., Chopra, S., Gabrieli, J. D., Gross, J. J., and Ochsner, K. N. (2010). The neural bases of distraction and reappraisal. *J. Cognitive Neurosci.* 22, 248–262. doi: 10.1162/jocn.2009.21243

Ochsner, K. N., Bunge, S. A., Gross, J. J., and Gabrieli, J. D. (2002). Re-thinking feelings: an fMRI study of the cognitive regulation of emotion. *J. Cognitive Neurosci.* 14, 1215–1229. doi: 10.1162/089892902760807212

Ochsner, K. N., and Gross, J. J. (2005). The cognitive control of emotion. *Trends Cogn. Sci.* 9, 242–249. doi: 10.1016/j.tics.2005.03.010

Ochsner, K. N., and Gross, J. J. (2008). Cognitive emotion regulation: insights from social cognitive and affective neuroscience. *Curr. Dir. Psychol. Sci.* 17, 153–158. doi: 10.1111/j.1467-8721.2008.00566.x

Ochsner, K. N., Ray, R. D., Robertson, E. R., Cooper, J. C., Chopra, S., Gabrieli, J. D. E., et al. (2004). For better or for worse: neural systems supporting the cognitive down- and up-regulation of negative emotion. *Neuroimage* 23, 483–499. doi: 10.1016/j.neuroimage.2004.06.030

Opitz, P. C., Rauch, L. C., Terry, D. P., and Urry, H. L. (2012). Prefrontal mediation of age differences in cognitive reappraisal. *Neurobiol. Aging* 33, 645–655. doi: 10.1016/j.neurobiolaging.2010.06.004

Phan, K. L., Fitzgerald, D. A., Nathan, P. J., Moore, G. J., Uhde, T. W., and Tancer, M. E. (2005). Neural substrates for voluntary suppression of negative affect: a functional magnetic resonance imaging study. *Biol. Psychiatry* 57, 210–219. doi: 10.1016/j.biopsych.2004.10.030

Raz, N., Gunning, F. M., Head, D., Rodrigue, K. M., Williamson, A., and Acker, J. D. (2004). Aging, sexual dimorphism, and hemispheric asymmetry of the cerebral cortex: replicability of regional differences in volume. *Neruobiol. Aging* 25, 377–396. doi: 10.1016/S0197-4580(03)00118-0

Salthouse, T. A. (1995). Influence of processing speed on adult age differences in learning. *Swiss J. Psychol.* 54, 102–112.

Scheibe, S., and Blanchard-Fields, F. (2009). Effects of regulating emotions on cognitive performance: what is costly for young adults is not so costly for older adults. *Psychol. Aging* 24, 217–223. doi: 10.1037/a0013807

Silvers, J. A., Buhle, J. T., and Ochsner, K. N. (2013). "The neuroscience of emotion regulation: basic mechanisms and their role in development, aging, and psychopathology," in *The Handbook of Cognitive Neuroscience, Vol. 1*, eds K. N. Oshsner and S. M. Kosslyn (New York, NY: Oxford University Press), 52–78. doi: 10.1093/oxfordhb/9780199988709.013.0004

Shiota, M., and Levenson, R. (2009). Effects of aging on experimentally instructed detached reappraisal, positive reappraisal, and emotional behavior suppression. *Psychol. Aging* 24, 890–900. doi: 10.1037/a0017896

Talairach, J., and Tournoux, P. (1988). *Co-planar Stereotaxic Atlas of the Human Brain: 3-D Proportional System: An Approach to Cerebral Imaging.* New York, NY: Thieme.

Tucker, A. M., Feuerstein, R., Mende-Siedlecki, P., Ochsner, K. N., and Stern, Y. (2012). Double dissociation: circadian off-peak times increase emotional reactivity; aging impairs emotion regulation via reappraisal. *Emotion* 12, 869–874. doi: 10.1037/a0028207

Urry, H. L., and Gross, J. J. (2010). Emotion regulation in older age. *Curr. Dir. Psychol. Sci.* 19, 352–357. doi: 10.1177/0963721410388395

Urry, H. L., van Reekum, C. M., Johnstone, T., and Davidson, R. (2009). Individual differences in some (but not all) medial prefrontal regions reflect cognitive demand while regulating unpleasant emotion. *Neuroimage* 47, 852–863. doi: 10.1016/j.neuroimage.2009.05.069

Urry, H. L., van Reekum, C. M., Johnstone, T., Kalin, N. H., Thurow, M. E., Schaefer, H. S., et al. (2006). Amygdala and ventromedial prefrontal cortex are inversely coupled during regulation of negative affect and predict the diurnal pattern of cortisol secretion among older adults. *J. Neurosci.* 26, 4415–4425. doi: 10.1523/JNEUROSCI.3215-05.2006

van Reekum, C. M., Johnstone, T., Urry, H. L., Thurow, M. E., Schaefer, H. S., Alexander, A. L., et al. (2007). Gaze fixations predict brain activation during the voluntary regulation of picture-induced negative affect. *Neuroimage* 36, 1041–1055. doi: 10.1016/j.neuroimage.2007.03.052

Wager, T. D., Davidson, M., Hughes, B. L., Lindquist, M. A., and Ochsner, K. N. (2008). Prefrontal-subcortical pathways mediating successful emotion regulation. *Neuron* 59, 1037–1050. doi: 10.1016/j.neuron.2008.09.006

Walter, B., Blecker, C., Kirsch, P., Sammer, G., Schienle, A., Stark, R., et al. (2003). "MARINA: an easy to use tool for the creation of masks for region of interest analyses [abstract]," in *Presented at the 9th International Conference on Functional Mapping of the Human Brain* (New York, NY), CD-Rom in *Neuroimage* 19.

Winecoff, A., LaBar, K. S., Madden, D. J., Cabeza, R., and Huettel, S. A. (2011). Cognitive and neural contributors to emotion regulation in aging. *Soc. Cogn. Affect. Neurosci.* 6, 165–176. doi: 10.1093/scan/nsq030

2

# A note on age differences in mood-congruent vs. mood-incongruent emotion processing in faces

**Manuel C. Voelkle[1]*, Natalie C. Ebner[2], Ulman Lindenberger[1] and Michaela Riediger[1]**

[1] Center for Lifespan Psychology, Max Planck Institute for Human Development, Berlin, Germany
[2] Department of Psychology, University of Florida, Gainesville, FL, USA

**Edited by:**
Hakan Fischer, Stockholm University, Sweden

**Reviewed by:**
Hakan Fischer, Stockholm University, Sweden
Mara Fölster, Humboldt-Universität zu Berlin, Germany
Marie Hennecke, University of Zurich, Switzerland

***Correspondence:**
Manuel C. Voelkle, Center for Lifespan Psychology, Max Planck Institute for Human Development, Lentzeallee 94, Berlin 14195, Germany
e-mail: voelkle@mpib-berlin.mpg.de

This article addresses four interrelated research questions: (1) Does experienced mood affect emotion perception in faces and is this perception mood-congruent or mood-incongruent? (2) Are there age-group differences in the interplay between experienced mood and emotion perception? (3) Does emotion perception in faces change as a function of the temporal sequence of study sessions and stimuli presentation, and (4) does emotion perception in faces serve a mood-regulatory function? One hundred fifty-four adults of three different age groups (younger: 20–31 years; middle-aged: 44–55 years; older adults: 70–81 years) were asked to provide multidimensional emotion ratings of a total of 1026 face pictures of younger, middle-aged, and older men and women, each displaying six different prototypical (primary) emotional expressions. By analyzing the likelihood of ascribing an additional emotional expression to a face whose primary emotion had been correctly recognized, the multidimensional rating approach permits the study of emotion perception while controlling for emotion recognition. Following up on previous research on mood responses to recurring unpleasant situations using the same dataset (Voelkle et al., 2013), crossed random effects analyses supported a mood-congruent relationship between experienced mood and perceived emotions in faces. In particular older adults were more likely to perceive happiness in faces when being in a positive mood and less likely to do so when being in a negative mood. This did not apply to younger adults. Temporal sequence of study sessions and stimuli presentation had a strong effect on the likelihood of ascribing an additional emotional expression. In contrast to previous findings, however, there was neither evidence for a change from mood-congruent to mood-incongruent responses over time nor evidence for a mood-regulatory effect.

**Keywords: emotion perception, mood-(in)congruent information processing, mood regulation, faces, crossed random effects analysis**

## INTRODUCTION

How does the way we feel influence the perception of the world around us, and how does this perception in turn affect our own feelings? As innocuous as it may seem, this question constitutes one of the most fundamental research objectives in psychology, ranging from basic research on attention and perception (e.g., Becker and Leinenger, 2011; Hunter et al., 2011) to research in clinical psychology and psychiatry (e.g., Elliott et al., 2002; Eizenman et al., 2003; Rinck et al., 2003; Stuhrmann et al., 2013). For example, cognitive theories of anxiety and depression suggest attentional and memory biases of patients suffering from anxiety or depression toward threatening, respectively dysphoric, stimuli, which in turn contributes to the maintenance or aggravation of the disorder (Clark et al., 1999; Beevers and Carver, 2003; Koster et al., 2010). In particular the question of mood-congruent vs. mood-incongruent information processing, its determinants and consequences, has sparked a lot of research. The present paper contributes to this literature by investigating the relationship between experienced mood and the perception of emotional expression in faces, which has been shown to be important for individuals' social interactions (e.g., Baron-Cohen et al., 2000; Adolphs, 2003). Special emphasis will be put on age-related differences in mood-(in)congruent information processing, the role of the temporal sequence of study sessions and stimuli presentation, and the question whether mood may not only affect emotion perception, but whether emotion perception may also serve a mood-regulatory function.

As will be outlined in the following, a number of different theoretical models have been proposed to explain the—in parts conflicting—empirical findings on mood-congruent vs. mood-incongruent information processing:

### MOOD-CONGRUENT INFORMATION PROCESSING

There exists ample evidence that information is often processed in a *mood-congruent* manner. For example, people in a positive mood are more likely to recall positive memories (Bower, 1981, 1991; Mayer et al., 1995), and report to be more satisfied with their lives (Schwarz and Clore, 1983). Mood congruency effects were also observed for emotion perception in faces. The pattern of findings, however, is somewhat mixed. For example, Coupland et al. (2004) demonstrated that low positive affect (anhedonia) decreased the identification of happy expressions, while negative affect increased the identification of disgust. Contrary to expectations, however, there was no increase in anger identification related to negative affect. Furthermore, Suzuki et al. (2007) found partial support for a mood-congruency effect by observing a positive correlation between negative affect and recognition of sadness. However, this effect did not generalize to other negative emotions. In addition, age-related decrease in sadness recognition was linked to an age-related decrease in negative affect. For similar findings on the relation between age-related decline in the perceived intensity of emotions in faces and age-related decrease in anxiety and depression see Phillips and Allen (2004).

At a more general level, the mood-congruency effect has been explained in terms of Bower's (1981) *associative network theory.* This theory refers to the idea that emotions serve as memory units and that activation of such a unit not only "aids retrieval of events associated with it [but... ] also primes emotional themata for use in free association, fantasies, and perceptual categorization" (Bower, 1981, p. 129). The effect has also been explained in terms of *mood as information* (Schwarz and Clore, 2003, p. 296), that is, the idea that mood may serve an informational function and may help in directing attention to possible sources of feelings (Wyer and Carlston, 1979; Schwarz and Clore, 1983, 2003). Although both approaches suggest mood-congruent information processing, the proposed mechanisms differ. According to the *associative network theory*, mood influences information processing *indirectly* by priming the encoding, retrieval, and use of information, for example by selectively attending to "activated" mood-congruent details in the environment, by selectively encoding information into a network of primed associations, or by selectively retrieving mood-congruent information. According to the *mood-as-information account*, mood influences information processing *directly*. By (implicitly) asking themselves "... how do I feel about this? [... people... ] misread their current feelings as a response to the object of judgment, resulting in more favorable evaluations under positive rather than negative moods, unless their informational value is discredited" (Schwarz and Clore, 2003, p. 299).

In an attempt to integrate these seemingly contradictory explanations, Forgas (1995) proposed the *affect infusion model (AIM),* which states the more general preconditions for mood-congruency effects in judgmental processes. According to the AIM, affect-priming, in the sense of Bower's (1981) associative network theory, is most likely to occur during *substantive processing,* that is, in situations with complex, atypical, and/or personally relevant targets. For example, when being in a happy mood, people evaluate others more favorably than when being in a sad mood, in particular when judging unusual, atypical, persons (Forgas, 1992).

In contrast, mood-as-information (Schwarz and Clore, 1983) is the major affect infusion mechanism during *heuristic processing,* that is, in situations involving typical targets of low personal relevance and/or in situations with limited processing capacity (e.g., due to time pressure or information overload; Forgas, 1995).

### MOOD-INCONGRUENT INFORMATION PROCESSING AS A MOOD-REGULATORY FUNCTION

In addition to the various findings on mood-congruency effects, a number of studies suggested that information may also be processed in a *mood-incongruent* manner (Morris and Reilly, 1987; Matt et al., 1992; Erber and Erber, 1994; Sedikides, 1994; Forgas and Ciarrochi, 2002; Isaacowitz et al., 2008, 2009b). For example, in two recent articles Isaacowitz and colleagues (Isaacowitz et al., 2008, 2009b) showed that older adults gazed toward positively valenced facial stimuli when in a bad mood. In contrast, a mood-congruency effect was observed in younger adults, in that they were more likely to look at positively valenced faces when in a good mood and more likely to look at negatively valenced faces when in a bad mood. Based on the observed age-differential relationship between mood and gazing pattern, Isaacowitz et al. (2008) concluded that "in older adults, gaze does not reflect mood, but rather is used to regulate it" (2008; p. 848). This interpretation is in line with socioemotional selectivity theory, which postulates that older adults—because of a shrinking time horizon—shift their motivational priorities toward emotion regulation (Carstensen et al., 1999; Carstensen, 2006). Furthermore, given that most studies on mood-(in)congruent information processing used college-student populations, this finding cautions generalizations to other populations and underscores the importance of studying different age groups.

Building upon the *first, congruency; then, incongruency* hypothesis postulated by Sedikides (1994, p. 163), Forgas and Ciarrochi (2002) showed, in a series of three experiments, that after an initial mood-congruency effect, people in a sad mood were more likely to generate positive person descriptions, positive personality trait adjectives, as well as positive self-descriptions. These findings were interpreted in terms of a spontaneous, homeostatic, mood management mechanism "that limit[s] affect congruence and thus allow[s] people to control and calibrate their mood states by selectively accessing more affect-incongruent responses over time" (Forgas and Ciarrochi, 2002, p. 337). Thus, the temporal sequence of information processing seems to play a crucial role in the interplay between experienced mood and information processing. This may also apply to the processing of emotional expressions in faces as investigated in the present study.

What the studies by Isaacowitz and colleagues and Forgas and colleagues have in common is that differences in mood-congruent vs. mood-incongruent information processing are explained in terms of mood regulation. That is, by focusing on stimuli of a certain valence, people attempt to manage their mood (e.g., they up-regulate their mood when previously in a bad mood). In contrast to work on mood-congruent attentional and memory biases for negatively valenced material, the mechanisms underlying a mood-incongruent bias toward positively valenced stimuli have been less clearly spelled out. However, given the functional relevance of mood-congruent information processing for dysphoria and depression (e.g., Clark et al., 1999; Beevers and Carver, 2003; Koster et al., 2010), it seems reasonable to assume that focusing on positively valenced stimuli when in a bad mood may help to counteract this effect. The underlying mechanism may either constitute a rather spontaneous, homeostatic mood management (Forgas and Ciarrochi, 2002) or active mood regulation.

While Isaacowitz and colleagues explained the mood-congruency vs. mood-incongruency effect *in terms of age* ("mood-congruent gaze in younger adults, positive gaze in older adults", Isaacowitz et al., 2008, p. 848), Forgas and Ciarrochi explained the effect *in terms of elapsed processing time* ("initially mood-congruent responses tend to be automatically corrected and reversed over time," Forgas and Ciarrochi, 2002, p. 344; see also Sedikides, 1994). Such mood-incongruent information processing is also in line with the AIM, which postulates that mood-congruency effects will be eliminated, or reversed, if a person is influenced by a strong motivational component, such as to improve mood when being in a bad mood (i.e., motivated processing; Erber and Erber, 1994; Forgas, 1995). In the absence of a strong motivational component, the AIM proposes the *direct access strategy* as another type of a low affect infusion strategy, that is, an information processing strategy that is unlikely to result in a mood-congruency effect. "Direct access processing is most likely when the target is well known or familiar and has highly prototypical features that cue an already-stored and available judgment, the judge is not personally involved, and there are no strong cognitive, affective, motivational, or situational forces mandating more elaborate processing" (Forgas, 1995, p. 46). We will get back to this strategy in the discussion. For a more detailed description of the AIM, and the four alternative processing strategies related to low affect infusion (motivated processing and direct access strategy) and high affect infusion (heuristic and substantive processing), we refer the reader to Forgas (1995).

To summarize, current research has provided ample support for mood-congruent, but also mood-incongruent, information processing. The AIM provides a general framework that predicts the degree of mood-(in)congruency in information processing (Forgas, 1995). According to this model, mood-congruency effects are most likely under *substantive processing* or *heuristic processing* which is in line with Bower's (1981) associative network theory, and Schwarz and Clore's (1983) theory of mood-as-information, respectively. In contrast, mood-congruency is least likely in case of *motivated processing* or the *direct access* strategy. Especially when in a bad mood, people may be motivated to change this state. As suggested by Isaacowitz et al. (2008), this motivation may be particularly strong in older adults. Furthermore, Forgas and Ciarrochi (2002) observed a shift from mood-congruent to mood-incongruent information processing, pointing to the role of homeostatic cognitive strategies in affect regulation. However, when explaining mood-incongruent information processing in terms of mood regulation, the crucial—and often untested—question is how effective is it in changing peoples' mood? In a recent eye-tracking study, Isaacowitz et al. (2009a,b) showed that older adults with good cognitive functioning showed less mood decline throughout the study when gazing toward positively valenced faces. This provides initial support for the notion that in some people mood-incongruent information processing may serve a mood-regulatory function.

Overall, the research reviewed so far indicates that effects of experienced mood on information processing are by no means simple, but influenced by multiple factors. With few exceptions (e.g., Mayer et al., 1995), most studies on mood-(in)congruent information processing involved active mood induction. Little is known about the extent to which these findings generalize to naturally occurring mood. Moreover, in real-life situations the various mechanisms underlying mood-(in)congruent information processing may work simultaneously and are likely to influence each other. For example, being in a moderately gloomy mood may prime the associative network toward the perception of negatively valenced features in the environment. This in turn may be perceived as more negative because of one's gloomy mood (mood-as-information). At the same time, this may increase the motivation to improve one's mood by selectively attending to positively valenced features in the environment, possibly eliminating or even reversing a mood-congruency effect. At present it is unclear which of these processes will prevail under less extreme conditions of natural mood, rather than experimentally induced mood.

## THIS STUDY

The purpose of the present study was to link naturally occurring fluctuations in mood to the perception of emotions in faces in order to provide new insights into mood-congruent vs. mood-incongruent information processing. To this end we (1) examined whether natural mood affects emotion perception in faces and to what extent this perception was mood-congruent or mood-incongruent. We (2) tested for age group differences in the interplay between emotion perception and experienced mood, and (3) investigated the role of temporal sequence in emotion processing. Finally, we (4) examined the extent to which emotion perception in faces may serve a mood-regulatory function.

Based on previous findings reviewed above, and independent of age, we expected mood-congruent processing of emotional expressions in faces—operationalized as a higher likelihood of perceiving a positively valenced emotional expression when in a good mood, and a negatively valenced emotional expression when in a bad mood (*Hypothesis 1*). In line with prior research, but competing with Hypothesis 1, we expected older adults to have a higher likelihood of perceiving positive emotions in facial expressions when in a bad mood (*Hypothesis 2*). In addition, we expected a shift from mood-congruent to mood-incongruent information processing as a function of processing time (*Hypothesis 3*). Based on prior research, we expected a positive relationship between the likelihood of perceiving positively valenced emotions in faces and subsequent improvements in mood (*Hypothesis 4*), supporting the notion of a mood-regulatory function of emotion perception.

To test these hypotheses, we asked young, middle-aged, and older adults to indicate the amount of happiness, sadness, fear, disgust, anger, and neutrality they perceived in photographs of faces displaying prototypical happy, sad, fearful, disgusted, angry, or neutral facial expressions. Of importance, using a multidimensional rating approach, participants had rated all six emotions for each prototypical facial expression. For example, although a face may have been correctly recognized as displaying anger (prototypical primary expression), participants could indicate that they also perceived some sadness, or any of the other emotion(s), in the same face. In terms of the AIM, recognizing a prototypical facial expression is likely the result of either a direct access or motivational processing strategy and thus unlikely to infuse affect

(Forgas, 1995). In addition, individuals differ in their ability to recognize prototypical facial expressions, with age as an important predictor of these differences (see Ruffman et al., 2008, for an overview)[1] . For these reasons we were *not* interested in emotion recognition, but in the likelihood of ascribing an *additional* emotional expression to a face, whose primary emotion had already been correctly recognized. This procedure controls[2] for differences in emotion recognition and maximizes the likelihood of affect infusion (i.e., a mood-congruency or mood-incongruency effect). Throughout the remainder of this paper, the term *emotion perception* thus refers to the perception of additional emotional expressions in a face (other than the primary expression), once its primary emotional expression had been correctly recognized (see Methods section for details).

The present article follows up on previous work with the same dataset in which we investigated anticipatory and reactive mood changes throughout the course of the study (Voelkle et al., 2013), age-of-perceiver and age-of-rater effects on multidimensional emotion perception (Riediger et al., 2011), and accuracy and bias in age estimation (Voelkle et al., 2012). Until now, however, we never linked participants' mood to the perception of emotion in others (faces), which is the primary aim of the present study.

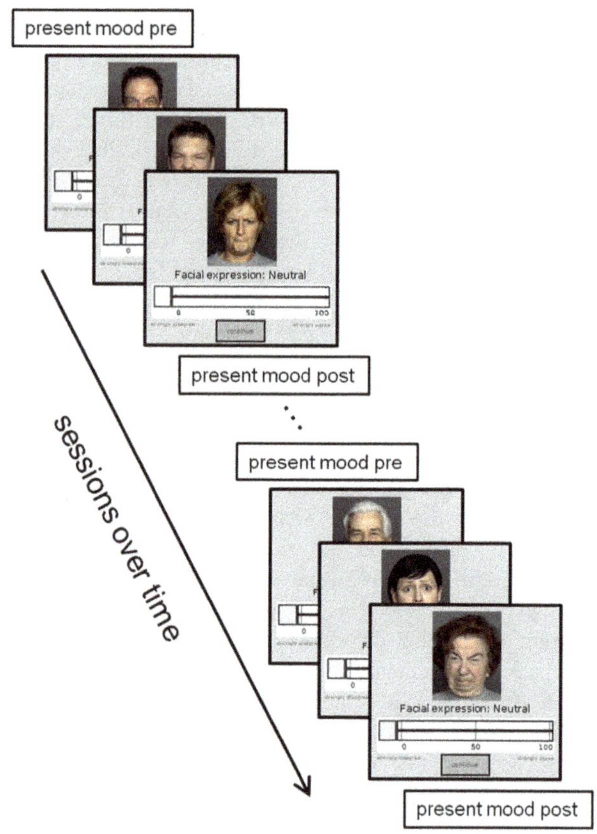


**FIGURE 1 | Illustration of the study procedure.** Present mood was assessed at the beginning and the end of each session. During each session, participants rated the emotional expression of different face pictures by adjusting a slider. In addition, the primary emotional expression (happiness, sadness, anger, disgust, fear, or neutrality) was assessed via categorical rating.

## METHODS

### PARTICIPANTS

One hundred fifty-four adults of three different age groups ($n = 52$ younger adults: 20–31 years; $n = 51$ middle-aged adults: 44–55 years; $n = 51$ older adults: 70–81 years) participated in the study. All of the 76 women and 78 men were Caucasian and German-speaking. Self-reported physical functioning was good, and visual-processing speed, as assessed by Wechsler's (1981) digit symbol substitution test, was comparable to typical performance levels in these age groups. For details about the demographic composition of the sample, see Ebner et al. (2010).

### PROCEDURE

The study was approved by the MPI ethics review board. **Figure 1** provides a graphical illustration of the study procedure. After giving informed consent, participants were randomly assigned to one of two sets of parallel face pictures, which were presented one at a time on a 19-inch monitor. For each picture, participants indicated in a self-paced fashion the degree of happiness, sadness, fear, disgust, anger, or neutrality perceived in the face on a scale from 0 (*does not apply at all*) to 100 (*applies completely*). After these continuous ratings, participants indicated which of the six emotions was primarily displayed in the face (categorical rating). This was followed by additional face-specific questions that are not of relevance for the present paper. Due to the large number of face stimuli, participants had to complete the ratings in several sessions. Each session lasted for 100 min and there was only one session per day. Although it took up to 24 sessions for the slowest participant to complete all ratings, we restricted our analyses to the first 10 sessions to maintain comparability with previous research and to avoid increasing sparseness of the data. Participants' mood was assessed at the beginning and at the end of each session.

### MEASURES

Positive and negative mood was assessed using Hampel's (1977) *Adjective Scales to Assess Mood.* For positive mood, participants

[1]For an analysis of age differences in emotional expression identification as a function of perceiver's and face model's age and facial expression with the present data, we refer the reader to Ebner et al. (2010).

[2]Although we disentangle the perception of additional emotional expressions from emotion recognition by analyzing only correctly recognized emotions, this does not preclude the possibility that people with higher recognition ability (and possible age differences therein) may be less likely to ascribe additional emotional expressions to a face after having identified the primary emotional expression. To control for this possibility, we repeated all analyses by including the person-specific recognition ability as an additional covariate. As a matter of fact, higher recognition ability decreased the likelihood of perceiving an additional emotional expression significantly (logit $= -10.750$; $p < 0.001$). In addition, the slightly lower (and non-significant at a 0.01 alpha level) likelihood of younger adults of perceiving an additional emotional expression disappeared after controlling for recognition ability. All other results, however, remained virtually unaffected by controlling for person-specific recognition ability. The additional analyses are provided as online Supplementary Materials A and B.

**Table 1 | Results of a crossed random effects analysis predicting the likelihood of perceiving an (additional but the primary) emotional expression in a face by type of emotion, positive mood, session number, stimulus number, and age group.**

| Parameter | Estimate | *SE* | *t*-value | *p*-value |
|---|---|---|---|---|
| **(A)** | | | | |
| Intercept (baseline: neutrality) | −1.9777 | 0.1230 | −16.07 | 0.000 |
| Happiness | −0.7191 | 0.018 | −39.94 | 0.000 |
| Anger | 1.0122 | 0.0147 | 69.03 | 0.000 |
| Disgust | 0.7639 | 0.0147 | 51.88 | 0.000 |
| Sadness | 0.7937 | 0.0147 | 53.90 | 0.000 |
| Fear | 0.9049 | 0.0147 | 61.53 | 0.000 |
| Session | −0.1340 | 0.0016 | −83.71 | 0.000 |
| Session squared | 0.0173 | 0.0006 | 29.25 | 0.000 |
| Younger adults (baseline: neutrality) | −0.3635 | 0.1727 | −2.10 | 0.035 |
| Older adults (baseline: neutrality) | 0.1622 | 0.1736 | 0.93 | 0.350 |
| Happiness × younger adults | −0.0446 | 0.025 | −1.78 | 0.075 |
| Happiness × older adults | −0.0179 | 0.0265 | −0.68 | 0.499 |
| Anger × younger adults | 0.0717 | 0.0202 | 3.55 | 0.000 |
| Anger × older adults | 0.0619 | 0.0216 | 2.87 | 0.004 |
| Disgust × younger adults | 0.1361 | 0.0203 | 6.72 | 0.000 |
| Disgust × older adults | 0.0318 | 0.0217 | 1.47 | 0.142 |
| Sadness × younger adults | 0.1819 | 0.0203 | 8.98 | 0.000 |
| Sadness × older adults | −0.0182 | 0.0217 | −0.84 | 0.403 |
| Fear × younger adults | 0.0727 | 0.0203 | 3.59 | 0.000 |
| Fear × older adults | 0.1388 | 0.0216 | 6.41 | 0.000 |
| **(B) MOOD–CONGRUENT vs. MOOD–INCONGRUENT INFORMATION PROCESSING IN FACES** | | | | |
| Positive mood (baseline: neutrality) | 0.0481 | 0.0155 | 3.11 | 0.002 |
| Positive mood × happiness | 0.1177 | 0.0207 | 5.69 | 0.000 |
| Positive mood × anger | −0.0365 | 0.0167 | −2.19 | 0.029 |
| Positive mood × disgust | −0.0595 | 0.0167 | −3.56 | 0.000 |
| Positive mood × sadness | −0.0560 | 0.0167 | −3.34 | 0.001 |
| Positive mood × fear | −0.1086 | 0.0167 | −6.50 | 0.000 |
| **(C) AGE GROUP DIFFERENCES IN MOOD–CONGRUENT vs. MOOD–INCONGRUENT INFORMATION PROCESSING** | | | | |
| Positive mood × younger adults (baseline: neutrality) | 0.0305 | 0.0204 | 1.50 | 0.135 |
| Positive mood × older adults (baseline: neutrality) | −0.1302 | 0.0236 | −5.53 | 0.000 |
| Positive mood × happiness × younger adults | −0.1567 | 0.0288 | −5.44 | 0.000 |
| Positive mood × happiness × older adults | 0.1512 | 0.0305 | 4.96 | 0.000 |
| Positive mood × anger × younger adults | −0.0128 | 0.0227 | −0.56 | 0.573 |
| Positive mood × anger × older adults | 0.0056 | 0.0244 | 0.23 | 0.818 |
| Positive mood × disgust × younger adults | −0.0580 | 0.0228 | −2.55 | 0.011 |
| Positive mood × disgust × older adults | 0.0764 | 0.0245 | 3.12 | 0.002 |
| Positive mood × sadness × younger adults | 0.0344 | 0.0228 | 1.51 | 0.131 |
| Positive mood × sadness × older adults | 0.0810 | 0.0246 | 3.29 | 0.001 |
| Positive mood × fear × younger adults | 0.0149 | 0.0228 | 0.65 | 0.513 |
| Positive mood × fear × older adults | −0.0291 | 0.0244 | −1.19 | 0.234 |
| **(D) TEMPORAL SEQUENCE IN MOOD–CONGRUENT vs. MOOD–INCONGRUENT INFORMATION PROCESSING** | | | | |
| Stimulus number (baseline: neutrality) | −0.0004 | 0.0004 | −1.05 | 0.295 |
| Happiness × stimulus number | −0.0028 | 0.0006 | −4.43 | 0.000 |
| Anger × stimulus number | −0.0026 | 0.0005 | −4.97 | 0.000 |
| Disgust × stimulus number | −0.0029 | 0.0005 | −5.63 | 0.000 |
| Sadness × stimulus number | −0.0016 | 0.0005 | −3.09 | 0.002 |
| Fear × stimulus number | −0.0017 | 0.0005 | −3.36 | 0.001 |
| Positive mood × stimulus number (baseline: neutrality) | −0.0008 | 0.0005 | −1.75 | 0.079 |
| Positive mood × happiness × stimulus number | 0.0011 | 0.0007 | 1.49 | 0.137 |
| Positive mood × anger × stimulus number | 0.0014 | 0.0006 | 2.36 | 0.018 |
| Positive mood × disgust × stimulus number | 0.0014 | 0.0006 | 2.44 | 0.015 |

*(Continued)*

**Table 1 | Continued**

| Parameter | Estimate | *SE* | *t*-value | *p*-value |
|---|---|---|---|---|
| Positive mood × sadness × stimulus number | 0.0006 | 0.0006 | 1.01 | 0.314 |
| Positive mood × fear × stimulus number | 0.0010 | 0.0006 | 1.63 | 0.102 |
| Random intercept face | Variance = 0.016; *SD* = 0.127 | | | |
| Random intercept participant | Variance = 2.289; *SD* = 1.513 | | | |
| AIC | 379620.8 | | | |
| BIC | 380192.4 | | | |
| Log-likelihood | −189758.4 | | | |
| Deviance | 379516.8 | | | |

*Type of emotion was dummy coded with perception of neutral emotional expression as baseline. Session = grand mean centered session number; Session squared = squared grand mean centered session number; Age group of participant (younger, middle-aged, older adults) was effect coded; Positive mood was group mean centered by subtracting the average positive mood at each study session; Stimulus number = individually centered position of stimulus in the sequence of stimuli within each session. Faces and participants were treated as two crossed random effects.*

indicated on a scale from one to five the extent to which they currently felt happy, cheerful, elated, in high spirits, relaxed, mellow, and exuberant. Negative mood was assessed using the seven items insecure, sorrowful, disappointed, hopeless, melancholic, downhearted, and helpless. Corrected item-scale correlations for positive mood at the first measurement time point ranged between 0.51 and 0.79 (Cronbach's $\alpha = 0.89$) and between 0.41 and 0.63 (Cronbach's $\alpha = 0.81$) for negative mood (see Voelkle et al., 2013).

### STIMULI

Face photographs of 58 younger (19–31 years), 56 middle-aged (39–55 years), and 57 older (69–80 years) adults were used as stimulus material. The photographs were taken from the FACES Lifespan Database of Facial Expressions (Ebner et al., 2010), which contains in two parallel sets a total of 2052 pictures, displaying each of the 171 target persons with a prototypical happy, angry, sad, disgusted, fearful, or neutral facial expression (i.e., the pictures were taken at the peak of the emotional expression, following a standardized production and selection procedure in line with the Affect Program Theory of facial expressions by Ekman, 1993). In line with the race and ethnicity of study participants and in order to reduce the design complexity (e.g., by avoiding possible race-biased in-group vs. out-group effects; cf. Meissner and Brigham, 2001) all face models were Caucasian. For details on the construction of the FACES database see Ebner et al. (2010).

### ANALYSIS

For each of the 1026 photographs (171 individuals times six emotions), $N = 154$ participants were asked to provide continuous emotion ratings on six different emotions, resulting in a theoretical maximum of $1026 \times 6 \times 154 = 948{,}024$ ratings (plus the categorical emotion ratings and other ratings as mentioned above). Given that the face pictures displayed maximally prototypical emotional expressions, with about 80%[3], the average recognition rate of the primary emotional expression was fairly high. As noted before, we were not interested in emotion recognition, but in the likelihood of ascribing an additional emotional expression to a face, for which the primary emotion had already been correctly recognized. Therefore, we controlled for interindividual differences in accuracy of emotion recognition, by including only ratings of those stimuli of which the primary emotional expression had been correctly identified (as indicated by the categorical ratings). Furthermore, we decided to analyze the *likelihood* with which an additional emotional expression was perceived in a face rather than the *intensity* of this perception. The reasons for this decision were twofold: First, the ratings of the additional emotions attributed to a face followed a highly right-skewed distribution. Despite correctly recognizing the primary facial expressions, some individuals indicated additional emotions of 100 (highest intensity of emotion expression) on a scale from 0 to 100. In addition, some people seemed to have used the middle of the rating scale as a reference point for some of their ratings. As a consequence, we could not find a meaningful transformation (such as a log-transform) that would have resulted in homoscedastic and normally distributed residuals. Second, in about 74% of the ratings, no additional continuous emotion ratings were provided resulting in a preponderance of zeros. Although models have been developed to deal with the combination of a zero-inflated and continuous or count part (Hall, 2000; Olsen and Schafer, 2001), we are not aware of any readily available integration with crossed random effects analyses employed in the present paper. Future research in this direction will be desirable.

Differences in the likelihood to perceive an emotion in addition to the primary emotion were modeled as a function of the type of *emotion* (happiness, sadness, fear, disgust, anger, neutrality; dummy coded with neutrality as baseline), *mood* at the beginning of the session (group mean centered at the average mood level prior to each session), study *session* (1–10; grand mean centered at 5.5), *age group* of perceiver (younger, middle-aged, older; effects coded), *stimulus number* (i.e., the relative position of a face photograph in the sequence of photographs presented to an individual participant, centered at the average number of stimuli rated by each individual in each session), and interactions

[3]The average recognition rate of emotional expressions differed across emotions and age groups. For a more detailed analysis, see Ebner et al. (2010).

**Table 2 | Results of a crossed random effects analysis predicting the likelihood of perceiving an (additional but the primary) emotional expression in a face by type of emotion, negative mood, session number, stimulus number, and age group.**

| Parameter | Estimate | *SE* | *t*-value | *p*-value |
|---|---|---|---|---|
| **(A)** | | | | |
| Intercept (baseline: neutrality) | −1.9633 | 0.1228 | −15.98 | 0.000 |
| Happiness | −0.7409 | 0.0190 | −39.06 | 0.000 |
| Anger | 0.9784 | 0.0151 | 64.99 | 0.000 |
| Disgust | 0.7296 | 0.0151 | 48.26 | 0.000 |
| Sadness | 0.7607 | 0.0151 | 50.32 | 0.000 |
| Fear | 0.8637 | 0.0151 | 57.13 | 0.000 |
| Session | −0.1331 | 0.0016 | −82.89 | 0.000 |
| Session squared | 0.0174 | 0.0006 | 29.29 | 0.000 |
| Younger adults (baseline: neutrality) | −0.3565 | 0.1724 | −2.07 | 0.039 |
| Older adults (baseline: neutrality) | 0.1484 | 0.1734 | 0.86 | 0.392 |
| Happiness × younger adults | −0.0519 | 0.0266 | −1.95 | 0.051 |
| Happiness × older adults | −0.0735 | 0.0286 | −2.56 | 0.010 |
| Anger × younger adults | 0.0529 | 0.021 | 2.52 | 0.012 |
| Anger × older adults | 0.0877 | 0.0221 | 3.96 | 0.000 |
| Disgust × younger adults | 0.0956 | 0.0211 | 4.53 | 0.000 |
| Disgust × older adults | 0.0631 | 0.0222 | 2.84 | 0.005 |
| Sadness × younger adults | 0.1713 | 0.0211 | 8.13 | 0.000 |
| Sadness × older adults | 0.0018 | 0.0223 | 0.08 | 0.936 |
| Fear × younger adults | 0.0169 | 0.0211 | 0.80 | 0.423 |
| Fear × older adults | 0.1773 | 0.0222 | 7.97 | 0.000 |
| **(B) MOOD–CONGRUENT vs. MOOD–INCONGRUENT INFORMATION PROCESSING IN FACES** | | | | |
| Negative mood (baseline: neutrality) | 0.0132 | 0.0265 | 0.50 | 0.618 |
| Negative mood × happiness | −0.2103 | 0.0396 | −5.31 | 0.000 |
| Negative mood × anger | −0.0520 | 0.0299 | −1.74 | 0.081 |
| Negative mood × disgust | 0.0514 | 0.0298 | 1.72 | 0.085 |
| Negative mood × sadness | −0.0500 | 0.0299 | −1.67 | 0.094 |
| Negative mood × fear | 0.1490 | 0.0297 | 5.03 | 0.000 |
| **(C) AGE GROUP DIFFERENCES IN MOOD–CONGRUENT vs. MOOD–INCONGRUENT INFORMATION PROCESSING** | | | | |
| Negative mood × younger adults (baseline: neutrality) | −0.0585 | 0.0314 | −1.86 | 0.063 |
| Negative mood × older adults (baseline: neutrality) | 0.0515 | 0.0422 | 1.22 | 0.222 |
| Negative mood × happiness × younger adults | 0.3286 | 0.0463 | 7.09 | 0.000 |
| Negative mood × happiness × older adults | −0.5495 | 0.0654 | −8.40 | 0.000 |
| Negative mood × anger × younger adults | 0.2393 | 0.0357 | 6.70 | 0.000 |
| Negative mood × anger × older adults | 0.0460 | 0.0459 | 1.00 | 0.316 |
| Negative mood × disgust × younger adults | 0.2511 | 0.0357 | 7.04 | 0.000 |
| Negative mood × disgust × older adults | −0.0853 | 0.046 | −1.86 | 0.063 |
| Negative mood × sadness × younger adults | 0.1920 | 0.0358 | 5.37 | 0.000 |
| Negative mood × sadness × older adults | −0.0669 | 0.0461 | −1.45 | 0.147 |
| Negative mood × fear × younger adults | 0.2346 | 0.0355 | 6.60 | 0.000 |
| Negative mood × fear × older adults | −0.0040 | 0.0458 | −0.09 | 0.931 |
| **(D) TEMPORAL SEQUENCE IN MOOD–CONGRUENT vs. MOOD–INCONGRUENT INFORMATION PROCESSING** | | | | |
| Stimulus number (baseline: neutrality) | −0.0005 | 0.0004 | −1.38 | 0.167 |
| Happiness × stimulus number | −0.0026 | 0.0006 | −4.31 | 0.000 |
| Anger × stimulus number | −0.0024 | 0.0005 | −4.70 | 0.000 |
| Disgust × stimulus number | −0.0028 | 0.0005 | −5.51 | 0.000 |
| Sadness × stimulus number | −0.0015 | 0.0005 | −3.03 | 0.002 |
| Fear × stimulus number | −0.0016 | 0.0005 | −3.13 | 0.002 |
| Negative mood × stimulus number (baseline: neutrality) | −0.0002 | 0.0007 | −0.36 | 0.720 |
| Negative mood × happiness × stimulus number | 0.0011 | 0.0010 | 1.06 | 0.289 |
| Negative mood × anger × stimulus number | 0.0005 | 0.0008 | 0.64 | 0.525 |

*(Continued)*

**Table 2 | Continued**

| Parameter | Estimate | *SE* | *t*-value | *p*-value |
|---|---|---|---|---|
| Negative mood × disgust × stimulus number | 0.0013 | 0.0008 | 1.53 | 0.126 |
| Negative mood × sadness × stimulus number | 0.0009 | 0.0008 | 1.04 | 0.297 |
| Negative mood × fear × stimulus number | 0.0002 | 0.0008 | 0.29 | 0.769 |
| Random intercept face | Variance = 0.016; *SD* = 0.127 | | | |
| Random intercept participant | Variance = 2.280; *SD* = 1.510 | | | |
| AIC | 379195.9 | | | |
| BIC | 379767.5 | | | |
| Log-likelihood | −189546.0 | | | |
| Deviance | 379091.9 | | | |

*Type of emotion was dummy coded with perception of neutral emotional expression as baseline. Session = grand mean centered session number; Session squared = squared grand mean centered session number; Age group of participant (younger, middle-aged, older adults) was effect coded; Negative mood was group mean centered by subtracting the average negative mood at each study session; Stimulus number = individually centered position of the stimulus in the sequence of stimuli within each session. Faces and participants were treated as two crossed random effects.*

between these factors[4]. Faces and participants were treated as two freely estimated crossed random effects in a generalized linear mixed effects model with a logit link function using the lme4 package 1.0.4 (Bates et al., 2013; see also Pinheiro and Bates, 2000) of R version 2.15.2 (R Core Team, 2012).

The possible role of emotion perception in faces as a mood-regulatory function was investigated by predicting the pre- to post-session *changes* in mood by how often a participant indicated perceiving a certain emotional expression out of the total number of ratings of this participant (i.e., the individual percentage of emotion perception in each session). In previous work we have demonstrated that changes in pre- to post-session mood decline significantly across the course of the entire study and that this change-in-change is almost perfectly captured by a logistic growth curve model (Voelkle et al., 2013). In order to control for this general trend we used the same model as in Voelkle et al. (2013) and added the interaction between age group and percentage of perceived emotional expression as time varying covariates with time varying effects[5]. To control for overall trends in emotion perception, session-mean centered scores were used.

## RESULTS

The results section is organized as follows: **Table 1** contains all parameter estimates of a single crossed random effects model as described above. In the following, we report results on the relationship between *positive* mood and emotion perception in faces. The corresponding results regarding *negative* mood and emotion perception are presented in **Table 2**. We will begin with discussing differences between displayed emotions, changes in emotion perception across study sessions, and age group differences in the perception of different emotions (**Tables 1, 2**, Part A). Next, we will turn to the question of *mood-congruent vs. mood-incongruent information processing in faces* by investigating the effect of present mood on the perception of different emotions in faces (*Hypothesis 1*; **Tables 1, 2**, Part B), as well as *age group differences in mood-congruent vs. mood-incongruent information processing* (*Hypothesis 2*; **Tables 1, 2**, Part C). After that we will focus on *the role of the temporal sequence in emotion processing* by analyzing the effect of stimulus position on emotion perception across the six different facial expressions along with a short discussion of possible three-way interactions of mood × stimulus position × emotion (*Hypothesis 3*; **Tables 1, 2**, Part D). Finally, we will investigate the *effectiveness of emotion perception in faces as a mood-regulatory function* (*Hypothesis* 4; **Figure 4**).

After recognizing the primary emotional expression, the average probability to perceive an additional neutral expression in a randomly selected face picture, presented after half of the stimuli had been rated within a given study session, and after half of the sessions had been completed was $[100 \cdot (1/(1 + e^{1.978}))] =$ 12.16% in a participant with an average within-session positive mood. However, there were large differences between the types of emotions: While the probability of perceiving an additional happy expression was significantly lower $[100 \cdot (1/(1 + e^{1.978+0.719}))] = 6.31\%$ (logit $= -0.719$; odds ratio $= 0.487$; $p < 0.001$), the probability of perceiving an additional angry expression was significantly higher (27.58%; logit $= 1.012$; odds ratio $= 2.751$; $p < 0.001$). The other emotions fell somewhere in between. Likewise, the likelihood of reporting an additional (neutral) emotional expression changed as a function of the number of sessions, with a significantly higher likelihood at the beginning of the study (20.82%) than after 10 sessions (6.79%). Note that the decline was not linear but leveled off toward the end of the study (i.e., a positive quadratic effect; $\text{logit}_{\text{Linear}} = -0.1340$, odds ratio $= 0.875$, $p < 0.001$; $\text{logit}_{\text{Quadratic}} = 0.017$, odds ratio $= 1.017$, $p < 0.001$). In contrast to the impact of session and type of emotion, age group differences in the perception of different emotions were smaller and somewhat mixed. As compared

[4] In a separate analysis, we included sex of participant as an additional predictor, which resulted in a non-significant improvement in model fit and did not change the pattern of results or any of the substantive conclusions ($2\text{Log-Likelihood}_{Diff} = 1.2$; $\text{df}_{Diff} = 1$). Because we had no prior expectations regarding sex effects, we report the analyses without sex.

[5] Missing values on the predictor variables due to study drop out were handled via Expectation Maximization (EM) imputation.

to the average age (age groups are effects coded[6]), the likelihood to perceive anger increased for both, younger ($\text{logit}_{\text{Younger}} = 0.072$, odds ratio $= 1.07$, $p < 0.001$) and older ($\text{logit}_{\text{Older}} = 0.062$, odds ratio $= 1.06$, $p < 0.001$) adults. The same applied to fear ($\text{logit}_{\text{Younger}} = 0.073$, odds ratio $= 1.08$, $p < 0.001$; $\text{logit}_{\text{Older}} = 0.139$, odds ratio $= 1.15$, $p < 0.001$). In addition, the likelihood of reporting disgust and sadness increased significantly in younger adults. However, with an odds ratio of $e^{0.182} = 1.20$ even the largest effect was rather small. See **Table 1**, Part A, for details.

## MOOD-CONGRUENT VS. MOOD-INCONGRUENT INFORMATION PROCESSING IN FACES

Turning to *Hypothesis 1*, and putting age aside for the moment, there was clear evidence for a mood-congruency effect in emotion perception. The more positive participants' mood, the more likely they were to perceive happiness in the presented faces. For example, someone in a maximally positive mood would have a probability of $[100 \cdot(1/(1 + e^{1.978+0.719-0.048\cdot 2-0.118\cdot 2}))] = 8.58\%$ of perceiving an additional happy expression, but only a probability of $[100 \cdot(1/(1 + e^{1.978+0.719-0.048\cdot -2-0.118\cdot -2}))] = 4.61\%$ if scoring at the lower end of the mood scale (logit $= 0.118$; odds ratio $= 1.125$; $p < 0.001$). Being in a positive mood also slightly increased the probability of perceiving an additional neutral expression (logit $= 0.048$; odds ratio $= 1.049$; $p < 0.01$). However, being in a positive mood consistently reduced the probability of perceiving an additional expression for all negatively valenced emotions (i.e., anger, disgust, sadness, and fear; see **Table 1**). See **Table 1**, Part B.

As apparent from **Table 2**, a similar pattern held for increasing negative mood. That is, higher levels of negative mood led to a lower probability of perceiving an additional happy expression (logit $= -0.210$; odds ratio $= 0.810$; $p < 0.001$), but an increase in the likelihood to perceive an additional fearful expression (logit $= 0.149$; odds ratio $= 1.161$; $p < 0.001$). All other emotions fell somewhere in between (none of them were significant at a 0.05 alpha level).

## AGE GROUP DIFFERENCES IN MOOD-CONGRUENT VS. MOOD-INCONGRUENT INFORMATION PROCESSING

Contradictory to *Hypothesis 2*, which predicted that older adults have a higher likelihood of perceiving positive emotions in facial expressions when being in a bad mood (i.e., mood-*in*congruency), a mood-congruency effect was primarily shown by older adults. Other than younger adults (logit $= -0.157$; odds ratio $= 0.855$; $p < 0.001$), older adults exhibited a significantly higher probability of perceiving happiness, when being in a good mood (logit $= 0.151$; odds ratio $= 1.163$; $p < 0.001$). **Figure 2** provides a graphical illustration of the model-predicted probabilities of perceiving an additional happy emotional expression in faces for younger and older adults with maximally high vs. low levels of positive mood. As compared to the baseline, higher levels of positive mood in older adults also increased the likelihood of perceiving disgust and sadness (logit $= 0.076$; odds ratio $= 1.079$; $p < 0.01$; logit $= 0.081$; odds ratio $= 1.084$; $p < 0.01$, respectively). In contrast, positive mood in older adults decreased the likelihood of perceiving neutrality (logit $= -0.130$; odds ratio $= 0.878$; $p < 0.001$). Although the results were somewhat mixed, the pronounced mood-congruency effect for older adults in the perception of happiness speaks against *Hypothesis 2*. See **Table 1**, Part C, for details. The effect for negative mood (**Table 2**) further bolstered the rejection of *Hypothesis 2*: Higher levels of negative mood in older adults *decreased* the probability of perceiving happiness (logit $= -0.550$; odds ratio $= 0.578$; $p < 0.001$), while no such decrease was found for younger adults (logit $= 0.329$; odds ratio $= 1.390$; $p < 0.001$). These results are illustrated in **Figure 3**.

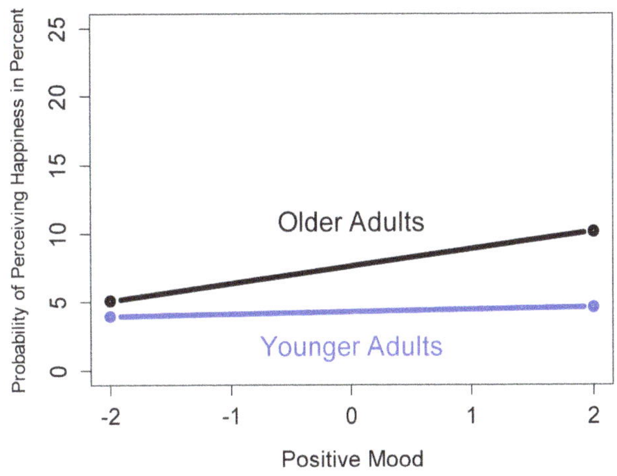


**FIGURE 2 | Predicted probability of perceiving an additional happy emotional expression in faces for younger and older adults with maximally high (right) vs. maximally low (left) levels of positive mood.**

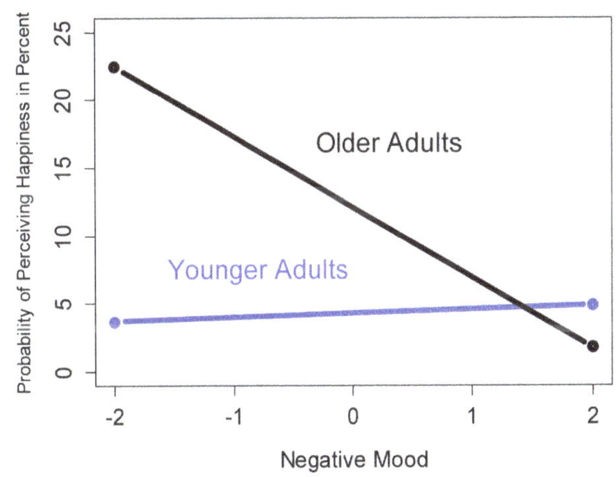


**FIGURE 3 | Predicted probability of perceiving an additional happy emotional expression in faces for younger and older adults with maximally high (right) vs. maximally low (left) levels of negative mood.**

[6]Middle-aged adults were chosen as the base group. As pointed out by Cohen et al. (2003), when using effects coding the base group is usually selected to be the group "for which comparisons to the mean are of *least* interest" (p. 322). This is because the analysis does not inform us *directly* about this group, but only indirectly. All information, however, is considered in the analysis. See Cohen et al. (2003) for more detailed information.

### THE ROLE OF THE TEMPORAL SEQUENCE IN EMOTION PROCESSING

The probability of perceiving an additional emotional expression decreased not only across study sessions, but also within each study session (i.e., with stimulus number; see **Table 1**, Part D). While the decrease was somewhat lower and non-significant for the perception of neutrality (logit $= -0.0004$; odds ratio $= 0.999$; $p = 0.295$), it was significant for all other emotions ($p < 0.01$). At the descriptive level, the downward trend in the likelihood of reporting an emotional expression, other than neutrality, was slightly weakened for participants in a positive mood, but none of the effects was significant at a 0.01 alpha level. Likewise, there were no three-way interactions with negative mood (see **Table 2**). Given the non-significant interaction of positive mood with stimulus number and negative mood with stimulus number, respectively, along with the uniform downward trend in the likelihood of perceiving an additional emotional expression, there was little evidence for a shift from mood-congruent to mood-incongruent information processing as a function of elapsed processing time in the present study. Thus, *Hypothesis 3* was rejected.

### EFFECTIVENESS OF EMOTION PERCEPTION IN FACES AS A MOOD-REGULATORY FUNCTION

In *Hypothesis* 4 we postulated a positive relationship between the likelihood of perceiving positively valenced emotions in faces and subsequent improvements in mood. This hypothesis was based on prior research suggesting that mood-incongruent information processing in older adults, or a shift from mood-congruent to mood-incongruent information processing as a function of processing time, may serve a mood-regulatory function—in particular if initial mood was bad. Given that we found no empirical support for Hypotheses 2 and 3 this seemed unlikely. To explicitly test the effect of emotion perception during a study session on mood changes from the beginning to the end of a session, we added the interaction between age group and percentage of perceived emotional expressions as time varying covariates to a logistic growth curve model of mood changes as described above. The results are presented in **Figure 4** which shows the standardized effects of emotion perception on pre- to post-session mood changes across the 10 study sessions, separated for younger, middle-aged, and older adults, and for all six emotional expressions. As apparent from the 95% confidence intervals, almost none of the effects were significant and there was no consistent pattern across time, across emotions, or across age groups. Rather, most effects varied around zero, providing no empirical support for *Hypothesis 4*.

## DISCUSSION

We began this work by asking how the way we feel influences the perception of the world around us, and how this perception may affect our own feelings. We approached this question by studying the relationship between natural mood (as opposed to experimentally induced mood) and the attribution of emotions to faces for which the primary emotional expression had been correctly identified.

Consistent with our expectations in Hypothesis 1, more positive mood increased the likelihood of perceiving a happy facial expression. In particular older adults had a higher likelihood of reporting the perception of happiness in faces when being in a positive mood, and a lower likelihood when being in a negative mood. Likewise, older adults were increasingly less likely to perceive happiness in faces when in a more negative mood. Both findings did not apply to younger adults. This stands in contrast to Hypothesis 2 which predicted that older adults have a higher likelihood of perceiving positive emotions in facial expressions when in a bad mood. In contrast to previous reports in the literature (Forgas and Ciarrochi, 2002; Isaacowitz et al., 2008, 2009a), we found neither evidence for a change from mood-congruent to mood-incongruent responses over time (Hypothesis 3) nor for a mood-regulatory effect of emotion processing in faces (Hypothesis 4). In the remainder of the discussion we will offer interpretations for our central findings.

### MOOD-CONGRUENT INFORMATION PROCESSING

Although partly in contrast to our expectations based on previous research using active mood induction in controlled laboratory settings, our results may be explained in terms of the AIM. The fact that older adults showed a mood-congruency effect in emotion perception suggests their use of a high affect infusion strategy such as heuristic or substantive processing. Unfortunately, the present study does not allow us to clearly disentangle the underlying mechanisms in terms of heuristic vs. substantive processing. Even though this remains an important topic to be addressed in future research, we believe that the observed mood-congruent information processing in older adults may even be due to a combination of the two processing strategies. On the one hand—and independent of present mood—older compared to younger adults were not only more likely to indicate the perception of an additional happy but also an additional neutral facial expression (see **Tables 1, 2**). This may reflect their higher personal involvement in the task, which suggests the use of a substantive processing strategy. On the other hand, reducing cognitive resources may have let older adults rely stronger on other sources of information, such as their current mood, supporting the notion of a heuristic (mood-as-information) processing strategy.

For younger adults in contrast, the increase in the perception of happiness almost completely disappeared (see **Figure 2**), suggesting their use of a low affect infusion strategy such as motivated processing or the direct access strategy. The motivation to increase one's mood—in particular when in a bad mood—should not only eliminate a mood-congruency effect, but should result in mood-incongruent information processing (i.e., an increased likelihood of perceiving happiness). The fact that we did not observe such an effect, rather suggests the use of a direct access strategy in younger adults. As described in the introduction, this strategy is particularly likely when "the judge is not personally involved, and there are no strong cognitive, affective, motivational, or situational forces mandating more elaborate processing" (Forgas, 1995, p. 46).

### MOOD-INCONGRUENT INFORMATION PROCESSING AS A MOOD-REGULATORY FUNCTION

As apparent from **Figure 4**, there was no empirical support that emotion perception in faces serves a mood-regulatory function

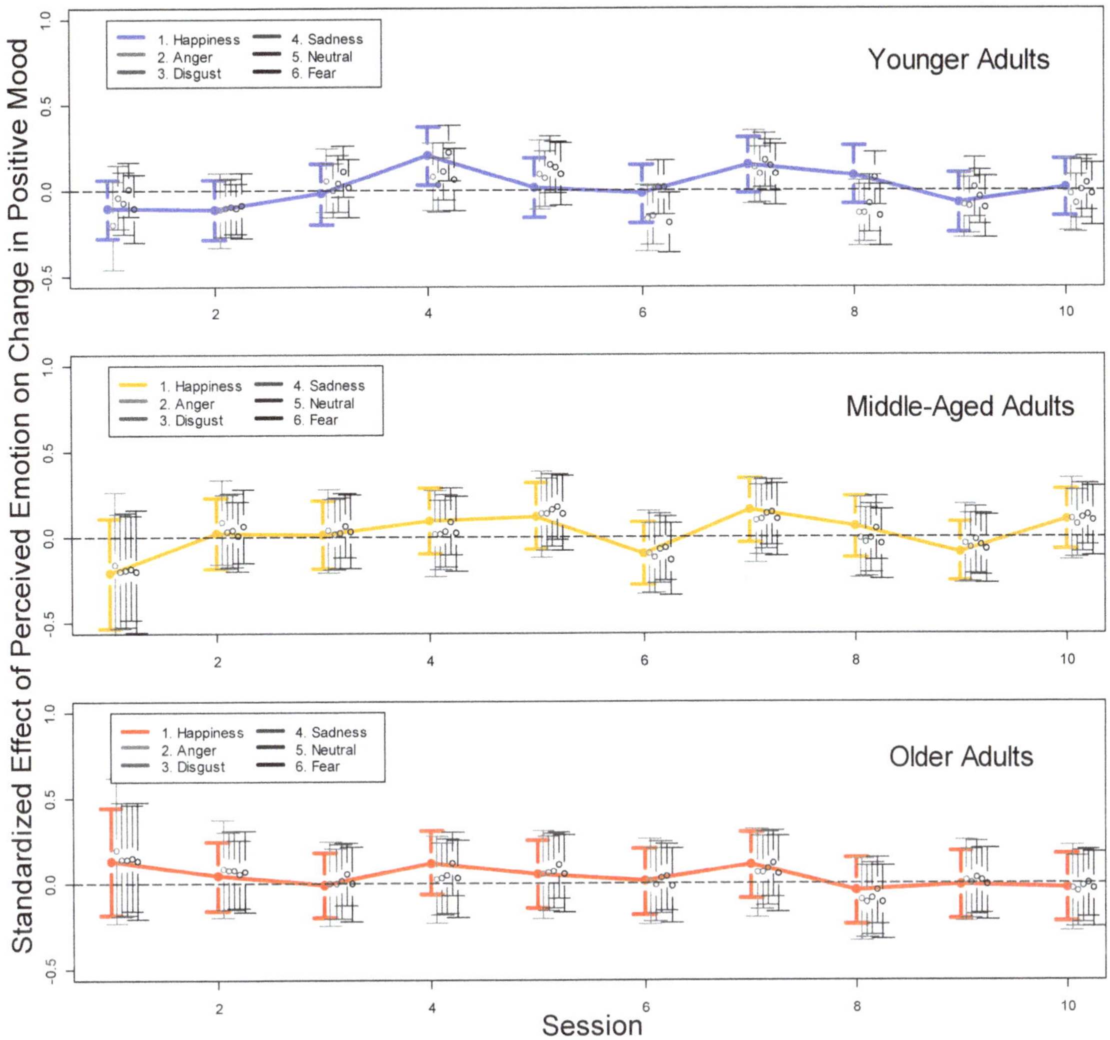


**FIGURE 4 | Standardized effects of perceived happiness, anger, disgust, sadness, neutrality, and fear on changes between pre- to post-session mood for younger, middle-aged, and older participants.** In six separate analyses (for the six emotions), the interaction between perceived emotional expression and age group was entered as a time-varying covariate with time-varying effects into a logistic growth curve model of changes in mood changes across the 10 study sessions (see Voelkle et al., 2013).

under conditions of natural occurring mood rather than actively induced mood. This stands in contrast to research using experimentally induced mood, which showed that the focus of older adults in a bad mood on positively valenced faces may help to regulate their mood. One reason for these different findings may be that the naturally occurring fluctuations in positive mood assessed in the present context were not sufficiently strong to reveal such an effect. Furthermore, ascribing an additional emotional expression to a face whose primary emotion had been correctly recognized is, of course, a much more subtle measure of mood-(in)congruent emotion processing as compared, for example, to gaze patterns toward prototypically positively or negatively valenced facial expressions as used in the study by Isaacowitz et al. (2008). In addition, the anticipatory (down)adjustment of positive mood may have further reduced the likelihood of discovering such an effect (Voelkle et al., 2013).

## LIMITATIONS AND FUTURE DIRECTIONS

We believe the general downward trend in the likelihood of reporting an emotional expression is likely due to participant's increasing fatigue and decreasing motivation. However, it is a shortcoming of the present study that these factors were not assessed in self-report, thus this belief remains speculative. Although we statistically controlled for the downward trend, the remaining variability in mood and emotion perception may have been too small to allow for additional mood regulation effects by means of emotion perception. After all, if an individual's mood is already perfectly adjusted to the situation at hand—or if fatigue effects are very strong—there is little room for additional regulation via mood-incongruent information processing.

This may be viewed as a shortcoming of the present study. However, it also shows that while natural mood (as opposed to experimentally induced mood) is likely to affect the perception of emotions in faces, a possible mood-regulatory effect of such perception seems negligible. In fact, we found that in particular for older adults, positive mood may rather increase the likelihood of perceiving positively valenced facial expressions.

The somewhat undifferentiated take on emotions and mood may be considered another weakness of the study. Future research may profit from more fine-grained distinctions between different aspects of positive and negative mood, including different aspects of valence and arousal, and a discrete emotion perspective as outlined by Kunzmann et al. (2014) in this issue. However, the primary purpose of the present paper was not to offer a comprehensive framework on age-related changes in the intricate interplay between specific aspects of affective experience and the perception (attribution) of additional emotions in faces whose primary emotion were correctly specified. Rather the focus was to place research on emotion perception in faces into the broader context on mood-congruent vs. mood-incongruent information processing. To accomplish this goal it is necessary to remain at a more general level, although we do report more detailed findings. In the same way we encourage future research to focus on more detailed aspects of experienced mood and the perception of emotional expression, we, thus, also encourage more integrative research linking these findings back to more general research on age-related changes in mood-(in)congruent information processing. We hope the present paper will contribute to both ends.

## ACKNOWLEDGMENTS

We thank Dulce Erdt, Colin Bauer, Philipp Möller, Luara Santos-Ferreira, Giorgi Kobakhidze, and the COGITO-Team for their assistance in study implementation, data collection, and data management. We thank Janek Berger for editorial assistance.

## REFERENCES

Adolphs, R. (2003). Cognitive neuroscience of human social behaviour. *Nat. Rev. Neurosci.* 4, 165–178. doi: 10.1038/nrn1056

Baron-Cohen, S. E., Tager-Flusberg, H. E., and Cohen, D. J. (2000). *Understanding Other Minds: Perspectives from Developmental Cognitive Neuroscience.* 2nd Edn. Oxford: Oxford Univeristy Press.

Bates, D., Maechler, M., Bolker, B., and Walker, S. (2013). *lme4: Linear Mixed-Effects Models using Eigen and S4 (Version 1.0-4) [R package].* Available online at: http://CRAN.R-project.org/package=lme4

Becker, M. W., and Leinenger, M. (2011). Attentional selection is biased toward mood-congruent stimuli. *Emotion* 11, 1248–1254. doi: 10.1037/a0023524

Beevers, C. G., and Carver, C. S. (2003). Attentional bias and mood persistence as prospective predictors of dysphoria. *Cogn. Ther. Res.* 27, 619–637. doi: 10.1023/A:1026347610928

Bower, G. H. (1981). Mood and memory. *Am. Psychol.* 36, 129–148. doi: 10.1037/0003-066X.36.2.129

Bower, G. H. (1991). "Mood congruity of social judgements," in *Emotion and Social Judgements,* ed J. P. Forgas (New York, NY: Pergamon), 31–53.

Carstensen, L. L. (2006). The influence of a sense of time on human development. *Science* 312, 1913–1915. doi: 10.1126/science.1127488

Carstensen, L. L., Isaacowitz, D. M., and Charles, S. T. (1999). Taking time seriously: a theory of socioemotional selectivity. *Am. Psychol.* 54, 165–181. doi: 10.1037/0003-066X.54.3.165

Clark, D. A., Beck, A. T., and Alford, B. A. (1999). *Scientific Foundations of Cognitive Theory and Therapy for Depression.* New York, NY: John Wiley and Sons.

Cohen, J., Cohen, P., West, S. G., and Aiken, L. S. (2003). *Applied Multiple Regression/Correlation Analysis for the Behavioral Sciences.* 3rd Edn. Hillsdale, NJ: Erlbaum.

Coupland, N. J., Sustrik, R. A., Ting, P., Li, D., Hartfeil, M., Singh, A. J., et al. (2004). Positive and negative affect differentially influence identification of facial emotions. *Depress. Anxiety* 19, 31–34. doi: 10.1002/da.10136

Ebner, N. C., Riediger, M., and Lindenberger, U. (2010). FACES—A database of facial expressions in young, middle-aged, and older women and men: development and validation. *Behav. Res. Methods* 42, 351–362. doi: 10.3758/BRM.42.1.351

Eizenman, M., Yu, L. H., Grupp, L., Eizenman, E., Ellenbogen, M., Gemar, M., et al. (2003). A naturalistic visual scanning approach to assess selective attention in major depressive disorder. *Psychiatry Res.* 118, 117–128. doi: 10.1016/S0165-1781(03)00068-4

Ekman, P. (1993). Facial expression and emotion. *Am. Psychol.* 48, 384–392. doi: 10.1037/0003-066X.48.4.384

Elliott, R., Rubinsztein, J. S., Sahakian, B. J., and Dolan, R. J. (2002). The neural basis of mood-congruent processing biases in depression. *Arch. Gen. Psychiatry* 59, 597–604. doi: 10.1001/archpsyc.59.7.597

Erber, R., and Erber, M. W. (1994). Beyond mood and social judgment: mood incongruent recall and mood regulation. *Eur. J. Soc. Psychol.* 24, 79–88. doi: 10.1002/ejsp.2420240106

Forgas, J. P. (1992). Mood and the perception of unusual people: affective asymmetry in memory and social judgments. *Eur. J. Soc. Psychol.* 22, 531–547. doi: 10.1002/ejsp.2420220603

Forgas, J. P. (1995). Mood and judgment: the affect infusion model (AIM). *Psychol. Bull.* 117, 39–66. doi: 10.1037/0033-2909.117.1.39

Forgas, J. P., and Ciarrochi, J. V. (2002). On managing moods: evidence for the role of homeostatic cognitive strategies in affect regulation. *Pers. Soc. Psychol. Bull.* 28, 336–345. doi: 10.1177/0146167202286005

Hall, D. B. (2000). Zero-Inflated poisson and binomial regression with random effects: a case study. *Biometrics* 56, 1030–1039. doi: 10.1111/j.0006-341X.2000.01030.x

Hampel, R. (1977). Adjektiv-Skalen zur Einschätzung der Stimmung (SES) [Adjective scales to assess mood]. *Diagnostica* 23, 43–60.

Hunter, P. G., Schellenberg, E. G., and Griffith, A. T. (2011). Misery loves company: mood-congruent emotional responding to music. *Emotion* 11, 1068–1072. doi: 10.1037/a0023749

Isaacowitz, D. M., Allard, E. S., Murphy, N. A., and Schlangel, M. (2009a). The time course of age-related preferences toward positive and negative stimuli. *J. Gerontol. B Psychol. Sci. Soc. Sci.* 64B, 188–192. doi: 10.1093/geronb/gbn036

Isaacowitz, D. M., Toner, K., Goren, D., and Wilson, H. R. (2008). Looking while unhappy: mood-congruent gaze in young adults, positive gaze in older adults. *Psychol. Sci.* 19, 848–853. doi: 10.1111/j.1467-9280.2008.02167.x

Isaacowitz, D. M., Toner, K., and Neupert, S. D. (2009b). Use of gaze for real-time mood regulation: Effects of age and attentional functioning. *Psychol. Aging* 24, 989–994. doi: 10.1037/a0017706

Koster, E. H. W., De Raedt, R., Leyman, L., and De Lissnyder, E. (2010). Mood-congruent attention and memory bias in dysphoria: exploring the coherence among information-processing biases. *Behav. Res. Ther.* 48, 219–225. doi: 10.1016/j.brat.2009.11.004

Kunzmann, U., Kappes, C., and Wrosch, C. (2014). Emotional aging: a discrete emotions perspective. *Front. Psychol.* 5:380. doi: 10.3389/fpsyg.2014.00380

Matt, G. E., Vázquez, C., and Campbell, W. K. (1992). Mood-congruent recall of affectively toned stimuli: a meta-analytic review. *Clin. Psychol. Rev.* 12, 227–255. doi: 10.1016/0272-7358(92)90116-P

Mayer, J. D., McCormick, L. J., and Strong, S. E. (1995). Mood-congruent memory and natural mood: new evidence. *Pers. Soc. Psychol. Bull.* 21, 736–746. doi: 10.1177/0146167295217008

Meissner, C. A., and Brigham, J. C. (2001). Thirty years of investigatin the own-race bias in memory for faces: a meta-analytic review. *Psychol. Public Policy Law* 7, 3–35. doi: 10.1037/1076-8971.7.1.3

Morris, W. N., and Reilly, N. P. (1987). Toward the self-regulation of mood: theory and research. *Motiv. Emot.* 11, 215–249. doi: 10.1007/BF01001412

Olsen, M. K., and Schafer, J. L. (2001). A two-part random-effects model for semicontinuous longitudinal data. *J. Am. Stat. Assoc.* 96, 730–745. doi: 10.2307/2670310

Phillips, L., and Allen, R. (2004). Adult aging and the perceived intensity of emotions in faces and stories. *Aging Clin. Exp. Res.* 16, 190–199. doi: 10.1007/BF03327383

Pinheiro, J. C., and Bates, D. M. (2000). *Mixed-Effects Models in S and S-Plus*. New York, NY: Springer. doi: 10.1007/978-1-4419-0318-1

R Core Team. (2012). *R: a Language and Environment for Statistical Computing.* Vienna: R Foundation for Statistical Computing. Available online at: http://www.R-project.org/

Riediger, M., Voelkle, M. C., Ebner, N. C., and Lindenberger, U. (2011). Beyond "happy, angry, or sad?": age-of-poser and age-of-rater effects on multidimensional emotion perception. *Cogn. Emotion* 25, 968–982. doi: 10.1080/02699931.2010.540812

Rinck, M., Becker, E. S., Kellermann, J., and Roth, W. T. (2003). Selective attention in anxiety: distraction and enhancement in visual search. *Depress. Anxiety* 18, 18–28. doi: 10.1002/da.10105

Ruffman, T., Henry, J. D., Livingstone, V., and Phillips, L. H. (2008). A meta-analytic review of emotion recognition and aging: implications for neuropsychological models of aging. *Neurosci. Biobehav. Rev.* 32, 863–881. doi: 10.1016/j.neubiorev.2008.01.001

Schwarz, N., and Clore, G. L. (1983). Mood, misattribution, and judgments of well-being: informative and directive functions of affective states. *J. Pers. Soc. Psychol.* 45, 513–523. doi: 10.1037/0022-3514.45.3.513

Schwarz, N., and Clore, G. L. (2003). Mood as information: 20 years later. *Psychol. Inq.* 14, 296–303. doi: 10.1080/1047840X.2003.9682896

Sedikides, C. (1994). Incongruent effects of sad mood on self-conception valence: it's a matter of time. *Eur. J. Soc. Psychol.* 24, 161–172. doi: 10.1002/ejsp.2420240112

Stuhrmann, A., Dohm, K., Kugel, H., Zwanzger, P., Redlich, R., Grotegerd, D., et al. (2013). Mood-congruent amygdala responses to subliminally presented facial expressions in major depression: associations with anhedonia. *J. Psychiatry Neurosci.* 38, 249–258. doi: 10.1503/jpn.120060

Suzuki, A., Hoshino, T., Shigemasu, K., and Kawamura, M. (2007). Decline or improvement? Age-related differences in facial expression recognition. *Biol. Psychol.* 74, 75–84. doi: 10.1016/j.biopsycho.2006.07.003

Voelkle, M. C., Ebner, N. C., Lindenberger, U., and Riediger, M. (2012). Let me guess how old you are: effects of age, gender, and facial expression on perceptions of age. *Psychol. Aging* 27, 265–277. doi: 10.1037/a0025065

Voelkle, M. C., Ebner, N. C., Lindenberger, U., and Riediger, M. (2013). Here we go again: anticipatory and reactive mood responses to recurring unpleasant situations throughout adulthood. *Emotion* 13, 424–433. doi: 10.1037/a0031351

Wechsler, D. (1981). *Wechsler Adult Intelligence Scale - Revised (WAIS-R)*. New York, NY: Psychological Corporation.

Wyer, R. S., and Carlston, D. E. (1979). *Social Cognition, Inference, and Attribution* Hillsdale, NJ: Lawrence Erlbaum Associates, Inc.

# 3

# Emotion and aging: evidence from brain and behavior

**Natalie C. Ebner[1]* and Håkan Fischer[2]**

[1] Psychology, Social-Cognitive and Affective Development Lab, Department of Psychology, University of Florida, Gainesville, FL, USA
[2] Department of Psychology, Stockholm University, Stockholm, Sweden

**Edited by:**
Marina A. Pavlova, Eberhard Karls Universität Tübingen, Germany

**Reviewed by:**
Nichole Lighthall, Duke University, USA
Antje Rauers, Max Planck Institute for Human Development, Germany

***Correspondence:**
Natalie C. Ebner, Psychology, Social-Cognitive and Affective Development Lab, Department of Psychology, University of Florida, Gainesville, FL 32611, USA
e-mail: natalie.ebner@ufl.edu

Emotions play a central role in every human life from the moment we are born until we die. They prepare the body for action, highlight what should be noticed and remembered, and guide decisions and actions. As emotions are central to daily functioning, it is important to understand how aging affects perception, memory, experience, as well as regulation of emotions. The Frontiers research topic *Emotion and Aging: Evidence from Brain and Behavior* takes a step into uncovering emotional aging considering both brain and behavioral processes. The contributions featured in this issue adopt innovative theoretical perspectives and use novel methodological approaches to target a variety of topics that can be categorized into three overarching questions: *How do cognition and emotion interact in aging in brain and behavior? What are behavioral and brain-related moderators of emotional aging? Does emotion-regulatory success as reflected in brain and behavior change with age?* In this perspective paper we discuss theoretical innovation, methodological approach, and scientific advancement of the 13 papers in the context of the broader literature on emotional aging. We conclude by reflecting on topics untouched and future directions to take.

**Keywords: emotional aging, brain-behavior links, cognition–emotion interactions, age-of-face effects, emotion regulation**

Emotions play a central role throughout human life. They highlight what is important and guide actions. As emotions are central to daily functioning, it is important to understand how aging affects them. An early scientific view argued that aging led to a deterioration of emotional function. This theory, represented by Carl Jung, claimed that old age is a period in life when people feel emotional sameness and the aging emotional landscape was described as bleached and barren. However, current psychological research shows that emotion is relatively unaffected by aging or even improves with age, in contrast to most cognitive functions (Scheibe and Carstensen, 2010). For example, aging is associated with improved emotional problem solving (Blanchard-Fields, 2007) and increased frequency of positive feelings (Carstensen et al., 2011). However, other emotional capacities, such as the ability to recognize other's emotions, decline with age (Ruffman et al., 2008). Such variations across emotional functional domains, and our limited understanding of mediating and moderating factors, call for more research. Given various representational levels of the phenomenon, an approach that combines brain and behavior in uncovering emotional aging seems promising.

The current Frontiers research topic takes a step into this direction. It comprises novel theoretical and methodological approaches and presents exciting new findings. The contributions evolve around three broader questions that have only recently received attention in the literature on emotional aging and answers to which will inform affective science research: (1) *How do cognition and emotion interact in aging in brain and behavior?* (2) *What are behavioral and brain-related moderators of emotional aging?* (3) *Does emotion-regulatory success as reflected in brain and behavior change with age?* Within those overarching questions, different emotion-related phenomena (emotion perception, emotion experience, attention and memory related to emotion, emotion regulation) will be addressed.

In the following, we will summarize the contributions. We will illustrate how they increase scientific understanding of emotional aging. In particular, we will emphasize how adoption of diverse theoretical and methodological approaches allow for a multifaceted study of emotional aging and we will lay out how adopting an aging brain-behavior prespective increases understanding of cognition–emotion interactions, moderators of emotion processing, and emotion-regulatory success. We will conclude by raising topics not yet covered for exploration in future research.

## NEW THEORETICAL AND METHODOLOGICAL APPROACHES IN THE STUDY ON EMOTION AND AGING

The research topic presents novel theoretical perspectives on emotional aging. Two of these are featured in perspective papers as summarized next. Other approaches are embedded in the context of the empirical paper contributions and integrated in the discussion below.

### A DISCRETE EMOTIONS APPROACH THAT CONSIDERS MULTI-DIRECTIONAL AGE DIFFERENCES IN SPECIFIC EMOTIONS OFFERS NEW DIRECTIONS OF RESEARCH

Complementing lifespan theories of developmental regulation that define negative affect and positive affect broadly (e.g., Baltes and Baltes, 1990), Kunzmann et al. (2014) propose a discrete emotions perspective on emotional aging. This approach links emotions to goals, emphasizing person–context interactions in their impact on adaptiveness of specific emotions (Haase et al., 2012). The approach is illustrated by delineating differential adult lifespan trajectories in the experience of anger and sadness. It sheds light on the mechanisms related to cognitive and physiological resources that underlie adaptive consequences of anger reactions in young adulthood and sadness reactions in old age and may prove particularly useful in understanding multi-directionality of affective responses across the adult lifespan. Extending this theoretical perspective to other emotions and across the entire lifespan will guide future research. English and Carstensen (2014) and Svärd et al. (2014) in this issue adopted a discrete emotions perspective. In contrast, Völkle et al. (2014) promote the usefulness of a multi-dimensional emotions approach, proposing that more than just one emotion is represented in a face. Other contributions differentiate broadly between positive and negative emotions (Pehlivanoglu et al., 2014; Petrican et al., 2014; Truong and Yang, 2014) and/or highlight the impact of the emotion dimension of arousal (Dolcos et al., 2014; English and Carstensen, 2014; Svärd et al., 2014; Truong and Yang, 2014).

### AGE OF THE FACE AFFECTS INTERPRETATION OF FACIAL EXPRESSIONS ACROSS THE ADULT LIFESPAN

The ability to read facial emotions in others declines with age (Ruffman et al., 2008). Fölster et al. (2014) propose that beyond effects of the age of the observer, effects of the age of the face, in interaction with the emotion expressed in the face, need to be considered in research on facial emotion perception. In particular, group differences in expressive style, higher familiarity with faces of in-group members (Elfenbein and Ambady, 2002) and increased motivation toward in-group faces (Thibault et al., 2006) may contribute to age-congruency effects. Fölster et al. (2014) importantly conclude that such effects are crucial in the context of face memory (Rhodes and Anastasi, 2012) but may play less of a role in facial emotion perception. The proposed perspective will facilitate future examination of how age stereotypes influence face recognition bias and how age differences in the frequency of experiencing certain emotions may affect change in facial features. Use of longitudinal approaches and ecologically valid stimuli, such as implemented in some contributions in this issue (Petrican et al., 2014; Riediger et al., 2014), appear particularly promising.

This issue is characterized by a wide selection of methodological approaches, reflecting the complexity of the emotional aging phenomenon. Employed approaches are experience sampling (English and Carstensen, 2014), subjective evaluations (Petrican et al., 2014; Riediger et al., 2014; Svärd et al., 2014; Völkle et al., 2014), cognitive-behavioral measures (Pehlivanoglu et al., 2014; Svärd et al., 2014; Truong and Yang, 2014), eye tracking (Pehlivanoglu et al., 2014), functional neuroimaging (Allard and Kensinger, 2014; Cassidy et al., 2014; Dolcos et al., 2014; Opitz et al., 2014), and electrophysiology (Opitz et al., 2014). Some of the contributions apply multiple methods to the same sample (Opitz et al., 2014; Pehlivanoglu et al., 2014), enabling integration of research findings. However, this research topic, as is characteristic of the current research field, also faces methodological heterogeneity between studies. While this allows for a multifaceted reflection on emotional aging, a direct comparison across studies is difficult. Innovatively, several contributions leverage new statistical advancements in multi-level modeling to decompose intra-individual from inter-individual variability (English and Carstensen, 2014; Opitz et al., 2014; Petrican et al., 2014).

## COGNITION–EMOTION INTERACTIONS IN AGING FROM A BRAIN-BEHAVIOR PERSPECTIVE

A growing number of studies are targeting cognition–emotion interactions. The majority of these studies examine behavioral age-related change (Isaacowitz and Riediger, 2011). Still little is known about the cognition–emotion interplay from an aging brain perspective (Fischer et al., 2010; Samanez-Larkin and Carstensen, 2011). Various contributions in this issue have addressed this research gap. As summarized next, Völkle et al. (2014) demonstrate a mood-emotion perception link across the adult lifespan. Svärd et al. (2014) show direct effects of emotion evaluations on emotion-related cognition. Cassidy et al. (2014), Pehlivanoglu et al. (2014), and Truong and Yang (2014) clarify age differences in working memory/source memory for information with emotional content.

### MOOD INFLUENCES YOUNG AND OLDER ADULTS' EMOTION PERCEPTION AND EMOTION PERCEPTION IN TURN AFFECTS MOOD

In Völkle et al. (2014) young, middle-aged, and older adults indicated their current mood before providing facial ratings along prototypical emotional expressions, using a multi-dimensional approach to emotions. Crossed-random effects analyses supported a mood-congruency effect: after controlling for accurate recognition of the primary facial expression, better mood increased the likelihood of perceiving additional facial happiness, while it reduced the likelihood of perceiving additional negative facial expressions. A reversed pattern held for negative mood. These effects were primarily shown by older adults. By assessing naturally occurring fluctuations in mood this study addresses cognition–emotion interactions in aging in a more ecologically valid way than experimental mood manipulation studies typically conducted in this domain.

### YOUNG AND OLDER ADULTS DIFFER IN SUBJECTIVE RATINGS OF EMOTIONAL FACES, WITH EFFECTS ON ATTENTION AND MEMORY FOR FACES

Svärd et al. (2014) adopted a three-dimensional approach to emotions by considering young and older adults' facial ratings of valence (pleasant/unpleasant), arousal (active/passive), and potency (weak/strong; Keil and Freund, 2009). They observed an age-related flattening of subjective impressions of facial emotions. Regression analyses confirmed a direct link between subjective ratings and task performance in that higher potency (but not arousal and valence) ratings of angry faces predicted better attention and memory for faces. This work contributes to the sparse knowledge on the interplay between subjective emotion ratings on emotion-related cognition in aging.

### EMOTIONAL INFORMATION BOTH FACILITATES AND DISRUPTS WORKING MEMORY IN AGING

Emotional content of information should affect working memory pronouncedly in older adults, given increased emotion orientation

(Carstensen, 2006) and preserved emotion processing (Ebner et al., 2012) with age. Using a working memory paradigm for target information in the presence of distraction, Truong and Yang (2014) systematically varied valence and arousal of word stimuli. For both age groups emotional targets facilitated working memory, while emotional distracters disrupted performance. Emotional disruptive effects were limited to negative words and occurred only in older adults. By identifying situations in which older adults' preserved emotional processing as a helpful "friend" versus a hindering "foe" for cognition, this work adds to the growing literature on the emotion-cognitive control interplay in aging (Dolcos et al., 2011). It supports recent frameworks on competitive advantage of emotional information in aging (Carstensen, 2006) and the role of goal relevance of emotion within specific task contexts (Pessoa, 2008).

### AGING IS ASSOCIATED WITH A DEFICIT IN UNBINDING IRRELEVANT EMOTIONAL INFORMATION FROM MEMORY

Pehlivanoglu et al. (2014) confirmed an age-related hyper-binding hypothesis according to which older compared to young adults show increased binding of task-irrelevant information (Campbell et al., 2010). This age-related deficit in unbinding task-irrelevant facial emotion information held beyond age-related differences in perception, attention, or short-term memory. Innovatively, the study employed pupil dilation and showed greater cognitive resource recruitment during attentional processing (Goldinger and Papesh, 2012) in older than young adults. Addition of neuroimaging data on the brain locus of the observed effects will further unwind the link between emotion and working memory in aging.

### AGE DIFFERENCES IN ENCODING OF SOURCE INFORMATION ARE AMELIORATED FOR SOCIOEMOTIONAL INFORMATION

In Cassidy et al. (2014) young and older adults encoded statements that varied in perceived truth value, as a type of socioemotional information. In line with work suggesting that socioemotional information reduces age-related source memory deficits (Cassidy and Gutchess, 2012), there was an age-related increase in encoding-related ventral relative to dorsal mPFC recruitment in older compared to young participants. This work importantly contributes to age-differential mPFC function in emotion-related source memory and suggests an increased focus on processing of emotionally relevant information, as opposed to knowledge acquistion, in aging.

## MODERATORS OF EMOTIONAL AGING FROM A BRAIN-BEHAVIOR PERSPECTIVE

Mechanisms underlying age deficits in the ability to read emotions in others are not well understood yet. The literature discusses age-related change in visual processing, brain structure and function, hormones, and neurotransmitters as possible explanations (Ruffman et al., 2008; Ebner et al., 2013). Recently, moderating factors such as arousal, emotion expressed, and face-age have received attention (Fölster et al., 2014). Accordingly, papers in this issue have taken up investigation of such moderating factors. As laid out next, Riediger et al. (2014) show moderator roles of age-of-face and genuineness of emotion in emotion perception. Studying proficiency in emotion perception as predictor of well-being, Petrican et al. (2014) provide evidence for a moderating function of neural degenerative disease. English and Carstensen (2014) demonstrate how specific emotions, variations in arousal, and variations in time of day moderate everyday life emotion experience.

In response to critique that the majority of studies on emotion perception use photographs of prototypic facial expressions (Isaacowitz and Stanley, 2011) and examine emotion in the artificial lab setting, several contributions in this issue increased the ecological validity of their stimuli by using dynamic emotion expressions (Riediger et al., 2014) and whole-body postures (Petrican et al., 2014), and by assessing emotion in everyday life (English and Carstensen, 2014) and with relevance in clinical-dyadic context (Petrican et al., 2014).

### YOUNG AND OLDER ADULTS DIFFER IN THEIR ABILITY TO IDENTIFY EMOTIONAL EXPERIENCES ACCOMPANYING SMILES, WITH VARIATIONS BY GENUINENESS OF SMILES AND AGE OF THE SMILING PERSON

People show similar facial expressions in disparate situations. Riediger et al. (2014) developed an extensive set of dynamic video episodes of positive-affective, negative-affective, and affectively neutral smiles of young and older adults. Contrasting previous work (Murphy et al., 2010), young participants outperformed older participants at identification of emotional experiences accompanying smiles. This improved performance in young relative to older adults was attenuated for older faces. Older adults were less likely than young adults to attribute positive emotions to smiles, and more likely to indicate a smile as posed. However, young adults more frequently attributed positive emotions to smiles in older than young faces. Use of dynamic, content-valid smile expressions provide a promising venue for studying age differences in emotion recognition and consideration of age-of-face moderation further informs the picture.

### PARTNER'S PROFICIENCY IN IDENTIFYING POSITIVE VERSUS NEGATIVE EMOTIONS IN OTHERS DIFFERENTIALLY PREDICTS WELL-BEING IN PARKINSON'S DISEASE (PD) PATIENTS VERSUS NEUROLOGICALLY INTACT AGE-MATCHED CONTROLS

Parkinson's disease is associated with reduced emotional expressivity (Simons et al., 2004). In a clinical-dyadic context, Petrican et al. (2014) used a pointlight walker paradigm that depicted emotions in whole-body postures. Spouses of PD patients were better in identifying positive emotions but worse in identifying negative emotions. Also, relative to controls, they underestimated the intensity in negative emotions, possibly as a compensatory mechanism. Greater expertise in identifying positive emotions was linked to greater spousal well-being in healthy elderly couples; for PD patients and their spouses greater proficiency in reading negative emotions predicted greater spousal well-being. This study is one of the few to shed light on the link between emotion recognition proficiency and close partner well-being in an intimate partnership (Gable et al., 2012), suggesting a moderating role of neurological status. The dynamic whole-body emotional stimuli were more naturalistic than the static facial emotional stimuli typically employed in this research field. Further scientific advancement will come from future implementation of longitudinal dyadic studies to assess emotion expressive habits of both spouses, their emotion expertise, and well-being over time.

### AGE DIFFERENCES IN EVERYDAY LIFE EMOTIONAL EXPERIENCE VARY ACROSS EMOTIONS AND TIME OF DAY

English and Carstensen (2014) used experience sampling to assess emotional experience twice a day across 10 days in community-dwelling young and older adults. Both age groups felt less positive and more negative in the evenings than in the mornings. Older compared to young adults reported relatively more positive emotions at both times of day. They also reported greater experience of positive emotions with the exception of the two high-arousal emotions excitement and pride. In contrast, age-related reductions in negative experience were observed only for reports of low-arousal negative emotions. For some emotions (relaxed) age differences were stronger in the mornings, whereas for other emotions (enthusiastic) age differences were more pronounced in the evenings. These findings underscore the importance of examining emotional aging in everyday life, thereby carefully considering the moderating roles of emotions sampled and assessment time.

## EMOTION-REGULATORY SUCCESS IN AGING FROM A BRAIN-BEHAVIOR PERSPECTIVE

Emotion regulation refers to promotion of helpful emotions while managing harmful emotions (Gross, 2013). Appropriately regulating one's feelings in favor of successful social interactions may become particularly relevant in old age, given increased dependency and social loss. There is behavioral evidence that older compared to young adults show improved emotion-regulatory capacity (Urry and Gross, 2010). Despite normative declines in various functional domains, improved emotion-regulatory capacities may contribute to high levels of life satisfaction in aging [English and Carstensen (2014) for qualification of these findings]. In contrast, neuroimaging evidence suggests that brain regions characterized by age-related decline in volumetric gray matter (Raz et al., 2004) are relevant for successful emotion regulation (Buhle et al., 2013). As summarized next, age-related change in emotion-regulatory success in brain and behavior were examined across three studies. Allard and Kensinger (2014) demonstrate age differences in efficient use of cognitive reappraisal. Dolcos et al. (2014) show emotion-regulatory benefits of spontaneous recruitment in emotion control regions in aging. Opitz et al. (2014) describe variations in emotion-regulatory success as a function of fluctuating resources across adulthood.

### OLDER COMPARED TO YOUNG ADULTS USE EMOTION-REGULATORY STRATEGIES LESS EFFICIENTLY

Allard and Kensinger (2014) engaged young and older adults in emotion-regulatory strategies in response to negative film clips. When comparing regulation (selective attention, cognitive reappraisal) to passive viewing, young adults showed greater regulation-related activity in lateral and medial PFC while older adults showed greater dorsolateral PFC activity. Activity in dorsolateral PFC was increased for reappraisal compared to selective attention in older but not young adults, possibly reflecting a compensation for less efficient cognitive control processing in aging. Consistent with this interpretation, the timing of reappraisal-related activity in ventrolateral PFC was delayed for older adults. This research constitutes a first step toward identification of emotion-regulatory strategies that are effective in aging. The authors emphasize adoption of trial-by-trial approaches to determine success for particular emotion-regulatory attempts as fruitful for future brain-behavior investigations.

### OLDER COMPARED TO YOUNG ADULTS SPONTANEOUS ENGAGEMENT OF EMOTION CONTROL BRAIN REGIONS RESULTS IN EMOTION-REGULATORY BENEFITS

Low-arousing negative stimuli engage controlled processes (Kensinger and Corkin, 2004), while high-arousing information captures attention automatically (Dolan, 2002), a process preserved in aging (Mather and Knight, 2006). In Dolcos et al. (2014) young and older participants viewed emotional pictures, that varied in arousal, and rated them for emotional content. Variations in amygdala and ventromedial PFC activity suggested that older adults engaged more automatic processes when evaluating high-arousing negative information, and more controlled processes in response to low-arousing negative information. Linking brain and behavior, spontaneous engagement of emotion control regions reduced subjective experience of low-arousing negative information in older adults, supporting the idea of chronic activation of emotion regulation in aging and delineating neural correlates underlying enhanced emotional well-being in aging.

### FLUID COGNITIVE ABILITY INCREASES EMOTION-REGULATORY SUCCESS IN YOUNG AND OLDER ADULTS

Successful cognitive reappraisal recruits brain areas involved in working memory (McRae et al., 2010) and is most effective when initiated early in the emotion-generative cycle (Sheppes and Meiran, 2007). Consequently, age-associated decline in fluid cognitive abilities should negatively impact cognitive reappraisal success. Opitz et al. (2014) showed that both young and older participants reinterpreted the meaning of sad pictures (versus passive viewing). Emotional responding was measured using a multiple-channel approach that integrated self-reported emotional intensity, expressive behavior, and autonomic physiology. Multi-level modeling showed that fluid (but not crystallized) cognitive abilities predicted emotion-regulatory success, independent of age. The research importantly supports the role of fluctuating resources across adulthood on emotion-regulatory success on brain-behavior levels.

## OPEN QUESTIONS AND FUTURE DIRECTIONS

The work discussed in this perspective paper provides novel insights into the study of emotional aging, providing responses to pressing research questions. However, various topics remain untouched, offering opportunities for exciting future research moving forward in this domain of inquiry. All articles in this issue adopted a cross-sectional approach. Longitudinal, lifespan research will allow examination of gradual quantitative and qualitative emotional change over the life-cycle, allowing to draw a comprehensive picture of emotional development. With one exception (Petrican et al., 2014), all papers used community-dwelling older research participants, prescreened to be free of serious affective or cognitive impairments. A promising future avenue is emotional aging research in clinical contexts such as in dementia, apathy, or social anxiety, pathologies with high relevance in aging (Goodkind et al., 2010). Expanding current research to more diverse samples coupled with continuous use of advanced methodology will move forward this emerging field. A thorough investigation of consequences of age-related emotional change on health and quality of social interactions is currently missing. Petrican et al. (2014) started exploring this territory and demonstrated an association between emotion recognition proficiency and well-being in elderly couples. Relatedly, a stronger research focus toward improvement of emotional aging is warranted such as through administration of medicinal products (Ebner et al., 2013; Campbell et al., 2014) or training of volitional brain activation associated with emotion-regulatory success (Caria et al., 2010). Several of the papers reflect a desirable development toward integration of positive and negative stimulus material (English and Carstensen, 2014; Riediger et al., 2014; Svärd et al., 2014; Völkle et al., 2014). Also, crucial to further advancement of the multi-faceted phenomenon of emotional aging will be an integration of brain-behavior links, thereby considering hormonal, genetic (Ebner et al., 2013) and contextual, motivational change (Carstensen, 2006). We look forward to integrative research advancements in this exciting domain.

## ACKNOWLEDGMENTS

While working on this manuscript, NCE was in parts supported by the NIH-funded Claude D. Pepper Older Americans Independence Center (P30AG028740). The authors wish to thank Devon Weir for assistance with preparation of the manuscript.

## REFERENCES

Allard, E. S., and Kensinger, E. A. (2014). Age-related differences in neural recruitment during the use of cognitive reappraisal and selective attention as emotion regulation strategies. *Front. Psychol.* 5:296. doi: 10.3389/fpsyg.2014.00296

Baltes, P. B., and Baltes, M. M. (1990). *Successful Aging: Perspectives From the Behavioral Sciences.* New York, NY: Cambridge University Press.

Blanchard-Fields, F. (2007). Everyday problem solving and emotion: an adult developmental perspective. *Curr. Dir. Psychol. Sci.* 16, 1, 26–31. doi: 10.1111/j.1467-8721.2007.00469.x

Buhle, J. T., Silvers, J. A., Wage, T. G., Lopez, R., Onyemekwu, O., Kober, H., et al. (2013). Cognitive reappraisal of emotion: a meta-analysis of human neuroimaging studies. *Cereb. Cortex* 1998, 1–10. doi: 10.1093/cercor/bht154

Campbell, A., Ruffman, T., Murray, J. E., and Glue, P. (2014). Oxytocin improves emotion recognition for older males. *Neurobiol. Aging* 35, 2246–2248. doi: 10.1016/j.neurobiolaging.2014.04.021

Campbell, K. L., Hasher, L., and Thomas, R. C. (2010). Hyper-binding: a unique age effect. *Psychol. Sci.* 21, 399–405. doi: 10.1177/0956797609359910

Caria, A., Sitaram, R., Veit, R., Begliomini, C., and Birbaumer, N. (2010). Volitional control of anterior insula activity modulates the response to aversive stimuli. A real-time functional magnetic resonance imaging study. *Biol. Psychiatry* 68, 425–432. doi: 10.1016/j.biopsych.2010.04.020

Carstensen, L. L. (2006). The influence of a sense of time on human development. *Science* 312, 1913–1915. doi: 10.1126/science.1127488

Carstensen, L. L., Turan, B., Scheibe, S., Ram, N., Ersner-Hershfield, H., Samanez-Larkin, G., et al. (2011). Emotional experience improves with age: evidence based on over 10 years of experience sampling. *Psychol. Aging* 26, 21–33. doi: 10.1037/a0021285

Cassidy, B. S., and Gutchess, A. H. (2012). Structural variation within the amygdala and ventromedial prefrontal cortex predicts memory for impressions in older adults. *Front. Psychol.* 3:319. doi: 10.3389/fpsyg.2012.00319

Cassidy, B. S., Hedden, T., Yoon, C., and Gutchess, A. H. (2014). Age differences in medial prefrontal activity for subsequent memory of truth value. *Front. Psychol.* 7:87. doi: 10.3389/fpsyg.2014.00087

Dolan, R. J. (2002). Emotion, cognition, and behavior. *Science* 298, 1191–1194. doi: 10.1126/science.1076358

Dolcos, S., Katsumi, Y., and Dixon, R. A. (2014). The role of arousal in the spontaneous regulation of emotions in healthy aging: an fMRI investigation. *Front. Psychol.* 5:681. doi: 10.3389/fpsyg.2014.00681

Dolcos, S., Sung, K., Denkova, E., Dixon, R. A., and Dolcos, F. (2011). Brain imaging investigation of the neural correlates of emotion regulation. *J. Vis. Exp.* 54, pii: 2430. doi: 10.3791/2430

Ebner, N. C., Johnson, M. K., and Fischer, H. (2012). Neural mechanisms of reading facial emotions in young and older adults. *Front. Psychol.* 3:223. doi: 10.3389/fpsyg.2012.00223

Ebner, N. C., Johnson, M. R., Rieckmann, A., Durbin, K. A., Johnson, M. K., and Fischer, H. (2013). Processing own-age vs. other-age faces: neuro-behavioral correlates and effects of emotion. *Neuroimage* 78, 363–371. doi: 10.1016/j.neuroimage.2013.04.029

Elfenbein, H. A., and Ambady, N. (2002). Is there an in-group advantage in emotion recognition? *Psychol. Bull.* 128, 243–249. doi: 10.1037/0033-2909.128.2.243

English, T., and Carstensen, L. L. (2014). Emotional experience in the mornings and evenings: consideration of age differences in specific emotions by time of day. *Front. Psychol.* 5:185. doi: 10.3389/fpsyg.2014.00185

Fischer, H., Nyberg, L., and Backman, L. (2010). Age-related differences in brain regions supporting successful encoding of emotional faces. *Cortex* 46, 490–497. doi: 10.1016/j.cortex.2009.05.011

Fölster, M., Hess, U., and Werheid, K. (2014). Facial age affects emotional decoding. *Front. Psychol.* 5:30. doi: 10.3389/fpsyg.2014.00030

Gable, S. L., Gosnell, C. L., Maisel, N. C., and Strachman, A. (2012). Safely testing the alarm: close others' responses to personal positive events. *J. Pers. Soc. Psychol.* 103, 963–981. doi: 10.1037/a0029488

Goldinger, S. D., and Papesh, M. H. (2012). Pupil dilation reflects the creation and retrieval of memories. *Curr. Dir. Psychol. Sci.* 21, 90–95. doi: 10.1177/0963721412436811

Goodkind, M. S., Gyurak, A., McCarthy, M., Miller, B. L., and Levenson, R. W. (2010). Emotion regulation deficits in frontotemporal lobar degeneration and Alzheimer's disease. *Psychol. Aging* 25, 30–37. doi: 10.1037/a0018519

Gross, J. J. (2013). Emotion regulation: taking stock and moving forward. *Emotion* 13, 359–365. doi: 10.1037/a0032135

Haase, C. M., Seider, B. H., Shiota, M. N., and Levenson, R. W. (2012). Anger and sadness in response to an emotionally neutral film: evidence for age-specific associations with well-being. *Psychol. Aging* 27, 305–317. doi: 10.1037/a0024959

Isaacowitz, D. M., and Riediger, M. (2011). When age matters: developmental perspectives on "cognition and emotion." *Cogn. Emot.* 25, 957–967. doi: 10.1080/02699931.2011.561575

Isaacowitz, D. M., and Stanley, J. T. (2011). Bringing an ecological perspective to the study of aging and recognition of emotional facial expressions: past, current, and future methods. *J. Nonverbal Behav.* 35, 261–278. doi: 10.1007/s10919-011-0113-6

Keil, A., and Freund, A. M. (2009). Changes in the sensitivity to appetitive and aversive arousal across adulthood. *Psychol. Aging* 24, 668–680. doi: 10.1037/a0016969

Kensinger, E. A., and Corkin, S. (2004). Two routes to emotional memory: distinct neural processes for valence and arousal. *Proc. Natl. Acad. Sci. U.S.A.* 101, 3310–3315. doi: 10.1073/pnas.0306408101

Kunzmann, U., Kappes, C., and Wrosch, C. (2014). Emotional aging: a discrete emotions perspective. *Front. Psychol.* 5:380. doi: 10.3389/fpsyg.2014.00380

Mather, M., and Knight, M. R. (2006). Angry faces get noticed quickly: threat detection is not impaired among older adults. *J. Gerontol. B Psychol. Sci. Soc. Sci.* 61, 54–57. doi: 10.1093/geronb/61.1.P54

McRae, K., Hughes, B., Chopra, S., Gabrieli, J. D. E., Gross, J. J., and Ochsner, K. N. (2010). The neural bases of distraction and reappraisal. *J. Cogn. Neurosci.* 22, 248–262. doi: 10.1162/jocn.2009.21243

Murphy, N. A., Lehrfeld, J. M., and Isaacowitz, D. M. (2010). Recognition of posed and spontaneous dynamic smiles in young and older adults. *Psychol. Aging* 25, 811–821. doi: 10.1037/a0019888

Opitz, P. C., Lee, I. A., Gross, J. J., and Urry, H. L. (2014). Fluid cognitive ability is a resource for successful emotion regulation in older and younger adults. *Front. Psychol.* 5:609. doi: 10.3389/fpsyg.2014.00609

Pehlivanoglu, D., Jain, S., Ariel, R., and Verhaeghen, P. (2014). The ties to unbind: age-related differences in feature (un)binding in working memory for emotional faces. *Front. Psychol.* 5:253. doi: 10.3389/fpsyg.2014.00253

Pessoa, L. (2008). On the relationship between emotion and cognition. *Nat. Rev. Neurosci.* 9, 148–158. doi: 10.1038/nrn2317

Petrican, R., Moscovitch, M., and Grady, C. (2014). Proficiency in positive vs. negative emotion identification and subjective well-being among long-term married elderly couples. *Front. Psychol.* 5:338. doi: 10.3389/fpsyg.2014.00338

Raz, N., Gunning-Dixon, F., Head, D., Rodrigue, K. M., Williamson, A., and Acker, J. D. (2004). Aging, sexual dimorphism, and hemispheric asymmetry of the cerebral cortex: replicability of regional differences in volume. *Neurobiol. Aging* 25, 377–396. doi: 10.1016/S0197-4580(03)00118-0

Rhodes, M. G., and Anastasi, J. S. (2012). The own-age bias in face recognition: a meta-analytic and theoretical review. *Psychol. Bull.* 138, 146–174. doi: 10.1037/a0025750

Riediger, M., Studtmann, M., Westphal, A., Rauers, A., and Weber, H. (2014). No smile like another: adult age differences in identifying emotions that accompany smiles. *Front. Psychol.* 5:480. doi: 10.3389/fpsyg.2014.00480

Ruffman, T., Henry, J. D., Livingstone, V., and Phillips, L. H. (2008). A meta-analytic review of emotion recognition and aging: implications for neuropsychological models of aging. *Neurosci. Biobehav. Rev.* 32, 863–881. doi: 10.1016/j.neubiorev.2008.01.001

Samanez-Larkin, G. R., and Carstensen, L. L. (2011). "Socioemotional functioning and the aging brain," in *The Handbook of Social Neuroscience*, eds J. T. Cacioppo and J. Decety (Oxford: Oxford University Press), 507–521.

Scheibe, S., and Carstensen, L. L. (2010). Emotional aging: recent findings and future trends. *J. Gerontol. B Psychol. Sci. Soc. Sci.* 65B, 135–144. doi: 10.1093/geronb/gbp132

Sheppes, G., and Meiran, N. (2007). Better late than never? On the dynamics of online regulation of sadness using distraction and cognitive reappraisal. *Pers. Soc. Psychol. Bull.* 33, 1518–1532. doi: 10.1177/0146167207305537

Simons, G., Pasqualini, M. C., Reddy, V., and Wood, J. (2004). Emotional and nonemotional facial expressions in people with parkinson's disease. *J. Int. Neuropsychol. Soc.* 10, 521–535. doi: 10.1017/S135561770410413X

Svärd, J., Fisher, H., and Lundgvist, D. (2014). Adult age-differences in subjective impression of emotional faces are reflected in emotion-related attention and memory tasks. *Front. Psychol.* 5:423. doi: 10.3389/fpsyg.2014.00423

Thibault, P., Bourgeois, P., and Hess, U. (2006). The effect of group-identification on emotion recognition: the case of cats and basketball players. *J. Exp. Soc. Psychol.* 42, 676–683. doi: 10.1016/j.jesp.2005.10.006

Truong, L., and Yang, L. (2014). Friend or foe? Decoding the facilitative and disruptive effects of emotion on working memory in younger and older adults. *Front. Psychol.* 5:94. doi: 10.3389/fpsyg.2014.00094

Urry, H. L., and Gross, J. J. (2010). Emotion regulation in older age. *Curr. Dir. Psychol. Sci.* 19, 352–357. doi: 10.1177/0963721410388395

Völkle, M. C., Ebner, N. C., Lindenberger, U., and Riediger, M. (2014). A note on age differences in mood-congruent versus mood-incongruent information processing in faces. *Front. Psychol.* 5:635. doi: 10.3389/fpsyg.2014.00635

# 4

# No smile like another: adult age differences in identifying emotions that accompany smiles

**Michaela Riediger[1]*, Markus Studtmann[1], Andrea Westphal[1†], Antje Rauers[1] and Hannelore Weber[2]**

[1] Max Planck Research Group "Affect Across the Lifespan," Max Planck Institute for Human Development, Berlin, Germany
[2] Institute for Psychology, University of Greifswald, Greifswald, Germany

**Edited by:**
Natalie Ebner, University of Florida, USA

**Reviewed by:**
Natalie Ebner, University of Florida, USA
Andrew E. Reed, Stanford University, USA
Tammy English, Washington University in St. Louis, USA

***Correspondence:**
Michaela Riediger, Max Planck Institute for Human Development, Lentzeallee 94, 14195 Berlin, Germany
e-mail: riediger@mpib-berlin.mpg.de

People smile in various emotional contexts, for example, when they are amused or angry or simply being polite. We investigated whether younger and older adults differ in how well they are able to identify the emotional experiences accompanying smile expressions, and whether the age of the smiling person plays a role in this respect. With this aim, we produced 80 video episodes of three types of smile expressions: positive-affect smiles had been spontaneously displayed by target persons as they were watching amusing film clips and cartoons. Negative-affect smiles had been displayed spontaneously by target persons during an interaction in which they were being unfairly accused. Affectively neutral smiles were posed upon request. Differences in the accompanying emotional experiences were validated by target persons' self-reports. These smile videos served as experimental stimuli in two studies with younger and older adult participants. In Study 1, older participants were less likely to attribute positive emotions to smiles, and more likely to assume that a smile was posed. Furthermore, younger participants were more accurate than older adults at identifying emotional experiences accompanying smiles. In Study 2, both younger and older participants attributed positive emotions more frequently to smiles shown by older as compared to younger target persons, but older participants did so less frequently than younger participants. Again, younger participants were more accurate than older participants in identifying emotional experiences accompanying smiles, but this effect was attenuated for older target persons. Older participants could better identify the emotional state accompanying smiles shown by older than by younger target persons. Taken together, these findings indicate that there is an age-related decline in the ability to decipher the emotional meaning of smiles presented without context, which, however, is attenuated when the smiling person is also an older adult.

**Keywords: smile expressions, age differences, emotion recognition, Duchenne, adulthood**

## INTRODUCTION

Facial expressions are a pivotal component of non-verbal communication. They can convey information about the emotional state of the expressive person (e.g., Ekman, 1972; Izard, 1994), and about accompanying behavioral intentions and action requests (e.g., Fridlund, 1994, 1997). Facial displays can thus help to coordinate and regulate social interactions, provided, of course, that the perceiver recognizes the emotional states associated with the expression and responds accordingly (Keltner et al., 2006). This, however, is not always easy because people can show similar facial expressions in disparate emotional situations. A prime example is smiling. Even though smiling is regarded in many cultures as a prototypical sign of pleasure (e.g., Ekman, 1972; Elfenbein and Ambady, 2002), people do not smile only when they are joyful or amused. They also smile when they experience negative affect, such as sadness (e.g., Bonanno and Keltner, 1997; Papa and Bonanno, 2008), and they also smile in the absence of intense feelings, for example, to be polite. The purpose of the present research was to investigate whether adults of different age groups differ in how well they are able to identify such diverse emotional experiences accompanying smiles, and whether the age of the smiling persons plays a role in this respect. Below, we elucidate the theoretical background for our investigation. We first review findings from previous research on adult age differences in the ability to interpret the emotional meaning of posed facial expressions and explain methodological criticisms that have been raised regarding this line of research. We then argue that studying age differences in the ability to understand the emotional meaning of authentic smile expressions can circumvent these criticisms. We briefly introduce the state of the art of research on smile expressions, and review the available evidence from age-comparative studies on identifying different types of smiles. Following that, we explain the steps we have taken in the present studies to further advance this line of research, and derive our research questions and predictions.

### RESEARCH ON AGE DIFFERENCES IN IDENTIFYING THE EMOTIONAL MEANING OF FACIAL EXPRESSIONS: THE TRADITIONAL PARADIGM

One might expect that as adults accumulate life experience with age, they should become better at identifying the emotional meaning of other people's facial expressions. Most of the empirical evidence available to date, however, speaks to the contrary. With few exceptions, the majority of these findings stem from a paradigm that we will refer to here as the traditional paradigm: participants were presented with photographs of individuals who pose prototypic expressions of highly intense basic emotions. Their task was to select the displayed emotion from a number of response options. A meta-analysis of 17 data sets demonstrated that younger adults outperform older participants in this task (Ruffman et al., 2008). This has been shown for recognizing posed facial expressions of fear, anger, sadness, and, with smaller effect sizes, also surprise and happiness. The only exception to this overarching pattern involved the recognition of posed disgust expressions, for which no significant differences between younger and older adults emerged. Overall, however, the performance advantage of younger adults in this traditional paradigm is undisputed. These findings suggest that older adults are less adept than younger adults in recognizing emotions from facial expressions. This interpretation has recently been challenged however by various authors who pointed out important limitations in the traditional approach. Two major points of criticism have been raised, pertaining to the limited age fairness and ecological validity of the traditional paradigm (Ruffman et al., 2008; Isaacowitz and Stanley, 2011; Richter et al., 2011; Richter and Kunzmann, 2011; Riediger et al., 2011).

The first criticism, limited age fairness, argues that the selection of expression stimuli may have often put older participants at a disadvantage compared to younger participants. Most studies in this research tradition have derived their stimuli from picture sets provided by Ekman and Friesen (1976) or Matsumoto and Ekman (1988). These picture sets were selected on the basis of prototypicality judgments by younger adults, which might disadvantage older study participants if such judgments vary with age. Furthermore, these stimulus sets include facial expressions shown by younger or middle-aged, but not older, posers. This, too, might have put older participants at a disadvantage. Empirical evidence shows that people are better at interpreting emotional expressions of individuals who are similar to themselves as opposed to individuals who are dissimilar. This has been demonstrated for similarity in terms of sharing the same interests, nationality, ethnicity, cultural group, or university affiliation (Elfenbein and Ambady, 2002; Thibault et al., 2006). Several explanations for these in-group effects have been proposed, such as that one has a better knowledge base for interpreting facial expressions shown by individuals belonging to a group with which one identifies, or that one has a higher motivation to attend to, and process, the expressions of such individuals. It has been argued that age-group membership might be relevant in this regard as well, although empirical evidence to date is still rare and inconclusive (e.g., Malatesta, 1987; Ebner and Johnson, 2009; Ebner et al., 2011; Riediger et al., 2011).

The second criticism, limited ecological validity, involves the argument that spontaneous emotional expressions in "real" life differ markedly from the stimuli used in the traditional paradigm. The experimental stimuli typically showcase photographs of prototypical displays, as proposed by the Affect Program Theory of facial expressions (APT, e.g., Ekman, 1972, 1993). Evidence is amounting, however, that facial expressions that are spontaneously shown while experiencing emotions are often more subtle, and typically comprise the activation of fewer and sometimes different muscular components (action units) than proposed by APT, even when the self-rated intensity of the emotional experience is high (for a review, see Reisenzein et al., 2013).

Another characteristic of the traditional paradigm that delimits its ecological validity is that still pictures of facial expressions are used as experimental stimuli. The spontaneous facial expressions that people encounter in their daily lives, however, are dynamic and rapidly changing. Evidence that partly different brain structures subserve the processing of static and dynamic stimuli underscores that the temporal dimension is an important characteristic of facial expressions (e.g., Adolphs et al., 2003; LaBar et al., 2003; Schultz and Pilz, 2009).

Like limited age fairness, the limited ecological validity may also have disadvantaged older adults more than younger adults because solving tasks that have not been practiced before appears to be more challenging for older than for younger adults. Age differences in various types of cognitive performance, for example, have been found to be more pronounced for unfamiliar or artificial problems and considerably smaller for ecologically valid problems that older adults encounter in their daily life contexts (e.g., Phillips et al., 2006; Kliegel et al., 2007). It seems reasonable to expect that this effect would generalize to differences between artificial and ecologically valid emotion-recognition tasks as well.

In essence, research on whether adults from different age groups differ in their ability to identify the emotional experiences accompanying facial expressions has a long tradition. The paradigm that has predominantly been used to date to investigate this question, however, has been criticized for various reasons. These criticisms have inspired researchers to search for alternative paradigms. One novel approach, which we consider promising and pursue further in the research reported here, is to investigate whether adults from various age groups differ in how well they are able to identify the emotional experiences accompanying smile expressions that were displayed in different emotional situations (McLellan, 2008; Murphy et al., 2010; Slessor et al., 2010a). Another approach to enhance ecological validity has been to study age differences in emotion recognition in naturalistic (e.g., Rauers et al., 2013) or semi-naturalistic situations (e.g., Richter and Kunzmann, 2011; Sze et al., 2012). In such situations, multiple information sources can be available (e.g., previously acquired knowledge about the interaction partner, the content of verbal communication, and other channels of nonverbal communication in addition to facial expressions, like pitch of voice, body posture and -movements). Therefore, this alternative research approach is well suited to examine age differences in the overarching ability to understand other people's emotional experiences—an ability that derives from integrating information from these multiple sources. In these studies, however, it is difficult to separate the specific components that contribute to this integrative ability. One of these specific skills is in the fore of the present paper: the ability to infer emotional states specifically from facial expressions.

## IDENTIFYING EMOTIONAL EXPERIENCES THAT ACCOMPANY SMILE EXPRESSIONS

Smiles are subtle facial displays that frequently occur in natural interactions. The smile expression involves lifting the corner of the mouth through contraction of the zygomaticus major muscle. It can, but need not, be accompanied by activation of other facial muscles as well (e.g., Ambadar et al., 2009). Smiling differs from laughing in that neither the characteristic laughing acoustic nor the typical laughing movements (e.g., rhythmically repeated head and shoulder movements) accompanies it.

Smile expressions are shown in different emotional situations. People often smile in positive emotional contexts, for example, when they feel happy or amused. In fact, smiling is regarded as a prototypical sign of pleasure in many cultures (e.g., Ekman, 1972; Elfenbein and Ambady, 2002). People also however occasionally smile in the absence of pleasant feelings, and even in the context of negative emotional experiences, such as feeling embarrassed (e.g., Keltner, 1995) or sad (Bonanno and Keltner, 1997; Papa and Bonanno, 2008). It has been argued that smiling in the absence of positive affect serves self-regulatory as well as social functions (Gross, 1999). It has been found, for example, that smiling can help to alleviate negative and enhance positive affect (Soussignan, 2002; Ansfield, 2007). People may also smile in the absence of positive affect to conform to social norms and expectations, for example, to conceal how they are feeling, or to appease their interaction partner (e.g., Keltner, 1995; Hecht and LaFrance, 1998; Keltner and Haidt, 1999).

The smile displays that accompany different emotional experiences are assumed to vary subtly in their expressive characteristics. What exactly these expressive differences are, is subject of an ongoing debate. Two types of smiles have been most extensively investigated in this regard, namely, those that are spontaneously shown when experiencing positive emotional states, and those that are deliberately posed in the absence of positive experiences (for overviews, see Ambadar et al., 2009; Johnston et al., 2010). An assumption that is still widely spread, but critically questioned today, traces back to the 19th century French physiologist Duchenne de la Boulogne. It pertains to the lateral part of the muscle surrounding the eye (i.e., the pars lateralize of the orbicularis oculi muscle, also referred to as the Duchenne marker), which has been proposed to contract during spontaneous smiles (thus narrowing the eyes and creating characteristic crow's feet), but not during deliberate smiles (e.g., Ekman et al., 1990; Soussignan, 2002). Empirical evidence, however, contradicts the assumption that the Duchenne marker indicates spontaneous, positive-affect smiles. Neither do positive-affect smiles reliably involve the presence, nor do non-positive smiles reliably involve the absence of the Duchenne marker (see overviews in Messinger et al., 1999; Krumhuber and Manstead, 2009). That is, contraction of the Duchenne marker also occurs at a considerable number of occasions when people deliberately pose smiles (Schmidt and Cohn, 2001; Schmidt et al., 2006, 2009; Krumhuber and Manstead, 2009), or when they smile while experiencing negative affect, such as embarrassment (e.g., Keltner, 1995; Papa and Bonanno, 2008). Also the proposal that spontaneous positive-affect smiles may be more symmetrical than posed smiles (e.g., Ekman et al., 1981) has not been supported by studies using precise measures of expression symmetry (e.g., Schmidt et al., 2006). Instead, evidence is accumulating that types of smiles may differ in their temporal characteristics (see overview in Schmidt et al., 2009). Compared to posed smiles, for example, spontaneous positive smiles have been found to involve longer onset and offset phases (Schmidt et al., 2006), and a smoother progression of muscle movements (Hess and Kleck, 1990). Overall, there is considerable agreement among smile researchers that there are expressive differences between smiles accompanying different emotional experiences. The exact nature of these expressive differences, however, still is an ongoing field of research.

Let us return to the question of whether adults from different age groups differ in their ability to identify emotional experiences accompanying facial expressions. One novel approach in this line of research, taken so far by three studies, has been to use the smile expressions that had been shown in different emotional situations as the experimental stimuli (as opposed to posed expressions of highly intense basic emotions in the traditional paradigm). Adults from different age groups were asked to choose among several response options the emotional context in which they believed that the specific smile expression had been shown (McLellan, 2008; Murphy et al., 2010; Slessor et al., 2010a). As described in more detail below, these studies suggest that the conclusion from studies with the traditional paradigm (namely, that the ability to identify emotions from facial expressions uniformly declines with age) needs to be modified. This novel approach is interesting because it circumvents shortcomings of the traditional paradigm, yet still maximizes experimental control: smile expressions are highly relevant in people's everyday life contexts and hence the requirement of ecological validity discussed above is fulfilled. In addition, smiles occur in different emotional contexts and therefore lend themselves as stimuli for the study of individual differences in the ability to identify emotional experiences accompanying facial expressions. Smile expressions thus do indeed appear to be well suited as experimental stimuli in studying adult age differences in the ability to identify emotional facial expressions. The smiles studies available to date, however, have had some limitations so that further evidence is necessary. The above review indicates that several requirements need to be met to fully exploit the potential advantages of using smile expressions as experimental stimuli. First, given the potential diagnostic value of the temporal characteristics in identifying the emotional experiences accompanying smile expressions, the smile stimuli should be dynamic rather than static. Second, because the research on mimic characteristics that reliably indicate the emotional experience during a smile episode is still evolving, the smiling persons' emotional experiences should not be determined on the basis of expression characteristics. In particular, the Duchenne criterion should be avoided, given accumulating evidence that it does not reliably differentiate between different types of smiles. An alternative approach to maximizing the content validity of smile types could be, for example, to establish that the smiling persons' self-reported emotional experiences correspond to the emotional nature of the situations in which they displayed the smile. Third, in light of previous evidence on in-group advantages in understanding emotional facial expressions, the age of the smiling person should be varied to enhance the age fairness of the task and to determine the role that the age of the smiling person plays for participants' recognition accuracy. Fourth, the range of emotional experiences that accompany the selected smile expressions should be wide and ideally include positive, negative, as well as emotionally neutral states. This latter stipulation is in line with the claim that to understand adult age differences in various aspects of emotional functioning, it is important to consider the valence dimension of emotional experiences. This claim derives from the assumption that as older adults become increasingly aware of their narrowing perspective of remaining life time, they should become progressively more motivated to optimize their emotional well-being in the here and now. This, in turn, should be reflected in an increasing preference to attend to and process positive rather than negative information from their surroundings (e.g., Carstensen et al., 2003). Indeed, there is ample evidence to support this claim, primarily in the domains of attention and memory (for overviews, see Carstensen and Mikels, 2005; Reed and Carstensen, 2012), but also in the ways how adults from different age groups interpret still pictures of emotional poses as used in the traditional paradigm (Riediger et al., 2011). It is possible that these preferences might also influence how individuals from different age groups interpret the emotional meaning of different type of smiles.

To the best of our knowledge, no previous study has been published thus far that fulfilled all of these requirements. We are aware of three previous publications on adult age differences in reading different types of smiles (McLellan, 2008; Murphy et al., 2010; Slessor et al., 2010a). All of these studies were interested in the ability to differentiate spontaneous, positive-affect smiles from posed, emotionally neutral smiles. None of these studies included smile expressions accompanying negative emotional experiences. The results of these studies indicated either no significant differences between younger and older adults in the ability to differentiate smile expressions (McLellan, 2008; Murphy et al., 2010, Study 1; Slessor et al., 2010a), or better performance in older as compared to younger adults (Murphy et al., 2010, Study 2). McLellan (2008) and Slessor et al. (2010a) used still pictures of smile expressions and thus did not provide the potentially diagnostic information of the smile dynamics. Furthermore, they included smile expressions only from young, but not older target persons, and used the Duchenne marker as a selection criterion for their smile stimuli, in addition to the targets' self-reported emotional experiences. Murphy et al. (2010) did use dynamic smile stimuli and also varied the age of the smiling person in one of the reported studies. They relied, however, exclusively on the Duchenne criterion to categorize their smile stimuli as positive-affect vs. posed smiles, without further verifying this, for example, with the smiling persons' self-reported experience or information on the emotional nature of the situation in which the smile was shown.

The purpose of the present research was to further advance this line of research by creating a content-valid set of dynamic smile stimuli that fulfills all of the requirements summarized above. This set of dynamic stimuli comprised smile expressions that were spontaneously displayed while experiencing elevated levels of either positive or negative affect, or that were displayed upon our request while being in an emotionally neutral state. We employed these stimuli in two studies. In Study 1, positive, negative, and neutral smile expressions displayed by younger targets were presented to younger and older adults. The participant's task was to identify the emotional experience accompanying the presented smile expressions. Because of their accumulated exposure to, and experience with, subtle emotional expressions of other persons, we expected older participants to be more accurate in their performance of this ecologically and content-valid smile emotion-recognition task than younger adults would be. We also explored whether this age effect would differ between positive-affect, negative-affect, and posed smiles. This exploration was motivated by prior evidence of age-related increases during adulthood in preferential attention toward positive and away from negative information (Carstensen and Mikels, 2005; Reed and Carstensen, 2012). We were interested in exploring whether these positivity effects would generalize to interpretations of smile expressions as well.

In Study 2, we presented positive and neutral smile expressions of younger and older targets to younger and older adults. Our aim was to investigate whether the age of the smiling person matters for the perceiver's accuracy in identifying emotional experiences accompanying smiles. Previous research suggests that people are better able to identify emotional experiences from facial expressions shown by individuals that belong to the same social group, broadly defined (Elfenbein and Ambady, 2002). We hypothesized that age-group membership may have similar effects on identifying the emotional meaning of dynamic smile expressions shown by target persons from different age groups. We are aware of only one prior study that investigated this possibility (Murphy et al., 2010). There was no indication of own-age effects in smile recognition in this study. This, however, could have been because the smile expressions in this study had been classified exclusively on the basis of the Duchenne criterion (i.e., without reference to the situations in which the smiles were shown or to the smiling persons' self-reported emotional experience). Because of previous evidence that the Duchenne marker is not a reliable indicator of emotional experiences accompanying smile expressions, we assumed that a different pattern might emerge in our study, which used smile stimuli that had been selected when the smiling person's self-reported emotional experience and the emotional nature of the situation in which the smile had been expressed corresponded with one another.

## PRE-STUDY: STIMULUS DEVELOPMENT

To fulfill the four requirements introduced above, we developed a new set of dynamic and content-valid smile expressions that were displayed in different emotional situations by target persons varying in age and gender whose self-reported emotional experiences matched the intended emotional context. The collection included negative-affect, positive-affect, and emotionally neutral smiles. The videos recorded the head and shoulders of the target persons. They started with the onset of the smile expression, ended with its offset, and did not include sound. Their average duration was 6.99 s ($SD = 2.27$). Smile duration differed neither between the three smile types, $F_{(2, 77)} = 0.031$, $p = 0.970$, partial $\eta^2 = 0.001$, nor between the two age groups of target persons, $F_{(1, 77)} = 0.385$, $p = 0.537$, partial $\eta^2 = 0.005$, and there was also no significant

Smile Type × Age Group interaction, $F_{(1, 77)} = 0.131, p = 0.718$, partial $\eta^2 = 0.002$.

Below, we describe the development and selection of these smile stimuli and demonstrate that the target persons' self-reported emotional experiences during the smile episodes matched the intended emotional situation and differed significantly between the three types of smiles. We also report the prevalence rates of the Duchenne marker, which confirm prior evidence that this marker is not suited to distinguish between different types of smiles.

## SELECTION OF NEGATIVE-AFFECT SMILES DISPLAYED BY YOUNGER TARGET PERSONS

Negative-affect smiles were extracted from video-recordings of a previously published anger-induction experiment with $N = 157$ non-psychology majors of the University of Greifswald, Germany, who had signed up to participate in a study allegedly investigating associations between personality and concentration (Weber and Wiedig-Allison, 2007). Of these participants, 34 persons were excluded because they reported suspicions during debriefing about the true study purposes, leaving recordings of 123 persons (60 female, $M = 22.9$ years of age, $SD = 3.0$) as material for the extraction of negative-affect smiles. Prior to the anger-induction phase, these target persons first completed, among other things, baseline measures of state anger and momentary negative affect. They were then instructed to work on a computerized task, and to only use certain keys for their responses. The task was programmed to break down after several minutes and trained experimenters accused the target persons of having caused the breakdown by pressing a wrong key. The experimenters also commented in a brusque and condescending way on the situation, implying that the participants had failed on a very simple task. After pretending that restarting the task had failed, the experimenter announced that the data had been lost due to the target person's fault and that he or she might therefore not receive the promised reimbursement. Following that, the target persons again completed, among other things, measures of momentary state anger and negative affect. Then they were debriefed about the true nature of the experiment and asked whether they still consented to be part of the study and whether they would permit their videotapes to be used in further studies and analyses (which all target persons did).

State anger was measured before and after the anger induction phase using four items from the German version of the State Anger Scale (Schwenkmezger et al., 1992). Items were responded to on a four-point rating scale. A sum score was determined as an indicator of the target person's momentary state anger and rescaled such that absence of anger was indicated by a value of zero. Negative affect was assessed with 10 items from the German version of the Positive and Negative Affect Schedule (Krohne et al., 1996), which were responded to on a five-point rating scale. A sum score of these items served as an indicator of momentary negative affect and was rescaled such that absence of negative affect was indicated by a value of zero.

In the video recordings, smile episodes during the anger-induction phase were identified as contractions of the zygomaticus major muscle (lip corner puller AU12 in the Facial Action Coding System FACS, Ekman and Friesen, 1978). From the resulting pool of 72 smile episodes, 16 negative-affect smiles (50% from female target persons) were selected that fulfilled the following criteria: (1) The smile was shown following insulting remarks by the experimenter; (2) The smile was displayed by target persons with an increase in momentary negative affect or an increase in state anger from baseline to post-induction, respectively; and (3) The smile expression was complete (i.e., included onset, apex, and offset phases) and unambiguous (i.e., included no more than one contraction of the zygomaticus major muscle). The average momentary state anger and the average momentary negative affect reported by the respective target persons after the anger induction phase are summarized in the first row of **Table 1** for the negative-affect smiles that were selected.

## SELECTION OF POSITIVE-AFFECT AND NEUTRAL SMILES DISPLAYED BY YOUNGER AND OLDER TARGET PERSONS

Episodes of positive-affect and neutral smiles were recorded at the Max Planck Institute for Human Development in Berlin during

**Table 1 | Self-reported emotional experiences accompanying the negative-affect, positive-affect, and neutral smile episodes selected as stimulus material for Studies 1 and 2.**

| Smile type | Age group of target | State anger[a] | | Negative affect[a] | | Amusement[b] | |
|---|---|---|---|---|---|---|---|
| | | *M* (POMP[c]) | *SD* | *M* (POMP[c]) | *SD* | *M* (POMP[c]) | *SD* |
| Negative-affect smile | Younger | 3.75 (31.25%) | 2.82 | 12.69 (31.73%) | 6.99 | – | – |
| | Older | – | – | – | – | – | – |
| Positive-affect smile | Younger | 0.00 (0.00%) | 0.00 | 0.69 (1.73%) | 1.25 | 80.42 (80.42%) | 12.46 |
| | Older | 0.00 (0.00%) | 0.00 | 0.94 (2.35%) | 1.06 | 79.38 (79.38%) | 12.06 |
| Neutral smile | Younger | 0.00 (0.00%) | 0.00 | 0.69 (1.73%) | 1.14 | 10.83 (10.83%) | 8.48 |
| | Older | 0.00 (0.00%) | 0.00 | 0.38 (0.95%) | 1.09 | 15.00 (15.00%) | 10.11 |

*Sixteen smile episodes per smile type and age group of targets.*

[a] *State anger and negative affect were assessed after the anger-induction phase, amusement-induction phase, and posing-instruction phase for negative-affect, positive-affect, and neutral smiles, respectively.*

[b] *Amusement was assessed immediately after each smile episode.*

[c] *POMP, percent of maximum possible score.*

an amusement-induction phase that was followed by a posing-instruction phase. The setting meticulously mirrored that of the negative-affect smile recordings with regard to furniture, background, and lighting. Contrast, depth of focus, brightness, and light temperature of the camera recordings were also matched to the negative-affect smile recordings, as were the clothing and movements of the target persons.

The sample of target persons included 42 younger adults ($M =$ 23.64 years, $SD = 2.36$, 21 female), and 48 older adults ($M =$ 74.25, $SD = 3.37$, 22 female). All target persons were residents of the Berlin area, Germany, and were recruited via the participant database of the Max Planck Institute for Human Development, Berlin. After giving their informed consent, they practiced various head and body movements that re-enacted those shown during the negative-affect smile interactions, where target persons had rarely sat still, but often had looked toward or away from the insulting experimenter. To ensure comparability between the three smile types with regard to the accompanying movements, we instructed the target persons to re-enact these movements (e.g., "Move your head to look at the red dot on the wall."). These instructed movements were practiced further while four emotionally neutral video clips were being watched. Following that, the target persons completed, among other things, baseline measures of momentary state anger and negative affect, using the same instruments as in the anger-induction experiment. Then, the target persons were video-recorded while watching funny video-clips ($n = 10$) and cartoons ($n = 5$) and performing the practiced movements upon request. Of the amusement stimuli, eleven were shown to all target persons, whereas four (3 cartoons and 1 clip) were selected to accommodate assumed differences in what younger and older persons might consider funny and thus differed between the two age groups. Following each amusement stimulus, target persons rated how amused, exhilarated, and cheerful they momentarily felt on a scale ranging from 0 (not at all) to 100 (very much). A mean score of these items served as an indicator of momentary amusement. Target persons also indicated after each amusement stimulus whether they had experienced any other feeling besides amusement. If yes, they reported the respectively most dominant feeling in an open response format (which was later content-coded by two independent coders) and rated its intensity on a scale from 0 to 100. This open-response item was included to ensure that the affective experience accompanying the smile expression was unequivocal in valence (and not, for example, also accompanied by feelings of awkwardness due to the experimental situation or the instructed movements). Following the amusement induction phase, participants again reported their momentary state anger and negative affect.

After that, participants were instructed to put themselves into an emotionally neutral state as much as possible. The experimenter described six to ten situations in which people smile without experiencing intense positive or negative feelings (e.g., "Imagine a friend telling a joke that you find neither funny nor juicy. To be polite, you smile.") The target persons' task was to display the smile expression they would show in such a situation and to also perform the movements practiced before upon request. The recording of the neutral smile expressions was scheduled last because, to do the recordings, we had to reveal our interest in smile expressions and we wished to avoid that the target persons' awareness of our interest in smile expressions might affect the genuineness of the positive-affect smiles they displayed while watching the amusing material.

After each posed smile, the target persons again rated their momentary amusement and potential other feelings, using the same items as in the amusement-induction phase. The experimenter ended the posing phase after six to ten posing attempts, when at least one suitable smile expression had been recorded. Following that, the target persons again rated their momentary state anger and negative affect.

Smile episodes during the amusement induction and posing instructions were identified from the video recordings as contractions of the zygomaticus major muscle (AU12). From the resulting pool of smile episodes, 16 positive-affect smiles from younger target persons (50% female) and 16 positive-affect smiles from older target persons (50% female) were selected that fulfilled the following criteria: (1) The smile was spontaneously shown in response to an amusing stimulus; (2) The smile was displayed by target persons (a) who reported intense amusement (at least 60 on a scale from 0 to 100) and no other feelings, and (b) who reported low negative affect (no more than 4 on a scale from 0 to 40) and no state anger after the amusement-induction phase; and (3) The smile expression was complete (i.e., included onset, apex, and offset phases) and unambiguous (i.e., included no more than one contraction of the zygomaticus major muscle).

We also selected 16 neutral smiles from younger target persons (50% female) and 16 neutral smiles from older target persons (50% female) according to the following criteria: (1) The smile was displayed in response to the experimenter's instruction to pose a smile; (2) The smile was displayed by target persons who reported little amusement (no more than 30 on a scale from 0 to 100) and no additional feelings after the smile episode, and who reported low negative affect (no more than 4 on a scale from 0 to 40) and no state anger after the posing-instruction phase; and (3) The smile expression was unambiguous, included onset, apex, and offset phases, but did not involve multiple contractions of the zygomaticus major muscle.

The second and third rows in **Table 1** summarize, for the positive-affect and neutral smiles chosen, the average momentary state anger and negative affect reported by the target persons after the amusement-induction and posing-instruction phases, respectively, and the average amusement reported immediately after the selected smile episodes.

## MANIPULATION CHECK: DIFFERENCES BETWEEN SMILE TYPES IN RELATION TO TARGET PERSONS' ACCOMPANYING EMOTIONAL EXPERIENCES

To statistically substantiate that the selected episodes for the three types of smiles significantly differed with regard to the targets' self-reported emotional experiences, we first compared the positive-affect and neutral smile episodes expressed by younger and older target persons. A multivariate analysis of variance on negative affect (reported after the amusement induction and the posing instruction, respectively) and amusement (reported immediately after each selected smile episode) confirmed a significant multivariate effect of smile type, $F_{(2, 59)} = 1298.12$, $p = 0.000$, partial $\eta^2 = 0.91$, according to Wilks Lambda, whereas neither the main effect of age group of target, $F_{(2,59)} = 0.17$, $p = 0.847$, partial $\eta^2 = 0.01$, nor the Age Group × Smile Type interaction, $F_{(2, 59)} = 0.92$, $p = 0.405$, partial $\eta^2 = 0.03$, reached statistical significance. (State anger was not included in this analysis because none of the targets reported any anger experiences for the positive and neutral smile episodes.) A multivariate main effect of smile type also emerged when we compared negative, positive, and neutral smile expressions by younger targets with regard to state anger and negative affect, $F_{(4, 88)} = 16.24$, $p = 0.000$, partial $\eta^2 = 0.43$, according to Wilks Lambda. (Older targets were not included in this analysis because no negative-affect smiles were available for them; amusement ratings were not included because they were not available for negative-affect smiles).

Pairwise comparisons confirmed that targets had experienced significantly higher state anger and negative affect when displaying negative-affect smiles than when displaying positive-affect smiles [state anger: $T_{(15)} = 3.75$, $p = 0.000$; negative affect: $T_{(15.41)} = 6.75$, $p = 0.000$] and neutral smiles [state anger: $T_{(15)} = 5.33$, $p = 0.000$; negative affect: $T_{(15.38)} = 6.91$, $p = 0.000$]. Positive-affect and neutral smiles did not differ with regard to state anger and negative affect (all $p > 0.05$). Compared to neutral smiles, however, positive-affect smiles were accompanied by significantly more intense amusement, $T_{(62)} = 24.74$, $p = 0.000$.

Overall, these analyses indicate that the aims of the stimulus development were met. The three smile types differed significantly in the target persons' self-reported emotional experiences, which in turn matched the intended emotional nature of the situation in which the smile expression was shown. There was no indication that this effect differed between younger and older target persons.

### DUCHENNE CODING OF SMILE SELECTION

The third author rated the presence/absence of the Duchenne marker (AU6, Ekman and Friesen, 1978) for the selected smile episodes. Coding was instructed and supervised by the second author who is an experienced FACS coder. Coding agreement with a second independent coder was satisfactory (across all smile episodes: $\kappa = 0.91$; across smile episodes from younger targets: $\kappa = 0.95$; across smile episodes from older targets: $\kappa = 0.76$; both coders were young adults). Of the 80 smile episodes, 10 (2 negative-affect smiles, 4 positive-affect smiles, and 4 neutral smiles) could not be reliably coded because hair or glasses partially obscured the eye region. Activation of the Duchenne marker was present in 57.1% of the remaining negative-affect smiles (younger targets only), in 57.1% of the remaining positive-affect smiles shown by younger targets; in 71.4% of the remaining positive-affect smiles shown by older targets; in 35.7% of the remaining neutral smiles shown by younger targets; and in 92.9% of the remaining neutral smiles shown by older targets. These findings are consistent with previous evidence that the Duchenne marker does not reliably distinguish between different emotional experiences accompanying smile expressions (see overviews in Messinger et al., 1999; Krumhuber and Manstead, 2009).

## STUDY 1

### METHODS

#### *Sample*

The sample consisted of $N = 100$ participants living in or around Berlin, Germany. Participants were recruited via a participant database of the Max Planck Institute for Human Development. Requirements for study participation were (a) that the participants were either between 20 and 30 years of age ($n = 48$, $M = 25.75$, $SD = 2.61$), or between 70 and 80 years of age ($n = 52$, $M = 74.53$, $SD = 3.05$); (b) that their mother tongue was German, (c) that they had sufficient (corrected) vision to see videos presented on a computer screen clearly; and (d) that they had not taken part in the Pre-Study for stimulus development. Both age groups were approximately stratified by gender (50 and 46.2% female in the younger and older age groups, respectively) and education (54.2% and 40.4% with German university-entrance qualification in the younger and older age groups, respectively). Informed consent was obtained from all participants, and the ethics committee of the Max Planck Institute for Human Development had approved of the study.

#### *Measures*

***Smiles task.*** Participants watched 48 videos of positive-affect smiles ($n = 16$), negative-affect smiles ($n = 16$), and neutral smiles ($n = 16$) expressed by younger targets. The presentation sequence of the videos was randomized. Prior to each video, participants saw a still picture of the start frame for 3 s, showing the target with a neutral expression that preceded the onset of the smile. It was presented so that participants could acquaint themselves with the physiognomy of the target before the smile task. After each video, participants completed the sentence stem "The person smiled in a situation ..." by selecting one of three response options: (a) "in which he or she experienced a pleasant feeling (e.g., amusement)," (b) "in which he or she experienced an unpleasant feeling (e.g., anger)," or (c) "in which he or she posed a smile without feeling anything." For the sake of simplicity, we will refer to these response categories as positive-affect, negative-affect, and neutral smiles below. The smiles task was programmed in DMDX (Forster and Forster, 2003).

Accuracy of categorization was determined as unbiased hit rate, following the procedure proposed by Wagner (1993). This measure accounts for the potentially distorting effects of response tendencies (which can be illustrated by the example of a blindfolded person who would obtain an uncorrected hit rate of 100% in one category without even looking at the stimuli if he always chose the same response). The unbiased hit rate is the joint probability that a smile type was correctly identified and that the response option was correctly used, and is thus insensitive to such a bias in responding. It is determined as the product of the conditional probability that a given smile type was correctly identified (i.e., the number of correctly identified stimuli from that smile type divided by the total number of stimuli from that smile type) and the conditional probability that a response category is correctly used, given that it is used (i.e., the number of correct uses of a response category divided by the total number of uses of that response category).

***Control variables.*** As control variables in the present research, we included measures of participants' education, as well as of crystallized cognitive, fluid cognitive, and visual abilities, all of which have been discussed as possible mechanisms that might underlie age-related differences in emotion recognition (e.g., Phillips et al., 2002; Keightley et al., 2006; Murphy et al., 2010). More specifically, participants indicated their *years of education* for the number of school years completed and the number of years in professional training. A sum score indicating the total number of years of education was used as a covariate. *Perceptual-motor speed* was measured using the Digit-Symbol Substitution Test of the Wechsler Intelligence Scales (Wechsler, 1981). Participants were given mappings of symbols and digits, and their task was to draw the corresponding symbols for a series of digits as fast as possible. The number of correct responses completed within 90 s served as an indicator of perceptual-motor speed. Participants' *vocabulary* was assessed with a test in which participants had to find real words among various pseudo-words (MWT-A, Lehrl et al., 1991). Participants' vision was assessed with two subtests of the computerized Freiburg Visual Acuity and Contrast Test (FrACT, Bach, 2007). In the Acuity Landolt C subtest of the FrACT assessing *visual acuity*, participants were presented with a series of 24 Landolt rings (i.e., rings that have a gap, thus looking similar to the letter C) varying in size. The position of the gap varied across stimuli. The participant's task was to choose, via button press, the gap's correct position out of eight possibilities. The size of the Landolt rings was varied depending on the participant's performance, and visual acuity was determined as decimal acuity (Snellen's fraction; higher values indicate better visual acuity). *Contrast sensitivity* was measured as the Michelson contrast using the subscale Contrast of the FrACT in which participants were presented with a series of 24 Landolt rings that varied in their luminance (smaller values indicate better contrast sensitivity).

In **Table 2** these control variables are compared for the younger and older subsamples. Compared to older participants, younger participants reported more years of school education, obtained higher scores in the perceptual-speed task, lower scores in the vocabulary task, and had better visual acuity and contrast sensitivity. Younger and older participants did not differ significantly with regard to years of professional training. Overall, this pattern of age-group differences is consistent with what is to be expected based on the developmental literature.

## RESULTS

In the following, we first report analyses of potential age-related differences in participants' response tendencies (irrespective of whether the responses were correct). Then we report age differences in the unbiased hit rates for identifying emotional experiences accompanying smiles and analyze whether the observed unbiased hit rates differed significantly from chance.

### *Response tendencies*

**Figure 1** shows the percentages with which younger and older participants chose each of the three response options for evaluating the emotional experience accompanying smiles, irrespective of whether or not the chosen responses were correct. Results of a multivariate analysis of variance on the percentage of chosen responses with age group (younger and older participants) as between-person factor, and response option (positive-affect smile, negative-affect smile, neutral smile) as within-person factor are summarized in **Table 3**. The significant interaction of Age Group × Response Option indicates younger and older participants varied in their response preferences. This underscores the importance of using the unbiased hit rate (Wagner, 1993) when analyzing how well participants from different age groups were able to identify emotional experiences accompanying smiles. Follow-up analyses of this interaction showed that in comparison to younger adults, older adults evaluated smile

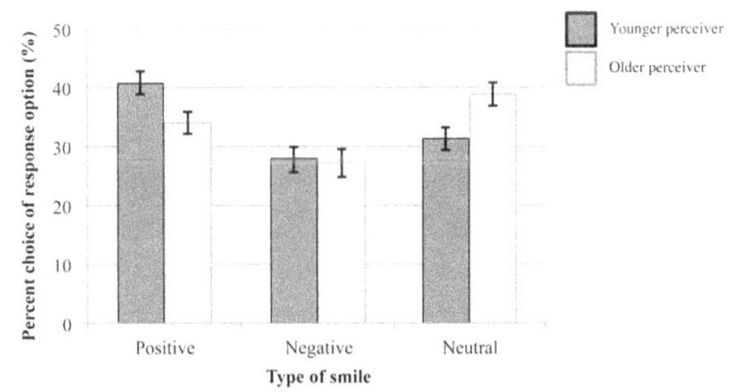


**FIGURE 1 | Use of response options in Study 1 (irrespective of whether response choice was correct).** Error bars represent ±1 standard errors from the mean.

**Table 2 | Descriptives of control variables in Study 1.**

| Construct | Younger participants (perceiver) | | Older participants (perceiver) | | | | |
|---|---|---|---|---|---|---|---|
| | *M* | *SD* | *M* | *SD* | *F* | *df* | *p* |
| Years of school education | 12.33 | 1.55 | 10.98 | 2.21 | 11.860 | 1, 96 | 0.001 |
| Years of professional training | 3.60 | 2.00 | 5.04 | 5.84 | 2.477 | 1, 94 | 0.119 |
| Perceptual-motor speed (Digit-Symbol) | 61.90 | 11.36 | 41.67 | 7.69 | 110.075 | 1, 98 | 0.000 |
| Vocabulary knowledge (MWT-A) | 28.94 | 2.95 | 32.52 | 1.75 | 55.462 | 1, 98 | 0.000 |
| Visual acuity (decimal acuity) | 1.47 | 0.28 | 0.83 | 0.39 | 87.808 | 1, 98 | 0.000 |
| Contrast sensitivity (Michelson contrast)[a] | 0.66 | 0.34 | 1.94 | 1.20 | 50.416 | 1, 98 | 0.000 |

*Multivariate age group effect according to Wilks Lambda: $F_{(6, 87)} = 41.68$, $p = 0.000$, partial $\eta^2 = 0.74$.*

[a] *Smaller values indicate better contrast sensitivity.*

expressions less frequently as being accompanied by positive affect, $F_{(1)} = 5.84$, $p = 0.018$, partial $\eta^2 = 0.06$, and more frequently as being emotionally neutral, $F_{(1)} = 7.64$, $p = 0.007$, partial $\eta^2 = 0.07$. Younger and older adults did not differ in the percentage with which they judged smile expressions as being accompanied by negative affect, $F_{(7)} = 0.07$, $p = 0.799$, partial $\eta^2 = 0.001$. Comparisons within age-group showed that younger adults chose the response option positive-affect smile significantly more frequently than each of the other two response options [negative-affect smile: $F_{(1)} = 13.00$, $p = 0.001$, partial $\eta^2 = 0.22$; neutral smile: $F_{(1)} = 7.49$, $p = 0.009$, partial $\eta^2 = 0.14$]. Their percentages of choosing the response options negative-affect smile and neutral smile did not differ significantly ($p > 0.05$). In contrast, older adults chose the response option neutral smile significantly more often than the response option negative-affect smile, $F_{(1)} = 8.55$, $p = 0.005$, partial $\eta^2 = 0.14$. All other pairwise comparisons of older adults' percentages of chosen response options were non-significant (all $p > 0.05$).

### *Age differences in unbiased hit rate of identifying emotional expressions accompanying smiles*

Solid bars in **Figure 2** represent the average unbiased hit rates of correctly identifying positive, negative, and neutral smiles for younger and older participants. Striped bars indicate the average expected chance levels of performance. In the following, we first analyze age-related differences in unbiased hit rates, and then investigate whether the observed unbiased hit rates were significantly different from chance-level performance.

**Table 3 | Predicting use of response options (irrespective of whether response was correct) in Study 1.**

| Effect | *F* | *df* | *p* | Partial eta squared |
|---|---|---|---|---|
| Response option[a] | 7.331 | 2, 97 | 0.001 | 0.131 |
| Response option × Age group of perceiver[a] | 4.901 | 2, 97 | 0.009 | 0.092 |
| Age group of perceiver | 0.055 | 1 | 0.816 | 0.001 |

[a] *Multivariate F-test based on Wilks Lambda.*

Results of a multivariate analysis of variance with age group of participants (younger and older) as between-person factor, and smile type (positive-affect smile, negative-affect smile, neutral smile) as within-person factor on unbiased hit rates are summarized in **Table 4.** Particularly important for our hypotheses is the significant main effect for age group of participant, which was qualified by the significant interaction of Age Group × Smile Type. Follow-up analyses on this interaction indicated that younger participants, contrary to our prediction, outperformed older participants in correctly identifying the accompanying emotional experiences for all three types of smile [positive-affect smiles: $F_{(1)} = 47.96$, $p = 0.000$, partial $\eta^2 = 0.33$; negative-affect smiles: $F_{(1)} = 8.59$, $p = 0.004$, partial $\eta^2 = 0.08$; neutral smiles: $F_{(1)} = 10.27$, $p = 0.002$, partial $\eta^2 = 0.10$], and this age difference was most pronounced for positive-affect smiles (see **Figure 2**)[1].

**Table 4 | Predicting unbiased hit rates in Study 1.**

| Effect | *F* | *df* | *p* | Partial eta squared |
|---|---|---|---|---|
| Type of smile[a] | 22.674 | 2, 97 | 0.000 | 0.319 |
| Type of smile × Age group of perceiver[a] | 5.545 | 2, 97 | 0.005 | 0.103 |
| Age group of perceiver | 49.519 | 1 | 0.000 | 0.336 |

[a] *Multivariate F-test based on Wilks Lambda.*

[1] This was due to differential patterns within age groups for the relative accuracies in identifying the different types of smiles. Younger adults' unbiased hit rates for identifying negative-affect smiles were significantly lower than those for identifying positive-affect [$F_{(1)} = 14.63$, $p = 0.000$, partial $\eta^2 = 0.24$] and neutral smiles [$F_{(1)} = 27.84$, $p = 0.000$, partial $\eta^2 = 0.37$], which did not differ significantly from each other ($p > 0.05$). Among older adults, the unbiased hit rate for negative-affect smiles did not differ significantly from that for positive-affect smiles ($p > 0.05$), and unbiased hit rates for both negative-affect and positive-affect smiles were significantly lower than the unbiased hit rate for neutral smiles [positive smile: $F(1) = 24.81$, $p = 0.000$, partial $\eta^2 = 0.33$]; negative smiles [$F_{(1)} = 18.04$, $p = 0.000$, partial $\eta^2 = 0.26$]. Note, however, that this age group × smile type interaction did not remain significant in our control analysis.

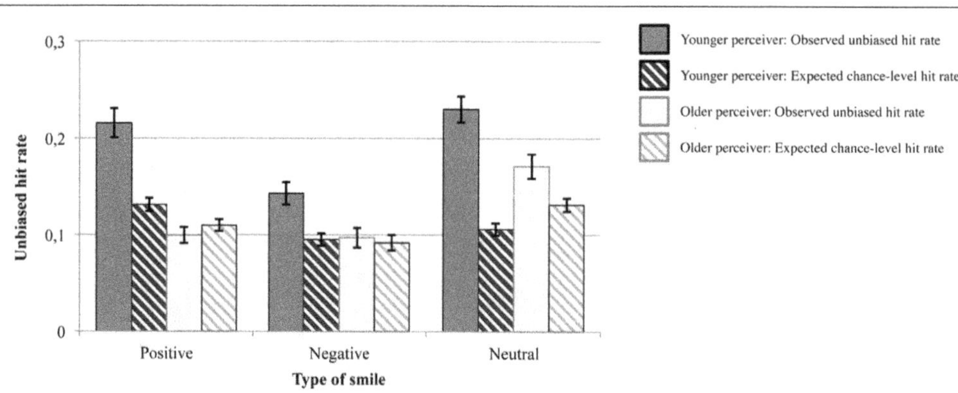


**FIGURE 2 | Observed unbiased hit rates and expected chance-level hit rates in Study 1.** Error bars represent ±1 standard errors from the mean.

The central finding of this analyses—the main effect of age group of participants remained—significant when we controlled for participants' years of education, processing speed, vocabulary knowledge, visual acuity, and visual contrast sensitivity, $F_{(1)} = 14.67$, $p = 0.000$, partial $\eta^2 = 0.14$. The main effect of type of smile as well as the interaction of Age Group × Smile Type no longer reached significance in this control analysis, $F_{(2, 92)} = 0.70$, $p = 0.502$, partial $\eta^2 = 0.02$, and $F_{(2, 92)} = 2.27$, $p = 0.109$, partial $\eta^2 = 0.05$, according to Wilks Lambda, respectively.

In a next step, we followed the procedure proposed by Wagner (1993, p. 18 f.) to investigate whether the observed unbiased hit rates differed significantly from chance-level performance. We first determined, separately for each participant, the unbiased hit rates that were to be expected by chance for each of the three smile types, given the participants' use of response options (i.e., we determined the probability with which a given participant would choose a correct response option by chance when a particular smile type was presented). This was achieved by multiplying the relative frequency of a given smile type (among all smile stimuli) with the relative frequency with which a given participant had chosen the corresponding response option (among all responses). The average resulting chance-level probabilities for correct responses are depicted as striped bars in **Figure 2**. To investigate statistically whether the observed unbiased hit rates were significantly different from these chance-level probabilities, we specified a multivariate analysis of variance with age group (younger and older participants) as between-person factor, and smile type (positive-affect smile, negative-affect smile, neutral smile) as well as type of hit rate (observed unbiased hit rate and chance-level hit rate) as within-person factors. This analysis yielded a significant three-way interaction of Age Group × Smile Type × Type of Hit Rate, $F_{(2, 97)} = 4.54$, $p = 0.013$, partial $\eta^2 = 0.09$, according to Wilks Lambda.

Follow-up analyses revealed that the unbiased hit rates of younger participants were significantly above chance levels for all three smile types [positive-affect smiles: $F_{(1, 47)} = 46.56$, $p = 0.000$, partial $\eta^2 = 0.50$; negative-affect smiles: $F_{(1, 47)} = 25.40$, $p = 0.000$, partial $\eta^2 = 0.35$; neutral smiles: $F_{(1, 47)} = 75.05$, $p = 0.000$, partial $\eta^2 = 0.62$]. Older adults' unbiased hit rates, however, were only significantly better than chance in correctly identifying neutral smiles [$F_{(1, 47)} = 14.30$, $p = 0.000$, partial $\eta^2 = 0.22$], but did not differ significantly from chance levels for positive-affect and negative-affect smiles (all $p > 0.05$).

### SUMMARY OF CENTRAL FINDINGS IN STUDY 1

Study 1 revealed that younger and older participants differed from each other in their tendencies to endorse the available response options for categorizing smile expressions, irrespective of whether the endorsed response was correct. Younger participants chose the category "positive-affect smile" significantly more frequently, and the category "neutral smile" significantly less frequently than older participants did. Younger and older participants did not differ from each other in the frequency of categorizing smile expressions as "negative-affect smile."

In addition, younger participants had higher unbiased hit rates than older adults for categorizing younger targets' smile expressions as positive-affect, negative-affect, or neutral smiles. In fact, older participants' unbiased hit rates for positive-affect and negative-affect smiles were not significantly different from performance levels that were to be expected by chance, given the participants' use of the response options. Younger participants' unbiased hit rates, in contrast, were significantly above chance-level performance for all three types of smiles. Control analyses showed that the age difference in unbiased hit rates was robust to simultaneously controlling for age-related differences in years of education, processing speed, vocabulary knowledge, and vision.

## STUDY 2

The purpose of Study 2 was to replicate findings from Study 1 and to investigate whether they were moderated by the age of the smiling persons. To fulfill this purpose, the smile task in Study 2 involved distinguishing between positive-affect and neutral smile expressions shown by younger and older targets. Negative-affect smiles were available only from younger targets and were thus not included in Study 2.

### SAMPLE

The sample consisted of $N = 97$ participants living in or around Berlin, Germany. Participants were recruited from a participant database of the Max Planck Institute for Human Development, Berlin. Requirements for participation were the same as in Study 1. In addition, we ensured that none of the participants had taken part in Study 1. Younger participants were between 20.2 and 30.9 years of age ($n = 48$, $M = 25.67$, $SD = 2.72$); older participants were between 70.0 and 78.8 years of age ($n = 49$, $M = 73.55$, $SD = 2.53$). Both participant age groups were approximately stratified by gender (50 and 51% female in the younger and older age groups, respectively) and education (52.1 and 38.8% with German university-entrance qualification in the younger and older age groups, respectively). Informed consent was obtained from all participants, and the ethics committee of the Max Planck Institute for Human Development had approved of the study.

### MEASURES

#### *Smiles task*

With two exceptions, the smiles task followed the same logic as in Study 1. The first difference involves the smile stimuli presented. In Study 2, participants watched 64 video recordings of positive-affect smiles shown by younger targets ($n = 16$) and older targets ($n = 16$), and of neutral smiles shown by younger targets ($n = 16$) and older targets ($n = 16$). The second difference involved the number of response options. This time, participants completed the sentence stem "The person smiled in a situation ..." by choosing one of two response options: (a) "in which he or she experienced a pleasant feeling (e.g., amusement)," or (b) "in which he or she posed a smile without feeling anything."

#### *Control variables*

Information on *years of education* (self report), *perceptual-motor speed* (Digit Symbol Substitution Test), *vocabulary knowledge* (MWT-A), and *visual contrast sensitivity* (FrACT) were obtained as covariates. The measures for these variables were the same as in Study 1. In **Table 5** the younger and older subsample are compared on these control variables. As in Study 1, the overall pattern of age differences is consistent with what would be expected based on the developmental literature. Younger participants reported fewer years of professional training, obtained higher scores in the perceptual-speed task, lower scores in the vocabulary task, and had better visual contrast sensitivity than older participants did. Younger and older participants did not differ significantly with regard to years of school education.

## RESULTS

We present the results of Study 2 following the same logic as in Study 1: First we report analyses on age-related differences in participants' response tendencies when evaluating the emotional experience accompanying smile expressions, irrespective of whether these responses were correct. Then we report age differences in the unbiased hit rates for identifying emotional experiences accompanying smiles, and analyze whether the observed unbiased hit rates were significantly different from chance-level performance.

### *Response tendencies*

**Figure 3** shows the percentages with which younger and older participants chose each response option in evaluating the emotional experience accompanying the smile expressions, irrespective of whether or not the chosen response was correct. The results of a multivariate analysis of variance on the percentage for choosing the response option "positive-affect smile," with age group of participants (younger and older) as between-person factor, and age group of target (younger and older smiling persons) as within-person factor are summarized in **Table 6**. (The pattern of findings for the other response option "neutral smile" is complementary.) Both main effects were significant, as was the Age of Target × Age of Participant interaction. Follow-up analyses indicated that both younger and older participants chose the response option "positive-affect smile" more often for smile expressions shown by older as compared to younger targets: $F_{(1, 47)} = 56.60$, $p = 0.000$, partial $\eta^2 = 0.55$ and $F_{(1, 48)} = 16.69$, $p = 0.000$, partial $\eta^2 = 0.26$, respectively. This effect,

**Table 6 | Predicting choice of response option "positive-affect smile" (irrespective of whether response choice was correct) in Study 2.**

| Effect | *F* | *df* | *p* | Partial eta squared |
|---|---|---|---|---|
| Age group of target[a] | 69.258 | 1, 95 | 0.000 | 0.422 |
| Age group of target × Age group of perceiver[a] | 8.034 | 1, 95 | 0.006 | 0.078 |
| Age group of perceiver | 5.733 | 1 | 0.019 | 0.057 |

[a] *Multivariate F-test based on Wilks Lambda.*

**Table 5 | Descriptives of control variables in Study 2.**

| Construct | Younger participants (perceiver) | | Older participants (perceiver) | | | | |
|---|---|---|---|---|---|---|---|
| | *M* | *SD* | *M* | *SD* | *F* | *df* | *p* |
| Years of school education | 11.81 | 1.55 | 11.04 | 2.29 | 3.674 | 1, 94 | 0.058 |
| Years of professional training | 3.34 | 2.02 | 8.16 | 9.78 | 10.431 | 1, 86 | 0.002 |
| Perceptual-motor speed (Digit-Symbol) | 58.94 | 10.67 | 41.80 | 10.19 | 65.467 | 1, 95 | 0.000 |
| Vocabulary knowledge (MWT-A) | 29.65 | 2.77 | 31.84 | 2.68 | 15.669 | 1, 95 | 0.000 |
| Contrast sensitivity (Michelson contrast)[a] | 0.67 | 0.31 | 2.82 | 3.13 | 22.444 | 1, 95 | 0.000 |

*Multivariate age group effect according to Wilks Lambda: $F_{(4, 81)} = 25.79$, $p = 0.000$, partial $\eta^2 = 0.61$.*
[a] *Smaller values indicate better contrast sensitivity.*

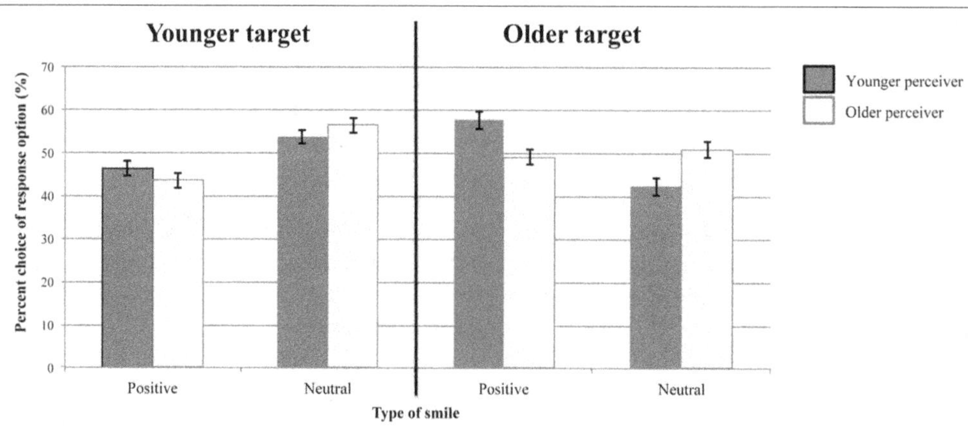


**FIGURE 3 | Use of response options in Study 2 (irrespective of whether response choice was correct).** Error bars represent ±1 standard errors from the mean.

however, was more pronounced for younger than for older participants (see **Figure 3**). Younger and older participants did not differ in how often they chose the response option "positive-affect smile" for expressions shown by younger targets, $F_{(1,\ 47)} = 1.30$, $p = 0.257$, partial $\eta^2 = 0.01$. They differed, however, with regard to their response preferences for older targets, with younger participants choosing the response option "positive-affect smile" more frequently than older participants, $F_{(1)} = 9.92$, $p = 0.002$, partial $\eta^2 = 0.10$. When judging smile expressions from younger target persons, both younger and older participants chose the response option "neutral smile" significantly more often than in 50% of the cases, and thus significantly more frequently than the response option "positive-affect smile," one-sample $T_{(47)} = 2.27$, $p = 0.028$ and one-sample $T_{(48)} = 3.64$, $p = 0.001$, respectively. When judging smile expressions from older target persons, however, younger participants chose the response option "positive-affect smile" more frequently than in 50% of the cases, and hence significantly more often than the response option "neutral smile," one-sample $T_{(47)} = 3.75$, $p = 0.000$. Older participants, in contrast, chose both response options about equally often when judging smile expressions of older target persons, one-sample $T_{(48)} = -0.49$, $p = 0.627$. These findings indicate differences between age group of participants in the preferential use of response categories and thus again underscore the importance of using the unbiased hit rate (Wagner, 1993) when analyzing how well participants from different age groups were able to identify emotional experiences accompanying smiles shown by targets of different age groups.

### *Age differences in unbiased hit rate for identifying emotional expressions accompanying smiles*

Solid bars in **Figure 4** represent the average unbiased hit rates in the younger and older participants for correctly identifying positive-affect and neutral smiles shown by younger and older targets. Striped bars in **Figure 4** indicate average expected chance levels of performance. In the following, we first analyze age-related differences in unbiased hit rates, and then investigate whether the observed unbiased hit rates were significantly different from chance-level performance.

**Table 7** summarizes the results of a multivariate analysis of variance on the unbiased hit rate with age group of participants (younger and older) as between-person factor, and smile type (positive-affect smile and neutral smile) and age group of target (younger and older) as within-person factors. This analysis yielded a significant Age Group of Target × Age Group of Participant × Type of Smile interaction. Consistent with our prediction, follow-up analyses revealed that the Age Group of Target × Age Group of Participant interaction was significant both for positive-affect smiles, $F_{(1,\ 95)} = 4.74$, $p = 0.032$, partial $\eta^2 = 0.048$, and for neutral smiles, $F_{(1,\ 95)} = 12.30$, $p = 0.001$, partial $\eta^2 = 0.12$. With regard to positive-affect smiles, older participants were more accurate in identifying positive-affect smiles shown by older as compared to those shown by younger targets, $F_{(1,\ 48)} = 21.27$, $p = 0.000$, partial $\eta^2 = 0.31$; whereas younger participants' unbiased hit-rates for identifying positive-affect smiles was independent of the age of the smiling person, $F_{(1,\ 47)} = 2.77$, $p = 0.103$, partial $\eta^2 = 0.06$. For the neutral smiles, older perceivers were again more accurate in identifying neutral smiles posed by older as opposed to by younger targets, $F_{(1,\ 48)} = 4.10$, $p = 0.049$, partial $\eta^2 = 0.08$; whereas younger perceivers were more accurate at identifying neutral smiles posed by younger than by older targets, $F_{(1,\ 47)} = 8.19$, $p = 0.006$, partial $\eta^2 = 0.15$.

Compared to older participants' unbiased hit rates, younger participants' unbiased hit rates were generally higher, which is contrary to our hypotheses and to results from previous studies, but consistent with the findings in Study 1. Corresponding to our prediction, however, the size of these age differences in unbiased hit rates was more pronounced for smile expressions shown by younger targets than for smile expressions shown by older targets (age-of-participant effect for positive-affect smiles shown by younger targets: $F_{(1)} = 66.67$, $p = 0.000$, partial $\eta^2 = 0.41$; for positive-affect smiles shown by older targets: $F_{(1)} = 37.06$, $p = 0.000$, partial $\eta^2 = 0.28$; for neutral smiles posed by younger targets: $F_{(1)} = 49.49$, $p = 0.000$, partial $\eta^2 = 0.34$; and for neutral smiles posed by older targets, $F_{(1)} = 11.17$, $p = 0.001$, partial $\eta^2 = 0.11$).

All effects of relevance for our predictions remained robust after controlling for participants' years of education, processing

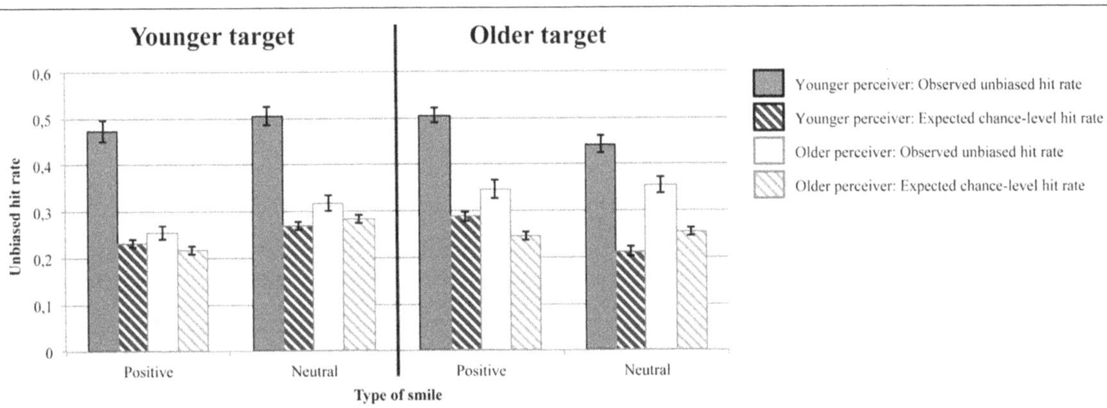


**FIGURE 4 | Observed unbiased hit rates and expected chance-level hit rates in Study 2.** Error bars represent ±1 standard errors from the mean.

speed, vocabulary knowledge, and visual contrast sensitivity. In other words, the main effect of age group of participants remained significant, $F_{(1)} = 41.65$, $p = 0.000$, partial $\eta^2 = 0.31$, as did the Age Group of Target × Age Group of Participant interaction, $F_{(1, 91)} = 4.91$, $p = 0.029$, partial $\eta^2 = 0.05$ according to Wilks Lambda, and the Type of Smile × Age Group of Participant interaction, $F_{(1, 91)} = 6.62$, $p = 0.012$, partial $\eta^2 = 0.07$ according to Wilks Lambda. The other significant effects shown in **Table 7** ceased to reach significance in this control analysis, all $p > 0.05$.

To investigate whether the observed unbiased hit rates differed significantly from chance-level performance, we again followed the procedure proposed by Wagner (1993). As in Study 1, we determined, separately for each participant, the unbiased hit rates that were to be expected by chance given the participant's use of response options. These chance probabilities for correct responses are depicted as striped bars in **Figure 4**. Observed unbiased hit rates for positive-affect smiles were significantly larger than the respective expected chance-level probabilities. This was the case in both age groups of participants and for positive-affect and neutral smile expressions shown by younger and older targets, respectively [effects of observed vs. chance-level hit rates for positive smiles by younger targets: $F_{(1, 47)} = 141.71$, $p = 0.000$, partial $\eta^2 = 0.75$ for younger and $F_{(1, 48)} = 7.69$, $p = 0.008$, partial $\eta^2 = 0.14$ for older participants, respectively; for positive smiles by older targets: $F_{(1, 47)} = 200.90$, $p = 0.000$, partial $\eta^2 = 0.81$ for younger and $F_{(1, 48)} = 33.10$, $p = 0.000$, partial $\eta^2 = 0.41$ for older participants, respectively; for neutral smiles by younger targets: $F_{(1, 47)} = 134.09$, $p = 0.000$, partial $\eta^2 = 0.74$ for younger and $F_{(1, 48)} = 7.21$, $p = 0.010$, partial $\eta^2 = 0.13$ for older participants, respectively; and for neutral smiles by older targets: $F_{(1, 47)} = 207.66$, $p = 0.000$, partial $\eta^2 = 0.82$ for younger and $F_{(1, 48)} = 34.27$, $p = 0.000$, partial $\eta^2 = 0.42$ for older participants, respectively; all according to Wilks Lambda].

### SUMMARY OF CENTRAL FINDINGS IN STUDY 2

Younger and older participants in Study 2 did not differ from each other in their response tendencies in evaluating smiles of younger target persons, and chose the response option "neutral smile" more frequently for younger targets' smile expressions than the response option "positive-affect smile." Furthermore, both younger and older participants ascribed positive-affective experiences more frequently to smile expressions shown by older as compared to younger target persons, but this age-of-target effect was particularly pronounced among younger participants. This was because younger participants in Study 2 chose the response option "positive-affect smile" more frequently and the response option "neutral smiles" less frequently than older participants did when evaluating the emotional nature of smile expressions displayed by older target persons.

Unbiased hit rates for younger and older participants were significantly above chance levels for all smile types. Having to choose between two categories of smile expressions in Study 2 was obviously an easier task than the three-fold categorization required in Study 1. (The similarity of both samples with regard to education, cognitive abilities, and vision that is evident in **Tables 2** and **5** renders the possibility unlikely that the difference in task performance is due to differences between the two samples tested.) Despite this difference in task difficulty, Study 2 replicated the better performance of younger participants for correctly identifying all types of smiles. It also indicated, however, that the size of this age difference was moderated by the age of the target person, such that age differences in unbiased hit rates were more pronounced for smile expressions from younger targets and less pronounced for those from older targets. As in Study 1, the age differences in unbiased hit rates were robust to simultaneously controlling for age-related differences in years of education, processing speed, vocabulary knowledge, and vision.

**Table 7 | Predicting unbiased hit rates in Study 2.**

| Effect | *F* | *df* | *p* | Partial eta squared |
|---|---|---|---|---|
| Age group of target[a] | 3.295 | 1, 95 | 0.073 | 0.034 |
| Type of smile[a] | 0.921 | 1, 95 | 0.340 | 0.010 |
| Age group of perceiver | 68.753 | 1 | 0.000 | 0.420 |
| Age group of target × Age group of perceiver[a] | 9.024 | 1, 95 | 0.003 | 0.087 |
| Type of smile × Age group of perceiver[a] | 5.977 | 1, 95 | 0.016 | 0.059 |
| Age group of target × Type of smile[a] | 72.971 | 1, 95 | 0.000 | 0.434 |
| Age group of target × Type of smile × Age group of perceiver[a] | 4.810 | 1, 95 | 0.031 | 0.048 |

[a]*Multivariate F-test based on Wilks Lambda.*

## DISCUSSION

Smile expressions can accompany diverse emotional experiences, such as amusement or anger, but can also occur in the absence of intense emotions. The current study contributes to an emerging line of research on adult age differences in the ability to identify the emotional meaning of other people's smile expressions. We compiled a set of 80 dynamic smile expressions displayed in different contexts by adults of different age groups whose self-reported affective experience matched the intended emotional nature of the situation. Comparisons of the target person's self-reported affective experiences while smiling in the three different contexts (i.e., while being the target of an unfair accusation, while watching amusing material, and while being instructed to pose a smile) demonstrated that we had successfully compiled groups of three emotionally distinct types of smile expressions (i.e., negative-affect, positive-affect, and neutral smiles).

FACS-coding of the Duchenne marker (AU6, Ekman and Friesen, 1978) confirmed prior evidence that contraction of the lateral part of the muscle surrounding the eyes does not reliably distinguish between the different emotional experiences that can accompany smile expressions (for overviews, see Messinger et al., 1999; Krumhuber and Manstead, 2009). Contrary to the assumption in many previous studies that activation of the Duchenne marker is an indicator of positive affect, we found that it was not reliably present in our selection of positive-affect smiles, and not reliably absent in our selection of negative-affect and neutral smiles. On the contrary, substantial proportions of the smile expressions in all three smile categories involved activation of the Duchenne marker. A limitation of our study was that only younger adults conducted the FACS-coding. In future studies it would be desirable to obtain FACS codings from older adult raters as well.

We used this newly developed set of content-valid and dynamic smile stimuli as stimulus material in two studies. In Study 1, we investigated potential differences between younger and older adults in their ability to distinguish positive-affect, negative-affect, and neutral smile expressions shown by younger target persons. In Study 2, we investigated the potential role of the target persons' age by investigating younger and older adults' ability to identify the emotional experiences accompanying positive-affect and neutral smile expressions shown by both younger and older targets.

## AGE DIFFERENCES IN USE OF RESPONSE OPTIONS (IRRESPECTIVE OF WHETHER RESPONSES WERE CORRECT)

In both studies, younger and older participants differed in their tendencies to endorse the available response options, irrespective of whether the endorsed response was correct. It is worth noting that the pattern of response preferences was different from previous findings of an age-related increase in preferential attention to and memory for positive over negative information (for overviews, see Carstensen and Mikels, 2005; Reed and Carstensen, 2012), which are also reflected in the ways how adults from different age groups interpret still pictures of posed expressions of highly intense basic emotions as used in the traditional paradigm (Riediger et al., 2011). The present studies demonstrate that such positivity effects do not generalize to how older adults interpret the emotional meaning of other people's dynamic smile expressions. In fact, the observed pattern for reading smile expressions was in part opposite to what has been found in the domain of attention and memory or the reading of emotional poses in the traditional paradigm: older participants ascribed *less* positive affective experiences to smile expressions than younger participants did. Of interest is also the observation that participants' response tendencies varied depending on the age of the smiling person. Both younger and older participants ascribed positive affective experiences more frequently to smile expressions shown by older target persons than to smile expressions shown by younger adults. The underlying causes remain to be investigated in future studies. They may include characteristics of the smiling persons, such as aging-related differences in skin texture and facial appearance, but also characteristics of the perceiving persons (participants), such as their subjective theories of cohort differences in emotional expressiveness (Otta, 1998). Indeed, social conventions for when smiling is appropriate and expected have changed throughout the 20th century. This is evident, for example, in a greater likelihood for younger as opposed to older cohorts to present themselves smiling in wedding or yearbook photographs (DeSantis and Sierra, 2000). The present results indicated that people were, in fact, more inclined to assume that a smile expression is emotionally neutral when it was displayed by a younger than by an older adult. This effect was particularly pronounced among the younger participants, which could reflect an age difference in subjective theories about the frequency with which older adults show emotionally neutral smile expressions, and possibly arises from differences in the frequency of contact with older individuals.

The observed age differences in response tendencies are interesting not only because they hint at possible age differences in people's subjective theories about the emotional nature of smile expressions. These results also underscore the importance of accounting for the potentially distorting effects of response tendencies on accuracy indices of smile categorizations, because the more often a particular response option is chosen, the higher the unbiased likelihood is to correctly categorize smile stimuli that belong to that smile type.

## AGE DIFFERENCES IN THE ACCURACY OF IDENTIFYING EMOTIONAL EXPERIENCES FROM FACIAL EXPRESSIONS

We determined participants' accuracy of smile categorizations as unbiased hit rates according to Wagner (1993). This indicator removes the potentially biasing effects of response tendencies by determining the joint probabilities that a given participant had correctly identified the smile type and that she had correctly used the respective response category. Contrary to our expectations and to evidence from previous studies on age differences in identifying the emotional meaning of smile expressions (McLellan, 2008; Murphy et al., 2010; Slessor et al., 2010a), younger participants outperformed older participants in both studies and with regard to all investigated types of smile. Corresponding to our hypotheses, however, older participants in Study 2 were more accurate in identifying the emotional meaning of smile expressions shown by older as compared to younger targets, which could have resulted from their better knowledge, or greater experience with smile expressions shown by older as opposed to younger individuals (e.g., Harrison and Hole, 2009). For younger participants, a corresponding own-age advantage was evident only in identifying neutral smiles; that is, younger participants were better at identifying neutral smile expressions stemming from younger target persons as opposed to older target persons. A limitation of the present research, which future studies should remedy, is that we were not able to investigate whether similar own-age advantages would also be evident for negative-affect smiles.

The observed own-age advantage for older participants' accuracy in identifying the emotional meaning of neutral and positive-affect smile expressions supports the argument that age differences in recognizing emotion from facial expressions are likely to be over-estimated in studies that only consider facial expressions from younger or middle-aged, but not older target persons. The unbiased hit rates of older participants were smaller than those of younger participants, however, even for smile expressions from the older targets. Overall, the present research thus supports the view that the ability to decipher emotional meaning from facial expressions alone, presented without the accompanying context, is not as good in older than for in younger adults. Control analyses in both studies showed that the age differences in unbiased hit rates were robust to simultaneously controlling for age-related differences in years of education, processing speed, vocabulary knowledge, and vision, showing that differences in these control variables did not account for the observed age differences in reading smiles. It thus remains an open question for future research to identify the mechanisms that underlie these effects. Future studies should examine, for example, the potential respective roles of age-related differences in subjective conceptions of when and by whom smile expressions are displayed, or in the ability to integrate information from various (e.g., structural and temporal) dimensions of smile expressions (Slessor et al., 2010b).

The results from the present studies are strikingly different from those of earlier studies that used smile stimuli. It seems likely that this is due to diverging strategies of compiling smile expressions. In contrast to the previous investigations, our collection of smile stimuli was both dynamic and content-valid in the sense that we selected smile expressions for different smile types based on the convergence between the affective nature of the situation in which the smile was shown (i.e., while being the target of an unfair accusation, watching amusing stimuli, or being asked to pose a smile) and the target persons' self-reported affective experiences in that situation. The earlier studies, in contrast, used the Duchenne marker either as the sole criterion for the categorization of smile expressions (Murphy et al., 2010), or as one criterion among several (McLellan, 2008; Slessor et al., 2010a). In replication of evidence from other studies, all categories of our content-valid selection of smile expressions included a substantial proportion of stimuli that involved the Duchenne marker, suggesting that the Duchenne marker is not a reliable criterion for distinguishing between different types of smiles. Another possible explanation for the disparity of findings could relate to the different cultural contexts (i.e., in Germany, the US, and the UK) in which the respective investigations had been conducted. An interesting task for future investigations remains to explore whether cultural differences in smile expressions, or in smile recognition, may have contributed to the observed differences in findings. Another open question for further studies is the identification of contexts in which the observed age differences in recognizing affective experiences that accompany smile expressions might be reduced (or perhaps even reversed). One might speculate, for example, that familiarity with the smiling person might play a moderating role in this regard.

Future research should also aim at overcoming some methodological limitations of the present research. Among the most notable of these is the present cross-sectional design. Future research should explore the extent to which the observed cross-sectional differences between age groups reflect cohort differences as opposed to aging-related changes within persons over time. Another important task for future research is closing the gap to real-life emotion-recognition demands: even though the smiles paradigm (in contrast to the traditional paradigm) employs expressions that participants frequently encounter in diverse emotional contexts of their daily lives, it is nevertheless still quite different from real-life emotion-recognition demands. One obvious difference is that real-life smile expressions occur within the context of a particular situation and that perceivers might have accumulated knowledge about the smiling person. Investigating potential age-related differences in the ability to decipher smile expressions when such contextual information is available remains an open task for future research. Another realm for future investigation would be to further increase the breadth of smile types under investigation, and to also consider the role of arousal. In the present study, we focused on smile expressions that accompanied emotional states that were unambiguous with regard to their valence (negative, positive, neutral); however, different elicitation methods were employed to obtain each of the three smile types, making it possible that the smile stimuli might differ in other factors than valence as well. Furthermore, the positive-affect and negative-affect smiles were recorded in potentially activating emotional contexts (i.e., anger and amusement). This leaves an open question as to whether the observed age differences would generalize to smile expressions accompanying other emotional states, for example, mixed emotional states (e.g., feeling joyful and sad at the same time) or low-arousal states (e.g., sadness or contentment).

### SUMMARY AND CONCLUSION

Two studies provided converging evidence that younger adult participants were better able to identify the emotional experiences accompanying different types of smile expressions than older participants were. Results further showed that these age differences were attenuated for smile expressions displayed by older target persons. Older adults were better able to identify the emotional meaning of smile expressions shown by older as compared to younger target persons. We conclude that dynamic and content-valid smile expressions provide a promising venue for studying age-differences in emotion recognition, and that it is important to vary the age of the expressing persons to further the understanding of adult age differences in the ability to recognize the emotional meaning of facial expressions.

## ACKNOWLEDGMENTS

We thank Dulce Erdt, Anne Böger, Laura Wolf, Lisa Thiele, Robert Neumann, Elisabeth Blanke, Teresa Holtfreter, Alexander Mielke, Doreen Müller, Caroline Cohrdes, Sandy Jahn, Anna Maria Jäger, Anika Schulz, Claudia Medel, and Manuela Meermann for their help with data collection and preparation, and Amy Michéle for editorial assistance.

## REFERENCES

Adolphs, R., Tranel, D., and Damasio, A. R. (2003). Dissociable neural systems for recognizing emotions. *Brain Cogn.* 52, 61–69. doi: 10.1016/S0278-2626(03)00009-5

Ambadar, Z., Cohn, J. F., and Reed, L. I. (2009). All smiles are not created equal: morphology and timing of smiles perceived as amused, polite, and embarrassed/nervous. *J. Nonverbal Behav.* 33, 17–34. doi: 10.1007/s10919-008-0059-5

Ansfield, M. E. (2007). Smiling when distressed: when a smile is a frown turned upside down. *Pers. Soc. Psychol. Bull.* 33, 763–775. doi: 10.1177/0146167206297398

Bach, M. (2007). The freiburg visual acuity test-variability unchanged by *post-hoc* reanalysis. *Graefe's Arch. Clin. Exp. Ophthalmol.* 245, 965–971. doi: 10.1007/s00417-006-0474-4

Bonanno, G. A., and Keltner, D. (1997). Facial expressions of emotion and the course of conjugal bereavement. *J. Abnorm. Psychol.* 106, 126–137. doi: 10.1037/0021-843X.106.1.126

Carstensen, L. L., Fung, H. H., and Charles, S. T. (2003). Socioemotional selectivity theory and the regulation of emotion in the second half of life. *Mot. Emot.* 27, 103–123. doi: 10.1023/A:1024569803230

Carstensen, L. L., and Mikels, J. A. (2005). At the intersection of emotion and cognition: aging and the positivity effect. *Curr. Dir. Psychol. Sci.* 14, 117–121. doi: 10.1111/j.0963-7214.2005.00348.x

DeSantis, M., and Sierra, N. (2000). Women smiled more often and openly than men when photographed for a pleasant, public occasion in 20th century United States society. *Psychol. A J. Hum. Behav.* 37, 21–31.

Ebner, N. C., He, Y., and Johnson, M. K. (2011). Age and emotion affect how we look at a face: visual scan patterns differ for own-age versus other-age emotional faces. *Cogn. Emot.* 25, 983–997. doi: 10.1080/02699931.2010.540817

Ebner, N. C., and Johnson, M. K. (2009). Young and older emotional faces: are there age group differences in expression identification and memory? *Psychol. Aging* 9, 329–339. doi: 10.1037/a0015179

Ekman, P. (1972). Universals and cultural differences in facial expressions of emotion. *Nebraska Symp. Mot.* 19, 207–283.

Ekman, P. (1993). Facial expression and emotion. *Am. Psychol.* 48, 384–392. doi: 10.1037/0003-066X.48.4.384

Ekman, P., Davidson, R. J., and Friesen, W. V. (1990). The Duchenne smile: emotional expression and brain physiology: II. *J. Pers. Soc. Psychol.* 58, 342–353. doi: 10.1037/0022-3514.58.2.342

Ekman, P., and Friesen, W. V. (1976). *Pictures of Facial Affect.* Palo Alto, CA: Consulting Psychologists Press.

Ekman, P., and Friesen, W. V. (1978). *Facial Action Coding System: A Technique for the Measurement of Facial Movement.* Palo Alto, CA: Consulting Psychologists Press.

Ekman, P., Hager, J. C., and Friesen, W. V. (1981). The symmetry of emotional and deliberate facial actions. *Psychophysiology* 18, 101–106. doi: 10.1111/j.1469-8986.1981.tb02919.x

Elfenbein, H. A., and Ambady, N. (2002). On the universality and cultural specificity of emotion recognition: a meta-analysis. *Psychol. Bull.* 128, 203–235. doi: 10.1037/0033-2909.128.2.203

Forster, K. I., and Forster, J. C. (2003). DMDX: a Windows display program with millisecond accuracy. *Behav. Res. Methods Instrum. Comput.* 35, 116–124. doi: 10.3758/BF03195503

Fridlund, A. J. (1994). *Human Facial Expression: an Evolutionary View.* San Diego, CA: Academic Press.

Fridlund, A. J. (1997). "The new ethology of human facial expressions," in *The Psychology of Facial Expression*, eds J. A. Russell and J. M. Fernandez-Dols (New York, NY; Paris: Cambridge University Press; Editions de la Maison des Sciences de l'Homme), 103–129.

Gross, J. J. (1999). "Emotion and emotion regulation," in *Handbook of Personality: Theory and Research, 2nd Edn*, eds L. A. Pervin and O. P. John (New York, NY: Guilford Press), 525–552.

Harrison, V., and Hole, G. J. (2009). Evidence for a contact-based explanation of the own-age bias in face recognition. *Psychon. Bull. Rev.* 16, 264–269. doi: 10.3758/PBR.16.2.264

Hecht, M. A., and LaFrance, M. (1998). License or obligation to smile: the effect of power and sex on amount and type of smiling. *Pers. Soc. Psychol. Bull.* 24, 1332–1342. doi: 10.1177/01461672982412007

Hess, U., and Kleck, R. E. (1990). Differentiating emotion elicited and deliberate emotional facial expressions. *Eur. J. Soc. Psychol.* 20, 369–385. doi: 10.1002/ejsp.2420200502

Isaacowitz, D. M., and Stanley, J. T. (2011). Bringing an ecological perspective to the study of aging and recognition of emotional facial expressions: past, current, and future methods. *J. Nonverbal Behav.* 35, 261–278. doi: 10.1007/s10919-011-0113-6

Izard, C. E. (1994). Innate and universal facial expressions: evidence from developmental and cross-cultural research. *Psychol. Bull.* 115, 288–299. doi: 10.1037/0033-2909.115.2.288

Johnston, L., Miles, L., and Macrae, C. (2010). Why are you smiling at me? Social functions of enjoyment and non-enjoyment smiles. *Br. J. Soc. Psychol.* 49, 107–127. doi: 10.1348/014466609X412476

Keightley, M., Winocur, G., Burianova, H., Hongwanishkul, D., and Grady, C. L. (2006). Age effects in social cognition: faces tell a different story. *Psychol. Aging* 21, 558–572. doi: 10.1037/0882-7974.21.3.558

Keltner, D. (1995). Signs of appeasement: evidence for the distinct displays of embarrassment, amusement, and shame. *J. Pers. Soc. Psychol.* 68, 441–454. doi: 10.1037/0022-3514.68.3.441

Keltner, D., and Haidt, J. (1999). Social functions of emotions at four levels of analysis. *Cogn. Emot.* 13, 505–521. doi: 10.1080/026999399379168

Keltner, D., Haidt, J., and Shiota, M. N. (2006). "Social functionalism and the evolution of emotions," in *Evolution and Social Psychology*, eds M. Schaller, J. A. Simpson, and D. T. Kenrick (Madison, CT: Psychosocial Press), 115–142.

Kliegel, M., Martin, M., McDaniel, M. A., and Phillips, L. H. (2007). Adult age differences in errand planning: the role of task familiarity and cognitive resources. *Exp. Aging Res.* 33, 145–161. doi: 10.1080/03610730601177395

Krohne, H. W., Egloff, B., Kohlmann, C. W., and Tausch, A. (1996). Untersuchungen mit einer deutschen Version der "Positive and Negative Affect Schedule" (PANAS) [Studies on a German version of the Positive and Negative Affect Schedule (PANAS)]. *Diagnostica* 42, 139–156.

Krumhuber, E. G., and Manstead, A. S. (2009). Can Duchenne smiles be feigned? New evidence on felt and false smiles. *Emotion* 9, 807–820. doi: 10.1037/a0017844

LaBar, K. S., Crupain, M. J., Voyvodic, J. T., and McCarthy, G. (2003). Dynamic perception of facial affect and identity in the human brain. *Cereb. Cortex* 13, 1023–1033. doi: 10.1093/cercor/13.10.1023

Lehrl, S., Merz, J., Burkhard, G., and Fischer, S. (1991). *Mehrfachwahl—Wortschatz—Intelligenztest, MWT-A [Multiple-choice Vocabulary Intelligence Test, MWT-A].* Göttingen: Hogrefe.

Malatesta, C. Z. (1987). Emotion communication skills in young, middle-aged, and older men and women. *Psychol. Aging* 2, 193–203. doi: 10.1037/0882-7974.2.2.193

Matsumoto, D., and Ekman, P. (1988). *Japanese and Caucasian Facial Expressions of Emotion and Neutral Faces (JACFEE and JACNeuF).* Available online at: http://www.davidmatsumoto.com/research.php

McLellan, T. L. (2008). *Sensitivity to Emotion Specified in Facial Expressions and the Impact of Aging and Alzheimer's Disease.* Doctoral thesis, University of Canterbury, Christchurch.

Messinger, D. S., Fogel, A., and Dickson, K. (1999). What's in a smile? *Dev. Psychol.* 35, 701–708. doi: 10.1037/0012-1649.35.3.701

Murphy, N. A., Lehrfeld, J. M., and Isaacowitz, D. M. (2010). Recognition of posed and spontaneous dynamic smiles in young and older adults. *Psychol. Aging* 25, 811–821. doi: 10.1037/a0019888

Otta, E. (1998). Sex differences over age groups in self-posed smiling in photographs. *Psychol. Rep.* 83, 907–913. doi: 10.2466/pr0.1998.83.3.907

Papa, A., and Bonanno, G. A. (2008). Smiling in the face of adversity: the interpersonal and intrapersonal functions of smiling. *Emotion* 8, 1–12. doi: 10.1037/1528-3542.8.1.1

Phillips, L. H., Kliegel, M., and Martin, M. (2006). Age and planning tasks: the influence of ecological validity. *Int. J. Aging Hum. Dev.* 62, 175–184. doi: 10.2190/EM1W-HAYC-TMLM-WW8X

Phillips, L. H., MacLean, R. D. J., and Allen, R. (2002). Age and the understanding of emotions: neuropsychological and sociocognitive perspectives. *J. Gerontol. Psychol. Sci.* 57B, P526–P530. doi: 10.1093/geronb/57.6.P526

Rauers, A., Blanke, E., and Riediger, M. (2013). Everyday empathic accuracy in younger and older couples: do you need to see your partner to know his or her feelings? *Psychol. Sci.* 24, 2210–2217. doi: 10.1177/0956797613490747

Reed, A. E., and Carstensen, L. L. (2012). The theory behind the age-related positivity effect. *Front. Psychol.* 3, 1–9. doi: 10.3389/fpsyg.2012.00339

Reisenzein, R., Studtmann, M., and Horstmann, G. (2013). Coherence between emotion and facial expression: evidence from laboratory experiments. *Emot. Rev.* 5, 16–23. doi: 10.1177/1754073912457228

Richter, D., Dietzel, C., and Kunzmann, U. (2011). Age differences in emotion recognition: the task matters. *J. Gerontol. B Psychol. Sci. Soc. Sci.* 66B, 48–55. doi: 10.1093/geronb/gbq068

Richter, D., and Kunzmann, U. (2011). Age differences in three facets of empathy: performance-based evidence. *Psychol. Aging* 26, 60–70. doi: 10.1037/a0021138

Riediger, M., Voelkle, M. C., Ebner, N. C., and Lindenberger, U. (2011). Beyond "happy, angry, or sad?" Age-of-poser and age-of-rater effects on multi-dimensional emotion perception. *Cogn. Emot.* 25, 968–982. doi: 10.1080/02699931.2010.540812

Ruffman, T., Henry, J. D., Livingstone, V., and Phillips, L. H. (2008). A meta-analytic review of emotion recognition and aging: implications for neuropsychological models of aging. *Neurosci. Biobehav. Rev.* 32, 863–881. doi: 10.1016/j.neubiorev.2008.01.001

Schmidt, K. L., Ambadar, Z., Cohn, J. F., and Reed, L. (2006). Movement differences between deliberate and spontaneous facial expressions: zygomaticus major action in smiling. *J. Nonverbal Behav.* 30, 37–52. doi: 10.1007/s10919-005-0003-x

Schmidt, K. L., Bhattacharya, S., and Denlinger, R. (2009). Comparison of deliberate and spontaneous facial movement in smiles and eyebrow raises. *J. Nonverbal Behav.* 33, 35–45. doi: 10.1007/s10919-008-0058-6

Schmidt, K. L., and Cohn, J. F. (2001). Human facial expressions as adaptations: evolutionary questions in facial expression research. *Am. J. Phys. Anthropol.* 116, 3–24. doi: 10.1002/ajpa.20001

Schultz, J., and Pilz, K. S. (2009). Natural facial motion enhances cortical responses to faces. *Exp. Brain Res.* 194, 465–475. doi: 10.1007/s00221-009-1721-9

Schwenkmezger, P., Hodapp, V., and Spielberger, C. D. (1992). *Das State-Trait-Ärgerausdrucks-Inventar (STAXI) [The State-Trait Anger Expression Inventory]*. Bern: Huber.

Slessor, G., Miles, L. K., Bull, R., and Phillips, L. H. (2010a). Age-related changes in detecting happiness: discriminating between enjoyment and nonenjoyment smiles. *Psychol. Aging* 25, 246–250. doi: 10.1037/a0 018248

Slessor, G., Phillips, L. H., and Bull, R. (2010b). Age-related changes in the integration of gaze direction and facial expressions of emotion. *Emotion* 10, 555–562. doi: 10.1037/a0019152

Soussignan, R. (2002). Duchenne smile, emotional experience, and autonomic reactivity: a test of the facial feedback hypothesis. [Empirical Study]. *Emotion* 2, 52–74. doi: 10.1037/1528-3542.2.1.52

Sze, J. A., Goodkind, M. S., Gyurak, A., and Levenson, R. W. (2012). Aging and emotion recognition: not just a losing matter. *Psychol. Aging* 27, 940–950. doi: 10.1037/a0029367

Thibault, P., Bourgeois, P., and Hess, U. (2006). The effect of group-identification on emotion recognition: the case of cats and basketball players. *J. Exp. Soc. Psychol.* 42, 676–683. doi: 10.1016/j.jesp.2005.10.006

Wagner, H. L. (1993). On measuring performance in category judgment studies on nonverbal behavior. *J. Nonverbal Behav.* 17, 3–28. doi: 10.1007/BF00987006

Weber, H., and Wiedig-Allison, M. (2007). Sex differences in anger-related behaviour: comparing expectancies to actual behaviour. *Cogn. Emot.* 21, 1669–1698. doi: 10.1080/02699930701202111

Wechsler, D. (1981). *Wechsler Adult Intelligence Scale-Revised (WAIS-R)*. New York, NY: Psychological Corporation.

# 5

# Proficiency in positive vs. negative emotion identification and subjective well-being among long-term married elderly couples

***Raluca Petrican*, Morris Moscovitch and Cheryl Grady***

*Department of Psychology and Psychiatry, Rotman Research Institute, University of Toronto, Toronto, ON, Canada*

***Edited by:***
*Natalie Ebner, University of Florida, USA*

***Reviewed by:***
*Tara L. Queen, University of Utah, USA*
*Natalie Ebner, University of Florida, USA*
*Hakan Fischer, Stockholm University, Sweden*

****Correspondence:***
*Raluca Petrican, Rotman Research Institute, 3560 Bathurst Street, Toronto, ON M6A 2E1, Canada*
*e-mail: raluca.petrican@gmail.com*

Evidence is accruing that positive emotions play a crucial role in shaping a healthy interpersonal climate. Inspired by this research, the current investigation sought to shed light on the link between proficiency in identifying positive vs. negative emotions and a close partner's well-being. To this end, we conducted two studies with neurologically intact elderly married couples (Study 1) and an age-matched clinical sample, comprising married couples in which one spouse had been diagnosed with Parkinson's Disease (Study 2), which tends to hinder emotional expressivity. To assess proficiency in identifying emotions from whole body postures, we had participants in both studies complete a pointlight walker task, featuring four actors (two male, two female) expressing one positive (i.e., happiness) and three negative (i.e., sadness, anger, fear) basic emotions. Participants also filled out measures of subjective well-being. Among Study 1's neurologically intact spouses, greater expertise in identifying positive (but not negative) emotions was linked to greater partner life satisfaction (but not hedonic balance). Spouses of PD patients exhibited increased proficiency in identifying positive emotions relative to controls, possibly reflective of compensatory mechanisms. Complementarily, relative to controls, spouses of PD patients exhibited reduced proficiency in identifying negative emotions and a tendency to underestimate their intensity. Importantly, all of these effects attenuated with longer years from PD onset. Finally, there was evidence that it was increased partner expertise in identifying negative (rather than positive) emotional states that predicted greater life satisfaction levels among the PD patients and their spouses. Our results thus suggest that positive vs. negative emotions may play distinct roles in close relationship dynamics as a function of neurological status and disability trajectory.

**Keywords: emotion recognition, well-being, marriage, Parkinson's Disease, point light walker, older adults**

## INTRODUCTION

Close relationships constitute a critical ingredient of psychological and physical health (e.g., Beach and O'Leary, 1993; Berscheid and Reis, 1998; Diener and Seligman, 2002). Perhaps unsurprisingly, numerous well-being theories identify fulfilling close relationships as a prerequisite for optimal hedonic balance (e.g., Ryff, 1995; Keyes, 1998; Diener and Biswas-Diener, 2008). Although traditionally relationship researchers focused on the role of negative emotions (e.g., Levenson and Gottman, 1983; Gottman, 1998), there is mounting evidence that positive emotions are crucial in shaping a healthy interpersonal environment (Gable et al., 2006, 2012). Inspired by this research, in the present studies, we sought to examine the link between proficiency in recognizing positive vs. negative emotions and spousal well-being among neurologically intact couples and couples where one partner has been diagnosed with Parkinson's Disease. To situate our present investigation in the literature, we begin by reviewing extant evidence on the role of close relationship quality in health and well-being, followed by a summary of the research on emotions within intimate partnerships, with a focus on social support and care giving circumstances. We conclude the Introduction with an overview of the literature on how emotion recognition proficiency—and thus the ability to provide responsive social support and effective care giving—may be impacted by normal aging and among couples, where one partner is afflicted by neurological conditions, typical of older age, such as Parkinson's Disease.

## CLOSE RELATIONSHIP QUALITY AND HEALTH

Most of the extant research focuses on the direct pathways through which poor close relationship—most often, marriage—quality can adversely impact well-being and health. For example, relationship turmoil has been found to contribute to psychopathological symptoms such as depression, anxiety, and substance abuse (e.g., Davila et al., 1997; Whisman, 2001; Whisman et al., 2010). Likewise, poorer marital quality and more hostile marital interactions have been linked to abnormal immune responses (Kiecolt-Glaser et al., 1993; Miller et al., 1999), greater cardiovascular reactivity (Morell and Apple, 1990; Ewart et al., 1991; Smith and Brown, 1991; Brown and Smith, 1992; Brown et al., 1998; Newton and Sanford, 2003), higher incidence of cardiac events (Orth-Gomer et al., 2000) and mortality (Eaker et al., 2007). Complementing these findings on the adverse health effects of poor marital quality, there is evidence on the beneficial consequences of greater marital adjustment, such as healthier physiological profiles (i.e., lower blood pressure, Holt-Lunstad et al., 2008), superior immune responses (Kiecolt-Glaser et al., 1987), better cardiovascular health (Baker et al., 2000), and lower mortality following cardiac incidents (among women; Hibbard and Pope, 1993; Rohrbaugh et al., 2006).

### SOCIAL SUPPORT IN CLOSE RELATIONSHIPS

Extending investigations on the direct consequences of marital adjustment on health, there is recent research on the role of marital quality in moderating the effects of non-relationship factors (e.g., work, disease) on physical and psychological well-being. The majority of these studies focused on the stress buffering function of positive marital environments and documented their beneficial effect on rehabilitation among cardiac patients (Wang et al., 2007), recovery from work-related stress (Saxbe et al., 2008) and reduced physiological reactivity to chronic problems at work (Ditzen et al., 2008).

One factor assumed to underlie the stress buffering function of happier marriages is the perception of social support availability, intrinsically linked to being part of a fulfilling intimate partnership (e.g., Kaul and Lakey, 2003). Indeed, there is extensive evidence that such perceptions of emotional support during stressful times constitute a pivotal determinant of physical and psychological health (Cohen and Wills, 1985; Cohen, 1988; Lakey and Cassady, 1990; Uchino et al., 1996; Sarason et al., 1997; Kaul and Lakey, 2003).

Intriguingly, though, perceptions of social support availability are only loosely based on the reality of actual support received during challenging times (e.g., Haber et al., 2007). Instead, they appear to be more heavily rooted in enacted support from others during propitious times (Gable et al., 2012). Moreover, it seems that only the latter is consistently linked to benign personal and relational outcomes (e.g., Gable et al., 2006, 2012), whereas enacted support from others during trying times is only sparsely associated with favorable outcomes, being occasionally even linked to adverse consequences (e.g., Collins et al., 1993; Bolger et al., 2000; Kaul and Lakey, 2003).

The apparent paradox of such findings has been illuminated by studies documenting that it is only provision of social support, perceived to be responsive by the recipient, that contributes to the latter's well-being and feeds his or her perceptions that a close other may be available for assistance during stressful times (Maisel and Gable, 2009; Gable et al., 2012). Provision of responsive support is reportedly easier during auspicious, rather than inauspicious, times, since any visible assistance during the latter periods may only augment the recipient's emotional turmoil by indirectly highlighting his/her inadequacy in coping with the stressor and rendering salient feelings of indebtedness to the support provider (Bolger et al., 2000; Gleason et al., 2003; Shrout et al., 2006). Taken together, the findings reviewed above thus imply that the stress buffering function of close relationships, instantiated in perceptions of emotional support availability during trying times, may be most dependent upon the intimates' ability to read each other's emotions accurately and thus provide each other with responsive support, particularly during favorable times.

### NEGATIVE EMOTIONS IN CARE GIVING AND RECEIVING

Spousal disease and disability create a dyadic environment in which negative emotions can flourish. Indeed, there is evidence that under such circumstances, it is not only the diseased who struggles with negative emotions, but also the care giver who must manage the challenges of both actively helping his/her ill spouse and dealing with potentially long "on-call" hours (Poulin et al., 2010). Importantly, though, the challenges of attending to an ill spouse are not the sole culprit for the significant hedonic and physical health costs incurred by prolonged care giving (Schulz et al., 2009). Instead, it has been proposed that the affective burden of care giving may be also rooted in the extensive exposure to the suffering of a close other and the intrinsic potential for emotion contagion between the care recipient and giver (for a review, see Monin and Schulz, 2009). Indeed, consistent with a suffering contagion model, several studies provided evidence of significant, positive associations in emotional distress between cancer patients and their caregivers (Given et al., 1993; Northouse et al., 2001). Moreover, longitudinal studies have documented the positive link between spousal suffering and subsequent decay in well-being or even development of depression and physical health problems (e.g., cardiovascular disease) in the care giving partner (Revenson and Majerovitz, 1990; Pakenham, 2001; Schulz et al., 2009).

Although witnessing the suffering of a close other may incur significant hedonic and physical health costs to the care givers, expression of negative emotions by care recipients is nonetheless a key component of effective care giving, because it conveys the need for support and thus enables the caregiver to be more responsive to a care recipient's needs (cf. Monin and Schulz, 2009). Consistent with this interpretation, there is evidence that expression of "vulnerable" negative emotions, such as fear, sadness, anxiety, predicts less caregiver stress (at least among female caregivers, Monin et al., 2009). Indeed, it seems plausible to posit that within a care giving context, the ability to accurately recognize negative emotions may be a critical asset for both the care giver and the care recipient. On one hand, accurate identification of a care recipient's negative emotions may enable the care giver to direct his/her efforts toward maximizing the patient's well-being. Complementarily, accurate identification of a caregiver's negative emotions may aid the care recipient in gauging the impact of his/her illness and adjust behavior (where possible) to reduce care giver burden and, thus, foster a more positive dyadic climate.

### EMOTION RECOGNITION AND AGING

An accumulating body of research suggests that, despite the increasing importance placed on emotions in older adulthood (Carstensen, 1992; Mather and Carstensen, 2005), the ability to decode them accurately decays with advancing age (e.g., Ruffman et al., 2009). The bulk of the investigations to date focused on the recognition of facial emotional cues and documented most consistent age-related deficits in the identification of negative emotions, specifically fear, anger, and sadness (Malatesta et al.,

1987; Moreno et al., 1993; MacDowell et al., 1994; Brosgole and Weisman, 1995; MacPherson et al., 2002, 2007; Phillips et al., 2002; Calder et al., 2003; Sullivan and Ruffman, 2004a,b; Wong et al., 2005; Keightley et al., 2006; Isaacowitz et al., 2007; Sullivan et al., 2007; Suzuki et al., 2007; Henry et al., 2008; Orgeta and Phillips, 2008; for a recent meta-analysis, see Ruffman et al., 2008).

More recent studies, using a broader array of stimuli, suggest that age-related deficits in emotion identification are not restricted to the decoding of facial cues, but also extend to auditory and postural affective cues (e.g., Brosgole and Weisman, 1995; Montepare et al., 1999; Wong et al., 2005; Ruffman et al., 2009). Moreover, beyond the well-documented global age-related decline in reading emotional expressions, there is also evidence of some modality-specific patterns of impairment. For example, although older adults are reportedly most impaired at recognizing negative emotions from facial cues (cf. Ruffman et al., 2008), they seem to experience greater difficulties with recognizing auditory cues of positive, rather than negative (e.g., fear), emotions (Wong et al., 2005). Similarly, whole-body cues of positive emotions are less legible to older, relative to younger, adults, although age-related deficits in deciphering postural cues have also been detected in response to negative emotions, most notably, sadness, and anger (Montepare et al., 1999; Ruffman et al., 2009).

## EMOTION EXPRESSION AND RECOGNITION IN PARKINSON'S DISEASE

Deficits in emotion recognition are also a hallmark of psychopathological conditions, typical of older age, such as Parkinson's Disease (PD). PD is a degenerative neurological disorder with a prevalence of 1/1000 (Peto et al., 1995). Uncommon before age 40, PD affects around 1% of people over 60 and around 2% of people over 80 (MacPhee and Stewart, 2007). The clinical signs of PD are primarily motor and include slowness of movement, rigidity, resting limb tremors, and postural and balance problems (Ferguson et al., 2008). Recently, though, there has been increasing recognition that despite their salience, motor symptoms are not the only clinical features of PD, which often also is characterized by cognitive deficits (Pillon et al., 1996) and affect dysregulation (Marsh, 2000).

Consistent with the clinical emphasis on motor symptoms, most of the extant empirical investigations on emotion in PD focused on the expressive deficits associated with the disorder. There is thus evidence that PD patients exhibit impairments in producing spontaneous (Buck and Duffy, 1980; Katsikitis and Pilowsky, 1988, 1991; Smith et al., 1996) and, to a somewhat lesser degree, voluntary (Simons et al., 2004) emotional expressions. Such expressive deficits constitute the likely cause of why they tend to be misunderstood and poorly evaluated by their interlocutors (Ellgring et al., 1993), even when the latter are health care professionals (Pentland et al., 1987, 1988). Of note, the motor difficulties associated with PD render the patients least apt at expressing positive emotions. Thus, in the laboratory, PD patients have been found to produce less legible voluntary facial expressions of happiness (Simons et al., 2004). Likewise, outside the laboratory, the facial movement difficulties, which typify PD, cause the patients' spontaneous smiles to be misread as "unfelt" (i.e., inauthentic because of a lack of accompanying cheek raises, Pitcairn et al., 1990).

Complementing the aforementioned investigations on the expressive deficits associated with PD, there is a recently growing body of research on the patients' impairments in decoding emotions. Most of these studies focused on recognition of facial or prosodic cues and provided evidence of marked deficits among PD patients, relative to controls (e.g., Kan et al., 2002; Pell and Leonard, 2003; Yip et al., 2003; Dujardin et al., 2004; Suzuki et al., 2006; Lawrence et al., 2007; Ariatti et al., 2008; Clark et al., 2008; Dara et al., 2008). Indeed, in a recent meta-analysis of the literature on emotion recognition in PD, Gray and Tickle-Degnen (2010) concluded that there is a robust link between PD and impaired recognition of both auditory and facial emotional cues, with deficits being particularly salient for negative emotions.

Despite compelling evidence that PD may incur significant emotion recognition deficits (Gray and Tickle-Degnen, 2010), some inconsistencies do exist in the literature. For example, although robust (adverse) effects of PD on (negative) emotion recognition have been documented among un-medicated, hence, somewhat paradoxically, early stage patients (Sprengelmeyer et al., 2003; Buxton et al., 2013), such impairments have been somewhat harder to detect among medicated patients in the later stages of PD (e.g., Adolphs et al., 1998; Assogna et al., 2010). Moreover, although the bulk of the evidence to date implies that PD may lead to most marked deficits in reading negative emotional cues (Gray and Tickle-Degnen, 2010), a recent study suggests that this may be an artifact of the affective stimuli used by prior research, since PD-related deficits in reading positive emotional cues have been detected when subtler affective expressions are employed (Buxton et al., 2013).

In sum, despite some inconsistencies, extant literature suggests that PD incurs significant deficits both in expressing and decoding affective cues. Interestingly, although deciphering of negative emotions may pose greatest difficulties to PD patients (cf. Gray and Tickle-Degnen, 2010, but see also Buxton et al., 2013), it appears that it is deficient expression of positive emotions that may afflict their social life the most (Pitcairn et al., 1990; Simons et al., 2004).

## PRESENT RESEARCH

The purpose of the present research was to investigate the link between individual differences in the ability to identify positive vs. negative emotions and a spouse's well-being among neurologically intact elderly couples (Study 1), as well as in an age- and marriage length-matched clinical sample, comprising married couples in which one spouse had been diagnosed with PD (Study 2).

Prior findings suggest that it is only provision of responsive support to a spouse during a positive event that is unambiguously linked to greater recipient well-being (cf. Gable et al., 2012). In contrast, provision of effective support to a spouse during negative events is not only difficult to enact, but even when perceived by the recipient to be highly responsive, it can still not buffer against the deleterious hedonic consequences associated with negative events (although responsive social support is associated with beneficial *relational* outcomes, see Study 2, Gable et al., 2012). Consequently, we hypothesized that among neurologically intact couples, higher levels of spousal well-being would be linked to greater proficiency in identifying positive, rather than negative, emotions. Indeed, we reasoned that those who are "experts" at recognizing positive emotions would be better skilled at reading their spouse's emotional reactions during a positive event and, thus, be in a better position to respond in a manner that would foster the spouse's well-being (cf. Maisel and Gable, 2009; Gable et al., 2012). In contrast, we reasoned that proficiency in identifying negative emotions, and, thus, presumably greater ability to respond effectively to a spouse during negative events, would evidence a weak (if any) relationship to the spouse's well-being.

Complementarily, prior research with couples, in which one partner struggles with a severe disease or disability, suggests that it is the ability to recognize and respond appropriately to negative emotions that may be a critical determinant of dyadic and individual well-being (cf. Monin et al., 2009). Indeed, on one hand, a care giver's ability to read accurately the patient's negative emotions may put him/her in a better position to provide the most responsive and efficient support (cf. Monin and Schulz, 2009). On the other hand, a care recipient's ability to recognize a care giver's negative emotions may allow him/her to adjust behavior (where possible) to minimize care giver burden. Thus, it seemed plausible that in our clinical sample, in which one of the spouses was evidencing increasing levels of disability and, thus, dependence on the care giving partner, the ability to identify accurately negative emotional cues may be as important (if not more important) a contributor to spousal well-being as the ability to identify positive emotions.

For our clinical sample, we opted to focus on PD patients and their spouses for several reasons. First, because it is a neurodegenerative disorder, PD challenges both patients and their spouses to cope with increasing (rather than stable) levels of patient disability, which, arguably, hinders both the patients' and their spouses' ability to habituate to their (ever changing) life circumstances. We thus reasoned that longer disease duration may render expression of negative emotions by the patients increasingly informative for their care givers because with increasing disability, patients become more dependent on their care givers to help them relieve their distress. Consequently, the PD sample allowed us to test the hypothesis that, consistent with the posited adaptive function of negative emotion expression by care recipients (Monin et al., 2009), spousal care givers would demonstrate increased proficiency in decoding negative emotional cues, an advantage that may accentuate with more years from disease onset and greater patient disability.

Second, PD is reportedly associated with deleterious effects on facial affective expressivity (Buck and Duffy, 1980; Katsikitis and Pilowsky, 1988, 1991; Smith et al., 1996), particularly the production of facial positive emotional cues (Pitcairn et al., 1990; Simons et al., 2004). Consequently, inclusion of the PD patients and their spouses allowed us to test whether, in line with our proposed critical role of positive emotion proficiency in fostering spousal well-being, a spouse's declining ability to produce positive emotional cues would be "compensated" by the other's spouse's increasing proficiency in decoding them. Although such effects may generalize across modalities, we reasoned that we may be particularly likely to find evidence of them in modalities that are relatively less affected by PD, such as the postural domain (see below). Finally, inclusion of the PD patients and their spouses in our research also allowed us to extend the literature on emotion perception in PD by examining whether the patients would exhibit deficits in reading postural emotional cues, similar to the ones previously documented for facial and auditory emotional cues (Gray and Tickle-Degnen, 2010).

To assess the cognitive and affective components of well-being, respectively, we had participants in both studies fill out two validated self-report measures (Diener et al., 1985; Gere et al., 2011). To assess individual differences in emotion recognition, we had them complete a point light walker task (Heberlein and Saxe, 2005; Atkinson et al., 2007). We chose this measure for a couple of reasons. First, there is recent evidence that individual differences in performance on this task may be a good indicator of social expertise, since they have been found to be uniquely predictive of individual differences in higher-order sociocogntive processes (e.g., false belief reasoning, Phillips et al., 2011), involved in extracting and updating multiple aspects of social information (Phillips et al., 2011). Second, to the best of our knowledge, despite accumulating evidence on the emotion recognition deficits associated with PD (Gray and Tickle-Degnen, 2010), there is still a dearth of research on the potential PD-associated impairments in decoding postural (rather than facial or auditory) emotional cues. Consequently, we reasoned that probing any potential deficits in reading whole-body emotional cues in PD may be a valuable extension of the literature.

## STUDY 1

### METHODS

#### Participants

Thirty-seven elderly couples, married between 18 and 56 years ($M = 42.22$, $SD = 9.09$, provided informed consent in accordance with the ethical guidelines of the Research Ethics Board at the University of Toronto [women's age: $M = 69.06$ ($SD = 5.67$); men's age: $M = 72.27$ years ($SD = 6.07$)]. All were native English speakers or had lived in Canada and used English as the primary language for at least 30 years. Prior to their laboratory visit, potential participants underwent a phone screening interview, conducted by a senior research assistant, associated with the study. Specifically, they were asked whether (a) they ever had a stroke, tumor, neurological disease, concussion, depression, seizure, head injury, aneurysm, learning disability, psychiatric illness, epilepsy; (b) they had ever been in a serious car accident and/or hit their head badly and/or been unconscious; and (c) what medication (if any) they take on a regular basis. Potential participants who responded "yes" to any of the questions at points "a" and "b" or reported that they were taking psychotropic medication on regular basis were excluded from participating (for the demographic information summary, see **Table 1**).

#### Measures

***Pointlight walker task.*** To assess participants' ability to read emotions from whole body postures, we presented them with a set of 38 movies, ranging in length from 4 to 14 s, obtained upon request from Andrea Heberlein (see also Heberlein and Saxe, 2005; Atkinson et al., 2007). According to Andrea Heberlein, this set of stimuli most consistently elicited emotionally valenced

**Table 1 | Demographic information for the Study 1 and 2 samples.**

| | Study 1 | Study 2 |
|---|---|---|
| 1. Marriage length | 42.22 ± 9.09 | 39.28 ± 11.67 years |
| 2. Females | Age = 69.06 ± 5.67 years | Age = 67.77 ± 9.95 years |
| 3. Males | Age = 72.27 ± 6.07 years | Age = 68.39 ± 10.22 years |
| 4. PD patients | | 12 males; Age = 69.75 ± 9.34 years<br>6 females; Age = 66.00 ± 10.99 years |
| 5. PD spouses | | 12 females; Age = 68.72 ± 9.76 years<br>6 males; Age = 65.67 ± 12.24 years |
| 6. Years from PD symptom onset | | 8.06 ± 3.89 years |

*The above information is based on data from 37 couples (Study 1) and 18 couples (Study 2).*

judgments from neurologically intact participants (i.e., the actor in the clip was perceived to express an emotion, rather than being neutral). The stimuli featured professional or student actors, 3 males and 3 females, who walked across the frame of a movie camera from left to right, with movement patterns intended to convey specific emotions (i.e., anger, fear, happiness, or sadness). Small lights were attached to the actors' wrists, ankles, knees, elbows, outer hip, waist, outer shoulder, and head; they were filmed in the dark, so that only the moving lights were visible. At the end of each movie clip, participants were requested to rate on a 7-point scale (from 1 not at all to 7 extremely) the extent to which the actor expressed each of the four emotions (i.e., fear, sadness, anger, happiness) or s/he was neutral (i.e., expressed no emotion at all). Taking our cue from Adolphs et al. (1998) and Dujardin et al. (2004), we chose to use the emotion rating profile, rather than categorical labeling of each movie within one emotion, to account for the fact that subtler, realistic cues are unlikely to be emotion-pure (i.e., other emotions are likely to be expressed together with the targeted one).

***Data scoring.*** For each clip, across all participants, we averaged separately the scores provided for each of the four emotions tested to create the sample's "agreed upon" ratings of each movie. Subsequently, for each participant and for each of the four scrutinized emotions, we created a "deviance" score as the absolute value of the difference between the sample's average rating of the movie on the given emotion and the respective participant's rating. Then, for each participant, we averaged these "deviance" scores across all movies, within each of the four tested emotions. For ease of interpretation, we then subtracted each "deviance" score from 1, so that for the resulting scores, greater values would reflect better recognition performance. Consequently, indicative of our ultimate interest in a participant's ability to accurately read his/her spouse's emotions, we have operationalized "accuracy" in emotion recognition as (greater) agreement between a participant's emotion ratings and the sample's mean emotion ratings. Our rationale was that, beyond any idiosyncratic effects, a significant predictor of whether a participant would successfully decode his/her spouse's emotions is his/her adherence to the affective vocabulary of those most demographically similar to his/her spouse. We also kept the raw values of the difference between a participant's rating of a movie on a given emotion and the sample's corresponding rating. These scores, averaged across all movies, indicated the direction of a participant's leaning on a given emotion judgment (i.e., over- or under-estimation of the intensity of an emotion, relative to the sample).

***Subjective well-being.*** Participants completed a 7-point Likert-type life satisfaction measure (e.g., "I am satisfied with my life."; Diener et al., 1985; $\alpha = 0.86$) and a positive and negative affect scale (e.g., "In general, I felt bad."; (Gere et al., 2011); $\alpha = 0.87$ and 0.90, respectively). To compute an index of hedonic balance, we subtracted participants' average score on the negative affect scale from their average score on the positive affect scale. Consistent with Diener's (1984) proposal that life satisfaction and hedonic balance constitute aspects—cognitive and affective, respectively—, of the same construct, i.e., subjective well-being, their indices were moderately correlated, $r_{(72)} = 0.45, p < 0.01$.

### Procedure

The study period was comprised of two 90-min sessions separated by a 30-min lunch break. Upon arriving at the lab, spouses were taken to separate testing rooms, where they remained for the duration of the two study sessions, reuniting during the break. At the beginning of the first session, partners were asked to fill out a larger questionnaire package that included the life satisfaction and affective well-being scales. During the second session, they completed the point light walker task. All measures and tasks were administered in this fixed order across all participants.

## RESULTS

### Data preparation

Due to the dependency in our couples' data, hierarchical linear regression models were regarded as the most appropriate statistical approach (HLM 7.01, Raudenbush et al., 2013). HLM produces essentially the same parameter estimates as simple linear regression, but uses more appropriate estimates of standard errors to test statistical significance. Following the recommendations of Campbell and Kashy (2002) for analysis of dyadic data in HLM, we investigated the interrelationships among our various measures by running fixed slopes regression models. As in simple regression, the outcome variable was uncentered. All predictors were mean-centered. In all the reported analyses, we included both actor and partner variables for all the predictors (all the reported results are unchanged if only the partner variables are introduced as predictors). Because the data violated normality assumptions, we report the robust standard error estimates for all the analyses conducted (cf. Hox, 2002).

### Preliminary analyses

***Gender effects.*** A One-Way ANOVA with gender as a fixed factor revealed that males exhibited lower accuracy in reading negative emotions ($M = 0.24$, $SD = 0.67$) relative to females ($M = 0.50$, $SD = 0.30$), $F_{(1, 73)} = 4.49$, $p < 0.05$, which was apparently due to their tendency to overperceive the amount of negative emotions portrayed in the clips ($M = 0.18$, $SD = 0.67$) relative to females ($M = -0.17$, $SD = 0.50$), $F_{(1, 73)} = 6.47$, $p < 0.05$. At the level of discrete emotions, this gender effect appeared to be driven by the males' tendency to overperceive sadness ($M = 0.35$, $SD = 1.07$), $F_{(1, 73)} = 10.75$, $p < 0.01$, and anger ($M = 0.38$, $SD = 1.14$), $F_{(1, 73)} = 8.07$, $p < 0.01$, relative to females ($M = -0.31$, $SD = 0.60$ for sadness and $M = -0.21$, $SD = 0.52$ for anger). In light of these gender differences, all the reported analyses controlled for gender, coded as −1 for males and 1 for females.

***Actor-partner correlations.*** Using a two-level HLM model with individuals (level-1) embedded in couples (level-2) and gender as a control variable, we found a significant positive association between the spouses' satisfaction with life, $b = 0.49$, $SE = 0.11$, $t_{(35)} = 4.45$, $p < 0.01$, but not hedonic balance levels, $b = 0.15$, $SE = 0.15$, $t_{(35)} = 1.05$, $p = 0.30$. Likewise, there was evidence that spouses tended to be similar not only with respect to their global ability to accurately identify the emotions portrayed in the movie clips, $b = 0.45$, $SE = 0.23$, $t_{(35)} = 1.96$, $p = 0.06$, but also with respect to their ability to accurately identify discrete emotions, specifically, happiness, $b = 0.42$, $SE = 0.14$, $t_{(35)} = 2.93$, $p < 0.01$, and fear, $b = 0.30$, $SE = 0.12$, $t_{(35)} = 2.47$, $p = 0.02$ (for the intercorrelations among the Study 1 measures, see **Table 3**).

#### Hypothesis testing

***Positive emotions and partner hedonic balance.*** Taking our cue from previous findings that provision of responsive support to a close partner during a positive event is a core contributor to the recipient's well-being (e.g., Gable et al., 2012), we tested whether accuracy in identifying positive emotions—and, thus, plausibly, superior ability to respond appropriately to circumstances giving rise to such affect—would predict a spouse's self-ratings of hedonic balance (i.e., the affective component of well-being, cf. Diener, 1984). Results of a regression analysis, predicting an actor's hedonic balance from his/her partner's ability to identify happiness, as well as the actor's own proficiency in detecting happiness disconfirmed our hypothesis, since neither predictor was found to exert a statistically significant effect, $b = 0.43$, $SE = 0.28$, $t_{(34)} = 1.57$, $p > 0.12$ (the partner's ability to identify happiness) and $b = 0.06$, $SE = 0.19$, $t_{(34)} = 0.30$, $p = 0.77$ (the actor's ability to identify happiness) (for the full model, see **Table 2**).

***Positive emotions and partner life satisfaction.*** In contrast, results of the analyses involving the cognitive component of well-being (i.e., life satisfaction, Diener, 1984) supported our hypothesis regarding the unique beneficial effect of a partner's proficiency in identifying positive emotions on an actor's well-being. Specifically, results of a regression analysis, predicting an actor's life satisfaction from his/her partner's ability to identify happiness, as well as the actor's own proficiency in detecting happiness revealed a significant effect of the former predictor, $b = 0.40$, $SE = 0.12$, $t_{(34)} = 3.31$, $p < 0.01$, but not the latter, $b = 0.23$, $SE = 0.19$, $t_{(34)} = 1.20$, $p = 0.24$ (for the full model, see **Table 2**). Indeed, further testifying to the specificity of this effect, a subsequent analysis revealed that a partner's proficiency in identifying happiness remained a significant predictor of an actor's satisfaction with life levels, even after accounting for the actor's hedonic balance, $b = 0.31$, $SE = 0.12$, $t_{(3)} = 2.50$, $p = 0.02$ (for the full model, see **Table 2**).

#### Post-hoc analyses

***Negative emotions and partner well-being.*** Since prior findings suggest that the partner's responsiveness to an actor's negative

**Table 2 | Parameter estimates for the HLM analyses predicting an actor's hedonic balance and life satisfaction from his/her partner's proficiency in identifying positive emotions in Study 1.**

| Fixed effect | Coefficient | SE | t-value (dfs) |
|---|---|---|---|
| **OUTCOME: ACTOR_HEDONIC_BALANCE** | | | |
| For overall INTERCEPT, $\beta_0$ | 2.71 | 0.17 | 16.00 (36)** |
| For ACTOR_GENDER slope, $\beta_1$ | 0.06 | 0.15 | 0.42 (34) |
| For PARTNER_HAPPINESS_RECOGNITION slope, $\beta_2$ | 0.43 | 0.27 | 1.57 (34) |
| For ACTOR_HAPPINESS_RECOGNITION slope, $\beta_3$ | 0.06 | 0.19 | 0.30 (34) |
| **OUTCOME: ACTOR_SATISFACTION_WITH_LIFE** | | | |
| For overall INTERCEPT, $\beta_0$ | 5.51 | 0.11 | 49.47 (36)** |
| For ACTOR_GENDER slope, $\beta_1$ | −0.04 | 0.07 | −0.55 (34) |
| For PARTNER_HAPPINESS_RECOGNITION slope, $\beta_2$ | 0.40 | 0.12 | 3.31 (34)** |
| For ACTOR_HAPPINESS_RECOGNITION slope, $\beta_3$ | 0.23 | 0.19 | 1.20 (34) |
| **OUTCOME: ACTOR_SATISFACTION_WITH_LIFE** | | | |
| For overall INTERCEPT, $\beta_0$ | 5.51 | 0.10 | 56.61 (36)** |
| For ACTOR_GENDER slope, $\beta_1$ | −0.05 | 0.07 | −0.75 (33) |
| For PARTNER_HAPPINESS_RECOGNITION slope, $\beta_2$ | 0.31 | 0.12 | 2.50 (33)* |
| For ACTOR_HAPPINESS_RECOGNITION slope, $\beta_3$ | 0.21 | 0.19 | 1.15 (33) |
| For ACTOR_HEDONIC_BALANCE slope, $\beta_4$ | 0.21 | 0.06 | 3.77 (33)** |

*$p < 0.05$; **$p < 0.01$.

**Table 3 | Intercorrelations among the Study 1 measures.**

| | 1 | 2 | 3 | 4 | 5 | 6 | 7 | 8 | 9 | 10 | 11 | 12 |
|---|---|---|---|---|---|---|---|---|---|---|---|---|
| 1. Spouse 1 happiness recognition | – | | | | | | | | | | | |
| 2. Spouse 1 fear recognition | 0.33** | – | | | | | | | | | | |
| 3. Spouse 1 sadness recognition | 0.24* | 0.55** | – | | | | | | | | | |
| 4. Spouse 1 anger recognition | 0.15 | 0.36** | 0.33* | – | | | | | | | | |
| 5. Spouse 2 happiness recognition | 0.42** | 0.32* | 0.17 | −0.03 | – | | | | | | | |
| 6. Spouse 2 fear recognition | 0.32* | 0.30* | 0.15 | 0.07 | 0.33** | – | | | | | | |
| 7. Spouse 2 sadness recognition | 0.17 | 0.15 | 0.07 | 0.10 | 0.24* | 0.55** | – | | | | | |
| 8. Spouse 2 anger recognition | −0.03 | 0.07 | 0.10 | 0.05 | 0.15 | 0.36** | 0.33* | – | | | | |
| 9. Spouse 1 SWLS | 0.15 | 0.21** | 0.12 | 0.07 | 0.26** | 0.19 | −0.04 | −0.06 | – | | | |
| 10. Spouse 1 AWB | 0.08 | 0.22 | 0.13 | 0.01 | 0.18 | 0.09 | −0.02 | −0.05 | 0.36** | – | | |
| 11. Spouse 2 SWLS | 0.26** | 0.19 | −0.04 | −0.06 | 0.15 | 0.21** | 0.12 | 0.07 | 0.49** | 0.12 | – | |
| 12. Spouse 2 AWB | 0.18 | 0.09 | −0.02 | −0.05 | 0.08 | 0.22 | 0.13 | 0.01 | 0.12 | 0.15 | 0.36** | – |

*$^{*}p < 0.05$; $^{**}p < 0.01$. $N = 74$ individuals embedded in 37 couples. To obtain standardized coefficients, correlations were computed using standardized variables in a two-level HLM model, which collapsed across all participants (Level-1), but controlled for gender and accounted for the interdependence in the data provided by the two spouses (Level-2: couple level). The coefficients and significance estimates in the table are based on the robust standard error estimates, provided by HLM. SWLS, satisfaction with life. AWB, hedonic balance.*

affective states may have some impact on the latter's well-being (Study 2, Maisel and Gable, 2009; Gable et al., 2012), we explored whether the partner's accuracy in reading negative emotions would predict an actor's subjective well-being levels. Results of this set of analyses provided no support for this conjecture with regards to either the actor's satisfaction with life, $b = 0.13$, $SE = 0.24$, $t_{(34)} = 0.55$, $p = 0.59$, or his/her hedonic balance, $b = -0.02$, $SE = 0.28$, $t_{(34)} = -0.07$, $p = 0.95$. Likewise, there was no evidence that an actor's greater accuracy in reading negative emotions would be a significant predictor of either his/her satisfaction with life, $b = 0.31$, $SE = 0.16$, $t_{(34)} = 1.91$, $p = 0.06$, or hedonic balance, $b = 0.39$, $SE = 0.38$, $t_{(34)} = 1.03$, $p = 0.31$. Because prior research suggested that expertise in recognizing distinct negative emotions may differentially impact social interactions (e.g., Niedenthal and Brauer, 2012), we investigated whether expertise in decoding fear vs. anger vs. sadness would be distinctly associated with partner well-being. Results of these analyses revealed only a significant link between an actor's proficiency in reading fear and his/her life satisfaction levels, $b = 0.31$, $SE = 0.12$, $t_{(34)} = 2.66$, $p = 0.01$ (all other $ps > 0.11$) (for standardized coefficients, see **Table 4**).

**Table 4 | Mean values of happiness and negative emotion recognition accuracy, as well as negative emotion leaning, among spouses of PD patients vs. controls as a function of years from PD symptom onset.**

| | Early PD spouses symptom onset < 5 years | Late PD spouses symptom onset > 11 years | Controls |
|---|---|---|---|
| 1. Happiness recognition accuracy | 0.60 | 0.26 | 0.36 |
| 2. Negative emotion recognition accuracy | 0.32 | 0.78 | 0.37 |
| 3. Negative emotion leaning | −0.73 | −0.19 | 0.00 |

*For Happiness and Negative Emotion Recognition Accuracy, respectively, higher coefficients indicate greater accuracy. For Negative Emotion Leaning, lower (i.e., more negative) values indicate greater under-estimation of the amount of negative emotion. The early and late PD groups comprise 4 couples each (8 in total), in which the number of years from PD symptom onset is 1 SD below and above, respectively, the PD sample's average number of years from PD onset.*

***Gender differences in the reported effects.*** Finally, we verified that there were no statistically significant gender differences in the relationship between an actor's proficiency in identifying positive vs. (global/discrete) negative emotions and his/her partner's either satisfaction with life (all $ps > 0.18$) or hedonic balance (all $ps > 0.05$).

In sum, Study 1 provided partial support to our hypothesis that greater expertise in identifying positive emotions would be linked to greater spousal well-being, conceivably because such expertise may render one better skilled at reading his/her spouse's emotional reactions during a positive event and, thus, be in a better position to respond in a manner that would foster the spouse's well-being (cf. Gable et al., 2012). Specifically, we found that a partner's proficiency in identifying positive emotions exhibited a significant association with an actor's life satisfaction, but not hedonic balance. Interestingly, this effect points to a potential interpersonal mechanism underlying the observed spousal similarity in life satisfaction (for similar findings, see Bookwala and Schulz, 1996; Schimmack and Lucas, 2010), since spouses were alike not only with respect to their cognitive well-being levels, but also with respect to their ability to identify positive emotions. Finally, Study 1 also revealed a potential intra-individual mechanism supporting spousal similarity on life satisfaction, since it provided evidence of spousal resemblance on fear recognition ability, which was, in turn, a significant intrapersonal predictor of life satisfaction. We will elaborate on the implications of these findings in the General Discussion.

## STUDY 2

The purpose of Study 2 was to investigate whether under circumstances that render negative emotions particularly salient and informative, such as spousal disability (Monin and Schulz, 2009; Monin et al., 2009), expertise in decoding negative (rather than positive) emotions would be a stronger predictor of spousal well-being. Moreover, we sought to replicate the Study 1 findings that it is an actor's cognitive, rather than affective, well-being levels that are most susceptible to the influence of spousal proficiency in (here, negative) emotion processing.

In a secondary vein, we also examined whether beyond any adverse effects of PD on the patients' ability to decode postural emotional cues, we would also detect any differences in emotion recognition performance between the patients' spouses and the controls, presumably reflective of the former's adaptations to living with PD. Specifically, we investigated whether in order to compensate for the PD patients' presumed deficits in producing facial expressions of positive emotions (cf. Pitcairn et al., 1990), their spouses would be particularly attuned and, thus, demonstrate increased accuracy in decoding expressions of happiness. Although it is plausible that such an adaptation effect (if it exists) may generalize across modalities, we reasoned that we may be particularly likely to detect it in a modality that is presumably less affected by PD (i.e., by using postural, rather than facial, cues of happiness). Finally, based on the assumption that proficiency in recognizing negative emotions may be a critical asset for care givers (i.e., to minimize care giver stress, cf. Monin et al., 2009), we examined whether relative to controls, PD spouses would also show increased expertise in reading negative emotions, specifically those indicative of vulnerability, such as fear and sadness. In all the reported analyses, the Study 1 participants served as the control group [$t$-test analyses confirmed that there were no significant differences in either age ($p > 0.10$) or marriage length ($p > 0.28$) between the Study 1 and 2 samples].

### METHODS

#### *Participants and procedure*

Eighteen PD patients and their spouses completed the same tasks and measures as the Study 1 participants. The patients were recruited through local newspaper advertisements or through their neurologist, who was affiliated with a teaching hospital associated with the University of Toronto. According to the patients' medical records (released with their consent by their neurologist following the patients' laboratory visit), they were all non-demented and not clinically depressed at the time of testing. Prior to their laboratory visit, the patients' spouses underwent the same phone screening interview as the Study 1 participants, in which they verified that they themselves had no known neurological or cognitive impairments. The patients [6 women, 12 men; mean age = 68.50 years ($SD = 11.67$)] averaged 2.56 (range 1.0–3.0) on the modified Hoehn and Yahr (1967) disability scale. On average, they had received the PD diagnosis 8.06 years ($SD = 3.89$ years; range 2–15 years) prior. Excepting one who developed intolerance to L-dopa six months prior, all were taking dopamine precursor treatments (i.e., L-dopa) to alleviate Parkinsonian symptoms. All patients were tested while on normal dosing schedules. They were tested late morning, approximately 3 h after taking their medication. The spouses' average age was 67.28 years ($SD = 10.23$). The couples had been married between 18 and 53 years ($M = 39.28$, $SD = 11.67$). All were native English speakers or had lived in Canada and used English as their primary language for at least 30 years (for the demographic information summary, see **Table 1**). Informed consent was obtained from both PD patients and their spouses in accordance with the ethical guidelines of the Research Ethics Boards at the University of Toronto and the University Health Network.

### RESULTS

Preliminary analyses confirmed that all the reported results were unchanged if the patient who became intolerant to L-dopa, and who was thus medication-free during the study period, was kept or eliminated from the sample. Consequently, we opted to keep this patient's data in the analyses. Two PD patients failed to fill out the positive/negative affect scale, whereas one PD spouse failed to complete the satisfaction with life scale. Consequently, all the reported well-being findings are based on data from 18 PD patients and 17 PD spouses (satisfaction with life), as well as 16 PD patients and 18 PD spouses (hedonic balance).

#### *Preliminary analyses*

Preliminary correlational analyses revealed no statistically significant association between the patients' and their spouses' satisfaction with life, $r_{(16)} = 0.39$, $p = 0.12$, hedonic balance, $r_{(15)} = -0.32$, $p = 0.24$, proficiency in recognizing positive, $r_{(16)} = 0.15$, $p = 0.56$, or negative, $r_{(16)} = -0.25$, $p = 0.33$, emotions.

#### *Hypothesis testing*

To test our hypotheses, we used the same two-level HLM model as in Study 1 and ran two sets of analyses, comparing the healthy controls to the PD patients and the patients' spouses, respectively. As in Study 1, we controlled for gender (coded as $-1$ for males and 1 for females) in all the reported analyses. For the comparisons involving the PD patients and the controls, two predictor variables were used: patient status, coded 0 for controls and 1 for PD patients and years from PD symptom onset, which had a value of 0 for controls and a number corresponding to the years from the symptom onset for patients. Likewise, for the comparisons involving the spouses of PD patients and controls, two predictors were employed: patient spouse status, coded 0 for controls and 1 for the spouses of the PD patients and years from PD symptom onset, which had a value of 0 for controls and a number corresponding to the years from the symptom onset for the patients' spouses. As in Study 1, we report the robust standard error estimates for all the analyses conducted.

***Well-being.*** As expected, PD patients exhibited significantly lower satisfaction with life levels compared to their age-matched controls, $b = -2.40$, $SE = 0.48$, $t_{(34)} = -4.97$, $p < 0.001$, although the discrepancy between the two groups diminished with more years from PD symptom onset, $b = 0.14$, $SE = 0.06$, $t_{(34)} = 2.46$, $p = 0.02$. Hedonic balance was also poorer among

PD patients, relative to their age-matched controls, $b = -2.11$, $SE = 0.93$, $t_{(34)} = -2.26$, $p = 0.03$, and this effect was impervious to the number of years from PD symptom onset, $b = 0.16$, $SE = 0.14$, $t_{(34)} = 1.13$, $p = 0.27$. In contrast, although spouses of PD patients tended to experience lower satisfaction with life as well, this effect failed to reach conventional levels of statistical significance, $b = -0.97$, $SE = 0.50$, $t_{(34)} = -1.96$, $p = 0.06$. Of note, there was no evidence that spouses of PD patients would exhibit poorer affective balance relative to their age-matched controls, $b = -1.08$, $SE = 0.93$, $t_{(34)} = -1.16$, $p = 0.25$, or that years from PD symptom onset would lead to any significant differences between the two groups in either satisfaction with life, $b = 0.06$, $SE = 0.07$, $t_{(34)} = 0.87$, $p = 0.39$, or hedonic balance, $b = 0.07$, $SE = 0.12$, $t_{(34)} = 0.60$, $p = 0.55$.

***Emotion recognition.***

*PD patients vs. controls.*

*Positive emotions*: We found no evidence that either patient status, $b = -0.09$, $SE = 0.21$, $t_{(34)} = -0.44$, $p = 0.66$, or years from PD symptom onset, $b = 0.00$, $SE = 0.02$, $t_{(34)} = 0.14$, $p = 0.89$, would impact significantly accuracy in identifying positive emotions.

*Negative emotions*: Likewise, there was no evidence that either patient status, $b = 0.16$, $SE = 0.18$, $t_{(34)} = 0.90$, $p = 0.37$, or years from PD symptom onset, $b = -0.02$, $SE = 0.01$, $t_{(34)} = 1.05$, $p = 0.30$, would affect significantly accuracy in identifying negative emotions. Subsequent analyses focused on accuracy in identifying discrete negative emotions yielded similar, non-significant results (all *ps* > 0.33).

*Spouses of PD patients vs. controls.*

*Positive emotions*: Results of this analysis revealed two significant main effects: Spouses of PD patients were more accurate than controls in identifying happiness, $b = 0.58$, $SE = 0.17$, $t_{(34)} = 3.46$, $p < 0.001$, but their advantage diminished with more years from PD symptom onset, $b = -0.05$, $SE = 0.02$, $t_{(34)} = 2.60$, $p = 0.01$ (see **Table 4**).

*Negative emotions*: Interestingly, we found evidence that spouses of PD patients tended to be somewhat less accurate than controls in identifying negative emotions, $b = -0.51$, $SE = 0.25$, $t_{(34)} = 2.05$, $p = 0.05$, although their "deficit" was reversed with more years from PD symptom onset, $b = 0.06$, $SE = 0.02$, $t_{(34)} = 2.45$, $p = 0.02$ (see **Table 4**). Follow-up analyses revealed that these effects were due to the PD spouses' tendency to underestimate the intensity of negative emotions (relative to controls), $b = -0.64$, $SE = 0.28$, $t_{(34)} = -2.31$, $p = 0.03$, a tendency that became weaker with longer years from PD symptom onset, $b = 0.07$, $SE = 0.03$, $t_{(34)} = 2.34$, $p = 0.03$ (see **Table 4**). Nevertheless, there was no evidence that the relatively poorer identification of negative emotions was specific to any of the discrete negative emotions under scrutiny (all *ps* > 0.09).

***Emotion recognition and partner well-being.*** Finally, we tested our hypothesis that among PD patients and their spouses, it would be expertise in decoding negative, rather than positive, emotions that would be a stronger predictor of partner well-being. To this end, we specified a two-level HLM model, with years from PD symptom onset as the level-2 (i.e., couple-level) variable, gender (coded as −1 for males and 1 for females), patient status (coded as −1 for PD patients' spouses and 1 for PD patients), and accuracy in identifying positive vs. negative emotions as the level-1 variables. Both level-1 and -2 continuous predictor variables were mean-centered. In all the reported analyses, we included both actor and partner variables for all the predictors (all the relevant results are unchanged if only the partner variables are introduced as predictors). Because of the small sample size (i.e., 35 and 34 individuals, respectively, embedded in 18 couples for the life satisfaction and hedonic balance analyses, respectively), we report the non-robust standard error regression coefficient estimates, which are preferred in this case for interpretational purposes (all the reported effects remain significant if using the robust standard error estimates).

*Hedonic balance.* Similar to Study 1, we found no evidence that an actor's proficiency in identifying positive or negative emotions would be a significant predictor of either his/her own or his/her partner's hedonic balance (all *ps* > 0.15).

*Satisfaction with life.* Results of two separate sets of analyses revealed that among PD patients and their spouses, greater proficiency in identifying positive emotions did not exert a significant effect on spousal satisfaction with life, $b = -0.30$, $SE = 0.51$, $t_{(9)} = -0.57$, $p = 0.58$, even when accounting for years from PD onset, $b = -0.23$, $SE = 0.14$, $t_{(9)} = -1.65$, $p = 0.13$. Instead, with more years from PD symptom onset, it was proficiency in identifying negative emotions that became an increasingly stronger predictor of spousal satisfaction with life, $b = 0.25$, $SE = 0.11$, $t_{(9)} = 2.22$, $p = 0.05$ (for the full model, see **Table 5**). Follow-up analyses focused on discrete negative emotions revealed that it was greater expertise in identifying sadness that constituted an increasingly reliable predictor of greater spousal life satisfaction with more years from PD symptom onset, $b = 0.22$, $SE = 0.06$, $t_{(9)} = 3.45$, $p < 0.01$ (for the full model, see **Table 6**). Results of similar analyses involving expertise in identifying fear or anger failed to reach traditional levels of statistical significance (all *ps* > 0.21). Likewise, there was no evidence that an actor's proficiency in identifying either positive or negative emotions would be a significant predictor of his/her own life satisfaction levels (all *ps* > 0.24).

*Patient-spouse differences.* Finally, we tested whether expertise in decoding positive vs. negative emotions would exert differential effects on spousal life satisfaction or hedonic balance, as a function of whether the spouse is the PD patient or not. To this end, we introduced the interaction between patient status and positive vs. negative emotion recognition scores as a level-1 predictor of partner well-being. Results of this set of analyses provided no support to the hypothesis that partner expertise in decoding positive vs. negative emotions would impact differentially either the life satisfaction or hedonic balance of the PD patients vs. that of their spouses (all *ps* > 0.37).

**Table 5 | Parameter estimates for the HLM analyses predicting an actor's hedonic balance and life satisfaction from his/her partner's proficiency in identifying negative emotions in Study 2.**

| Fixed effect | Coefficient | *SE* | *t*-value (dfs) |
|---|---|---|---|
| OUTCOME: ACTOR_SATISFACTION_WITH_LIFE | | | |
| **For overall INTERCEPT, $\beta_0$** | | | |
| Intercept2, $B_{00}$ | 4.66 | 0.19 | 24.87(16)$^{**}$ |
| PD_Symptom_Onset, $B_{01}$ | 0.09 | 0.05 | 1.73(16) |
| **For ACTOR_GENDER slope, $\beta_1$** | | | |
| Intercept2, $B_{10}$ | −0.33 | 0.12 | −2.78(9)$^{*}$ |
| PD_Symptom_Onset, $B_{11}$ | −0.05 | 0.03 | −1.85(9) |
| **For ACTOR_PATIENT_STATUS slope, $\beta_2$** | | | |
| Intercept2, $B_{20}$ | −0.48 | 0.13 | −3.78(9)$^{**}$ |
| PD_Symptom_Onset, $B_{21}$ | 0.09 | 0.03 | 3.09(9)$^{*}$ |
| **For PARTNER_NEGATIVE_EMOTIONS_RECOGNITION slope, $\beta_3$** | | | |
| Intercept2, $B_{30}$ | 0.34 | 0.39 | 0.89(9) |
| PD_Symptom_Onset, $B_{31}$ | 0.25 | 0.11 | 2.22(9)* |
| **For ACTOR__NEGATIVE_EMOTIONS_RECOGNITION slope, $\beta 4$** | | | |
| Intercept2, $B_{40}$ | 0.48 | 0.39 | 1.23(9) |
| PD_Symptom_Onset, $B_{41}$ | −0.03 | 0.11 | −0.31(9) |

*$^{*}p < 0.05$; $^{**}p < 0.01$. The estimates are the non-robust error estimates (since they are preferred for interpretative purposes).*

**Table 6 | Parameter estimates for the HLM analyses predicting an actor's hedonic balance and life satisfaction from his/her partner's proficiency in identifying sadness in Study 2.**

| Fixed effect | Coefficient | *SE* | *t*-value (dfs) |
|---|---|---|---|
| OUTCOME: ACTOR_SATISFACTION_WITH_LIFE | | | |
| **For overall INTERCEPT, $\beta_0$** | | | |
| Intercept2, $B_{00}$ | 4.61 | 0.17 | 27.71(16)$^{**}$ |
| PD_Symptom_Onset, $B_{01}$ | 0.08 | 0.05 | 1.68(16) |
| **For ACTOR_GENDER slope, $\beta_1$** | | | |
| Intercept2, $B_{10}$ | −0.21 | 0.09 | −2.38(9)$^{*}$ |
| PD_Symptom_Onset, $B_{11}$ | −0.07 | 0.02 | −3.27(9)$^{**}$ |
| **For ACTOR_PATIENT_STATUS slope, $\beta_2$** | | | |
| Intercept2, $B_{20}$ | −0.41 | 0.09 | −4.37(9)$^{**}$ |
| PD_Symptom_Onset, $B_{21}$ | 0.08 | 0.02 | 3.34(9)$^{**}$ |
| **For PARTNER_SADNESS_RECOGNITION slope, $\beta_3$** | | | |
| Intercept2, $B_{30}$ | 0.44 | 0.23 | 1.95(9) |
| PD_Symptom_Onset, $B_{31}$ | 0.22 | 0.06 | 3.45(9)$^{**}$ |
| **For ACTOR_SADNESS_PERCEPTIONRECOGNITION slope, $\beta 4$** | | | |
| Intercept2, $B_{40}$ | 0.41 | 0.23 | 1.82(9) |
| PD_Symptom_Onset, $B_{41}$ | 0.04 | 0.06 | 0.65(9) |

*$^{*}p < 0.05$; $^{**}p < 0.01$. The estimates are the non-robust error estimates (since they are preferred for interpretative purposes).*

## GENERAL DISCUSSION

The present research investigated the link between expertise in reading postural cues of positive vs. negative emotions and spousal well-being among neurologically intact elderly couples (Study 1) and a sample of PD patients and their spouses (Study 2). Study 1 provided evidence that among healthy controls, greater expertise in identifying positive, rather than negative, emotions is linked to greater spousal cognitive, but not affective, well-being. Despite its specificity (see discussion below), such an association is broadly in line with our hypothesis that greater expertise in decoding positive emotional cues renders one better skilled at reading his/her spouse's emotional reactions during positive events and, thus, better able to provide adequate support to the spouse, which, in turn, is a well-documented contributor to spousal well-being (cf. Gable et al., 2012).

Study 2 extended the Study 1 findings regarding the unique link between spousal proficiency in emotion processing and an actor's cognitive, rather than affective, well-being levels. Specifically, in line with our hypotheses, Study 2 documented that under conditions that may render a close partner's negative emotions particularly informative for adjusting behavior to protect the dyadic environment, it is proficiency in reading negative, but not positive, emotions that predicts greater spousal life satisfaction. Thus, with more years from PD symptom onset, and, thus, conceivably, greater patient disability and care giver burden, it was proficiency in recognizing negative emotions, most importantly, sadness, that predicted greater spousal life satisfaction among PD patients and their partners. Moreover, although we did not detect any deficits in deciphering postural emotional cues among PD patients, we found suggestive evidence of PD-induced adaptation effects among the patients' spouses. Specifically, complementing earlier findings on the PD patients' deficits in producing facial expressions of positive emotions (Pitcairn et al., 1990; Simons et al., 2004), we found evidence of greater proficiency in decoding whole-body cues of happiness among PD spouses, relative to controls. Given the significance of positive emotion recognition for spousal well-being, documented in Study 1, it seems plausible that the PD spouses' advantage in identifying happiness would reflect a compensation mechanism, whose function would be to preserve the dyadic homeostasis. Further evidence suggestive of adaptation effects among PD spouses is provided by our findings that although in earlier stages, PD spouses may be somewhat less skilled than controls at negative emotion recognition, this deficit reverses with more years from PD symptom onset. Such an effect is indeed noteworthy, since among PD patients and their spouses, proficiency in identifying negative emotions becomes an increasingly reliable predictor of spousal satisfaction with life with more years from symptom onset.

Our present findings suggest several venues for future research on affective proficiency and well-being among married couples. First, the unique role of superior positive emotion recognition in spousal life satisfaction needs to be probed in future studies. For example, a spouse who is better skilled at decoding positive emotions may provide more effective support during propitious times and thus foster an actor's life satisfaction because s/he is better able to facilitate meaning-making processes that integrate an isolated positive event in the context of an actor's broader life goals and strivings. Complementarily, any beneficial effects of spousal positive emotion expertise on an actor's hedonic balance may be only indirect, mediated by changes in the actor's life satisfaction. To the best of our knowledge, there have been no investigations of the unique effects of effective social support on spousal affective vs. cognitive well-being. Consequently, future studies, assessing individual differences not only in well-being and positive emotion processing, but also in reappraisal and meaning making within a dyadic context, are needed to test the viability of our proposed hypotheses.

Second, the mechanisms underlying our observed association between performance on a point light walker task and spousal life satisfaction deserve further investigation. Prior research suggested that individual differences in decoding postural emotional cues are predictive of broader sociocognitive functioning (e.g., false belief reasoning, Phillips et al., 2011). Consequently, the question arises whether the observed link between spousal well-being and performance on the point light walker task is merely due to the fact that the latter is a good indicator of social cue understanding and utilization or whether indeed the ability to read whole-body (rather than facial or auditory, for example) emotional cues is particularly relevant to interpersonal functioning. With respect to the latter hypothesis, it seems indeed plausible that postural affective cues may be more informative to social exchanges than facial cues, because the latter may be easier to control and thus be used to conceal one's inner experience from others. Future studies using a comprehensive sociocognitive assessment package and individual differences or situational manipulations of emotional expression are needed to shed light on this issue.

Third, future studies should examine the implications of our findings that spouses are assorted not only on life satisfaction (cf. Bookwala and Schulz, 1996; Schimmack and Lucas, 2010), but also on traits predictive of life satisfaction, either on the interpersonal (i.e., happiness recognition) or intrapersonal (i.e., fear recognition) level (cf. Study 1). Indeed, in Study 1, we documented the association between expertise in identifying positive emotions and spousal life satisfaction, whereas others provided evidence that fear recognition plays an important role in determining prosocial behavior (for a review, see Niedenthal and Brauer, 2012). It thus seems plausible that the previously documented spousal matching on life satisfaction may be (partly) due to spousal assortment on dispositions that predict behaviors conducive to close others' happiness (i.e., proficiency in positive emotion recognition) or are linked to more fulfilling interpersonal exchanges (i.e., proficiency in fear recognition) and, thus, indirectly, contribute to one's own satisfaction with life. Future studies, examining the early acquaintanceship stages of potential romantic partners, may be required to test this hypothesis.

Fourth, additional research is needed to elucidate the underlying mechanisms and functionality of the PD spouses' proficiency in reading postural cues of positive emotions, as documented in Study 2 of the present manuscript. One venue for future research would be to shed light on whether PD spouses exhibit proficiency in decoding positive emotions across all modalities, or whether their advantage is more modality-specific (i.e., only detectable for non-facial forms of positive emotion expression). Such a distinction is important to be made, since it may also elucidate the pattern of expressive deficits associated for PD. Indeed, support for a more modality-specific (rather than modality-general) advantage in decoding positive affective cues among the PD spouses may suggest that, at least in the earlier stages of the disease, PD patients' ability to express emotions through non-facial cues may be relatively less affected. Nevertheless, future studies are needed to test these hypotheses by incorporating more modality-diverse emotional stimuli and by assessing PD patients' ability to produce and their spouses' proficiency in decoding positive emotional cues across multiple modalities. Likewise, future research should examine the mechanisms underlying the PD spouses' decreasing accuracy in decoding positive emotional cues and increasing accuracy in identifying negative emotional cues with more years from PD symptom onset. For example, one possibility may be that these effects are due to the decreased motivational salience of positive and increased relevance of negative emotional cues (cf. Study 2's link between spousal life satisfaction and proficiency in identifying negative emotions). Alternatively or additionally, in line with the documented PD-related impairments in producing positive emotional cues (Pitcairn et al., 1990; Simons et al., 2004), these effects may arise due to the PD spouses' diminishing exposure to positive emotional cues and relatively heightened exposure to negative emotional cues with more years from PD symptom onset.

Finally, the link between positive vs. negative emotion proficiency and spousal well-being deserves further investigation in more demographically diverse samples. Specifically, it is worth pointing out that our neurologically intact sample was exclusively comprised of older adults, who have been previously shown to exhibit greater sensitivity to positive, and lower sensitivity to negative, emotional stimuli, relative to younger adults (for a review, see Mather and Carstensen, 2005). Consequently, it may be the case that the null effect of proficiency in negative emotion recognition on spousal well-being may be partly due to older adults' superior ability to fend off negative emotions on their own, thereby minimizing the impact of any spousal aide, and/or their reduced tendency to allow negative emotions, evoked by external stressors, to permeate their marital interactions (for evidence on more positive marital interactions in older adulthood, see Levenson et al., 1994). In contrast, among younger adults, who presumably exhibit higher sensitivity to negative emotional stimuli (Mather and Carstensen, 2005), significantly greater interpersonal costs may be incurred by poorer negative emotion recognition and, thus, arguably, poorer ability to provide adequate support to a close partner during inauspicious times. Thus, although extant research suggests that social support provision to a close partner during propitious, rather than adverse, periods is a stronger contributor to the latter's well-being (Study 2, Gable et al., 2012), reduced ability to identify negative emotions and, consequently, respond appropriately to a partner during negative events may still result in significant hedonic damage, among younger, rather than elderly, social support recipients.

## LIMITATIONS

Inevitably, our present research has a few limitations. First, our correlational design precludes any conclusions regarding the causal direction of the link between proficiency in identifying positive vs. negative emotions and spousal life satisfaction. For example, in Study 1, it is plausible that individuals with higher, relative to lower, life satisfaction levels may express positive emotions more frequently. Thus, their spouses may have greater exposure to positive emotional cues and, consequently, gain greater expertise in decoding them. Nevertheless, if that were to be the case, then we would expect a stronger relationship between an actor's proficiency in decoding happiness and spousal hedonic balance, rather than life satisfaction. Importantly, this is not what we found in Study 1, where, in fact, the association between a partner's hedonic balance and an actor's ability to read happiness failed to reach conventional levels of statistical significance. Moreover, if frequency of exposure to a spouse's positive/negative emotional cues accounts for the link between an actor's proficiency in decoding emotional cues and spousal life satisfaction, then the Study 2 findings would suggest that among PD patients and their spouses, higher life satisfaction individuals express negative emotions more frequently, thereby fostering their spouses' expertise in deciphering them. Although we argued that expression of negative emotions is informative within a care giving context (cf. Monin and Schulz, 2009; Monin et al., 2009), we would find it difficult to contend that more frequent expression of such emotions is the hallmark of greater happiness among PD patients and their spouses. Nevertheless, future longitudinal studies, assessing the emotion expressive habits of both spouses, as well as their emotion expertise and well-being, are needed to elucidate the causal direction of the link between emotion recognition expertise and spousal well-being.

Second, we did not find any evidence of deficits in reading postural emotional cues among PD patients. To the best of our knowledge, there are no reports of PD-induced impairments in decoding whole-body affective cues in the literature, which renders our present null findings rather uncontroversial. Moreover, even deficits in facial emotion recognition have not been consistently documented among PD patients. Indeed, studies using subtler facial emotional cues and more advanced PD patients, tested on regular dosing schedules—as in our research—either failed to document any impairments (Adolphs et al., 1998; Sprengelmeyer et al., 2003) or documented impairments in disgust recognition (Suzuki et al., 2006; Assogna et al., 2010), an emotion not assessed in our study. Future studies with larger and more diverse PD samples, tested both on and off medication, may be required to elucidate the nature of any potential deficits in deciphering postural emotional cues among PD patients.

Third, although we posited that emotion recognition abilities are crucial to an individual's capacity to provide responsive support to a spouse, our research did not include any social support measures. Future studies, incorporating indicators of both enacted and perceived support during positive and negative events, are needed to characterize the hypothesized link between proficiency in identifying emotional cues and responsive support provision in close relationships.

Fourth, our research focused on a patient population exhibiting irreversibly increasing levels of disability. Future studies, examining care recipients with reversible or stable impairments, are warranted to shed light on any differential effects of spousal expertise in positive vs. negative emotion recognition as a function of disability type.

Fifth, in our present research, we used a rather narrowly defined standard of emotion recognition accuracy, specifically, the mean ratings provided by the neurologically intact sample in response to the point light walker clips. We regarded our operationalization of accuracy as justifiable because, beyond any idiosyncratic effects, a significant predictor of whether an actor would successfully decode his/her spouse's emotions is, arguably, his/her adherence to the affective vocabulary of those most demographically similar to his/her spouse. Nevertheless, future studies, using a broader affective vocabulary, based on the judgments of more demographically diverse samples, are certainly warranted to elucidate the nature of the association between an actor's emotion recognition proficiency and his/her spouse's well-being.

Finally, although the dynamic whole-body emotional stimuli, used in the present research, are more naturalistic than the static facial emotional stimuli, often employed in emotion recognition studies, they still fall short of the affective richness that typifies numerous interpersonal exchanges. For example, in each point light walker clip, the actor was requested to portray a specific emotion (see Heberlein and Saxe, 2005; Atkinson et al., 2007). Such affective "single-mindedness" is probably seldom characteristic of social actor's experiences in real life. Consequently, future studies are needed to elucidate the effect of proficiency in decoding emotions from realistic social interactions on spousal and dyadic well-being.

In conclusion, our present research suggests that expertise in decoding emotional cues may have wide-ranging implications for dyadic well-being. Moreover, our results imply that positive vs. negative emotions may play distinct roles in close relationship dynamics as a function of the spouses' neurological status and disability trajectory. Research is now needed to shed light on the mechanisms underlying the observed links between emotion recognition proficiency and close partner well-being across the lifespan of an intimate partnership.

## ACKNOWLEDGMENTS

This research was partially supported by a Canadian Institutes of Health Research doctoral fellowship awarded to Raluca Petrican.

## REFERENCES

Adolphs, R., Schul, R., and Tranel, D. (1998). Intact recognition of facial emotion in Parkinson's disease. *Neuropsychology* 12, 253–258. doi: 10.1037/0894-4105.12.2.253

Ariatti, A., Benuzzi, F., and Nichelli, P. (2008). Recognition of emotions from visual and prosodic cues in Parkinson's disease. *Neurol. Sci.* 29, 219–227. doi: 10.1007/s10072-008-0971-9

Assogna, F., Pontieri, F. E., Cravello, L., Peppe, A., Pierantozzi, M. A., Stefani, A., et al. (2010). Intensity-dependent facial emotion recognition and cognitive functions in Parkinson's disease. *J. Int. Neuropsychol. Soc.* 16, 867–876. doi: 10.1017/S1355617710000755

Atkinson, A. P., Heberlein, A. S., and Adolphs, R. (2007). Spared ability to recognise fear from static and moving whole-body cues following bilateral amygdala damage. *Neuropsychologia* 45, 2772–2782. doi: 10.1016/j.neuropsychologia.2007.04.019

Baker, B., Paquette, M., Szalai, J., Driver, H., Perger, T., Helmers, K., et al. (2000). The influence of marital adjustment on 3-year left ventricular mass and ambulatory blood pressure in mild hypertension. *Arch. Int. Med.* 160, 3453–3458. doi: 10.1001/archinte.160.22.3453

Beach, S. R., and O'Leary, K. D. (1993). Marital discord and dysphoria: for whom does the marital relationship predict depressive symptomatology? *J. Soc. Pers. Relat.* 10, 405–420.

Berscheid, E., and Reis, H. T. (1998). "Interpersonal attraction and close relationships," in *Handbook of Social Psychology, 4th Edn.*, eds D. T. Gilbert, S. T. Fiske, and G. Lindzey (New York, NY: Random House), 193–281.

Bolger, N., Zuckerman, A., and Kessler, R. C. (2000). Invisible support and adjustment to stress. *J. Pers. Soc. Psychol.* 79, 953–961. doi: 10.1037/0022-3514.79.6.953

Bookwala, J., and Schulz, R. (1996). Spousal similarity in subjective well-being: the cardiovascular health study. *Psychol. Aging* 11, 582–590. doi: 10.1037/0882-7974.11.4.582

Brosgole, L., and Weisman, J. (1995). Mood recognition across the ages. *Int. J. Neurosci.* 82, 169–189. doi: 10.3109/00207459508999800

Brown, P. C., and Smith, T. W. (1992). Social influence, marriage, and the heart: cardiovascular consequences of interpersonal control in husbands and wives. *Health Psychol.* 11, 88–96. doi: 10.1037/0278-6133.11.2.88

Brown, P. C., Smith, T. W., and Benjamin, L. S. (1998). Perceptions of spouse dominance predict blood pressure reactivity during marital interactions. *Ann. Behav. Med.* 20, 294–301. doi: 10.1007/BF02886378

Buck, R., and Duffy, R. J. (1980). Nonverbal communication of affect in brain-damaged patients. *Cortex* 16, 351–362. doi: 10.1016/S0010-9452(80)80037-2

Buxton, S. L., MacDonald, L., and Tippett, L. J. (2013). Impaired recognition of prosody and subtle emotional facial expressions in Parkinson's Disease. *Behav. Neurosci.* 127, 193–203. doi: 10.1037/a0032013

Calder, A. J., Keane, J., Manly, T., Sprengelmeyer, R., Scott, S., Nimmo-Smith, I., et al. (2003). Facial expression recognition across the adult life span. *Neuropsychologia* 41, 195–202. doi: 10.1016/S0028-3932(02)00149-5

Campbell, L., and Kashy, D. A. (2002). Estimating actor, partner, and interaction effects for dyadic data using PROC MIXED and HLM: a guided tour. *Pers. Relat.* 9, 327–342. doi: 10.1111/1475-6811.00023

Carstensen, L. L. (1992). Social and emotional patterns in adulthood: support for socioemotional selectivity theory. *Psychol. Aging* 7, 331–338. doi: 10.1037/0882-7974.7.3.331

Clark, U. S., Neargarder, S., and Cronin-Golomb, A. (2008). Specific impairments in the recognition of emotional facial expressions in Parkinson's disease. *Neuropsychologia* 46, 2300–2309. doi: 10.1016/j.neuropsychologia.2008.03.014

Cohen, S. (1988). Psychosocial models of the role of social support in the etiology of physical disease. *Health Psychol.* 7, 269–297. doi: 10.1037/0278-6133.7.3.269

Cohen, S., and Wills, T. A. (1985). Stress, social support, and the buffering hypothesis. *Psychol. Bull.* 98, 310–357. doi: 10.1037/0033-2909.98.2.310

Collins, N. L., Dunkel-Schetter, C., Lobel, M., and Scrimshaw, S. C. (1993). Social support in pregnancy: psychosocial correlates of birth outcomes and postpartum depression. *J. Pers. Soc. Psychol.* 65, 1243–1258. doi: 10.1037/0022-3514.65.6.1243

Dara, C., Monetta, L., and Pell, M. D. (2008). Vocal emotion processing in Parkinson's disease: reduced sensitivity to negative emotions. *Brain Res.* 1188, 100–111. doi: 10.1016/j.brainres.2007.10.034

Davila, J., Bradbury, T. N., Cohan, C. L., and Tochluk, S. (1997). Marital functioning and depressive symptoms: evidence for a stress generation model. *J. Pers. Soc. Psychol.* 73, 849–861. doi: 10.1037/0022-3514.73.4.849

Diener, E. (1984). Subjective well-being. *Psychol. Bull.* 95, 542–575. doi: 10.1037/0033-2909.95.3.542

Diener, E., and Biswas-Diener, R. (2008). *Happiness: Unlocking the Mysteries of Psychological Wealth.* Malden, MA: Blackwell Publishing. doi: 10.1002/9781444305159

Diener, E., Emmons, R. A., Larsen, R. J., and Griffin, S. (1985). The satisfaction with life scale. *J. Pers. Assess.* 49, 71–75. doi: 10.1207/s15327752jpa4901_13

Diener, E., and Seligman, M. E. P. (2002). Very happy people. *Psychol. Sci.* 13, 81–84. doi: 10.1111/1467-9280.00415

Ditzen, B., Hoppmann, C., and Klumb, P. (2008). Positive couple interactions and daily cortisol: on the stress-protecting role of intimacy. *Psychosom. Med.* 70, 883–889. doi: 10.1097/PSY.0b013e318185c4fc

Dujardin, K., Blairy, S., Defebvre, L., Duhem, S., Noel, Y., Hess, U., et al. (2004). Deficits in decoding emotional facial expressions in Parkinson's disease. *Neuropsychologia* 42, 239–250. doi: 10.1016/S0028-3932(03)00154-4

Eaker, E. D., Sullivan, L. M., Kelly-Hayes, M., D'Agostino, R. B., and Benjamin, E. J. (2007). Marital status, marital strain, and risk of coronary heart disease or total mortality: the Framingham offspring study. *Psychosom. Med.* 69, 509–513. doi: 10.1097/PSY.0b013e3180f62357

Ellgring, H., Seiler, S., Perleth, B., Frings, W., Gasser, T., and Oertel, W. (1993). Psychosocial aspects of Parkinson's disease. *Neurology* 43 (Suppl. 6), S41–S44.

Ewart, C. K., Taylor, C. B., Kraemer, H. C., and Agras, W. S. (1991). High blood pressure and marital discord: not being nasty matters more than being nice. *Health Psychol.* 10, 155–163. doi: 10.1037/0278-6133.10.3.155

Ferguson, L. W., Rajput, M. L., Muhajarine, N., Shah, S. M., and Rajput, A. (2008). Clinical features at first visit and rapid disease progression in Parkinson's disease. *Parkinsonism Relat. Disord.* 14, 431–435. doi: 10.1016/j.parkreldis.2007.10.012

Gable, S. L., Gonzaga, G., and Strachman, A. (2006). Will you be there for me when things go right? Supportive responses to positive event disclosures. *J. Pers. Soc. Psychol.* 91, 904–917. doi: 10.1037/0022-3514.91.5.904

Gable, S. L., Gosnell, C. L., Maisel, N. C., and Strachman, A. (2012). Safely testing the alarm: close others' responses to personal positive events. *J. Pers. Soc. Psychol.* 103, 963–981. doi: 10.1037/a0029488

Gere, J., Schimmack, U., Pinkus, R., and Lockwood, P. (2011). The effects of romantic partners' goal congruence on affective well-being. *J. Res. Pers.* 45, 549–559. doi: 10.1016/j.jrp.2011.06.010

Given, C. W., Stommel, M., Given, B., Osuch, J., Kurtz, M. E., and Kurtz, J. C. (1993). The influence of cancer patients' symptoms and functional states on patients' depression and family caregivers' reaction and depression. *Health Psychol.* 12, 277–285. doi: 10.1037/0278-6133.12.4.277

Gleason, M. E. J., Iida, M., Bolger, N., and Shrout, P. E. (2003). Daily supportive equity in close relationships. *Pers. Soc. Psychol. Bull.* 29, 1036–1045. doi: 10.1177/0146167203253473

Gottman, J. M. (1998). Psychology and the study of marital processes. *Annu. Rev. Psychol.* 49, 169–197. doi: 10.1146/annurev.psych.49.1.169

Gray, H. M., and Tickle-Degnen, L. (2010). A meta-analysis of performance on emotion recognition tasks in Parkinson's disease. *Neuropsychology* 24, 176–191. doi: 10.1037/a0018104

Haber, M. G., Cohen, J. L., Lucas, T., and Baltes, B. B. (2007). The relationship between self-reported received and perceived social support: a meta-analytic review. *Am. J. Commun. Psychol.* 39, 133–144. doi: 10.1007/s10464-007-9100-9

Heberlein, A. S., and Saxe, R. (2005). Dissociation between emotion and personality judgments: convergent evidence from functional neuroimaging. *Neuroimage* 28, 770–777. doi: 10.1016/j.neuroimage.2005.06.064

Henry, J. D., Ruffman, T., McDonald, S., Peek O'Leary, M.-A., Phillips, L. H., Brodaty, H., et al. (2008). Recognition of disgust is selectively preserved in Alzheimer's disease. *Neuropsychologia* 46, 1363–1370. doi: 10.1016/j.neuropsychologia.2007.12.012

Hibbard, J. H., and Pope, C. R. (1993). The quality of social roles as predictors of morbidity and mortality. *Soc. Sci. Med.* 36, 217–225. doi: 10.1016/0277-9536(93)90005-O

Hoehn, M. M., and Yahr, M. D. (1967). Parkinsonism: onset, progression, and mortality. *Neurology* 17, 427–442. doi: 10.1212/WNL.17.5.427

Holt-Lunstad, J., Birmingham, W., and Jones, B. Q. (2008). Is there something unique about marriage? The relative impact of marital status, relationship quality, and network social support on ambulatory blood pressure and mental health. *Ann. Behav. Med.* 35, 239–244. doi: 10.1007/s12160-008-9018-y

Hox, J. (2002). *Multilevel Analysis Techniques and Applications. Quantitative methodology series.* Mahwah, NJ: Lawrence Erlbaum Associates.

Isaacowitz, D. M., Lockenhoff, C. E., Lane, R. D., Wright, R., Sechrest, L., Riedel, R., et al. (2007). Age differences in recognition of emotion in lexical stimuli and facial expressions. *Psychol. Aging* 22, 147–159. doi: 10.1037/0882-7974.22.1.147

Kan, Y., Kawamura, M., Hasegawa, Y., Mochizuki, S., and Nakamura, K. (2002). Recognition of emotion from facial, prosodic and written verbal stimuli in Parkinson's disease. *Cortex* 38, 623–630. doi: 10.1016/S0010-9452(08)70026-1

Katsikitis, M., and Pilowsky, I. (1988). A study of facial expression in Parkinson's disease using a novel microcomputer-based method. *J. Neurol. Neurosurg. Psychiatry* 51, 362–366. doi: 10.1136/jnnp.51.3.362

Katsikitis, M., and Pilowsky, I. (1991). A controlled quantitative study of facial expression in Parkinson's disease and depression. *J. Nerv. Ment. Dis.* 179, 683–688. doi: 10.1097/00005053-199111000-00006

Kaul, M., and Lakey, B. (2003). Where is the support in perceived support? The role of generic relationship satisfaction and enacted support in perceived support's relation to low distress. *J. Soc. Clin. Psychol.* 22, 59–78. doi: 10.1521/jscp.22.1.59.22761

Keightley, M. L., Winocur, G., Burianova, H., Hongwanishkul, D., and Grady, C. L. (2006). Age effects on social cognition: faces tell a different story. *Psychol. Aging* 21, 558–572. doi: 10.1037/0882-7974.21.3.558

Keyes, C. L. M. (1998). Social well-being. *Soc. Psychol. Q.* 61, 121–140. doi: 10.2307/2787065

Kiecolt-Glaser, J. K., Fisher, L. D., Ogrocki, P., Stout, J. C., Speicher, C. E., and Glaser, R. (1987). Marital quality, marital disruption, and immune function. *Psychosom. Med.* 49, 13–34.

Kiecolt-Glaser, J. K., Malarkey, W. B., Chee, M., Newton, T., Cacioppo, J. T., Mao, H., et al. (1993). Negative behavior during marital conflict is associated with immunological down-regulation. *Psychosom. Med.* 55, 395–409.

Lakey, B., and Cassady, P. B. (1990). Cognitive processes in perceived social support. *J. Pers. Soc. Psychol.* 59, 337–343. doi: 10.1037/0022-3514.59.2.337

Lawrence, A. D., Goerendt, I. K., and Brooks, D. J. (2007). Impaired recognition of facial expressions of anger in Parkinson's disease patients acutely withdrawn from dopamine replacement therapy. *Neuropsychologia* 45, 65–74. doi: 10.1016/j.neuropsychologia.2006.04.016

Levenson, R. W., Carstensen, L. L., and Gottman, J. M. (1994). The influence of age and gender on affect, physiology, and their interrelations: a study of long-term marriages. *J. Pers. Soc. Psychol.* 67, 56–68. doi: 10.1037/0022-3514.67.1.56

Levenson, R. W., and Gottman, J. M. (1983). Marital interaction: physiological linkage and affective exchange. *J. Pers. Soc. Psychol.* 45, 587–597. doi: 10.1037/0022-3514.45.3.587

MacDowell, C. L., Harrison, D. W., and Demaree, H. A. (1994). Is right hemisphere decline in the perception of emotion a function of aging? *Int. J. Neurosci.* 79, 1–11.

MacPhee, G. J. A., and Stewart, D. A. (2007). Parkinson's disease. *Rev. Clin. Gerontol.* 16, 1–21. doi: 10.1017/S0959259806002073

MacPherson, S. E., Phillips, L. H., and Della Sala, S. (2002). Age, executive function, and social decision making: a dorsolateral prefrontal theory of cognitive aging. *Psychol. Aging* 17, 598–609. doi: 10.1037/0882-7974.17.4.598

MacPherson, S. E., Phillips, L. H., and Della Sala, S. (2007). Age related decline in the ability to perceive sad facial expressions. *Aging Clin. Exp. Res.* 18, 418–424. doi: 10.1007/BF03324838

Maisel, N. C., and Gable, S. L. (2009). The paradox of received social support. *Psychol. Sci.* 20, 928 –932. doi: 10.1111/j.1467-9280.2009.02388.x

Malatesta, C. Z., Izard, C. E., and Culver, C. (1987). Emotion communication skills in young, middle-aged, and older women. *Psychol. Aging* 2, 193–202. doi: 10.1037/0882-7974.2.2.193

Marsh, L. (2000). Neuropsychiatric aspects of Parkinson's disease. *Psychosomatics* 41, 15–23. doi: 10.1016/S0033-3182(00)71169-8

Mather, M., and Carstensen, L. L. (2005). Aging and motivated cognition: the positivity effect in attention and memory. *Trends Cogn. Sci.* 9, 496–502. doi: 10.1016/j.tics.2005.08.005

Miller, G. E., Dopp, J. M., Myers, H. F., Stevens, S. Y., and Fahey, J. L. (1999). Psychosocial predictors of natural killer cell mobilization during marital conflict. *Health Psychol.* 18, 262–271. doi: 10.1037/0278-6133.18.3.262

Monin, J., Martire, L., Schulz, R., and Clark, M. (2009). Willingness to express emotions to caregiving spouses. *Emotion* 9, 101–106. doi: 10.1037/a0013732

Monin, J. K., and Schulz, R. (2009). Interpersonal effects of suffering in older adult caregiving relationships. *Psychol. Aging* 24, 681–695. doi: 10.1037/a0016355

Montepare, J., Koff, E., Zaitchik, D., and Albert, M. (1999). The use of body movements and gestures as cues to emotions in younger and older adults. *J. Nonverb. Behav.* 23, 133–152. doi: 10.1023/A:1021435526134

Morell, M. A., and Apple, R. F. (1990). Affect expression, marital satisfaction, and stress reactivity among premenopausal women during a conflictual marital discussion. *Psychol. Women Quart.* 14, 387–402. doi: 10.1111/j.1471-6402.1990.tb00027.x

Moreno, C., Borod, J., Welkowitz, J., and Alpert, M. (1993). The perception of facial emotion across the adult life span. *Dev. Neuropsychol.* 9, 305–319. doi: 10.1080/87565649309540559

Newton, T. L., and Sanford, J. M. (2003). Conflict structure moderates associations between cardiovascular reactivity and negative marital interactions. *Health Psychol.* 22, 270–278. doi: 10.1037/0278-6133.22.3.270

Niedenthal, P. M., and Brauer, M. (2012). Social functionality of human emotion. *Annu. Rev. Psychol.* 63, 259–285. doi: 10.1146/annurev.psych.121208.131605

Northouse, L., Templin, T., and Mood, D. (2001). Couples' adjustment to breast disease during the first year following diagnosis. *J. Behav. Med.* 24, 115–136. doi: 10.1023/A:1010772913717

Orgeta, V., and Phillips, L. H. (2008). Effects of age and emotional intensity on the recognition of facial emotion. *Exp. Aging Res.* 34, 63–79. doi: 10.1080/03610730701762047

Orth-Gomer, K., Wamala, S. P., Horsten, M., Schenck-Gustafsson, K., Schneiderman, N., and Mittleman, M. A. (2000). Marital stress worsens prognosis in women with coronary heart disease: the stockholm female coronary risk study. *JAMA* 284, 3008–3014. doi: 10.1001/jama.284.23.3008

Pakenham, K. I. (2001). Application of a stress and coping model to caregiving in multiple sclerosis. *Psychol. Health Med.* 6, 13–27. doi: 10.1080/13548500125141

Pell, M. D., and Leonard, C. L. (2003). Processing emotional tone from speech in Parkinson's disease: a role for the basal ganglia. *Cogn. Affect. Behav. Neurosci.* 3, 275–288. doi: 10.3758/CABN.3.4.275

Pentland, B., Gray, J. M., Riddle, W. J. R., and Pitcairn, T. K. (1988). The effects of reduced non-verbal communication in Parkinson's disease. *Br. J. Disord. Commun.* 23, 31–34. doi: 10.3109/13682828809019874

Pentland, B., Pitcairn, T. K., Gray, J. M., and Riddle, W. J. R. (1987). The effects of reduced expression in Parkinson's disease on impression formation by health professionals. *Clin. Rehabil.* 1, 307–313. doi: 10.1177/026921558700100410

Peto, V., Jenkinson, C., Fitzpatrick, R., and Greenhall, R. (1995). The development and validation of a short measure of functioning and well being for individuals with Parkinson's disease. *Qual. Life Res.* 4, 241–248. doi: 10.1007/BF02260863

Phillips, L. H., Bull, R., Allen, R., Insch, P., Burr, K., and Ogg, W. (2011). Lifespan aging and belief reasoning: influences of executive function and social cue decoding. *Cognition* 120, 236–247. doi: 10.1016/j.cognition.2011.05.003

Phillips, L. H., MacLean, R. D. J., and Allen, R. (2002). Age and the understanding of emotions: neuropsychological and sociocognitive perspectives. *J. Gerontol. B Psychol. Sci. Soc. Sci.* 57, P526–P530. doi: 10.1093/geronb/57.6.P526

Pillon, B., Dubois, B., and Agid, Y. (1996). Testing cognition may contribute to the diagnosis of movement disorders. *Neurology* 46, 324–334. doi: 10.1212/WNL.46.2.329

Pitcairn, T. K., Clemie, S., Gray, J. M., and Pentland, B. (1990). Nonverbal cues in the self-presentation of Parkinsonian patients. *Br. J. Clin. Psychology* 29, 177–184. doi: 10.1111/j.2044-8260.1990.tb00867.x

Poulin, M. J., Brown, S. L., Ubel, P. A., Smith, D. M., Jankovic, A., and Langa, K. M. (2010). Does a helping hand mean a heavy heart? Helping behavior and well-being among spouse caregivers. *Psychol. Aging* 25, 108–117. doi: 10.1037/a0018064

Raudenbush, S., Bryk, A., and Congdon, R. (2013). *HLM 7.01 for Windows [Hierarchical Linear and Nonlinear Modeling Software]*. Lincolnwood, IL: Multivariate Software, Inc.

Revenson, T. A., and Majerovitz, S. D. (1990). Spouses' support provision to chronically ill patients. *J. Soc. Pers. Relat.* 7, 575–586. doi: 10.1177/0265407590074013

Rohrbaugh, M. J., Shoham, V., and Coyne, J. C. (2006). Effect of marital quality on eight-year survival of patients with heart failure. *Am. J. Cardiol.* 98, 1069–1072. doi: 10.1016/j.amjcard.2006.05.034

Ruffman, T., Henry, J. D., Livingstone, V., and Phillips, L. H. (2008). A meta-analytic review of emotion recognition and aging: implications for neuropsychological models of aging. *Neurosci. Biobehav. Rev.* 32, 863–881. doi: 10.1016/j.neubiorev.2008.01.001

Ruffman, T., Sullivan, S., and Dittrich, W. (2009). Older adults' recognition of bodily and auditory expressions of emotion. *Psychol. Aging* 24, 614–622. doi: 10.1037/a0016356

Ryff, C. D. (1995). Psychological well-being in adult life. *Curr. Direct. Psychol. Sci.* 4, 99–103. doi: 10.1111/1467-8721.ep10772395

Sarason, B. R., Sarason, I. G., and Gurung, R. A. R. (1997). *Close Personal Relationships and Health Outcomes: A Key to The Role of Social Support.* Hoboken, NJ: Wiley.

Saxbe, D., Repetti, R. L., and Nishina, A. (2008). Marital satisfaction, recovery from work, and diurnal cortisol among men and women. *Health Psychol.* 27, 15–25. doi: 10.1037/0278-6133.27.1.15

Schimmack, U., and Lucas, R. E. (2010). Environmental influences on well-being: a dyadic latent panel analysis of spousal similarity. *Soc. Indic. Res.* 98, 1–21. doi: 10.1007/s11205-009-9516-8

Schulz, R., Beach, S. R., Hebert, R. S., Martire, L. M., Monin, J. K., Thompkins, C. A., et al. (2009). Spousal suffering and partner depression and cardiovascular disease: the cardiovascular health study. *Am. J. Geriatr. Psychiatry* 17, 246–254. doi: 10.1097/JGP.0b013e318198775b

Shrout, P. E., Herman, C. M., and Bolger, N. (2006). The costs and benefits of practical and emotional support on adjustment: a daily diary study of couples experiencing acute stress. *Pers. Relat.* 13, 115–134. doi: 10.1111/j.1475-6811.2006.00108.x

Simons, G., Pasqualini, M. C. S., Reddy, V., and Wood, J. (2004). Emotional and nonemotional facial expressions in people with Parkinson's disease. *J. Int. Neuropsychol. Soc.* 10, 521–535. doi: 10.1017/S135561770410413X

Smith, M. C., Smith, M. K., and Ellgring, H. (1996). Spontaneous and posed facial expression in Parkinson's disease. *J. Int. Neuropsychol. Soc.* 2, 383–391. doi: 10.1017/S1355617700001454

Smith, T. W., and Brown, P. C. (1991). Cynical hostility, attempts to exert social control, and cardiovascular reactivity in married couples. *J. Behav. Med.* 14, 581–592. doi: 10.1007/BF00867172

Sprengelmeyer, R., Young, A. W., Mahn, K., Schroeder, U., Woitalla, D., Büttner, T., et al. (2003). Facial expression recognition in people with medicated and unmedicated Parkinson's disease. *Neuropsychologia* 41, 1047–1057. doi: 10.1016/S0028-3932(02)00295-6

Sullivan, S., and Ruffman, T. (2004a). Emotion recognition deficits in the elderly. *Int. J. Neurosci.* 114, 403–432. doi: 10.1080/00207450490270901

Sullivan, S., and Ruffman, T. (2004b). Social understanding: how does it fare with advancing years? *Br. J. Psychol.* 95, 1–18. doi: 10.1348/000712604322779424

Sullivan, S., Ruffman, T., and Hutton, S. (2007). Age differences in emotion recognition skills and the visual scanning of emotion faces. *J. Gerontol. B Psychol. Sci. Soc. Sci.* 62, P53–P60. doi: 10.1093/geronb/62.1.P53

Suzuki, A., Hoshino, T., and Shigemasu, K. (2007). Decline or improvement? Age-related differences in facial expression recognition. *Biol. Psychol.* 74, 75–84. doi: 10.1016/j.biopsycho.2006.07.003

Suzuki, A., Hoshino, T., Shigemasu, K., and Kawamura, M. (2006). Disgust-specific impairment of facial expression recognition in Parkinson's disease. *Brain J. Neurol.* 129, 707–717. doi: 10.1093/brain/awl011

Uchino, B. N., Cacioppo, J. T., and Kiecolt-Glaser, J. K. (1996). The relationship between social support and physiological processes: a review with emphasis on underlying mechanisms and implications for health. *Psychol. Bull.* 119, 488–531. doi: 10.1037/0033-2909.119.3.488

Wang, H. X., Leineweber, C., Kirkeeide, R., Svane, B., Schenck-Gustafsson, K., Theorell, T., et al. (2007). Psychosocial stress and atherosclerosis: family and work stress accelerate progression of coronary disease in women. The stockholm female coronary angiography study. *J. Int. Med.* 261, 245–254. doi: 10.1111/j.1365-2796.2006.01759.x

Whisman, M. A. (2001). "The association between depression and marital dissatisfaction," in *Marital and Family Processes in Depression: A Scientific Foundation for Clinical Practice*, ed S. R. H. Beach (Washington, DC: American Psychological Association), 3–24. doi: 10.1037/10350-001

Whisman, M. A., Uebelacker, L. A., and Settles, T. D. (2010). Marital distress and the metabolic syndrome: linking social functioning with physical health. *J. Family Psychol.* 24, 367–370. doi: 10.1037/a0019547

Wong, B., Cronin-Golomb, A., and Neargarder, S. (2005). Patterns of visual scanning as predictors of emotion identification in normal aging. *Neuropsychology* 19, 739–749. doi: 10.1037/0894-4105.19.6.739

Yip, J. T., Lee, T. M., Ho, S. L., Tsang, K. L., and Li, L. S. (2003). Emotion recognition in patients with idiopathic Parkinson's disease. *Mov. Disord.* 18, 1115–1122. doi: 10.1002/mds.10497

6

# Emotional experience in the mornings and the evenings: consideration of age differences in specific emotions by time of day

***Tammy English[1]* and Laura L. Carstensen[2]***

[1] *Department of Psychology, Washington University in St. Louis, St. Louis, MO, USA*
[2] *Department of Psychology, Stanford University, Stanford, CA, USA*

***Edited by:***
*Natalie Ebner, University of Florida, USA*

***Reviewed by:***
*Hakan Fischer, Stockholm University, Sweden*
*Didem Pehlivanoglu, Georgia Institute of Technology, USA*
*Jennifer Tehan Stanley, University of Akron, USA*

****Correspondence:***
*Tammy English, Department of Psychology, Washington University in St. Louis, Campus Box 1125, One Brookings Drive, St. Louis, MO 63130-4899, USA*
*e-mail: tenglish@ wustl.edu*

Considerable evidence points to age-related improvements in emotional well-being with age. In order to gain a more nuanced understanding of the nature of these apparent shifts in experience, we examined age differences in a range of emotional states in the mornings and evenings in a sample of 135 community-residing participants across 10 consecutive days. Participants ranged in age from 22 to 93 years. Each participant completed a diary in the morning and again in the evening every day for the study period. During each of the assessments, participants reported the degree to which they experienced emotions sampled from all four quadrants of the affective circumplex. Overall, participants felt less positive and more negative in the evenings than in the mornings. As expected, older adults reported a relatively more positive emotional experience than younger adults at both times of day. Importantly, however, age effects varied based on emotion type and time of day. Older adults reported experiencing more positive emotion than relatively younger adults across a range of different positive states (although age differences emerged most consistently for low arousal positive states). Age-related reductions in negative experience were observed only for reports of low arousal negative emotions. There were no age differences in anger, anxiety, or sadness. For some emotions, age differences were stronger in the mornings (e.g., relaxed) whereas for other emotions age differences were more pronounced in the evenings (e.g., enthusiastic). Findings are discussed in the context of adulthood changes in motivation and emotional experience.

**Keywords: affect, emotional experience, discrete emotions, aging, circumplex model**

## INRODUCTION

Emotional well-being appears to improve with age (see reviews by Consedine and Magai, 2006; Scheibe and Carstensen, 2010; Charles and Carstensen, 2013) and, importantly, age differences do not appear to be due to cohort effects since longitudinal evidence also points to improvements in emotional experience within individuals as they grow older (Charles et al., 2001; Carstensen et al., 2011). In order to gain a more nuanced understanding of age-differences in everyday life, in the present study we examined whether age differences in emotional experience are apparent across a range of emotions and at different points in the day.

One of the first reports of age-related improvements in emotional functioning was published by Mroczek and Kolarz (1998). Based on a cross-sectional comparison in a large representative sample of Americans, they observed that age was associated with more reported positive experience and less negative experience. Many replications of overall improvements in emotional experience have followed, although findings have been less consistent concerning the emotional changes that drive improvements in emotional well-being. Some studies find that age differences are driven by reductions in negative emotional experience (e.g., Carstensen et al., 2000) whereas others observe the differences to be due to increases in positive emotional experience (e.g., Riediger et al., 2009). In a very large scale cross-sectional study based on yesterday interviews [1], Stone et al. (2010) observed a peak in happiness in early old age, followed by relative constancy into more advanced ages, while negative emotions showed linear declines. A handful of large-scale studies have found small age-related increases in depressive symptoms (Fiske et al., 2003; Davey et al., 2004) and negative emotional experiences (Diener and Suh, 1998); however, studies that have controlled for physical health typically eliminate these effects suggesting that illness more than age is responsible for such findings (Gatz et al., 1996; Kunzmann et al., 2000; although see Fiske et al., 2003).

One explanation for differences in the published literature reflects the fact that researchers use a wide range of measures and procedures, which tap different aspects of emotional experience. While the variety in approaches adds support for the contention that emotional well-being improves with age, the same variability may account for discrepancies across studies in patterns of findings. Global measures, for example, tap deliberative evaluations

[1] Yesterday interviews asked respondents "Did you experience [emotions] a lot yesterday?"

of life more than emotional experience *per se*. Experience sampling, in contrast, typically considered the gold standard in the measurement of emotion in daily life, does an excellent job of characterizing daily life yet often misses low base rate emotions like surprise and anger. Thus, though experience sampling characterizes the emotional tone of daily life very well (most people are not routinely surprised, for example), it can downplay the role of short-lived but powerful emotional experiences. These types of low frequency emotional states might be better detected by global assessments or daily diary studies that ask individuals to reflect on specific experiences across an entire day. Memory based measures, such as, yesterday interviews, are susceptible to motivated reconstructions and can be influenced differentially by motivated processes (e.g., positivity effect, Mather and Carstensen, 2005; Reed and Carstensen, 2012).

The measures researchers adopt also vary in the degree to which they tap high and low arousal. Affective states have been found to vary along two independent dimensions: valence and arousal (Watson and Tellegen, 1985; Larsen and Diener, 1992). Excitement, for example, is both positive and arousing whereas contentment is positive and low in arousal. Traditionally, widely used measures of experience developed for use with young populations have focused mostly on high arousal emotional states, especially in regard to positive emotion (e.g., excitement, enthusiasm), creating an inadvertent conflation of arousal and valence.

These measurement issues are particularly troublesome because increasingly findings point to arousal as a key aspect of emotional development. Powell Lawton et al. (1992) observed many years ago that older adults are less likely to report high arousal or surgent emotions. Consistent with this observation, Kessler and Staudinger (2009) recently reported findings from a study comparing younger and older adults where age differences were observed when emotional composites were broken down by valence and arousal. Specifically, older adults only reported more low arousal positive states (e.g., relaxed), whereas they reported less negative emotion regardless of valence. In an experience sampling study, Scheibe et al. (2013) also observed age-related increases in the daily experience of low arousal positive emotion but no age differences for high arousal positive states.

One potential explanation for these findings comes from the strengths and vulnerabilities integration model (SAVI; Charles, 2010), which suggests that older adults avoid situations that elicit high arousal states because they are less able to recover from disruptions of physiological homeostasis. Therefore, as individuals age they may come to focus their emotional goals more on activities that engender low positive arousal states (e.g., calm) and avoid high arousal states, regardless of valence. Indeed, Scheibe et al. (2013), noted above, found that older adults reported a greater preference for low arousal positive emotions relative to high arousal positive emotions than younger adults. In addition, age-related decreases in negative emotions have been found consistently for high arousal negative states (e.g., anger, rage, despair; Lawton et al., 1992; Schieman, 1999; Phillips et al., 2008; Ross and Mirowsky, 2008; Stone et al., 2010), but it is less clear whether there are similar declines in the experience of low arousal negative states such as sadness. Thus, in order to better understand how emotional experience changes with age, it will be necessary to decompose emotion composites into more fine grained emotional states. Based on the extant literature, emotional benefits associated with age seem to come primarily in the form of increased experience of low arousal positive affective states coupled with a decrease in negative emotions, particularly those that are arousing (e.g., anger; Stone et al., 2010).

Another potential source of inconsistency in the literature on age differences in emotion is time of day. Studies have typically focused on either global reports of emotional experience (typically or on a given day) or momentary emotional experience averaged across various time points (in a day or a series of days). It is conceivable that age differences are stronger in the mornings than evening. Prior research suggests that cognitive performance varies by time of day, such that older adults perform better early in the day whereas younger adults perform better later in the day (Yoon et al., 1999; Knight and Mather, 2013). Emotion regulation, like many goal-directed processes, often demands cognitive resources (Muraven et al., 1998; Ochsner et al., 2012), so if emotion regulation plays a role in older adults relatively more positive emotional experience, then time of day may influence age differences in emotional experience as well. That is, it is conceivable that widely documented emotional advantages of older adults are strongest in the mornings. To our knowledge, however, although older people are more likely to describe themselves as "morning types" than younger adults (Biss and Hasher, 2012), age differences in emotion per se have not been examined as a function of time of day.

In order to gain a clearer picture of age differences in emotional life, we examined a range of specific emotions representing all four quadrants in the affective circumplex, in the mornings and in the evenings across a 10-day period. We hypothesized that older adults would show a more positive affective profile overall and, based on prior research, that older adults would report relatively more low arousal positive emotion and less high arousal negative emotion. We also hypothesized that age differences in emotional experience would be more pronounced in the mornings, consistent with prior research on cognitive performance. In addition, we examined two potential sources of differential age differences in morning versus evening emotional experience: sleep and individual differences in morningness. Older adults may report relatively more positive emotional experience in the morning because they are more likely to be "morning types" or have different sleep patterns than younger adults.

## METHODS

### PARTICIPANTS

The sample consisted of 135 participants (50% female) ranging in age from 22 to 93 years ($M = 53.87$, $SD = 19.23$). Participants were roughly evenly distributed across this age range. Sixty-seven percent of the participants were European American, 30% were African American, and 3% identified with multiple ethnicities. Socioeconomic status (SES) was determined by a survey research firm based on answers to questions about income, education and occupation. Thirty-two percent of participants were blue-collar workers, 64% were white-collar workers, and 4% were pink-collar workers. Gender, ethnicity, and SES were stratified across age.

## PROCEDURE

After providing informed consent, participants completed a number of measures, including assessments of health, cognition, and morningness. The experimenter then explained the format and schedule of the daily diaries. For 10 consecutive days, participants completed an online diary in the morning and again in the evening. Participants were asked to complete the diaries as soon as they woke up and just before bedtime in the evening. Emotional experience was assessed at both time points (morning and evening) each day; sleep the previous night was assessed only in the morning. Reminder emails were sent each day around the time participants would be completing the diaries. Participants accessed the online diaries by logging into a secure website where they were presented with a series of questions. Prior to recruitment, this study was approved by the Institutional Review Board (IRB) at Stanford University.

## MATERIALS

### Daily emotional experience

In each of the morning and evening diaries, participants rated on a 7-point scale that ranged from *not at all* to *extremely* the degree to which they were currently feeling each of 14 emotions. The list of emotions included terms commonly used in emotion research and covered each quadrant of the affective circumplex. Specifically, there were 7 positive emotions, including happiness (a prototypical pleasant emotion), 3 high arousal states (enthusiastic, excited, proud), and 3 low arousal states (calm, content, relaxed), as well as 7 negative emotions, including sadness (a prototypical unpleasant emotion), 2 high arousal states (angry and anxious/worried), 2 low arousal states (bored and fatigued), and 2 other states of particular interest in old age (lonely and regretful). These emotion terms were presented together on one screen in a randomized order at each assessment point.

### Daily sleep

At each morning assessment, participants rated the quality of their sleep the previous night (1 = *very bad* to 7 = *very good*) and indicated their subjective sleep quantity by rating how much they slept the previous night (1 = *not at all* to 5 = *a lot*). They also listed the number of hours they slept the previous night.

### Physical health

Participants completed a comprehensive health questionnaire (Hultsch et al., 1993) that assessed multiple facets of physical health, including self-rated overall health ($M = 3.15, SD = 1.22$), illness episodes ($M = 2.41$, $SD = 1.82$), instrumental health ($M = 1.28$, $SD = 2.63$), chronic illnesses (weighted by severity rating, $M = 1.92, SD = 2.15$), and number of medications ($M = 1.51$, $SD = 1.54$). An index of physical health was computed by averaging scores across these five dimensions (alpha = 0.70). Higher scores indicate poorer physical health.

### Verbal fluency

To assess verbal fluency, participants were asked to verbally list as many animals as possible in 90 s. This is a widely used measure that has been shown to be strongly associated with general intellectual ability (Lindenberger et al., 1993).

### Morningness

Individual differences in morningness were assessed using the 5-item brief Morningness-Eveningness Questionnaire (MEQ; Adan and Almirall, 1991). This scale is well-validated and has been extensively used in younger and older adults samples. An example item is, "At what time of the day do you think that you reach your "feeling best" peak?" To determine overall ratings of morningness-eveningness, each question is given a scaled score and then these scores are summed. Higher scores indicate greater morningness.

## RESULTS

## DATA REDUCTION AND ANALYTIC APPROACH

### Emotion indices

The data we report represent the intensity of emotion reports[2]. In addition to examining specific emotions, we computed composites to represent the degree to which participants reported positive and negative emotional experience on each occasion. The positive emotion composite was created by averaging momentary ratings across calm, content, enthusiastic, excited, happy, proud, and relaxed (alpha= 0.89). The negative emotion composite was created by averaging momentary ratings across angry, anxious/worried, bored, fatigued, sad, regretful, and lonely (alpha= 0.83). Descriptive statistics for these emotion composites and the specific emotions appear in **Table 1**.

### Analytic approach

To examine age differences in daily emotion, we conducted multilevel modeling using the linear MIXED MODELS function in SPSS. We tested a three-level model, in which time of day (AM or PM) was nested within days and days were nested within persons. Maximum likelihood (ML) estimation was used to account for missing data. Age effects were tested with linear and quadratic age terms. Time of day (morning = 0, evening = 1) and its interaction with each of the age components were also included as predictors. Age was correlated with poorer physical health ($r = 0.25$, $p < 0.05$) and lower verbal fluency ($r = -0.20$, $p < 0.05$), so health and fluency were included in the models as time invariant covariates. Results are reported as unstandardized MLM coefficients in **Table 2**.

To better understand potential interactions between time of day and age, we also fit a model with random intercept, linear age, and quadratic age components separately for morning and evening emotion (controlling for physical health and verbal fluency). Results are reported as unstandardized MLM coefficients in **Table 3**.

---

[2]In our prior experience sampling work we report frequencies based on endorsements greater than 1 for specific emotions (Carstensen et al., 2000, 2011). A relatively similar pattern of findings emerged when using this frequency index rather than the intensity based one we focus on here. The most notable difference was fewer interactions between Age and Time of Day (the only one that remained significant was for enthusiasm). In addition, there were no longer Time of Day effects for pride, sadness, and anxiety, but all the other Time of Day effects remained significant and a new one emerged, namely contentment was reported more often in the morning than in the evening ($\gamma = -0.0125$, $p < 0.05$). Importantly, all the age effects remained significant except for happiness ($p = 0.16$).

**Table 1 | Descriptive statistics for emotional experience in the morning and the evening.**

| | Intensity of experience | | | | Frequency of experience | | | |
|---|---|---|---|---|---|---|---|---|
| | Mean | *SD* | Min. | Max. | Mean | *SD* | Min. | Max. |
| **AM POSITIVE** | **4.36** | **0.94** | **1.74** | **6.77** | **0.94** | **0.10** | **0.46** | **1.00** |
| Happy | 4.74 | 1.13 | 1.33 | 7.00 | 0.97 | 0.11 | 0.22 | 1.00 |
| Content | 4.88 | 1.08 | 1.50 | 7.00 | 0.98 | 0.08 | 0.30 | 1.00 |
| Calm | 4.88 | 1.01 | 2.10 | 7.00 | 0.98 | 0.06 | 0.60 | 1.00 |
| Relaxed | 4.71 | 1.09 | 2.07 | 7.00 | 0.98 | 0.05 | 0.71 | 1.00 |
| Enthusiastic | 3.98 | 1.29 | 1.00 | 7.00 | 0.92 | 0.19 | 0.00 | 1.00 |
| Excited | 3.56 | 1.26 | 1.00 | 6.80 | 0.87 | 0.23 | 0.00 | 1.00 |
| Proud | 3.79 | 1.52 | 1.00 | 7.00 | 0.87 | 0.25 | 0.00 | 1.00 |
| **AM NEGATIVE** | **1.76** | **0.63** | **1.00** | **3.99** | **0.35** | **0.27** | **0.00** | **1.00** |
| Sad | 1.48 | 0.66 | 1.00 | 4.10 | 0.26 | 0.32 | 0.00 | 1.00 |
| Bored | 1.46 | 0.67 | 1.00 | 3.70 | 0.25 | 0.32 | 0.00 | 1.00 |
| Fatigued | 2.47 | 1.16 | 1.00 | 6.10 | 0.61 | 0.37 | 0.00 | 1.00 |
| Anxious | 2.37 | 1.16 | 1.00 | 5.60 | 0.57 | 0.37 | 0.00 | 1.00 |
| Angry | 1.32 | 0.54 | 1.00 | 4.00 | 0.17 | 0.27 | 0.00 | 1.00 |
| Lonely | 1.59 | 0.78 | 1.00 | 4.90 | 0.31 | 0.34 | 0.00 | 1.00 |
| Regretful | 1.62 | 0.98 | 1.00 | 5.30 | 0.29 | 0.37 | 0.00 | 1.00 |
| **PM POSITIVE** | **4.30** | **0.92** | **2.06** | **6.57** | **0.93** | **0.11** | **0.49** | **1.00** |
| Happy | 4.84 | 1.10 | 1.60 | 6.90 | 0.98 | 0.07 | 0.44 | 1.00 |
| Content | 4.90 | 1.06 | 1.30 | 7.00 | 0.98 | 0.08 | 0.30 | 1.00 |
| Calm | 4.86 | 1.04 | 2.22 | 7.00 | 0.98 | 0.07 | 0.60 | 1.00 |
| Relaxed | 4.74 | 1.04 | 1.78 | 7.00 | 0.98 | 0.06 | 0.56 | 1.00 |
| Enthusiastic | 3.57 | 1.31 | 1.00 | 6.60 | 0.88 | 0.22 | 0.00 | 1.00 |
| Excited | 3.24 | 1.22 | 1.00 | 6.40 | 0.83 | 0.26 | 0.00 | 1.00 |
| Proud | 3.93 | 1.47 | 1.00 | 7.00 | 0.89 | 0.23 | 0.00 | 1.00 |
| **PM NEGATIVE** | **1.89** | **0.68** | **1.00** | **4.04** | **0.38** | **0.26** | **0.00** | **1.00** |
| Sad | 1.56 | 0.81 | 1.00 | 5.36 | 0.27 | 0.33 | 0.00 | 1.00 |
| Bored | 1.58 | 0.81 | 1.00 | 4.20 | 0.30 | 0.35 | 0.00 | 1.00 |
| Fatigued | 3.23 | 1.39 | 1.00 | 6.60 | 0.76 | 0.32 | 0.00 | 1.00 |
| Anxious | 2.17 | 1.08 | 1.00 | 6.00 | 0.53 | 0.37 | 0.00 | 1.00 |
| Angry | 1.41 | 0.61 | 1.00 | 3.71 | 0.20 | 0.28 | 0.00 | 1.00 |
| Lonely | 1.69 | 1.05 | 1.00 | 5.40 | 0.30 | 0.38 | 0.00 | 1.00 |
| Regretful | 1.60 | 0.82 | 1.00 | 4.70 | 0.30 | 0.35 | 0.00 | 1.00 |

*AM indicates the morning assessment and PM indicates the evening assessment. Intensity of experience represents average emotion ratings across the 10-day sampling period. Frequency of emotion represents the percent of occasions that participants reported experiencing an emotion to any degree (i.e., greater than the 1 on the rating scale) across the 10-day sampling period.*

In preliminary analyses, we tested for effects of gender, SES and ethnicity on positive and negative emotion. There were no main effects of these demographic variables in predicting emotional experience, nor did they moderate the effects of age on emotion. However, there were gender differences in the effects of Time of Day for both positive emotion (Gender × Time of Day = $-0.1674$, $p < 0.05$) and negative emotion (Gender × Time of Day = 0.1899, $p < 0.01$). Compared to the morning, women reported feeling less positive emotion ($\gamma = -0.2196$, $p < 0.01$) and more negative emotion in the evening ($\gamma = 0.2220$, $p < 0.01$); however, there were no Time of Day effects for men (positive emotion: $\gamma = -0.0521$, $p = 0.24$; negative emotion: $\gamma = 0.0321$, $p = 0.35$). In addition, for negative emotion, the interaction between age and time of day varied based on gender (Gender × $Age^2$ × Time of Day: $\gamma = -0.0004$, $p < 0.05$; $Age^2$ × Time of Day for men: $\gamma = 0.0002$, $p < 0.01$; $Age^2$ × Time of Day for women: $\gamma = -0.0002$, $p < 0.05$), as well as based on SES (SES × Age × Time of Day: $\gamma = -0.0056$, $p < 0.01$) and ethnicity (Ethnicity × Age × Time of Day: $\gamma = 0.0058$, $p < 0.01$). Age moderated the effect of Time of Day on negative emotion among African-Americans ($\gamma = -0.0045$, $p < 0.05$) and blue collar workers ($\gamma = -0.0047$, $p < 0.01$), but not among European-Americans ($\gamma = 0.0002$, $p = 0.86$) and white collar workers ($\gamma = 0.0009$, $p = 0.39$); specifically, the tendency for participants to feel more negative emotion in the evening than in the morning was attenuated among older African-Americans and older blue-collar workers.

## AGE EFFECTS

Age was linearly associated with more overall positive emotion ($\gamma = 0.0141, p < 0.01$) and less negative emotion ($\gamma = -0.0061$,

**Table 2 | Results of multilevel analyses testing the effects of age and time of day on daily emotion.**

| Fixed effects estimates | Intercept | Age | Age$^2$ | Time of Day | Time × Age | Time × Age$^2$ | Health | Fluency |
|---|---|---|---|---|---|---|---|---|
| **POSITIVE** | | | | | | | | |
| Happy | 4.7056 (0.1309) | 0.0140 (0.0048)** | 0.0000 (0.0003) | −0.0063 (0.0496) | −0.0005 (0.0018) | 0.0003 (0.0000)** | −0.5137 (0.1347)** | −0.1205 (0.0886) |
| Content | 4.8204 (0.1281) | 0.0153 (0.0047)** | 0.0002 (0.0003) | −0.0716 (0.0525) | −0.0027 (0.0019) | 0.0002 (0.0001)* | −0.4009 (0.1315)** | 0.0078 (0.0865) |
| Calm | 4.9099 (0.1225) | 0.0151 (0.0045)** | 0.0000 (0.0002) | −0.0903 (0.0575) | −0.0023 (0.0020) | 0.0002 (0.0001)$^+$ | −0.3326 (0.1248)** | 0.0381 (0.0821) |
| Relaxed | 4.8582 (0.1267) | 0.0205 (0.0047)** | −0.0004 (0.0003) | −0.0944 (0.0591) | −0.0086 (0.0021)** | 0.0004 (0.0001)** | −0.3029 (0.1291)* | 0.0262 (0.0850) |
| Enthusiastic | 4.0590 (0.1472) | 0.0225 (0.0054)** | −0.0002 (0.0003) | −0.5139 (0.0576)** | 0.0050 (0.0020)* | 0.0003 (0.0001)* | −0.4827 (0.1513)** | −0.0713 (0.0995) |
| Excited | 3.5770 (0.1492) | 0.0048 (0.0055) | 0.0000 (0.0003) | −0.3560 (0.0587)** | 0.0040 (0.0021)$^+$ | 0.0000 (0.0001) | −0.4265 (0.1534)** | −0.1834 (0.1009)$^+$ |
| Proud | 3.9011 (0.1827) | 0.0062 (0.0067) | −0.0003 (0.0004) | 0.1625 (0.0410)** | −0.0044 (0.0018)* | 0.0000 (0.0001) | −0.2324 (0.1897) | −0.3412 (0.1248)* |
| **NEGATIVE** | | | | | | | | |
| Sad | 1.5833 (0.0912) | −0.0022 (0.0034) | −0.0003 (0.0002) | 0.1346 (0.0423)** | −0.0027 (0.0015)$^+$ | −0.0002 (0.0000)$^+$ | 0.0761 (0.0930) | 0.0432 (0.0612) |
| Bored | 1.4836 (0.0919) | −0.0068 (0.0034)* | 0.0000 (0.0002) | 0.1050 (0.0390)** | −0.0021 (0.0014) | 0.0000 (0.0000) | 0.0268 (0.0941) | −0.0327 (0.0619) |
| Fatigued | 2.4868 (0.1453) | −0.0145 (0.0053)** | 0.0000 (0.0003) | 0.6548 (0.0705)** | −0.0006 (0.0025) | 0.0003 (0.0001)* | 0.5508 (0.1478)** | 0.1630 (0.0972)$^+$ |
| Anxious | 2.3964 (0.1396) | −0.0065 (0.0051) | 0.0000 (0.0003) | −0.1869 (0.0573)** | 0.0017 (0.0020) | 0.0000 (0.0001) | 0.0250 (0.1432) | −0.0698 (0.0942) |
| Angry | 1.3914 (0.0703) | −0.0047 (0.0026)$^+$ | −0.0002 (0.0001) | 0.1341 (0.0420)** | −0.0015 (0.0015) | −0.0001 (0.0000) | 0.1044 (0.0703) | −0.0590 (0.0463) |
| Lonely | 1.6722 (0.1276) | −0.0029 (0.0047) | −0.0001 (0.0003) | 0.0540 (0.0427) | −0.0011 (0.0015) | 0.0000 (0.0000) | 0.0802 (0.1319) | −0.0626 (0.0868) |
| Regretful | 1.7191 (0.1002) | −0.0052 (0.0037) | −0.0004 (0.0002)$^+$ | 0.0021 (0.0431) | −0.0005 (0.0015) | 0.0000 (0.0000) | 0.1490 (0.1026) | −0.0062 (0.0675) |

*Unstandardized estimates are presented with standard errors in parentheses. Age is centered at age 54 years; Time of day coded 0 for morning, and 1 for evening; Physical health and verbal fluency Z-scored.*

*$^+p < 0.10$; $^*p < 0.05$; $^{**}p < 0.01$.*

$p < 0.05$). In terms of positive specific emotions, older adults reported feeling more happy ($\gamma = 0.0140, p < 0.01$) and more of each of the low arousal positive emotions, including content ($\gamma = 0.0153, p < 0.01$), calm ($\gamma = 0.0151, p < 0.01$), and relaxed ($\gamma = 0.0205, p < 0.01$). In addition, there was an age-related increase in enthusiasm ($\gamma = 0.0225, p < 0.01$), but there were not significant age differences for the two other higher arousal positive emotions (excitement: $\gamma = 0.0048, p = 0.39$; pride: $\gamma = 0.0062, p = 0.36$). In terms of specific negative emotions, older adults only reported feeling less bored ($\gamma = -0.0068, p < 0.05$) and less fatigued ($\gamma = -0.0145, p < 0.01$) than did younger adults. Age was unrelated to reports of sadness ($\gamma = -0.0022, p = 0.51$), loneliness ($\gamma = -0.0029, p = 0.54$), and regret ($\gamma = -0.0052, p = 0.16$), as well as high arousal negative emotions, anxiety ($\gamma = -0.0065, p = 0.21$) and anger ($\gamma = -0.0047, p = 0.069$). There were no significant quadratic effects of age.

### TIME OF DAY EFFECTS

Participants reported less positive emotion ($\gamma = -0.1372, p < 0.01$) and more negative emotion ($\gamma = 0.1288, p < 0.01$) in the evenings compared to mornings. Specifically, compared to the mornings, in the evenings participants' reported less enthusiasm ($\gamma = -0.5139, p < 0.01$) and excitement ($\gamma = -0.3560, p < 0.01$), as well as more sadness ($\gamma = 0.1346, p < 0.01$), boredom ($\gamma = 0.1050, p < 0.01$), fatigue ($\gamma = 0.6549, p < 0.01$), and anger ($\gamma = 0.1341, p < 0.01$). Two exceptions to the general pattern of reduced well-being at the end of the day were pride and anxiety. Pride was experienced more ($\gamma = 0.1625, p < 0.01$) and anxiety was experience less ($\gamma = -0.1869, p < 0.01$) in the evenings than in the mornings. Happiness ($\gamma = -0.0063, p = 0.90$) and low arousal positive emotions (content: $\gamma = -0.0716, p = 0.17$; calm: $\gamma = -0.0903, p = 0.12$; relaxed: $\gamma = -0.0944, p = 0.11$) did not differ by time of day, nor did loneliness ($\gamma = 0.0540, p = 0.21$) or regret ($\gamma = 0.0021, p = 0.96$).

### MODERATION OF AGE EFFECTS BY TIME OF DAY

The effect of age on emotional experience varied somewhat as a function of when emotion as assessed, especially for positive states. There were significant interactions between time of day and age for all of the positive emotions (although the effects were only marginal for calm and excited). However, the nature of this interaction varied across the specific emotions. For instance, as shown in **Figure 1**, older adults enhanced experience of relaxation was greater in the morning than the evening (Time of Day × Age: $\gamma = -0.0086, p < 0.01$), whereas their increased experience of enthusiasm showed the reverse pattern (i.e., it was stronger in the evening; Time of Day × Age: $\gamma = 0.0050, p < 0.05$). Notably, as shown in **Table 3**, at both times of day older adults reported feeling significantly more relaxed (morning: $\gamma = 0.0201, p < 0.01$; evening: $\gamma = 0.0123, p < 0.05$) and enthusiastic (morning: $\gamma = 0.0224, p < 0.01$; evening: $\gamma = 0.0275, p < 0.05$) than younger people. Time also moderated the effect of age on happiness (Time of Day × Age$^2$: $\gamma = 0.0003, p < 0.01$) and contentment (Time of Day × Age$^2$: $\gamma = 0.0002, p < 0.05$), such that there was more of a quadratic (accelerated) age effect in the evening than in the morning (see **Figure 2**). However, there were significant linear effects of age on happiness and contentment at both time points

**Table 3 | Results of multilevel analyses testing the effects of age on morning and evening emotion.**

| Fixed effects estimates | Intercept | Age | Age$^2$ | Health | Fluency |
|---|---|---|---|---|---|
| **AM POSITIVE** | | | | | |
| Happy | 4.7033 (0.1332) | 0.0136 (0.0049)** | 0.0001 (0.0003) | −0.5104 (0.1396)** | −0.1597 (0.0919)+ |
| Content | 4.8159 (0.1308) | 0.0144 (0.0048)** | 0.0002 (0.0003) | −0.3684 (0.1371)** | −0.0542 (0.0902) |
| Calm | 4.9092 (0.1219) | 0.0152 (0.0045)** | 0.0000 (0.0002) | −0.3459 (0.1278)** | 0.0234 (0.0841) |
| Relaxed | 4.8576 (0.1282) | 0.0201 (0.0047)** | −0.0004 (0.0003) | −0.3032 (0.1344)* | −0.0024 (0.0885) |
| Enthusiastic | 4.0589 (0.1510) | 0.0224 (0.0056)** | −0.0002 (0.0003) | −0.4996 (0.1583)** | −0.0846 (0.1042) |
| Excited | 3.5805 (0.1547) | 0.0046 (0.0057) | 0.0000 (0.0003) | −0.4338 (0.1621)** | −0.1849 (0.1067)+ |
| Proud | 3.9012 (0.1853) | 0.0058 (0.0068) | −0.0003 (0.0004) | −0.2404 (0.1943) | −0.3898 (0.1278)** |
| **AM NEGATIVE** | | | | | |
| Sad | 1.5829 (0.0825) | −0.0024 (0.0030) | −0.0003 (0.0002)+ | 0.0666 (0.0864) | 0.0223 (0.0569) |
| Bored | 1.4816 (0.0832) | −0.0063 (0.0031)* | 0.0000 (0.0002) | −0.0048 (0.0872) | −0.0241 (0.0574) |
| Fatigued | 2.4868 (0.1410) | −0.0137 (0.0052)* | 0.0000 (0.0003) | 0.4161 (0.1478)** | 0.0954 (0.0973) |
| Anxious | 2.3930 (0.1463) | −0.0064 (0.0054) | 0.0000 (0.0003) | −0.0142 (0.1534) | −0.1155 (0.1009) |
| Angry | 1.3929 (0.0676) | −0.0045 (0.0025)+ | −0.0002 (0.0001) | 0.0713 (0.0709) | −0.0565 (0.0467) |
| Lonely | 1.6725 (0.1247) | −0.0025 (0.0046) | −0.0001 (0.0003) | 0.0526 (0.1307) | −0.0518 (0.0860) |
| Regretful | 1.7168 (0.0974) | −0.0051 (0.0036) | −0.0004 (0.0002)+ | 0.1317 (0.1021) | −0.0179 (0.0672) |
| **PM POSITIVE** | | | | | |
| Happy | 4.7009 (0.1299) | 0.0139 (0.0048)** | 0.0004 (0.0003) | −0.5158 (0.1361)** | −0.0812 (0.0896) |
| Content | 4.7525 (0.1269) | 0.0135 (0.0047)** | 0.0004 (0.0003) | −0.4309 (0.1330)** | 0.0689 (0.0875) |
| Calm | 4.8197 (0.1270) | 0.0128 (0.0047)** | 0.0001 (0.0003) | −0.3149 (0.1331)* | 0.0529 (0.0876) |
| Relaxed | 4.7633 (0.1275) | 0.0123 (0.0047)* | 0.0000 (0.0003) | −0.2975 (0.1338)* | 0.0561 (0.0880) |
| Enthusiastic | 3.5436 (0.1511) | 0.0275 (0.0056)** | 0.0000 (0.0003) | −0.4644 (0.1584)** | −0.0572 (0.1042) |
| Excited | 3.2169 (0.1486) | 0.0089 (0.0055) | 0.0000 (0.0003) | −0.4192 (0.1557)** | −0.1818 (0.1025)+ |
| Proud | 4.0631 (0.1817) | 0.0023 (0.0067) | −0.0004 (0.0004) | −0.2238 (0.1905) | −0.2921 (0.1254)* |
| **PM NEGATIVE** | | | | | |
| Sad | 1.7190 (0.1004) | −0.0047 (0.0037) | −0.0004 (0.0002)* | 0.0848 (0.1052) | 0.0645 (0.0693) |
| Bored | 1.5902 (0.1007) | −0.0093 (0.0037)* | 0.0000 (0.0002) | 0.0584 (0.1055) | −0.0410 (0.0695) |
| Fatigued | 3.1408 (0.1633) | −0.0158 (0.0060)* | 0.0002 (0.0003) | 0.6816 (0.1711)** | 0.2306 (0.1126)* |
| Anxious | 2.2126 (0.1371) | −0.0048 (0.0051) | −0.0001 (0.0003) | 0.0631 (0.1437) | −0.0228 (0.0946) |
| Angry | 1.5247 (0.0752) | −0.0065 (0.0028)* | −0.0003 (0.0002)+ | 0.1365 (0.0787)+ | −0.0611 (0.0519) |
| Lonely | 1.7270 (0.1325) | −0.0044 (0.0049) | −0.0001 (0.0003) | 0.1071 (0.1390) | −0.0734 (0.0914) |
| Regretful | 1.7227 (0.1028) | −0.0057 (0.0038) | −0.0003 (0.0002) | 0.1638 (0.1077) | 0.0054 (0.0709) |

*Unstandardized estimates are presented with standard errors in parentheses. Age is centered at age 54 years; Physical health and verbal fluency Z-scored.*
*+p < 0.10; *p < 0.05; **p < 0.01.*

(no quadratic age effects): older adult felt happier and more content than relatively younger adults in both the mornings (happy: $\gamma = 0.0136$, $p < 0.01$; content: $\gamma = 0.0144$, $p < 0.01$) and in the evenings (happy: $\gamma = 0.0139$, $p < 0.01$; content: $\gamma = 0.0135$, $p < 0.01$). For pride, the effect of age was weaker in the evening than in the morning ($\gamma = -0.0044$, $p < 0.05$), but there were not significant age differences at either point in the day (morning: $\gamma = 0.0058$, $p = 0.40$; evening: $\gamma = 0.0023$, $p = 0.74$). Both younger and older people experienced more pride in the evenings than mornings.

Age differences in negative emotion varied less based on time of assessment. There was only a significant interaction for fatigue (Time × Age$^2$: $\gamma = 0.0003$, $p < 0.05$). As shown in **Figure 2**, the age-related decrease in fatigue flattened at advanced ages for evening emotion more so than for morning emotion (although there were significant linear age effects at both time points). For sadness, age effects were somewhat stronger in the evening: there was a significant quadratic effect of age in the evening (Age$^2$: $\gamma = -0.0004$, $p < 0.05$) but this effect was not significant in the morning (Age$^2$: $\gamma = -0.0003$, $p = 0.09$). However, there was not a significant interaction between time of day and age for sadness (Time × Age: $\gamma = -0.0027$, $p = 0.07$; Time × Age$^2$: $\gamma = -0.0002$, $p = 0.07$). Regardless of age and time of day, individuals reported relatively low levels of sadness (see **Figure 2**). There were not significant interactions between time of day and age for the other negative emotions either, including the higher arousal negative states (anger and anxiety).

## ANCILLARY ANALYSES: SLEEP AND MORNINGNESS

We ran additional models that included the measures of sleep (quantity and quality the previous night) and individual differences in morning along with the core predictors (i.e., linear and quadratic age terms, Time of Day, and the interaction between Time of Day and each of the age components) to test whether

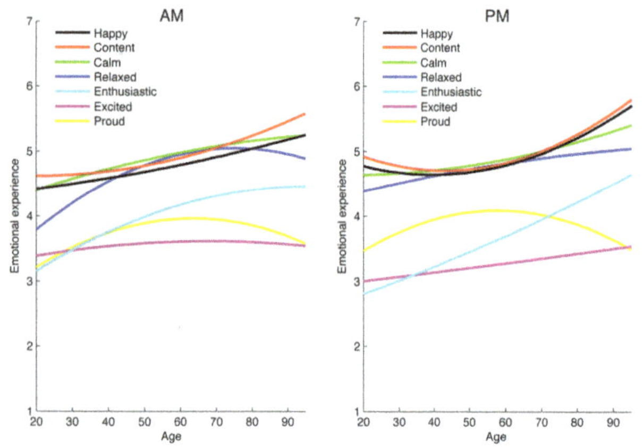


**FIGURE 1 | Age differences in positive emotional experience in the morning (AM) and evening (PM).**

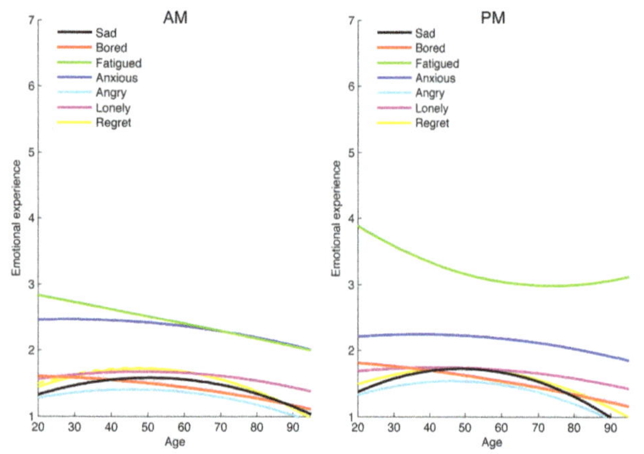


**FIGURE 2 | Age differences in negative emotional experience in the morning (AM) and evening (PM).**

these variables might explain the effects of Age or the interaction between Age and Time of Day. The sleep variables were included together as day-level predictors; morningness was included as a person-level predictor along with its interaction with Time of Day.

Older adults reported better subjective sleep quantity (Age: $\gamma = 0.0091, p < 0.001$) and quality (Age: $\gamma = 0.0109, p < 0.01$); for number of hours slept, there was a quadratic age effect indicating that middle-aged adults slept fewer hours than did relatively younger and older adults (Age: $\gamma = -0.0049$, $p = 0.27$; Age$^2$: $\gamma = 0.0008$, $p < 0.01$). Individuals who reported better sleep quality the previous night felt more of each of the positive emotions (happy: $\gamma = 0.0795$, $p < 0.01$; content: $\gamma = 0.0849, p < 0.01$; calm: $\gamma = 0.1062, p < 0.001$; relaxed: $\gamma = 0.0867$, $p < 0.01$; enthusiastic: $\gamma = 0.0882$, $p < 0.01$; excited: $\gamma = 0.0920, p < 0.01$; pride: $\gamma = 0.0592, p < 0.05$) and less of each of the negative emotion (sadness: $\gamma = -0.1059, p < 0.001$; anger: $\gamma = -0.0442, p < 0.05$; boredom: $\gamma = -0.0398, p < 0.05$; fatigue: $\gamma = -0.1713, p < 0.001$; lonely: $\gamma = -0.0572, p < 0.01$; regret: $\gamma = -0.0732$, $p < 0.01$) except anxiety ($\gamma = -0.0474$, $p = 0.083$). Importantly, however, the effects of Age and the Age × Time of Day interactions remained intact when the sleep variables were included as covariates. Only the age effect for boredom became marginal when controlling for sleep ($\gamma = -0.0065$, $p = 0.059$).

As expected, older adults scored higher on morningness ($r = 0.40$). However, when both Age and Morningness were included as predictors of emotional experience, all the effects of Age and the Age × Time of Day interactions remained significant. The only significant main effect of Morningness was for anger: individuals higher on morningness reported feeling less angry ($\gamma = -0.1052$, $p < 0.05$). There were also significant Morningness × Time of Day interactions for calm ($\gamma = 0.1135, p < 0.01$), relaxed ($\gamma = 0.1013, p < 0.05$), and enthusiastic ($\gamma = -0.0861, p < 0.05$): individuals higher in morningness reported feeling relatively more calm and relaxed in the evening (compared to the morning) and more enthusiastic in the morning (compared to the evening). Overall, these findings suggest that sleep patterns and individual differences in morningness do not explain the age differences in emotional experience observed in this study.

## DISCUSSION

Consistent with previous findings, older adults in the present study reported relatively more positive daily emotional experiences than did younger adults. Older adults characterized their emotional experiences as more positive and less negative in both the mornings and evenings. This finding contributes to a compelling literature on age-related improvements in the emotion domain. Older adults' relatively greater emotional well-being has been observed across a wide range of samples and in studies using a wide variety of methods. Whether emotions are sampled randomly throughout the course of a week, studied in the laboratory or recalled at the end of the day or from the day before, age advantages reliably appear. Evidence about the specific motions that drive these age differences is far more mixed. In some studies, greater positive experience accounts for age differences. In others, less negative experience accounts for differences. Findings from several recent studies suggest that these variations may be due to differences in methodological approaches and the measures used to assess emotion.

In the present study, we aimed to capture a more differentiated view of emotional experience across specific positive and negative emotions early and late in the day. We expected that age differences would be more pronounced for low arousal emotions, given previous findings (Kessler and Staudinger, 2009; Scheibe et al., 2013) and theory (Charles, 2010), specifically contentions stemming from the strengths and vulnerabilities integration model (SAVI) that high arousal states may be unpleasant for older adults. Sampling a range of emotions that represented all four quadrants of the affective circumplex, we asked participants spanning in age from young adulthood to very old age to describe how calm, content, enthusiastic, excited, happy, proud, relaxed, angry, anxious/worried, bored, fatigued, sad, regretful, and lonely they felt every morning and evening across ten days. The hypothesis that age differences would be most apparent for low arousal positive emotions was largely supported. Of the seven positive emotions sampled, older people reported greater experience of all of them except two high arousal emotions, namely excitement and pride. However, among negative emotions, only two distinguished age: older adults reported feeling less bored and less fatigued. No differences by age were observed for any of the high arousal negative emotions (viz., anger, anxiety/worry). We expect that this may be due, in part, to a relatively lesser reports of negative emotions. Notably, these age differences in emotional experience held when taking into account physical health and cognition, as well as sleep patterns and individual difference in morningness.

Considering time of day, even more complexity was observed. Participants generally felt more negative and less positive in the evenings than they did in the mornings. However, interactions between age and time of day did not follow a conceptually meaningful pattern. The age benefit for relaxation was stronger in the mornings than evenings, for example, but this interaction was not observed for calm or content. In addition, older adults were more likely to report increased enthusiasm compared to younger adults in the evening, but other high arousal positive emotions did not show this same trajectory. The time of day effects also varied somewhat based on demographic factors. Only women showed a decline in emotional well-being across the day (i.e., less positive emotion and more negative emotion in the evening than in the morning). In addition, the increase in negative emotional experience at the end of the day was attenuated in old age for African Americans and blue-collar workers, but not for European Americans and white collar workers. Thus, the present set of findings leave answers to many questions about time of day equivocal. Still, they suggest that some of the seeming inconsistencies across findings related to aging and emotion might be at least partially be explained by the specific emotions sampled and time of day. Measures that focus exclusively on high arousal terms (e.g., PANAS) can be expected to find weaker age differences, missing important age-related increases in lower arousal positive emotion, perhaps especially so if sessions are run later in the day.

Past work based on experience sampling suggested that age differences are weaker for emotional intensity than emotion frequency (e.g., Carstensen et al., 2000, 2011). Carstensen et al. concluded that although older adults may experience negative emotions less often, when they do experience these emotions they are felt just as intensely. In the present study, however, we observed differences in intensity of emotional experience in the mornings and evenings and the pattern of findings did not change when we analyzed frequency instead of intensity. Unlike Carstensen et al.'s experience sampling project, in the present study, we compared only two time points: emotional experience upon waking in the morning and immediately before bedtime. One of the advantages of focusing on waking and bedtime is that age differences in environmental factors are likely smaller than in the middle of day (when younger and older adults engage in very different types of activities). Still, many interesting experiences in life occur in between mornings and evenings (indeed, the most intense emotional experiences likely occur then), and age differences may be more pronounced mid-day (when older adults have relatively more opportunities to be selective).

Differences in findings as a function of sample size and related statistical power also merit thoughtful consideration. Studies that rely on very large samples (e.g., Mroczek and Kolarz, 1998; Stone et al., 2010) are more likely to find significant age differences because they have the statistical power to detect very small effects. For instance, the widely reported increase in positive emotion observed by Mroczek and Kolarz (1998) was not meaningfully different from the non-significant increase reported by Carstensen et al. (2000, 2011). Thus, some apparent difference in findings about age-related shifts in emotion reflect statistical power. Similarly, in the present study and prior experience sampling research from our group, we observe very low rates of high arousal negative emotions regardless of age. Non-significant findings in frequency and intensity may mask other potential differences in the nature and influence of such emotions in daily life.

In the present study, age was largely unrelated to the experience of high arousal states, regardless of valence. For instance, age differences in negative emotional experience were driven by less intense, low arousal emotions, rather than declines in anger or anxiety. Reasoning from the vantage point of SAVI (Charles, 2010), low arousal emotions may be easier to manage and, thus, older adults are more successful in regulating them. This interpretation is also consistent with findings that suggest a lack of age differences in high arousal positive emotions (Lawton et al., 1992; Kessler and Staudinger, 2009; Scheibe et al., 2013). Scheibe et al. (2013), for example, found that older adults reported a greater preference for experiencing low arousal positive emotion relative to high arousal positive emotion than did younger adults. Whether or not high and low arousal emotions show distinct developmental trajectories and, if confirmed, the reasons for such differences remains highly speculative and demands targeted investigation.

Overall, the findings from the present study underscore the importance of carefully considering the emotions sampled and the time of assessment when examining emotional experience. Age-related changes in emotional well-being may be more pronounced for certain emotional states and at certain times of day.

## ACKNOWLEDGMENTS

This research was supported by National Institute on Aging grant R37 AG008816 awarded to Laura L. Carstensen and F32 AG034783 awarded to Tammy English. The content is solely the responsibility of the authors and does not necessarily represent the official views of the National Institute on Aging or the National Institutes of Health.

## REFERENCES

Adan, A., and Almirall, H. (1991). Horne and ostberg morningness-eveningness questionnaire: a reduced scale. *Pers. Individ. Dif.* 12, 241–253. doi: 10.1016/0191-8869(91)90110-W

Biss, R. K., and Hasher, L. (2012). Happy as a lark: Morning-type younger and older adults are higher in positive affect. *Emotion* 12, 437–441. doi: 10.1037/a0027071

Carstensen, L. L., Pasupathi, M., Mayr, U., and Nesselroade, J. R. (2000). Emotional experience in everyday life across the adult life span. *J. Pers. Soc. Psychol.* 79, 644–655. doi: 10.1037/0022-3514.79.4.644

Carstensen, L. L., Turan, B., Scheibe, S., Ram, N., Ersner-Hershfield, H., Samanez-Larkin, G. R., et al. (2011). Emotional experience improves with age: evidence based on over 10 years of experience sampling. *Psychol. Aging* 26, 21–33. doi: 10.1037/a0021285

Charles, S. T. (2010). Strength and vulnerability integration: a model of emotional well-being across adulthood. *Psychol. Bull.* 136, 1068–1091. doi: 10.1037/a0021232

Charles, S. T., and Carstensen, L. L. (2013). "Emotion regulation and aging," in *Handbook of Emotion Regulation, 2nd Edn.,* ed J. J. Gross (New York, NY: Guilford Press), 203–218.

Charles, S. T., Reynolds, C. A., and Gatz, M. (2001). Age-related differences and change in positive and negative affect over 23 years. *J. Pers. Soc. Psychol.* 80, 136–151. doi: 10.1037/0022-3514.80.1.136

Consedine, N. S., and Magai, C. (2006). "Emotional development in adulthood: a developmental functionalist review and critique," in *Handbook of Adult Development and Learning,* ed C. Hoare (New York, NY: Oxford University Press), 123–148.

Davey, A., Halverson, C. F., Jr., Zonderman, A. B., and Costa, P. T. Jr. (2004). Change in depressive symptoms in the baltimore longitudinal study of aging. *J. Gerontol. Ser. B Psychol. Sci. Soc. Sci.* 59, P270–P277. doi: 10.1093/geronb/59.6.P270

Diener, E., and Suh, E. M. (1998). "Subjective well-being and age: an international analysis," in *Annual Review of Gerontology and Geriatrics, Vol. 17, Focus on Emotion and Adult Development,* eds K. W. Schaie and M. P. Lawton (New York, NY: Springer), 304–324.

Fiske, A., Gatz, M., and Pedersen, N. (2003). Depressive symptoms and aging: the effects of illness and non-health-related events. *J. Gerontol. Ser. B Psychol. Sci. Soc. Sci.* 58, P320–P328. doi: 10.1093/geronb/58.6.P320

Gatz, M., Kasl-Godley, J. E., and Karel, M. J. (1996). "Aging and mental disorders," in *Handbook of the Psychology of Aging, 4th Edn.,* eds J. E. Birren and K. W. Schaie (San Diego, CA: Academic Press), 365–382.

Hultsch, D. F., Hammer, M., and Small, B. J. (1993). Age differences in cognitive performance in later life: relationships to self-reported health and activity life style. *J. Gerontol. Psychol. Sci.* 48, 1–11. doi: 10.1093/geronj/48.1.P1

Kessler, E. M., and Staudinger, U. M. (2009). Affective experience in adulthood and old age: the role of affective arousal and perceived affect regulation. *Psychol. Aging* 24, 349–362. doi: 10.1037/a0015352

Knight, M., and Mather, M. (2013). Look out—it's your off-peak time of day! Time of day matters more for alerting than for orienting or executive attention. *Exp. Aging Res.* 39, 305–321. doi: 10.1080/0361073X.2013.779197

Kunzmann, U., Little, T. D., and Smith, J. (2000). Is age-related stability of subjective well-being a paradox? Cross-sectional and longitudinal evidence from the Berlin Aging Study. *Psychol. Aging* 15, 511–526. doi: 10.1037/0882-7974.15.3.511

Larsen, R. J., and Diener, E. (1992). "Promises and problems with the circumplex model of emotion," in *Review of Personality and Social Psychology: Emotion,* ed M. S. Clark (Newbury Park, CA: Sage), 25–59.

Lawton, M. P., Kleban, M. H., Rajagopal, D., and Dean, J. (1992). Dimensions of affective experience in three age groups. *Psychol. Aging* 7, 171–184. doi: 10.1037/0882-7974.7.2.171

Lindenberger, U., Mayr, U., and Kliegl, R. (1993). Speed and intelligence in old age. *Psychol. Aging* 8, 207–220. doi: 10.1037/0882-7974.8.2.207

Mather, M., and Carstensen, L. L. (2005). Aging and motivated cognition: the positivity effect in attention and memory. *Trends in Cognitive Science,* 9, 496–502. doi: 10.1016/j.tics.2005.08.005

Mroczek, D. K., and Kolarz, C. M. (1998). The effect of age on positive and negative affect: a developmental perspective on happiness. *J. Pers. Soc. Psychol.* 75, 1333–1349. doi: 10.1037/0022-3514.75.5.1333

Muraven, M., Tice, D. M., and Baumeister, R. F. (1998). Self-control as a limited resource: regulatory depletion patterns. *J. Pers. Soc. Psychol.* 74, 774–789. doi: 10.1037/0022-3514.74.3.774

Ochsner, K. N., Silvers, J. A., and Buhle, J. T. (2012). Functional imaging studies of emotion regulation: a synthetic review and evolving model of the cognitive control of emotion. *Ann. N.Y. Acad. Sci.* 1251, E1–E24. doi: 10.1111/j.1749-6632.2012.06751.x

Phillips, L. H., Henry, J. D., Hosie, J. A., and Milne, A. B. (2008). Effective regulation of the experience and expression of negative affect in old age. *J. Gerontol. Psychol. Sci.* 63B, 138–145. doi: 10.1093/geronb/63.3.P138

Reed, A. E., and Carstensen, L. L. (2012). The theory behind the age-related positivity effect. *Front. Psychol.* 3:339. doi: 10.3389/fpsyg.2012.00339

Riediger, M., Schmiedek, F., Wagner, G. G., and Lindenberger, U. (2009). Seeking pleasure and seeking pain: differences in prohedonic and contra-hedonic motivation from adolescence to old age. *Psychol. Sci.* 20, 1529–1535. doi: 10.1111/j.1467-9280.2009.02473.x

Ross, C. E., and Mirowsky, J. (2008). Age and the balance of emotions. *Soc. Sci. Med.* 66, 2391–2400. doi: 10.1016/j.socscimed.2008.01.048

Scheibe, S., and Carstensen, L. L. (2010). Emotional aging: recent findings and future trends. *J. Gerontol. Psychol. Sci.* 65B, 135–144. doi: 10.1093/geronb/gbp132

Scheibe, S., English, T., Tsai, J. L., and Carstensen, L. L. (2013). Striving to feel good: ideal affect, actual affect, and their correspondence across adulthood. *Psychol. Aging* 28, 160–171. doi: 10.1037/a0030561

Schieman, S. (1999). Age and anger. *J. Health Soc. Behav.* 40, 273–289. doi: 10.2307/2676352

Stone, A. A., Schwartz, J. E., Broderick, J. E., and Deaton, A. (2010). A snapshot of the age distribution of psychological well-being in the United States. *Proc. Natl. Acad. Sci. U.S.A.* 107, 9985–9990. doi: 10.1073/pnas.1003744107

Watson, D., and Tellegen, A. (1985). Toward a consensual structure of mood. *Psychol. Bull.* 98, 219–235. doi: 10.1037/0033-2909.98.2.219

Yoon, C., May, C. P., and Hasher, L. (1999). "Aging, circadian arousal patterns, and cognition," in *Cognition, Aging, and Self-reports,* eds N. Schwarz, D. C. Park, B. Knaulper, and S. Sudman (Hove: Psychology Press/Erlbaum (UK) Taylor & Francis), 117–143.

# 7

# The role of arousal in the spontaneous regulation of emotions in healthy aging: a fMRI investigation

**Sanda Dolcos[1]*, Yuta Katsumi[1] and Roger A. Dixon[2]**

[1] Department of Psychology, University of Illinois at Urbana-Champaign, Champaign, IL, USA
[2] Department of Psychology, University of Alberta, Edmonton, AB, Canada

**Edited by:**
Natalie Ebner, University of Florida, USA

**Reviewed by:**
Hakan Fischer, Stockholm University, Sweden
Heather L. Urry, Tufts University, USA
Anne Krendl, Indiana University Bloomington, USA

***Correspondence:**
Sanda Dolcos, Department of Psychology, University of Illinois at Urbana-Champaign, 603 E. Daniel Street, Champaign, IL 61820, USA
e-mail: sdolcos@illinois.edu

Despite ample support for enhanced affective well-being and emotional stability in healthy aging, the role of potentially important dimensions, such as the emotional arousal, has not been systematically investigated in neuroimaging studies. In addition, the few behavioral studies that examined effects of arousal have produced inconsistent findings. The present study manipulated the arousal of pictorial stimuli to test the hypothesis that preserved emotional functioning in aging is modulated by the level of arousal, and to identify the associated neural correlates. Young and older healthy participants were presented with negative and neutral pictures, which they rated for emotional content, while fMRI data were recorded. There were three main novel findings regarding the neural mechanisms underlying the processing of negative pictures with different levels of arousal in young and older adults. First, the common engagement of the right amygdala in young and older adults was driven by high arousing negative stimuli. Second, complementing an age-related reduction in the subjective ratings for low arousing negative pictures, there were opposing patterns of activity in the rostral/ventral anterior cingulate cortex (ACC) and the amygdala, which showed increased vs. decreased responses, respectively, to low arousing negative pictures. Third, increased spontaneous activity in the ventral ACC/ventromedial prefrontal cortex (vmPFC) in older adults was linked to reduced ratings for low arousing negative pictures. Overall, these findings advance our understanding of the neural correlates underlying processing of negative emotions with different levels of arousal in the context of enhanced emotional functioning in healthy aging. Notably, the results support the idea that older adults have emotion regulation networks chronically activated, in the absence of explicit induction of the goal to regulate emotions, and that this effect is specific to low arousing negative emotions.

**Keywords: emotion control, spontaneous emotion regulation, brain imaging**

## INTRODUCTION

Aging is associated with well-known co-morbidities and losses, but also with relatively high levels of emotional well-being. The idea of relatively well-preserved emotional processing in aging is supported by evidence showing that older adults tend to (a) pay attention to and remember more positive information (Charles et al., 2003; Mather and Carstensen, 2003; Isaacowitz et al., 2006) and (b) show reduced processing of negative information compared to young adults (Wood and Kisley, 2006; Gruhn et al., 2007).

Prominent models of emotion identify valence and arousal as fundamental components of emotion (see Bradley and Lang, 2000, for a review). Valence refers to the direction of an emotional response (positive or negative), whereas arousal refers to the magnitude of the response (exciting, agitating, or calming, subduing; Russell, 1980). Empirical evidence shows that these two emotional dimensions are not independent of each other (Ito et al., 1998; Lang et al., 1998; Libkuman et al., 2007; but see Ribeiro et al., 2007). Rather, they form a V ("boomerang")-shaped function, with the unpleasant pictures tending to be more highly arousing than pleasant stimuli, and both pleasant and unpleasant pictures being more arousing than neutral stimuli. Considerable evidence supports the "boomerang" shape in averaged data on arousal and valence ratings of people's reactions to affective visual stimuli, such as the International Affective Picture System (IAPS) (e.g., Lang et al., 1992, 1998; Lang, 1995; Bradley and Lang, 2007). Despite substantial support for the preserved emotional function in aging, the role of emotional arousal has not been systematically investigated in neuroimaging studies. Moreover, the few behavioral studies that included examinations of arousal have produced inconsistent findings. For instance, a study investigating age-differences in memory for arousing and non-arousing words (Kensinger, 2008) showed that older adults remembered more positive than negative low-arousing words, whereas young adults showed the reverse pattern. There were no differences in the ratio of high-arousing positive vs. negative words remembered by young and older adults. A study examining age-differences in the relation between valence and arousal ratings

(Keil and Freund, 2009) showed that in young adults both pleasantness and unpleasantness increased with emotional arousal, whereas in older adults low-arousing stimuli were experienced as most pleasant, and the high-arousing ones as most unpleasant. Finally, a study investigating age-differences in emotional reactions to stimuli differing in arousal and age-relevance (Streubel and Kunzmann, 2011) showed that older adults rated unpleasant low-arousing pictures as less unpleasant compared to young adults, while there were no age-related differences in unpleasant ratings for unpleasant pictures that were high in arousal. Despite these inconsistent findings, these behavioral studies indicate that age-related changes are more likely to influence the response to stimuli low in arousal. This idea is also suggested by recent neuroimaging evidence (St. Jacques et al., 2010) showing that older adults tend to rate some negative pictures as neutral more frequently than young adults (thus suggesting a negative-to-neutral shift in older adults). However, the latter study did not explicitly manipulate the level of arousal.

Previous evidence has shown that processing of low and high arousing emotional stimuli relies on distinct processes. On the one hand, low arousing negative stimuli activate more goal-driven processes, which tend to engage controlled, resource-demanding processes (Kensinger and Corkin, 2004) and the prefrontal cortex (PFC). On the other hand, high arousing information activates more stimulus-driven processes (Mather and Knight, 2006), which tend to capture attention automatically and require reduced cognitive effort (Dolan, 2002). There is evidence for the idea that the automatic processing of high-arousing stimuli is relatively preserved in older adults (Mather and Knight, 2006). One structure typically associated with the relatively automatic processing of emotional information is the amygdala. Amygdala, a region involved in basic emotion processing, is involved in two related and important abilities: (a) to rapidly detect emotional information presented with a rapid stream of stimuli (Anderson and Phelps, 1998) and (b) to detect emotional stimuli even when attentional resources are drained (reviewed by Dolan and Vuilleumier, 2003). These observations suggest that the role of the amygdala in emotional processing is not heavily dependent on the availability of extensive cognitive resources. Despite a relative structural preservation of the amygdala in healthy aging (Allen et al., 2005; Brabec et al., 2010), functional magnetic resonance imaging (fMRI) evidence reveals different patterns of activation in the amygdala. For instance, some fMRI studies have found an age-related decrease in activation in response to negative stimuli (Iidaka et al., 2002; Gunning-Dixon et al., 2003; Mather et al., 2004; Tessitore et al., 2005; Erk et al., 2008). One study reported robust amygdala activity in both young and older adults during the perception of novel fearful faces (vs. familiar neutral ones) (Wright et al., 2006), while another study found enhanced amygdala activity to negative compared to neutral stimuli in both young and older adults (St. Jacques et al., 2010). Importantly, the latter study also showed that the amygdala activation in older adults involved overlapping areas with young adults, thus suggesting that amygdala functions similarly in healthy young and older adults. This makes it unlikely that an age-related decline in the amygdala (as suggested by the aging-brain model: Cacioppo et al., 2011) would account for the reduced amygdala activity to negative stimuli in older adults reported in some of the previous studies.

A more probable explanation for the inconsistent findings regarding age-related differences in amygdala activation to negative stimuli may be that the pictures used in those studies differed in emotional arousal. This explanation is in line with previous evidence in older adults showing (a) preserved amygdala responses to positive (Mather et al., 2004) or novel stimuli (Moriguchi et al., 2011), (b) reduced responses selectively to negative stimuli, and (c) decreased amygdala activity for the trials in which older participants subjectively experienced negative pictures as neutral (negative-to-neutral shift), but not for the negative pictures subjectively rated as negative (St. Jacques et al., 2010). Taken together, these findings suggest the possibility of age-related differential engagement of the amygdala by stimuli with different levels of arousal, but again such manipulation has not been previously used in conjunction with brain imaging recordings.

Decreased amygdala activity, combined with increased activity in emotion control regions, such as the medial PFC and the adjacent anterior cingulate cortex (ACC), might also be the result of a greater focus on emotion regulation goals. According to the Socioemotional Selectivity Theory (SST; Scheibe and Carstensen, 2010), older adults tend to prioritize social and emotional well-being goals over other goals, potentially as a result of shrinking time horizons. The increased salience of emotional goals may enhance older adults' motivation to regulate the emotions experienced in everyday life, either by selecting stimuli and situations that minimize negative emotions (Blanchard-Fields et al., 2004) or by using emotion regulation strategies (Gross et al., 1997). The "cognitive-control model" extension of the SST (Mather and Knight, 2005; Kryla-Lighthall and Mather, 2009) posits that such negativity avoidance is the result of older adults' greater chronic focus on emotion regulation goals. Consistent with the cognitive control model, a number of studies reported increased activity in the medial PFC/ACC to negative compared to neutral stimuli in older compared to young adults (Gunning-Dixon et al., 2003; Williams et al., 2006; Leclerc and Kensinger, 2008; Roalf et al., 2011). Moreover, studies also showed that the increased activity in medial PFC/ACC was accompanied by decreased activity in the amygdala in older, but not in young adults, during the anticipation of monetary loss (Larkin et al., 2007) and during evaluation of negative stimuli (St. Jacques et al., 2010). Notably, functional connectivity between these regions was greater in older compared to young adults, thus suggesting that medial PFC and ACC might be involved more generally in subcortical emotion regulation.

This interpretation is consistent with studies showing interactions between similar medial PFC/ACC regions and the amygdala, when older adults voluntarily decreased emotional responses to negative stimuli (Urry et al., 2006; Winecoff et al., 2011). Given that medial PFC shows stronger activity when adults (a) are told to up-regulate positive emotion and down-regulate negative emotion (Ochsner et al., 2004) and (b) spontaneously regulate their emotions (e.g., Drabant et al., 2009), the increased medial PFC/ACC activity seen in older adults while processing emotional stimuli might reflect their spontaneous engagement of emotion regulation operations. Moreover, negative correlations between the ventral ACC and amygdala when evaluating negative pictures (according to IAPS standardized norms) as neutral (negative-to-neutral shift; St. Jacques et al., 2010) suggest that the spontaneous emotion regulation in older adults might be limited to low arousing stimuli.

The present event-related fMRI study used a broader range of negative emotional stimuli (low, medium, and high arousing) to test the hypothesis that emotional functioning in aging is modulated by the level of arousal, and to identify the associated neural correlates. The focus was on the ACC/vmPFC and the amygdala. Participants were presented with negative and neutral pictures, which they rated for emotional content, while fMRI data were recorded. Based on the above review, we made the following four predictions. First, from the evidence showing a negative-to-neutral shift in older adults' ratings, we predicted lower ratings to the low arousing negative pictures in older adults. Second, we predicted that common engagement of the amygdala in young and older adults would be specific to high arousing pictures, reflecting preserved responses to high arousing stimuli in older adults. Third, we predicted that opposing patterns of response in the ACC/vmPFC (increased) vs. amygdala (decreased) would be specific to low arousing stimuli. Finally, consistent with a role of the vACC/vmPFC in spontaneous emotional regulation, we explored the possibility that increased activity in this region would be linked to reduced ratings for low arousing negative stimuli in older adults.

## METHODS

### PARTICIPANTS

The subject sample comprised 18 young adults between the ages of 18 and 32 years (10 females, mean age = 23.61, *SD* = 4.19) and 16 older adults between the ages of 59 and 84 years (11 females, mean age = 68.56, *SD* = 6.98). Participants were healthy, right-handed, native English speakers. As part of the initial screening, participants completed a number of questionnaires and cognitive measures. However, in the present study, these were used only for inclusion/exclusion purposes. Also as part of the initial screening, people with history of psychiatric and/or neurological conditions, uncontrolled hypertension, and subjects with history of alcohol or drug abuse were excluded from participation. It has been estimated that fMRI data from 18 subjects are needed to detect reasonable effect sizes with a power of 0.8 and an alpha of 0.05 (Huettel and McCarthy, 2001; Desmond and Glover, 2002). We collected data from more participants, but due to data attrition (e.g., ratings not recorded, response box problems, participants feeling uncomfortable in the scanner) only data from 18 young and 16 older participants are used for analyses. The age groups were matched on demographic variables, including education (see **Table 1**). All participants provided written informed consent under a protocol approved by the Institutional Ethics Review Board.

### MATERIALS

Stimuli presented during the scanning session consisted of 180 pictures (90 negative and 90 neutral) selected from the IAPS (Lang et al., 1997). Additional neutral pictures were selected from other sources (Yamasaki et al., 2002), to equate the emotional pictures for visual complexity and human content. The negative picture set was further divided into equal numbers of low, medium, and high arousing negative pictures, based on their normative scores. Valence has not been held constant across the three levels of arousal in the negative pictures. Information about the pictures could be received from the corresponding author.

**Table 1 | Summary of demographic characteristics for young and older groups.**

| | Younger | Older | *p* |
|---|---|---|---|
| *n* | 18 | 16 | |
| Male/Female | 8/10 | 5/11 | |
| Age range | 18–32 | 59–84 | |
| Mean age (*SD*) | 23.61 (4.19) | 68.56 (6.98) | <0.001 |
| Years of education (*SD*) | 14.11 (2.22) | 14.19 (2.97) | 0.99 |

*SD, standard deviation.*

The focus on negative emotional pictures in the present study was justified by the following reasons. First, previous evidence shows that the influence of arousal on age differences is more pronounced for negative than for positive stimuli (Kensinger, 2008). Second, previous behavioral results show that positive stimuli are generally more difficult to interpret, due to the lack of consistency of subjective ratings for positive pictures with the normative ratings in the older participants (St. Jacques et al., 2010). Such inconsistencies are even more evident when considering arousal, as older adults tend to rate low-arousing pleasant pictures as more pleasant than high-arousing pleasant pictures (Streubel and Kunzmann, 2011). Thus, it would be difficult to meaningfully interpret the fMRI data based on the behavioral results. Third, to match the level of arousal in negative stimuli, the positive stimuli should have included a large number of pictures with radical sport and erotic content, which are processed differently in older adults (see Backs et al., 2005).

### PROCEDURE

The pool of 180 pictures was divided into sets of 30 pictures (15 negative and 15 neutral pictures in each set), which were randomly assigned to six study blocks. The block orders were randomly assigned to the participants. To avoid mood induction, pictures were pseudo-randomized so that no more than three pictures of the same valence were consecutively presented. Functional MR images were recorded while participants viewed and rated negative and neutral images. Each picture was presented on the screen for 4 s, and then was removed to minimize confounding effects of eye movements associated with prolonged scanning of images. Participants were asked to watch the pictures and rate their subjective emotional experience triggered by the pictures on an 8-point scale (1 = neutral, 8 = extremely negative). The rating scale was presented at the bottom of each picture. The screen containing the picture and rating scale was followed by a fixation cross, presented on the screen for 12 s. Participants were instructed to rate the pictures only after they were aware of the content of the picture and of their emotional response to the picture. Participants were encouraged to try and rate the pictures while they were on the screen. However, participants were also told to respond during the fixation screen if they needed more time to rate the picture. Participants first completed a run in which they were instructed to experience any feelings or thoughts the pictures might trigger. The first run was intended to collect data on participants' spontaneous processing and evaluation of negative information with varying degrees of arousal. The following runs were intended to collect data on participants' responses following the induction of the goal to regulate emotion (Dolcos et al., 2011). Given the present focus on spontaneous processing of emotional information in young and older adults, the results reported here resulted from analyses performed on the data collected during the first run, before the induction of the goal to regulate emotions. The results of the emotion regulation manipulation are the focus of a different report.

## SCANNING

fMRI data were recorded using a 1.5 Tesla Siemens Sonata scanner. The anatomical images were 3D MPRAGE anatomical series (repetition time, $TR = 1600$ ms; echo time $TE = 3.82$ ms; field of view, FOV $= 256 \times 256$ mm; number of slices $= 112$; voxel size $= 1 \times 1 \times 1$ mm), and the functional images consisted of series of images acquired axially using an echoplanar sequence ($TR = 2000$ ms; $TE = 40$ ms; FOV $= 256 \times 256$ mm; number of slices $= 28$; voxel size $= 4 \times 4 \times 4$ mm; flip angle $= 90°$; T2*-weighted images), thus allowing for full-brain coverage. Stimuli were projected on a screen directly behind the participant's head within the scanner, which participants viewed through a mirror. Responses were recorded using a 4-button response box placed under the participant's right hand; ratings 5–8 were indicated by the participants with double-clicks on buttons 1–4, respectively. Double-clicking to rate the higher-arousing negative pictures (to indicate a rating of 5–8) might lead to higher activation in motor areas, compared to the lower-arousing pictures, which required only one button click (ratings of 1–4). However, analyses looking at this issue showed no significant differences in the motor areas between the high and low arousing pictures in the two groups.

## fMRI DATA ANALYSIS

Standard pre-processing steps included quality assurance, TR alignment, motion correction, co-registration, normalization and smoothing (8 mm full-width half maximum isotropic kernel). Motion parameters calculated during the realignment were included as parameters of no interest to control for movement artifacts. For individual analyses, each event was modeled by the canonical hemodynamic response function (hrf) and its temporal derivative. The hemodynamic response can potentially show age-related differences (for review, see Dennis and Cabeza, 2008), but in the present study these differences were not problematic because we examined the effects of relative activity between task conditions (Buckner et al., 2000; Huettel et al., 2001; St. Jacques et al., 2010). The general linear model, as implemented in SPM2, was used to model the effects of interest and other confounding effects (e.g., magnetic field drift). Individual analyses produced whole-brain activation maps for the contrasts of interest. These individual contrasts were then entered into group-level random-effects analyses, which allowed investigation of the common and dissociating effects of negative and neutral pictures on brain activity engaged by young and older adults.

The main goal of the study was to investigate age-related differences in the neural correlates of evaluating emotional information with different levels of arousal. The focus was on the role of regions involved in basic emotion processing (amygdala) and emotion control (ACC/vmPFC). To accomplish this goal, analyses were performed to identify the common set of brain regions engaged by both young and older adults, through conjunction analyses. To examine our a priori hypothesis regarding the amygdala, we used anatomical ROI masks derived from the Wake Forest University Pick Atlas toolbox (Dolcos et al., 2004). For the amygdala, an intensity threshold of $p < 0.05$ uncorrected and an extent threshold of five contiguous voxels were used. The conjunction map for the amygdala was defined as $[(\text{Negative}_{\text{Old}} > \text{Neutral}_{\text{Old}}) \cap (\text{Negative}_{\text{Young}} > \text{Neutral}_{\text{Young}})]$, and calculated using the ImCalc feature in SPM. Thus, the conjoint probability of the conjunction map for the amygdala was 0.0025 (Fisher, 1950). In this context, we would like to emphasize the advantages of using the conjunction procedures. The conjunction procedure was performed using the Minimum Statistic compared to the Conjunction Null (MS/CN; Nichols et al., 2005), where a voxel/cluster only survives if it is significant in each independent map included in the conjunction analysis. While corrections for multiple comparisons, such as false discovery rate (FDR) and family-wise error rate (FWER), offer conservative approaches to controlling for Type I errors, they are (especially FWER) prone to Type II errors (Lieberman and Cunningham, 2009). Therefore, when used in conjunction, the statistical and extent thresholds used for the current analyses offer the best balance between Type I and II errors and result in a statistical value that is within the acceptable criterion for publication (Forman et al., 1995; Lieberman and Cunningham, 2009).

Further analyses were performed to identify dissociable sets of brain regions showing greater sensitivity to negative than to neutral pictures across groups, using ANOVAs and two-sample $t$-tests. Analyses were also performed separately for the low, medium and high arousing negative stimuli. Finally, to further elucidate the role of the brain regions showing age-related differences in response to negative and neutral stimuli, brain-behavior relations were investigated by examining co-variations of their neural responses with behavioral ratings. Behavioral measures were correlated with mean statistics after identifying clusters of activation at the group level. For all analyses, an intensity threshold of $p < 0.005$ uncorrected and an extent threshold of 10 contiguous voxels were used, except for the amygdala where an intensity threshold of $p < 0.05$ and an extent threshold of five contiguous voxels were used. An intensity threshold of $p < 0.005$ uncorrected coupled with an extent threshold of 10 voxels is typically considered a good trade-off between Type I and Type II errors (Lieberman and Cunningham, 2009). We also corrected for multiple comparisons in two ways. We applied two levels of FDR corrections: one corresponding to a $p$-value of 0.05 for each anatomical ROI (see **Table 3**), and the other corresponding to a $p$-value of 0.05 for each functional cluster.

## RESULTS

### BEHAVIORAL RESULTS

#### *Reduced ratings to low arousing negative pictures in older adults*

First, a Valence (Negative and Neutral) × Age Group (Young and Older) repeated-measures ANOVA with Valence as a within-subject factor and Age Group as a between-subjects factor revealed a main effect of Valence [$F_{(1, 32)} = 247.38, p < 0.001$]. The Valence × Age Group [$F_{(1, 32)} = 1.66$, $p = 0.21$] interaction was not significant. Second, separate analyses showed the expected effect of valence, with the negative pictures being rated as more negative than the neutral pictures, both by the young ($t = 17.28, p < 0.001$) and the older ($t = 7.97, p < 0.001$) adults. Third, an Arousal (Negative Low, Medium, and High) × Age Group (Young and Older) repeated-measures ANOVA with Arousal as a within-subject factor and Age Group as a between-subjects factor revealed a main effect of Arousal [$F_{(1, 32)} = 46.86$, $p < 0.001$]. The Arousal × Age Group [$F_{(1, 32)} = 0.77, p = 0.47$] interaction was not significant. Fourth, planned comparisons revealed a trend in the age-related comparison of low-arousing negative pictures, consistent with our first prediction that the ratings for low-arousing negative pictures will be lower in the older ($M = 3.88, SD = 1.19$) than in the young ($M = 4.62, SD = 1.29$) adults ($t = 1.72$, $p = 0.096$; one-tailed $p = 0.048$). There were no age-related differences in the ratings for the high and medium arousing negative pictures, nor in the ratings for the neutral pictures (see **Table 2**). Analyses also showed no age-related differences in the ratings for Negative High vs. Negative Low, and Negative Medium vs. Negative Low.

### fMRI RESULTS

#### *Common engagement of the amygdala in young and older groups driven by high arousing stimuli*

Conjunction analyses of brain activity associated with the evaluation of negative and neutral pictures identified an area in the right amygdala that was commonly engaged by both age groups (see **Table 3**; **Figure 1**). Consistent with previous evidence showing common engagement of the amygdala to negative compared to neutral stimuli by both age-groups (St. Jacques et al., 2010), we did not find significant differences in this region in an ANOVA examining Valence (Negative and Neutral) × Age Group (Young and Older) interaction. Analyses looking at the effect of arousal revealed that the common engagement of the right amygdala in the two age-groups was driven by the high arousing negative stimuli, which also activated left amygdala in both groups. Further analyses identified amygdala activation to low, medium, and high arousing negative stimuli in younger adults, but only to high and medium arousing negative stimuli in older adults. However, there were no overlapping areas in the brain regions engaged by the low and medium arousing pictures. The Arousal (NegLo vs. NeuAll, NegMed vs. NeuAll, and NegHi vs. NeuAll) × Age Group (Young and Older) interaction was not significant in the amygdala region commonly engaged by young and older adults in response to negative compared to neutral pictures, but it was significant ($F = 4.55$, $p < 0.05$) for the peak voxel showing decreased amygdala activity to low-arousing stimuli in the older compared to young adults (discussed below). Although the interaction was not significant in the amygdala region commonly

**Table 2 | Behavioral ratings for young and older groups.**

| | Age group | | $t$ | $p$ |
|---|---|---|---|---|
| | Young ($n = 18$) | Older ($n = 16$) | | |
| NegHi | 6.55 (1.08) | 5.68 (1.82) | 1.68 | 0.106 |
| NegMed | 5.58 (1.38) | 5.18 (1.59) | 0.80 | 0.425 |
| NegLo | 4.62 (1.29) | 3.89 (1.19) | 1.72 | 0.096 |
| *NegAll* | *5.59 (1.11)* | *4.91 (1.39)* | 1.56 | 0.128 |
| *NeuAll* | *1.88 (0.55)* | *1.77 (0.60)* | 0.55 | 0.584 |

*Values before parentheses indicate the means. Values in parentheses indicate standard deviations. Reported p-values are two-tailed.*

**Table 3 | Common amygdala activity for negative vs. neutral stimuli.**

| Brain region | *H* | Voxels | Talairach coordinates | | | *t* |
|---|---|---|---|---|---|---|
| | | | *x* | *y* | *z* | |
| **YOUNG ∩ OLDER (NegAll vs. NeuAll)** | | | | | | |
| Amygdala | R | 6 | 28 | −1 | −20 | **3.86** |
| **YOUNG ∩ OLDER (NegHi vs. NeuAll)** | | | | | | |
| Amygdala | L | 6 | −20 | −5 | −17 | **3.98** |
| Amygdala | R | 22 | 16 | −5 | −17 | **3.11*** |
| | | | 28 | −1 | −20 | **2.86*** |

*H, Hemisphere. t-values represent the multiplied score from the conjunction analysis of young and older groups. Bolded t-values indicate the voxels surviving a voxel-level threshold of p < 0.05 (FDR-corrected). *Denotes significant difference at a cluster-level threshold of p < 0.05 (FDR-corrected).*

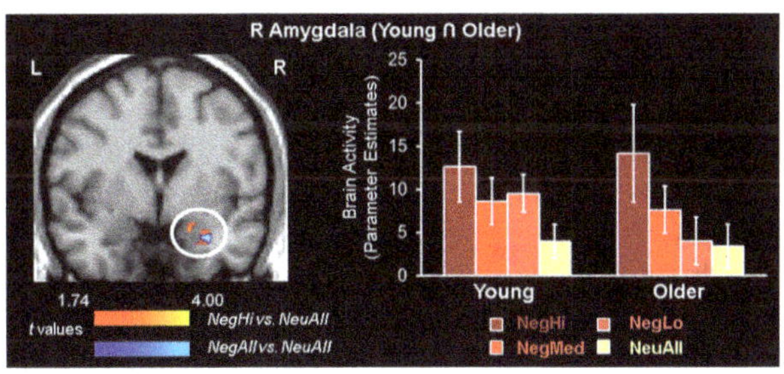


**FIGURE 1 | Common amygdala activation for high arousing stimuli in young and older adults.** Common engagement of the right amygdala by young and older groups was identified using conjunction analysis based on a region of interest approach, where both young and older groups showed common activity for negative vs. neutral (blue area) and high arousing negative vs. neutral (red area) stimuli ($p = 0.0025$). The bar graph illustrates the parameter estimates corresponding to the peak voxel in the area of R AMY commonly activated by young and older adults for NegAll vs. NeuAll contrast. L, left; R, right; NegHi, Negative High Arousal; NegMed, Negative Medium Arousal; NegLo, Negative Low Arousal; NegAll, Negative All; NeuAll, Neutral All.

engaged by young and older adults in response to negative compared to neutral pictures, our findings are still consistent with the idea that the overlap is more likely to occur in high-arousing stimuli, and with our prediction that amygdala activity will be associated with minimal age-related differences for high arousing negative stimuli, but will show age-related differences for the low-arousing negative stimuli. This differential impact is also reflected in the results of the follow-up pairwise comparisons showing age-related differences in the amygdala to low, but not to medium and high arousing negative pictures. *T*-tests comparing amygdala activation to high arousing negative stimuli revealed reduced activity to the high arousing negative pictures in temporal, occipital, parietal, and cingulate areas, and to the medium arousing pictures in occipital areas (see **Table 4**) in older compared to the young adults. In addition to the right amygdala, high arousing stimuli also engaged a common area in the extra striate cortex (Talairach coordinates: $x = 48$, $y = -74$, $z = 7$), in both young and older adults. As described below, low arousing pictures were associated with different patterns of activity in young and older adults.

#### *Opposing spontaneous responses in rostral/ventral ACC and amygdala activity in older adults driven by low-arousing pictures*

Confirming our third prediction, targeted two-sample *t*-tests revealed an age-related increase to low arousing stimuli in the rostral/ventral ACC (**Tables 4, 5**). In older adults this region showed activation, whereas in young adults it showed deactivation. Deactivation in this area is not surprising, as a variety of previous fMRI studies have shown that deactivation in medial frontal areas is rather common during tasks that entail goal-directed behavior (Frankenstein et al., 2003). Deactivations in this region typically occur when resources are allocated to other brain regions, possibly to facilitate task-relevant processing (Frankenstein et al., 2003). Importantly, this region partially overlapped with the ACC region showing a significant Arousal × Age Group interaction ($F = 12.70$, $p < 0.005$). Targeted two-sample *t*-tests also revealed an age-related decrease in the bilateral amygdala activity, for the low arousing pictures (see **Figure 2**). Moreover, the peak voxel showing decreased amygdala activity to low arousing stimuli in older compared to the young adults also survived the Arousal × Age Group interaction ($F = 4.55$, $p < 0.05$). As illustrated in **Figure 2**, rostral/ventral ACC activation was significant only for the older group, whereas the amygdala activation was significant only for the young group. In addition, young adults showed increased activity in frontal, temporal, and occipital areas (see **Table 4**).

#### *Age-related increased activity in ventral ACC/ventromedial PFC was linked to lower ratings for low arousing negative stimuli*

Co-variations of activity in the vACC/vmPFC with the behavioral ratings further elucidated the role played by this region in the evaluation of low arousing stimuli in older adults (see **Figure 3**). As illustrated in the figure, the vACC/vmPFC (Talairach coordinates: $x = 0$, $y = 38$, $z = -9$) activity was negatively correlated with the ratings for low arousing negative pictures in the older adults ($r = -0.72$, $p < 0.005$). That is, older participants who engaged this region when processing low arousing negative pictures also rated those pictures as less negative. Of note, portions of the vACC/vmPFC showing the negative co-variation with ratings for low arousing pictures in older adults partially overlapped with the vACC/vmPFC area showing stronger response to low arousing negative stimuli in older, compared to the young adults. The correlation between vACC/vmPFC and ratings was specific to ratings for low arousing negative pictures in older adults, as indicated by the significant difference between this correlation and the similar correlation for the young group (using the *r* to *z* transformation, $z = -4.06$, $p < 0.0001$). There were no other significant correlations between the vACC/vmPFC and ratings. The significant co-variations between other brain areas and behavioral ratings are presented in **Table 6**.

## DISCUSSION

Despite substantial evidence supporting the idea of enhanced affective well-being and emotional stability in healthy aging, relatively little is known about the role of emotional arousal in this effect and the underlying brain mechanisms. The current study addressees this gap in the emotional aging literature by investigating the effect of emotional arousal on behavioral and neural responses in young and older adults. There were three main novel findings regarding the neural correlates. First, we showed that the common engagement of the right amygdala in young and older adults was driven by high arousing stimuli. Second, we showed that the opposing spontaneous pattern of increased activity in the rostral/ventral ACC and decreased activity in the right amygdala is specific to low arousing stimuli. Third, we linked the increased spontaneous activity in the vACC/vmPFC to older adults' reduced ratings for low arousing stimuli. These findings are discussed below.

### COMMON ENGAGEMENT OF THE AMYGDALA IN YOUNG AND OLDER GROUPS DRIVEN BY HIGH AROUSING STIMULI

The present study revealed that right amygdala activation in older adults had overlapping areas with that from younger adults, thus showing that both groups involve the same amygdala regions to process negative stimuli. Moreover, the present study advances previous findings (St. Jacques et al., 2010) by showing that the common engagement of the right amygdala is driven by high arousing stimuli. Decreased amygdala activity to low arousing stimuli in older adults might be attributed to a potential deterioration of this brain structure with age. However, our finding showing similar amygdala engagement by high arousing stimuli in both age groups provides evidence against such a hypothesis and confirms previous evidence showing that amygdala activity is preserved with age. Increased amygdala activation by high arousing negative emotional stimuli is consistent with previous behavioral findings suggesting that emotion processing is not impaired in aging (Mather and Knight, 2006), and with brain imaging evidence showing that aging is associated with robust functional activation of the amygdala (Wright et al., 2006; St. Jacques et al., 2010). Increased amygdala activation in response to high arousing stimuli is also consistent with previous behavioral evidence (Kensinger, 2008) showing minimal age-differences for high arousing stimuli (but identifying age-related differences for low arousing stimuli).

**Table 4 | Dissociable brain activity for negative vs. neutral stimuli by arousal levels in young and older adults.**

| Contrast | Brain region | BA | *H* | Voxels | Talairach coordinates | | | *t* |
|---|---|---|---|---|---|---|---|---|
| | | | | | *x* | *y* | *z* | |
| **YOUNG > OLDER** | | | | | | | | |
| **High arousal (NegHi vs. NeuAll)** | | | | | | | | |
| | Cuneus | 18 | R | 26 | 12 | −85 | 19 | 4.26 |
| | | | | | 8 | −92 | 19 | 3.71 |
| | Precuneus | 19 | R | 12 | 28 | −60 | 36 | 3.94 |
| | Middle temporal gyrus | 19 | R | 21 | 48 | −61 | 14 | 3.85 |
| | Cingulate gyrus | 32 | L | 17 | −4 | 17 | 32 | 3.69 |
| | Postcentral gyrus | 2 | R | 10 | 51 | −21 | 42 | 3.66 |
| | Middle temporal gyrus | 19 | L | 18 | −44 | −61 | 14 | 3.60 |
| | Middle temporal gyrus | 37 | | | −51 | −62 | 3 | 2.83 |
| **Medium arousal (NegMed vs. NeuAll)** | | | | | | | | |
| | Middle occipital gyrus | 18 | L | 21 | −32 | −89 | 4 | 3.47 |
| | | | | | −24 | −89 | 15 | 3.38 |
| **Low arousal (NegLo vs. NeuAll)** | | | | | | | | |
| | Amygdala | 34 | L | 11 | −20 | −1 | −10 | 2.49* |
| | | | | | −32 | −5 | −17 | 2.10* |
| | Amygdala | 28 | R | 18 | 16 | −4 | −10 | 2.44* |
| | | 34 | | | 28 | 3 | −14 | 1.96* |
| | Inferior frontal gyrus | 47 | R | 34 | 44 | 11 | −4 | 4.81 |
| | Superior temporal gyrus | 41 | R | 13 | 40 | −35 | 9 | 4.02 |
| | | | | | 48 | −31 | 5 | 3.17 |
| | | | | | 40 | −38 | 16 | 2.82 |
| | Middle temporal gyrus | 39 | R | 23 | 48 | −61 | 21 | 3.85 |
| | | | | | 44 | −54 | 14 | 3.31 |
| | | | | | 48 | −62 | 10 | 2.99 |
| | Superior frontal gyrus | 9 | R | 26 | 40 | 40 | 31 | 3.79 |
| | | | | | 16 | 52 | 38 | 3.78 |
| | | | | | 4 | 56 | 38 | 3.67 |
| | Superior frontal gyrus | 9 | L | 22 | −28 | 52 | 34 | 3.77 |
| | | | | | −12 | 52 | 38 | 3.62 |
| | Middle occipital gyrus | 19 | L | 14 | −28 | −77 | 11 | 3.75 |
| | | | | | −32 | −85 | 8 | 3.43 |
| | | | | | −24 | −89 | 15 | 3.09 |
| | Inferior frontal gyrus | 47 | L | 20 | −48 | 42 | −9 | 3.75 |
| | | | | | −51 | 30 | −5 | 2.94 |
| | | | | | −55 | 35 | 2 | 2.86 |
| | Middle frontal gyrus | 8 | R | 32 | 36 | 22 | 47 | 3.68 |
| | | | | | 48 | 21 | 39 | 3.67 |
| | | | | | 32 | 6 | 58 | 3.25 |
| | Superior temporal gyrus | 38 | L | 40 | −44 | 11 | −14 | 3.64 |
| | | | | | −40 | 23 | −11 | 3.47 |
| | | | | | −51 | 7 | −7 | 3.32 |
| **OLDER > YOUNG** | | | | | | | | |
| **Low arousal (NegLo vs. NeuAll)** | | | | | | | | |
| | Anterior cingulate gyrus | 32 | L | 39 | −16 | 36 | 13 | **4.22** |
| | | | | | −12 | 43 | −2 | 2.42 |
| | | 32 | R | 8 | 8 | 40 | 16 | 1.88 |

*BA, Brodmann's area; H, Hemisphere. A threshold of $p < 0.005$ (uncorrected) was used. Bolded t-values indicate the voxels surviving a cluster-level threshold of $p < 0.05$ (FDR-corrected). *Denotes significant difference at $p < 0.05$ (uncorrected).*

**Table 5 | Mean parameter estimates for peak voxel activity in anterior cingulate cortex (ACC) and amygdala (AMY) for young and older groups.**

| Brain region | | Age group | |
|---|---|---|---|
| | | Young ($n$ = 18) | Older ($n$ = 16) |
| ACC | NegHi | 1.35 (1.42) | −4.93 (2.27) |
| | NegMed | −4.91 (2.08) | −3.08 (1.98) |
| | NegLo | −4.29 (1.48) | 2.39 (1.35) |
| | NeuAll | −1.78 (1.83) | −4.68 (1.60) |
| AMY | NegHi | 22.93 (7.18) | 12.88 (4.92) |
| | NegMed | 15.18 (5.07) | 2.34 (4.34) |
| | NegLo | 15.83 (4.44) | −0.93 (3.96) |
| | NeuAll | 6.74 (2.29) | 4.12 (3.20) |

*Values before parentheses indicate the means. Values in parentheses indicate the standard errors of the means. The mean parameter estimates were extracted in each of the four conditions against the baseline activity for each age group at the coordinates corresponding to the peak voxels for each of the ACC and AMY regions showing overlapping activity between (1) the Arousal × Age Group interaction and (2) the two-sample t-test targeting low arousing stimuli.*

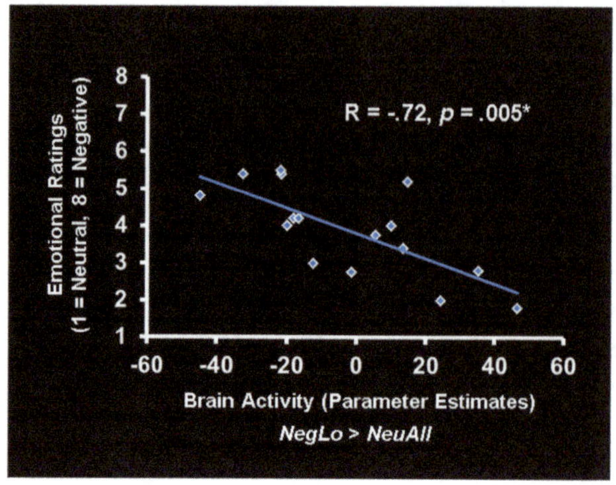


**FIGURE 3 | Activity in the ACC was linked to reduced ratings for low-arousing stimuli in older adults.** In older adults, increased activity in the ventral anterior cingulate cortex (vACC)/ventro-medial prefrontal cortex (vmPFC) correlated negatively with the ratings for low arousing negative stimuli. The scatterplot is based on the parameter estimates corresponding to the peak voxel in the area of vACC/vmPFC showing negative correlation with the behavioral ratings. NegLo, Negative Low Arousal; NeuAll, Neutral All.

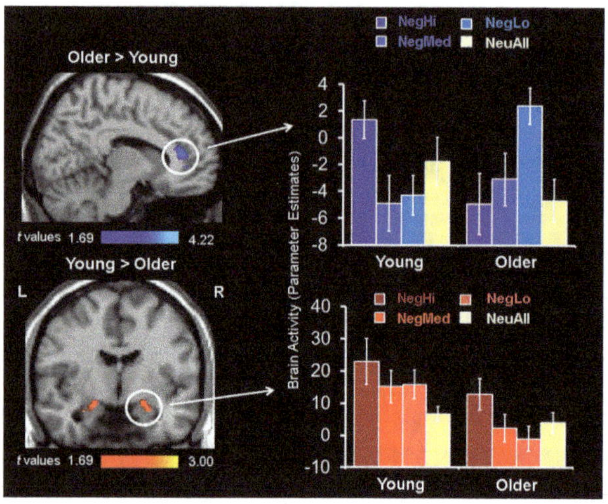


**FIGURE 2 | Opposing patterns of response in rostral/ventral ACC and AMY for low arousing stimuli.** Increased activity in rostral/ventral ACC (top sagittal image), and decreased activity in the amygdala (bottom coronal image) in older compared to young adults was identified using two-sample $t$-tests between activation maps for NegLo vs. NeuAll contrast in the two groups. The bar graphs on the right illustrate the parameter estimates corresponding to the peak voxels in the area of ACC and AMY showing increased activity to low arousing negative stimuli in the young and older groups. L, left; R, right; NegHi, Negative Hi Arousal; NegMed, Negative Medium Arousal; NegLo, Negative Low Arousal; NeuAll, Neutral All.

The present results are also in line with more recent theories of emotional aging (cognitive control model: Mather and Carstensen, 2005), which suggest that the relatively preserved emotional well-being in older adults is the result of age-related differences in the controlled processing of emotional information, and that processing of high arousing stimuli is less dependent on controlled processing compared to low arousing stimuli (Kensinger, 2008). Therefore, if the emotional well-being is caused by age-related declines in the controlled processing of emotional information, evaluation of low arousing stimuli, which relies more on controlled processes, would be more affected than the evaluation of the high arousing stimuli, which relies more on automatic processes. Given that (a) amygdala is involved in processing stimulus relevance for the goals and motivations of the perceiver (Cunningham and Brosch, 2012) and (b) right amygdala is involved in the initial, rapid, possibly automatic detection of an emotional stimulus (Gläscher and Adolphs, 2003), then (c) our results showing bilateral amygdala engagement in the evaluation of high arousing stimuli by both age groups suggest that this type of stimuli are automatically detected by both groups because of their increased personal relevance. The present findings showing dissociable responses in the commonly activated amygdala based on the level of arousal suggest that the age-related differences identified in previous studies may not be caused by an overall decline in the amygdala functioning, but rather by age-related changes in the intensity of the emotional stimuli to which amygdala is more receptive.

### OPPOSING SPONTANEOUS RESPONSES IN ROSTRAL/VENTRAL ACC AND AMYGDALA ACTIVITY IN OLDER ADULTS SPECIFIC TO LOW-AROUSING PICTURES

The present study also advances previous findings by showing that the age-related differences in the engagement of amygdala and rostral/ventral ACC are specific to low arousing negative stimuli. Older adults' reduced amygdala activation to low arousing negative pictures can be the consequence of many factors,

**Table 6 | Co-variations between brain activity and the ratings of negative pictures by young and older adults.**

| (Contrast) × Ratings | *r* value | Brain region | BA | *H* | Voxels | Talairach coordinates | | | *t* |
|---|---|---|---|---|---|---|---|---|---|
| | | | | | | *x* | *y* | *z* | |
| **YOUNG** | | | | | | | | | |
| (NegHi vs. NeuAll) × NegHi | −0.668 | Inferior frontal gyrus | 47 | L | 10 | −20 | 31 | −5 | 3.59 |
| (NegLo vs. NeuAll) × NegLo | −0.726 | Parahippocampal gyrus | 35 | L | 14 | −20 | −35 | −5 | 4.22 |
| **OLDER** | | | | | | | | | |
| (NegHi vs. NeuAll) × NegHi | +0.803 | Precuneus | 7 | L | 56 | −4 | −53 | 43 | 5.04 |
| | +0.770 | | | | | 0 | −45 | 28 | 4.52 |
| | +0.705 | | 7 | R | | 12 | −52 | 43 | 3.72 |
| | +0.778 | Precentral gyrus | 9 | L | 12 | −36 | 21 | 39 | 4.64 |
| | +0.769 | Superior parietal lobule | 7 | R | 16 | 28 | −68 | 44 | 4.50 |
| | +0.746 | Precuneus | 7 | L | 10 | −12 | −59 | 55 | 4.19 |
| | +0.722 | | | | | −12 | −68 | 51 | 3.90 |
| | +0.707 | Medial frontal gyrus | 8 | | 12 | 0 | 45 | 38 | 3.74 |
| | +0.707 | | | | | 0 | 56 | 30 | 3.74 |
| | +0.669 | Medial frontal gyrus | 9 | L | | −4 | 40 | 31 | 3.37 |
| | +0.690 | Superior frontal gyrus | 9 | L | 14 | −8 | 60 | 26 | 3.57 |
| | +0.679 | | | R | | 8 | 63 | 15 | 3.45 |
| (NegMed vs. NeuAll) × NegMed | −0.819 | Inferior parietal lobule | 40 | L | 11 | −40 | −29 | 42 | 5.34 |
| | −0.686 | | | | | −28 | −37 | 42 | 3.52 |
| | −0.797 | Precentral gyrus | 6 | R | 10 | 32 | −9 | 56 | 4.94 |
| | −0.783 | Precentral gyrus | 6 | L | 26 | −24 | −10 | 52 | 4.70 |
| | −0.699 | | | | | −16 | −1 | 55 | 3.65 |
| | −0.699 | | | | | −24 | −1 | 48 | 3.65 |
| | −0.777 | Precentral gyrus | 6 | L | 13 | −55 | −2 | 41 | 4.62 |
| | −0.774 | Precuneus | 7 | R | 26 | 8 | −59 | 62 | 4.58 |
| | −0.668 | | | | | 4 | −56 | 51 | 3.35 |
| | −0.751 | Precuneus | 7 | L | 11 | −28 | −71 | 55 | 4.25 |
| | −0.749 | Caudate nucleus | | R | 20 | 4 | 8 | 0 | 4.23 |
| | −0.711 | | | L | | −4 | 4 | −4 | 3.79 |
| | −0.739 | Lentiform nucleus | | R | 19 | 20 | −4 | 8 | 4.11 |
| | −0.712 | Inferior parietal lobule | 40 | L | 21 | −44 | −36 | 57 | 3.79 |
| | −0.700 | | | | | −40 | −47 | 61 | 2.67 |
| | −0.710 | Superior temporal gyrus | 22 | R | 10 | 60 | −7 | 8 | 3.77 |
| | −0.708 | | | | | 51 | 4 | 7 | 3.75 |
| | −0.675 | | | | | 48 | 5 | 15 | 3.43 |
| (NegLo vs. NeuAll) × NegLo | +0.750 | Insula | 13 | R | 12 | 28 | −26 | 23 | 4.24 |
| | +0.743 | | | | | 36 | −45 | 28 | 4.22 |
| | +0.767 | | | | | 32 | −34 | 24 | 4.04 |
| | +0.711 | Supramarginal gyrus | 40 | L | 11 | −44 | −45 | 32 | 4.16 |
| | +0.653 | Superior frontal gyrus | 8 | R | 10 | 4 | 37 | 46 | 3.53 |
| (NegLo vs. NeuAll) × NegLo | −0.577 | Anterior cingulate | 32 | R | 7 | 0 | 38 | −9 | 4.11 |

*BA, Brodmann's area; H, Hemisphere. A threshold of $p < 0.005$ (uncorrected) was used.*

including an age-related atrophy in neural systems important for processing negative stimuli, age-related decreases in psychophysiological responses to arousing stimuli (Tsai et al., 2000), or an age-related decline in the amygdala, which selectively diminishes emotional arousal in response to negative stimuli and decreases the experienced negative affect (the aging brain model; Cacioppo et al., 2011). However, in the present study, the decreased bilateral amygdala activity was accompanied by increased activity in the rostral/ventral ACC in older compared to the young adults. This opposing pattern of brain activity is consistent with previous findings showing decreased amygdala activity coupled with increased activity in cortical control regions during the perception and evaluation of negative stimuli (anterior ventral insula; Fischer et al., 2005; ventral and medial PFC; Tessitore et al., 2005), and with greater functional connectivity between the right amygdala and ACC in older compared to young adults (St. Jacques et al., 2010). Moreover, a similar region has shown a negative correlation with right amygdala on trials in which older adults subjectively experienced negative pictures (according to the IAPS standardized norms) as neutral, but not for negative pictures subjectively rated as negative (St. Jacques et al., 2010). This suggests a role of this region in reducing amygdala activity when regulation is successful. This evidence, together with our findings, indicate that older adults' reduced amygdala activation to low arousing pictures may be the result of their successful emotion regulation of this type of stimuli.

Taken together, our findings show enhanced activity in an emotional control region, the rostral/ventral ACC, coupled with decreased bilateral amygdala activity to low arousing negative stimuli, in a task in which participants were not explicitly instructed to down-regulate their emotional responses. This may reflect older adults' spontaneous engagement of emotion control regions to down-regulate low arousing negative emotions. Moreover, the negative association between vACC/vmPFC and behavioral ratings for low arousing stimuli, discussed below, reflects their success in regulating low arousing negative emotions. These results support the idea that older adults may have emotion regulation chronically activated (Mather and Carstensen, 2005; Nashiro et al., 2012), and that this effect is specific to low arousing negative emotions.

### AGE-RELATED INCREASED ACTIVITY IN VENTRAL ACC/VENTROMEDIAL PFC LINKED TO LOWER RATINGS FOR LOW AROUSING STIMULI

Ventromedial PFC and the ACC play an important role in processing emotional information, and are particularly involved in the automatic regulation of emotional responses (for reviews see Bush et al., 2000; Phillips et al., 2003) during incidental emotion regulation paradigms, such as affect labeling and self-distraction from a fear-conditioning stimulus (Lieberman et al., 2007). Unlike other frontal regions, which thin dramatically with aging (Fjell et al., 2009), vmPFC/ACC maintain their cortical thickness in normal aging, which suggests that some of the neural circuitry critical for emotion regulation is well preserved in older adults. In the present study, evaluation of low arousing negative stimuli was associated with increased vACC/vmPFC activity in older compared to the young adults. Moreover, activity in these areas was negatively associated with the behavioral ratings for low arousing stimuli in older adults, further supporting a role of this region in effective spontaneous regulation of this type of emotions.

Although our study contributes important novel information, it also has some limitations. One limitation concerns the size of our subject sample in the older group, which although allowed identification of robust findings, was slightly smaller than the optimal fMRI sample size of 18 suggested for investigations of brain-behavior relations (Lieberman et al., 2009). However, the size of our samples was comparable to that involved in other investigations of age-related differences (e.g., St. Jacques et al., 2010). Although we took measures to minimize multiple comparisons, we recognize the importance of replicating the findings in a larger sample. There were also different age-spans in the young (14 years) and the older (25 years) groups, which potentially could have led to greater variance in the older adults group. Finally, involving only negative stimuli and manipulating only the level of arousal limits the generalizability of our results to negative stimuli with different degrees of arousal. Future studies should investigate whether the effects identified in the present study are confirmed for positive stimuli and in investigations that manipulate independently emotional valence and arousal.

## CONCLUSION

In the present study, we examined the effect of arousal as a potential factor influencing the enhanced affective well-being and emotional stability commonly associated with healthy aging. There were three novel findings regarding the neural correlates of emotion processing: (a) right amygdala was commonly engaged by young and older adults only during the evaluation of high arousing stimuli, (b) amygdala and rostral/ventral ACC showed an opposing pattern of activity for low arousing stimuli in older compared to young adults, and (c) the engagement of the ventral ACC/vmPFC in older adults reflected successful regulation of low arousing negative stimuli. These findings highlight the important effect of arousal on age-related emotional processing, suggesting that aging is associated with preserved emotional processing of high arousing negative information, and with altered processing of low arousing negative information. By showing that older adults engage more automatic processes when evaluating high arousing negative information, and more controlled, resource-demanding processes in response to low arousing negative information, the present study advances our understanding of the neural correlates underlying the enhanced emotional well-being in healthy aging. Moreover, by linking the spontaneous engagement of the emotion control regions in older adults to reduced subjective experiencing of low arousing negative information, the present study provides further evidence supporting the idea that emotion regulation is chronically activated in healthy aging, and clarifies that this effect is specific to low arousing negative information. This new evidence highlights the need of adopting a comprehensive approach that takes into consideration both the valence and arousal in examining emotional aging.

## ACKNOWLEDGMENTS

This research was supported by funds from the Brain & Behavior Research Foundation (formerly NARSAD), Healthy Minds Canada (formerly CPRF), and the University of Alberta. The authors were supported by NIH R01 grant AG008235 from the National Institutes of Health (National Institute on Aging) (Roger A. Dixon and Sanda Dolcos), the Canada Research Chairs program (Roger A. Dixon), the University of Alberta (Sanda Dolcos and Roger A. Dixon), and the University of Illinois (Sanda Dolcos). The authors wish to thank Keen Sung, Trisha Chakrabarty, and Kristina Suen for assistance with data collection and analysis, and to Florin Dolcos for feedback on an earlier version of the manuscript.

## REFERENCES

Allen, J. S., Bruss, J., Brown, C. K., and Damasio, H. (2005). Normal neuroanatomical variation due to age: the major lobes and a parcellation of the temporal region. *Neurobiol. Aging* 26, 1245–1260. doi: 10.1016/j.neurobiolaging.2005.05.023

Anderson, A. K., and Phelps, E. A. (1998). Intact recognition of vocal expressions of fear following bilateral lesions of the human amygdala. *Neuroreport* 9, 3607–3613.

Backs, R. W., da Silva, S. P., and Han, K. (2005). A comparison of younger and older adults' self-assessment manikin ratings of affective pictures. *Exp. Aging Res.* 31, 421–440. doi: 10.1080/03610730500206808

Blanchard-Fields, F., Stein, R., and Watson, T. L. (2004). Age differences in emotion-regulation strategies in handling everyday problems. *J. Gerontol. B Psychol. Sci. Soc. Sci.* 59, 261–269. doi: 10.1093/geronb/59.6.P261

Brabec, J., Rulseh, A., Hoyt, B., Vizek, M., Horinek, D., Hort, J., et al. (2010). Volumetry of the human amygdala—an anatomical study. *Psychiatry Res.* 182, 67–72. doi: 10.1016/j.pscychresns.2009.11.005

Bradley, M. M., and Lang, P. J. (2000). "Measuring emotion: behavior, feeling, and physiology," in *Cognitive Neuroscience of Emotion*, eds R. D. Lane and L. Nadel (New York, NY: Oxford University Press), 242–276.

Bradley, M. M., and Lang, P. J. (2007). "Emotion and motivation," in *Handbook of Psychophysiology*, 3rd Edn., eds J. T. Cacioppo, L. G. Tassinary, and G. Berntson (New York, NY: Cambridge University Press), 581–607.

Buckner, R. L., Snyder, A. Z., Sanders, A. L., Raichle, M. E., and Morris, J. C. (2000). Functional brain imaging of young, nondemented, and demented older adults. *J. Cogn. Neurosci.* 12, 24–34. doi: 10.1162/089892900564046

Bush, G., Luu, P., and Posner, M. I. (2000). Cognitive and emotional influences in anterior cingulate cortex. *Trends Cogn. Sci.* 4, 215–222. doi: 10.1016/S1364-6613(00)01483-2

Cacioppo, J. T., Berntson, G. G., Bechara, A., Tranel, D., and Hawkley, L. C. (2011). "Could an aging brain contribute to subjective well-being? The value added by a social neuroscience perspective," in *Social Neuroscience: Toward Understanding the Underpinnings of the Social Mind*, eds A. Todorov, S. Fiske, and D. Prentice (New York, NY: Oxford University Press), 249–262.

Charles, S. T., Mather, M., and Carstensen, L. L. (2003). Aging and emotional memory: the forgettable nature of negative images for older adults. *J. Exp. Psychol. Gen.* 132, 310–324. doi: 10.1037/0096-3445.132.2.310

Cunningham, W. A., and Brosch, T. (2012). Motivational salience: amygdala tuning from traits, needs, values, and goals. *Curr. Dir. Psychol. Sci.* 21, 54–59. doi: 10.1177/0963721411430832

Dennis, N. A., and Cabeza, R. (2008). "Neuroimaging of healthy cognitive aging," in *The Handbook of Aging and Cognition*, 3rd Edn., eds F. I. M. Craik and T. A. Salthouse (Mahwah, NJ: Lawrence Erlbaum Associates), 1–54.

Desmond, J. E., and Glover, G. H. (2002). Estimating sample size in functional MRI (fMRI) neuroimaging studies: statistical power analyses. *J. Neurosci. Methods* 118, 115–128. doi: 10.1016/S0165-0270(02)00121-8

Dolan, R. J. (2002). Emotion, cognition, and behavior. *Science* 298, 1191–1194. doi: 10.1126/science.1076358

Dolan, R. J., and Vuilleumier, P. (2003). Amygdala automaticity in emotional processing. *Ann. N.Y. Acad. Sci.* 985, 348–355. doi: 10.1111/j.1749-6632.2003.tb07093.x

Dolcos, F., LaBar, K. S., and Cabeza, R. (2004). Interaction between the amygdala and the medial temporal lobe memory system predicts better memory for emotional events. *Neuron* 42, 855–863. doi: 10.1016/S0896-6273(04)00289-2

Dolcos, S., Sung, K., Denkova, E., Dixon, R. A., and Dolcos, F. (2011). Brain imaging investigation of the neural correlates of emotion regulation. *J. Vis. Exp.* 54:2430. doi: 10.3791/2430

Drabant, E. M., McRae, K., Manuck, S. B., Hariri, A. R., and Gross, J. J. (2009). Individual differences in typical reappraisal use predict amygdala and prefrontal responses. *Biol. Psychiatry* 65, 367–373. doi: 10.1016/j.biopsych.2008.09.007

Erk, S., Walter, H., and Abler, B. (2008). Age-related physiological responses to emotion anticipation and exposure. *Neuroreport* 19, 447–452. doi: 10.1097/WNR.0b013e3282f5d92f

Fischer, H., Sandblom, J., Gavazzeni, J., Fransson, P., Wright, C. I., and Backman, L. (2005). Age-differential patterns of brain activation during perception of angry faces. *Neurosci. Lett.* 386, 99–104. doi: 10.1016/j.neulet.2005.06.002

Fisher, R. A. (1950). *Statistical Methods for Research Workers.* London: Oliver and Boyd.

Fjell, A. M., Westlye, L. T., Amlien, I., Espeseth, T., Reinvang, I., Raz, N., et al. (2009). High consistency of regional cortical thinning in aging acrossmultiple samples. *Cereb. Cortex* 19, 2001–2012. doi: 10.1093/cercor/bhn232

Forman, S. D., Cohen, J. D., Fitzgerald, M., Eddy, W. F., Mintun, M. A., and Noll, D. C. (1995). Improved assessment of significant activation in functional magnetic resonance imaging (fMRI): use of a cluster-size threshold. *Magn. Reson. Med.* 33, 636–647. doi: 10.1002/mrm.1910330508

Frankenstein, U., Wennerberg, A., Richter, W., Bernstein, C., Morden, D., Rémy, F., et al. (2003). Activation and deactivation in blood oxygenation level dependent functional magnetic resonance imaging. *Concept. Magnetic Res. Educ. J.* 16A, 63–70. doi: 10.1002/cmr.a.10054

Gläscher, J., and Adolphs, R. (2003). Processing of the arousal of subliminal and supraliminal emotional stimuli by the human amygdala. *J. Neurosci.* 23, 10274–10282. Available online at: http://www.jneurosci.org/content/23/32/10274.full

Gross, J. J., Carstensen, L. L., Pasupathi, M., Tsai, J., Skorpen, C. G., and Hsu, A. Y. C. (1997). Emotion and aging: experience, expression, and control. *Psychol. Aging* 12, 590–599. doi: 10.1037/0882-7974.12.4.590

Gruhn, D., Scheibe, S., and Baltes, P. B. (2007). Reduced negativity effect in older adults' memory for emotional pictures: the heterogeneity-homogeneity list paradigm. *Psychol. Aging* 22, 644–649. doi: 10.1037/0882-7974.22.3.644

Gunning-Dixon, F. M., Gur, R. C., Perkins, A. C., Schroeder, L., Turner, T., Turetsky, B. I., et al. (2003). Age-related differences in brain activation during emotional face processing. *Neurobiol. Aging* 24, 285–295. doi: 10.1016/S0197-4580(02)00099-4

Huettel, S. A., and McCarthy, G. (2001). The effects of single-trial averaging upon the spatial extent of fMRI activation. *Neuroreport* 12, 2411–2416. doi: 10.1097/00001756-200108080-00025

Huettel, S. A., Singerman, J. D., and McCarthy, G. (2001). The effects of aging upon the hemodynamic response measured by functional MRI. *Neuroimage* 13, 161–175. doi: 10.1006/nimg.2000.0675

Iidaka, T., Okada, T., Murata, T., Omori, M., Kosaka, K., Sadato, N., et al. (2002). Age-related differences in the medial temporal lobe responses to emotional faces as revealed by fMRI. *Hippocampus* 12, 352–362. doi: 10.1002/hipo.1113

Isaacowitz, D. M., Wadlinger, H. A., Goren, D., and Wilson, H. R. (2006). Selective preference in visual fixation away from negative images in old age? An eye-tracking study. *Psychol. Aging* 21, 40–48. doi: 10.1037/0882-7974.21.1.40

Ito, T. A., Cacioppo, J. T., and Lang, P. J. (1998). Eliciting affect using the international affective picture system: trajectories through evaluative space. *Pers. Soc. Psychol. Bull.* 24, 855–879. doi: 10.1177/0146167298248006

Keil, A., and Freund, A. M. (2009). Changes in the sensitivity to appetitive and aversive arousal across adulthood. *Psychol. Aging* 24, 668–680. doi: 10.1037/a0016969

Kensinger, E. A. (2008). Age differences in memory for arousing and nonarousing emotional words. *J. Gerontol. Psychol. Sci.* 63, P13–P18. doi: 10.1093/geronb/63.1.P13

Kensinger, E. A., and Corkin, S. (2004). Two routes to emotional memory: distinct neural processes for valence and arousal. *Proc. Natl. Acad. Sci. U.S.A.* 101, 3310–3115. doi: 10.1073/pnas.0306408101

Kryla-Lighthall, N., and Mather, M. (2009). "The role of cognitive control in older adults' emotional well-being," in *Handbook of Theories of Aging*, eds V. Berngtson, D. Gans, N. Putney, and M. Silverstein (New York, NY: Springer Publishing), 323–344.

Lang, P. J. (1995). The emotion probe: studies of motivation and attention. *Am. Psychol.* 50, 372. doi: 10.1037/0003-066X.50.5.372

Lang, P. J., Bradley, M. M., and Cuthbert, B. N. (1992). A motivational analysis of emotion: reflex-cortex connections. *Psychol. Sci.* 3, 44–49. doi: 10.1111/j.1467-9280.1992.tb00255.x

Lang, P. J., Bradley, M. M., and Cuthbert, B. N. (1997). *International Affective Picture System (IAPS): Technical Manual and Affective Ratings.* Gainesville, FL: NIMH, The center for the study of emotion and attention, University of Florida.

Lang, P. J., Bradley, M. M., and Cuthbert, B. N. (1998). Emotion, motivation, and anxiety: brain mechanisms and psychophysiology. *Biol. Psychiatry* 44, 1248–1263. doi: 10.1016/S0006-3223(98)00275-3

Larkin, G. R., Gibbs, S. E., Khanna, K., Nielsen, L., Carstensen, L. L., and Knutson, B. (2007). Anticipation of monetary gain but not loss in healthy older adults. *Nat. Neurosci.* 10, 787–791. doi: 10.1038/nn1894

Leclerc, C. M., and Kensinger, E. A. (2008). Age-related differences in medial prefrontal activation in response to emotional images. *Cogn. Affect. Behav. Neurosci.* 8, 153–164. doi: 10.3758/CABN.8.2.153

Libkuman, T. M., Otani, H., Kern, R., Viger, S. G., and Novak, N. (2007). Multidimensional normative ratings for the international affective picture system. *Behav. Res. Methods* 39, 326–334. doi: 10.3758/BF03193164

Lieberman, M. D., Berkman, E. T., and Wager, T. D. (2009). Correlations in social neuroscience aren't voodoo: a reply to Vul, et al. *Perspect. Psychol. Sci.* 4, 299–307. doi: 10.1111/j.1745-6924.2009.01128.x

Lieberman, M. D., and Cunningham, W. A. (2009). Type I and Type II error concerns in fMRI research: re-balancing the scale. *Soc. Cogn. Affect. Neurosci.* 4, 423–428. doi: 10.1093/scan/nsp052

Lieberman, M. D., Eisenberger, N. I., Crockett, M. J., Tom, S. M., Pfeifer, J. H., and Way, B. M. (2007). Putting feelings into words: affect labeling disrupts amygdala activity to affective stimuli. *Psychol. Sci.* 18, 421–428. doi: 10.1111/j.1467-9280.2007.01916.x

Mather, M., Canli, T., English, T., Whitfield, S., Wais, P., Ochsner, K., et al. (2004). Amygdala responses to emotionally valenced stimuli in older and younger adults. *Psychol. Sci.* 15, 259–263. doi: 10.1111/j.0956-7976.2004.00662.x

Mather, M., and Carstensen, L. L. (2003). Aging and attentional biases for emotional faces. *Psychol. Sci.* 14, 409–415. doi: 10.1111/1467-9280.01455

Mather, M., and Carstensen, L. L. (2005). Aging and motivated cognition: the positivity effect in attention and memory. *Trends Cogn. Sci.* 9, 496–502. doi: 10.1016/j.tics.2005.08.005

Mather, M., and Knight, M. (2005). Goal-directed memory: the role of cognitive control in older adults' emotional memory. *Psychol. Aging* 20, 554–570. doi: 10.1037/0882-7974.20.4.554

Mather, M., and Knight, M. R. (2006). Angry faces get noticed quickly: threat detection is not impaired among older adults. *J. Gerontol. B Psychol. Sci. Soc. Sci.* 61, P54–P57. doi: 10.1093/geronb/61.1.P54

Moriguchi, Y., Negreira, A., Weierich, M., Dautoff, R., Dickerson, B. C., Wright, C. I., et al. (2011). Differential hemodynamic response in affective circuitry with aging: an FMRI study of novelty, valence, and arousal. *J. Cogn. Neurosci.* 23, 1027–1041. doi: 10.1162/jocn.2010.21527

Nashiro, K., Sakaki, M., and Mather, M. (2012). Age differences in brain activity during emotion processing: Reflections of age-related decline or increased emotion regulation? *Gerontology* 58, 156–163. doi: 10.1159/000328465

Nichols, T., Brett, M., Andersson, J., Wager, T., and Poline, J. B. (2005). Valid conjunction inference with the minimum statistic. *Neuroimage* 25, 653–660. doi: 10.1016/j.neuroimage.2004.12.005

Ochsner, K. N., Ray, R. D., Cooper, J. C., Robertson, E. R., Chopra, S., Gabrieli, J. D., et al. (2004). For better or for worse: neural systems supporting the cognitive down- and up-regulation of negative emotion. *Neuroimage* 23, 483–499. doi: 10.1016/j.neuroimage.2004.06.030

Phillips, M. L., Drevets, W. C., Rauch, S. L., and Lane, R. (2003). Neurobiology of emotion perception I: the neural basis of normal emotion perception. *Biol. Psychiatry* 54, 504–514. doi: 10.1016/S0006-3223(03)00168-9

Ribeiro, R. L., Teixeira-Silva, F., Pompéia, S., and Bueno, O. F. A. (2007). IAPS includes photographs that elicit low-arousal physiological responses in healthy volunteers. *Physiol. Behav.* 91, 671–675. doi: 10.1016/j.physbeh.2007.03.031

Roalf, D. R., Pruis, T. A., Stevens, A. A., and Janowsky, J. S. (2011). More is less: emotion induced prefrontal cortex activity habituates in aging. *Neurobiol. Aging* 32, 1634–1650. doi: 10.1016/j.neurobiolaging.2009.10.007

Russell, J. A. (1980). A circumplex model of affect. *J. Pers. Soc. Psychol.* 39, 1161. doi: 10.1037/h0077714

Scheibe, S., and Carstensen, L. L. (2010). Emotional aging: recent findings and future trends. *J. Gerontol. Psychol. Sci.* 65, 135–144. doi: 10.1093/geronb/gbp132

St. Jacques, P., Dolcos, F., and Cabeza, R. (2010). Effects of aging on functional connectivity of the amygdala during negative evaluation: a network analysis of fMRI data. *Neurobiol. Aging* 31, 315–331. doi: 10.1016/j.neurobiolaging.2008.03.012

Streubel, B., and Kunzmann, U. (2011). Age differences in emotional reactions: arousal and age-relevance count. *Psychol. Aging* 26, 966–978. doi: 10.1037/a0023424

Tessitore, A., Hariri, A. R., Fera, F., Smith, W. G., Das, S., Weinberger, D. R., et al. (2005). Functional changes in the activity of brain regions underlying emotion processing in the elderly. *Psychiatry Res.* 139, 9–18. doi: 10.1016/j.pscychresns.2005.02.009

Tsai, J. L., Levenson, R. W., and Carstensen, L. L. (2000). Autonomic, subjective, and expressive responses to emotional films in older and younger Chinese Americans and European Americans. *Psychol. Aging* 15, 684–693. doi: 10.1037/0882-7974.15.4.684

Urry, H. L., van Reekum, C. M., Johnstone, T., Kalin, N. H., Thurow, M. E., Schaefer, H. S., et al. (2006). Amygdala and ventromedial prefrontal cortex are inversely coupled during regulation of negative affect and predict the diurnal pattern of cortisol secretion among older adults. *J. Neurosci.* 26, 4415–4425. doi: 10.1523/JNEUROSCI.3215-05.2006

Williams, L. M., Brown, K. J., Palmer, D., Liddell, B. J., Kemp, A. H., Olivieri, G., et al. (2006). The mellow years? Neural basis of improving emotional stability over age. *J. Neurosci.* 26, 6422–6430. doi: 10.1523/JNEUROSCI.0022-06.2006

Winecoff, A., Labar, K. S., Madden, D. J., Cabeza, R., and Huettel, S. A. (2011). Cognitive and neural contributors to emotion regulation in aging. *Soc. Cogn. Affect. Neurosci.* 6, 165–176. doi: 10.1093/scan/nsq030

Wood, S., and Kisley, M. A. (2006). The negativity bias is eliminated in older adults: age-related reduction in event-related brain potentials associated with evaluative categorization. *Psychol. Aging* 21, 815–820. doi: 10.1037/0882-7974.21.4.815

Wright, C. I., Wedig, M. M., Williams, D., Rauch, S. L., and Albert, M. S. (2006). Novel fearful faces activate the amygdala in healthy young and elderly adults. *Neurobiol. Aging* 27, 361–374. doi: 10.1016/j.neurobiolaging.2005.01.014

Yamasaki, H., LaBar, K. S., and McCarthy, G. (2002). Dissociable prefrontal brain systems for attention and emotion. *Proc. Natl. Acad. Sci. U.S.A.* 99, 11447–11451. doi: 10.1073/pnas.182176499

# 8

# Fluid cognitive ability is a resource for successful emotion regulation in older and younger adults

**Philipp C. Opitz[1†], Ihno A. Lee[2], James J. Gross[2] and Heather L. Urry[1*]**

[1] Department of Psychology, Tufts University, Medford, MA, USA
[2] Department of Psychology, Stanford University, Stanford, CA, USA

**Edited by:**
Natalie Ebner, University of Florida, USA

**Reviewed by:**
Hakan Fischer, Stockholm University, Sweden
Sanda Dolcos, University of Illinois at Urbana-Champaign, USA
Susanne Scheibe, University of Groningen, Netherlands

***Correspondence:**
Heather L. Urry, Department of Psychology, Tufts University, 490 Boston Avenue, Medford, MA 02155, USA
e-mail: heather.urry@tufts.edu

The Selection, Optimization, and Compensation with Emotion Regulation (SOC-ER) framework suggests that (1) emotion regulation (ER) strategies require resources and that (2) higher levels of relevant resources may increase ER success. In the current experiment, we tested the specific hypothesis that individual differences in one internal class of resources, namely cognitive ability, would contribute to greater success using cognitive reappraisal (CR), a form of ER in which one reinterprets the meaning of emotion-eliciting situations. To test this hypothesis, 60 participants (30 younger and 30 older adults) completed standardized neuropsychological tests that assess fluid and crystallized cognitive ability, as well as a CR task in which participants reinterpreted the meaning of sad pictures in order to alter (increase or decrease) their emotions. In a control condition, they viewed the pictures without trying to change how they felt. Throughout the task, we indexed subjective emotional experience (self-reported ratings of emotional intensity), expressive behavior (corrugator muscle activity), and autonomic physiology (heart rate and electrodermal activity) as measures of emotional responding. Multilevel models were constructed to explain within-subjects variation in emotional responding as a function of ER contrasts comparing increase or decrease conditions with the view control condition and between-subjects variation as a function of cognitive ability and/or age group (older, younger). As predicted, higher fluid cognitive ability—indexed by perceptual reasoning, processing speed, and working memory—was associated with greater success using reappraisal to alter emotional responding. Reappraisal success did not vary as a function of crystallized cognitive ability or age group. Collectively, our results provide support for a key tenet of the SOC-ER framework that higher levels of relevant resources may confer greater success at emotion regulation.

**Keywords: emotion regulation, cognitive reappraisal, working memory, cognitive ability, SOC-ER, older adults**

## INTRODUCTION

Emotions are frequently helpful in achieving adaptive goals. However, our emotions can at times be either the wrong intensity or duration, thereby impeding rather than facilitating goal achievement. When this happens, it is useful to regulate our emotions. Gross' (1998) process model of emotion regulation (ER) describes five families of ER strategies, namely, situation selection, situation modification, attentional deployment, cognitive change, and response modulation. Research has shown that people differ with regard to the strategies they habitually choose to regulate their emotions (Gross and John, 2003) and there are individual differences in success at implementing specific ER strategies as well (for example, as a function of older vs. younger age; Shiota and Levenson, 2009; Opitz et al., 2012a).

Although ER has been linked to important adaptive outcomes (Appleton et al., 2013; Gross, 2014), we know very little about the factors that explain these individual differences. The Selection, Optimization, and Compensation with Emotion Regulation (SOC-ER) framework (Urry and Gross, 2010; Opitz et al., 2012b) offers a set of factors that may help explain individual differences in ER.

According to the SOC-ER framework, successful ER depends on three factors: (1) choosing ER strategies for which resources are available at sufficient levels (Selection), (2) devoting time, practice, and effort to using these strategies successfully (Optimization), and (3) choosing alternate ER strategies when the ER strategy one chose initially is unsuccessful, perhaps as a result of insufficient resources (Compensation) (Urry and Gross, 2010; Opitz et al., 2012b). The cornerstone of this framework is the notion that successful ER requires resources—internal abilities and/or environmental affordances that promote the use of a given ER strategy. From this perspective, as resource levels vary within individuals (i.e., from one situation to the next, or from one phase of the life span to the next) or across individuals (i.e., from one person to another), ER success should vary accordingly. In the present study, we test this cornerstone SOC-ER idea with respect to individual differences in one class of resources—cognitive ability—and one ER strategy, cognitive reappraisal (CR).

CR refers to altering one's emotional response by reinterpreting the emotion-eliciting situation or one's response to it. Neuroimaging studies have shown that successful CR recruits brain areas involved in working memory, suggesting that successful CR may depend on the ability to hold information in mind (Ochsner et al., 2002, 2004; McRae et al., 2010). Additionally, CR has been shown to be most effective when initiated early in the emotion-generative cycle (Sheppes and Meiran, 2007), signifying that the ability to process information quickly may be beneficial, too. These observations hint at two cognitive abilities—working memory capacity (WMC) and processing speed (PS)—that may be resources for CR and thus contribute to CR success. Providing partial support for this idea, cross-sectional research suggests that older adults (OA), who exhibit deficits in WMC and PS (e.g., Salthouse et al., 2003; Hedden and Gabrieli, 2004), are less successful using some forms of CR compared to younger adults (YA), like detached reappraisals aimed at decreasing negative emotions (Shiota and Levenson, 2009). Of course, the observation of an age difference provides only indirect support for the role of cognitive ability as a resource for CR. To clarify our understanding of the relationship between these putative resources and CR, research directly assessing relations between cognitive abilities and CR success is needed.

Schmeichel et al. (2008) presented the first direct assessment of the role of cognitive ability as a resource for successful CR in a between-subjects design. These authors demonstrated that higher levels of WMC were correlated with reduced experience of unpleasant emotion in a group of participants who were assigned to adopt neutral, nonemotional appraisals of disgusting film clips. In another between-subjects design, Malooly et al. (2013) assessed relations between affective and nonaffective cognitive flexibility and successful CR. In both cases, cognitive flexibility was operationalized as reaction time costs of switching between rules regarding how to process different features of target stimuli. In the nonaffective flexibility task, neither the rules nor the target stimuli were emotional; in the affective flexibility task, both were emotional. Results of this study suggested that higher levels of affective cognitive flexibility were associated with reduced experience of sad emotion in a group of participants who were assigned to reappraise sad film clips by adopting a neutral, analytic, objective mindset. Finally, McRae et al. (2012) examined the relationship between CR and WMC, as well as other components of cognitive ability, in a within-subjects context. Results indicated moderate positive correlations between the ability to use CR to decrease unpleasant emotions and WMC and set-shifting costs; a similar trend was observed for perceptual reasoning. By contrast, verbal fluency and response inhibition were uncorrelated with reappraisal ability.

Together, these findings from Schmeichel et al. (2008); McRae et al. (2012); Malooly et al. (2013) and provide convergent, direct support for the role of cognitive ability—particularly, WMC and cognitive flexibility—as a resource for successful CR. These studies further suggest that not all cognitive abilities are resources for CR, pointing to a certain degree of specificity regarding the role of cognitive resources in CR. Still, with only these three studies in hand, important questions remain.

In the present paper, our primary goal is to address the following questions: First, are as-of-yet unexamined cognitive abilities resources for successful CR? Here, we examine PS, an index of cognitive ability that also has promise as a resource for CR. We also examine working memory, verbal ability, and perceptual reasoning to conceptually replicate previous findings. Second, are associations between cognitive ability and CR success dependent on whether one's CR goal is to decrease or increase one's emotional response? The two previous studies found that some aspects of cognitive ability were associated with the ability to use CR to *decrease* unpleasant emotional experience. Here we examine the ability to *increase* unpleasant emotion too. This is important methodologically because it provides an active, effortful comparison. In addition, this is important conceptually since ER efforts are sometimes directed in pursuit of contrahedonic feeling states (Ford and Tamir, 2012; Tamir and Ford, 2012; Tamir et al., 2013).

To achieve our primary goal, we recruited both younger and OA. In light of aforementioned age differences in cognitive abilities of interest, recruiting younger and OA allowed us to maximize meaningful variation in cognitive abilities in our sample. This also allowed us to address a secondary goal, which was to assess whether older age—normatively associated with decrements in cognitive resources including WM and PS—impacts CR success. Previous research has demonstrated mixed results, with some indicating age-related decrements for reappraisals aimed at decreasing unpleasant emotions (Opitz et al., 2012a) and detached reappraisals (Shiota and Levenson, 2009), and others indicating age-related sparing for reappraisals aimed at increasing unpleasant emotions (Opitz et al., 2012a) and positive reappraisals (Shiota and Levenson, 2009; Lohani and Isaacowitz, 2013). However, these mixed results may reflect variation across studies in emotional load and task demands. OA may perform less well only when CR tasks include highly potent negative images and require excessive shifting from one condition to the next. Here we examine CR success in a task that keeps emotional load and task demands to a minimum.

In pursuit of our primary and secondary goals, our younger and older participants completed well-validated, standardized neuropsychological measures of fluid and crystallized cognitive ability and a CR task. In the CR task, participants used CR to increase or decrease their emotional response to sad pictures. We chose sad stimuli specifically as previous research suggests sadness to be among the most frequently regulated emotions (Gross et al., 2006), thus maximizing the likelihood that participants would want to regulate emotions elicited by the pictures and have some experience doing so. These two conditions were compared to a view control condition in which participants responded naturally to the pictures without trying to change how they felt. We used a gaze-directed variant of the CR task validated in previous studies (Urry, 2010; Opitz et al., 2012a). The gaze direction manipulation enabled us to maximize the extent to which deployment of attention to arousing and non-arousing information was equivalent across the increase, view, and decrease CR instructions. This may be particularly important when studying OA because OA are more apt to deploy greater attention to positive than negative emotional information in some contexts (Isaacowitz et al., 2008, 2009).

During the CR task, we recorded subjective emotional experience (self-reported ratings of intensity), expressive behavior (corrugator muscle activity), and autonomic physiology [heart rate (HR) and electrodermal activity (EDA)] as measures of emotional responding. Multilevel models were constructed to explain within-subjects variation in emotional responding as a function of the CR manipulations and between-subjects variation as a function of cognitive ability or age. Our comprehensive approach offers several benefits. First, we are capturing trial-by-trial variation in emotional responding in three components of emotion. Past studies suggest that components of emotional responding cohere to some degree (Mauss et al., 2005), but this coherence is imperfect. This means one cannot measure just one component and make strong inferences about other, unmeasured components. This also means some components of emotional responding may show predicted effects while others may not. Second, our measures of expressive behavior and autonomic physiology are less subject to demand characteristics than self-report evaluations of emotional experience. Thus, were we to find predicted effects for expressive behavior and/or autonomic physiology, this would bolster the interpretation that differences between the CR conditions of interest reflect emotion regulatory success and not just demand characteristics of the experiment. Third, the continuous nature of our peripheral physiological measures provided a moment-to-moment index of responses during the task, allowing us to separately model pre-instruction and post-instruction activity. This allowed us to account for initial emotion reactivity (for which there often are age differences).

With these design features in place, we tested the hypothesis that higher levels of fluid (perceptual reasoning, PS, and working memory) and perhaps crystallized (verbal ability) cognitive abilities would predict greater CR success.

## METHODS

### PARTICIPANTS

Thirty younger (20 female, 18–22 years, $M = 19.5$, $SD = 1.18$) and 30 older (17 female, 55–71 years, $M = 61.9$, $SD = 5.14$) adults were recruited via internet (e.g., http://www.craigslist.com), local newspaper, and community e-mailing list advertisements. Participants endorsed the following non-exclusive racial categories: Asian: 11 (18.3%); White: 46 (76.7%); Declined to respond: 3 (5%). Two participants (3.4%) endorsed being of Hispanic origin, and two participants declined to report ethnicity. See **Table 1** for additional participant characteristics.

No participants reported any history of psychiatric or neurological disorders, or current use of any psychoactive medications. Before completing the experiment, participants completed a hearing test (WWW Hearing Test, Digital Recordings, Halifax, NS, Canada) and two vision tests (Arditi, 2005; Dougherty et al., 2005) to ensure they could hear and see the stimuli. All procedures were approved by the Social, Behavioral, and Educational Research Institutional Review Board at Tufts University. Participants provided written informed consent prior to participating.

**Table 1 | Characteristics of the sample.**

| Measure | Younger | Older | Significant age difference? |
|---|---|---|---|
| Mean (*SD*) age in years | 19.45 (1.18) | 61.90 (5.14) | $t_{(30.96)} = -42.44$, $p < 0.001$ |
| Total *N* | 30 | 30 | |
| Men | 10 (33%) | 13 (43%) | $\chi^2(1) = 0.648$, $p = 0.421$ |
| Women | 19 (67%) | 16 (57%) | |
| **HIGHEST LEVEL OF EDUCATION** | | | |
| High school diploma | 11 (36%) | 1 (3%) | $\chi^2(3) = 30.21$, $p < 0.001$ |
| Some college | 16 (53%) | 6 (20%) | |
| College diploma | 2 (6%) | 10 (33%) | |
| Graduate degree | 0 | 12 (40%) | |
| **MARITAL STATUS** | | | |
| Never married | 29 (97%) | 3 (10%) | $\chi^2(4) = 47.13$, $p < 0.001$ |
| Married | 0 | 12 (40%) | |
| Separated | 0 | 1 (3%) | |
| Divorced | 0 | 11 (36%) | |
| Widowed | 0 | 2 (6%) | |

*Demographic data for two participants (one younger) were not collected, and are therefore not included (except in total N).*

### MATERIALS

#### Cognitive ability

To assess cognitive ability, participants completed four subtests of the Wechsler Adult Intelligence Scale IV (WAIS IV, Pearson, San Antonio, TX).

We assessed working memory using the Digit Span (DS) task, in which participants hear and verbally reproduce an increasing number of digit strings (two trials per digit string length) in forward order (DS Forward), backward order (DS Backward), or in ascending order (Sequencing). The task continues until both trials of a given digit string length are incorrect or until the last item of the task is reached.

We assessed verbal ability using the Vocabulary (VC) task, in which participants provide definitions for increasingly difficult words presented orally. For instance, on an early (easy) trial, participants defined "APPLE," whereas on a later (hard) trial, participants defined "PALLIATE." For the purposes of this paper, we report scores based on one half of the VC task. The other difficulty-matched half was subject to a manipulation of no relevance to this paper.

We assessed perceptual reasoning using the Block Design (BD) task, in which participants are given a set of nine red-and/or-white cubes, which they have to assemble to reproduce two-dimensional patterns of increasing difficulty. The task continues until two consecutive trials are incorrect or until the last item of the task is reached.

Lastly, we assessed PS using the Coding (CD) task, in which participants are given a sheet of paper containing a "key" that links numbers one through nine with simple non-alphanumeric symbols. Participants are asked to draw the correct symbol (according to the key) below each of multiple rows of numbers on the sheet below until 2 min has elapsed or until the last item of the task is reached. Data for one older participant were not available for CD due to participant misunderstanding of instructions.

OA tend to perform less well than YA on the DS, BD, and CD subtests, which are indicators of fluid cognitive ability; OA perform similarly or better than YA on the VC subtest, an indicator of crystallized cognitive ability (Salthouse et al., 2003; Hedden and Gabrieli, 2004).

#### *Picture stimuli*

In the CR task, which is described below, participants viewed a set of 120 digital color pictures (800 × 600 pixels). Most were selected from the International Affective Picture System (IAPS; Lang et al., 2008) using normative valence ratings provided by Mikels et al. (2005). Specifically, we used those images that Mikels et al. (2005) categorized as sad on a scale from 1 to 7, where 1 corresponded to *not at all* sad, and 7 corresponded to *very sad*; our set was moderately sad on average ($M = 4.09$, $SD = 0.85$). To have enough sad pictures to avoid repetition, we supplemented the IAPS pictures with pictures selected from stock photo libraries (Shutterstock and the Wellcome Image Collection). These pictures, for which no normative ratings exist, were selected for content similar to those selected from the IAPS. The final set of 120 sad pictures mostly depicted withdrawn, lonely, or sad older and YA and/or injured, solitary, or apparently sad animals. We purposefully sought content that is relevant to participants in both age groups.

#### *Cognitive reappraisal task*

The pictures were presented in the context of a gaze-directed CR task, a variant of the task validated by Urry (2010) and also used with both younger and OA by Lang et al. (2008); Opitz et al. (2012b). This task comprised 120 trials described by crossing two within-subjects factors, CR condition (increase, view, decrease, no CR) and gaze direction condition (arousing, free/no gaze direction, non-arousing). Prior to completing the CR task, participants received in-depth training to ensure that they understood the CR and gaze direction manipulations (described below) as well as how to rate the intensity of their emotional response on each trial.

For the CR manipulation, participants were trained to increase or decrease their emotional response to the pictures by considering the personal relevance of the depicted situation (self-focused reappraisal) or imagining alternative outcomes (situation-focused reappraisal). Cues to begin using CR were presented via single-word audio recording, "increase" or "decrease" 3 s after picture onset. As part of their training, participants saw a picture of a man lying in a hospital bed, seemingly in pain. For the "increase" instruction, participants were told they could imagine that "you yourself or a loved one are the person in this picture, or that you are present and are witnessing the man's pain and struggle." Conversely, for the "decrease" instruction, participants were told that they could imagine that "you are simply observing the man objectively, or that he will get better soon." A third audio recording, "view," served as a cue to respond naturally without trying to change how they felt. A fourth CR condition, "no CR," entailed viewing the picture with no instruction, which enabled us to determine whether the simple instruction to "view" would alter emotional responding. For all four conditions, participants were instructed not to think of the pictures as fake or unreal.

For the gaze direction manipulation, participant gaze was directed to an emotionally arousing or non-arousing (neutral) area of the picture beginning 4 s after picture onset, or participant gaze was not directed, i.e., allowed to vary freely. This gaze direction manipulation enabled us to control the ways in which participants deployed their visual attention to the emotional information in the pictures during the 8-s regulation period of interest (c.f., Isaacowitz et al., 2008, 2009). As validated in prior work (Urry, 2010), eye tracking data (not shown) confirmed that the present sample of participants followed the gaze direction instruction equally across the CR conditions, increasing looking time in the designated areas of interest following the manipulation onset. These data also suggested that older and YA did not differ in their gaze behavior.

The CR task was programmed using E-Prime version 1.2.1.8 (Psychology Software Tools, Inc., Sharpsburg, PA) in 10 blocks of 12 trials each. Pictures were presented on a TFT display (1280 × 1204 maximum resolution) while auditory instructions were delivered via speakers in a sound- and RF-shielded experiment booth. Half of the blocks included the "increase," "view," and "no CR" conditions, while the other half included the "decrease," "view," and "no CR" conditions. We blocked increase and decrease CR trials in this manner to reduce the mental set shifting demands of the experiment. CR conditions, gaze directions, and pictures were otherwise randomly assigned to each trial. The gaze-directed CR task trial structure is depicted in **Figure 1**.

### DEPENDENT VARIABLES

Three measures of emotional responding were recorded during the CR task. Self-report ratings of emotional intensity were collected at the end of each trial. Expressive behavior (corrugator muscle activity via facial electromyography) and autonomic physiology (HR and EDA) were collected continuously using an MP150 system (Biopac, Goleta, CA) and processed offline using ANSLAB (Wilhelm and Peyk, 2005).

#### *Self-report ratings of intensity*

Self-report ratings of emotional intensity ranging from 1 (not very intense) to 9 (very intense) were collected at the end of each trial. This 9-point numeric scale was illustrated with five figures based on the arousal scale of the Self-Assessment Manikin (Lang et al., 2008). Figures ranged from a relaxed, sleepy figure at the left (not at all intense) to an excited, wide-eyed figure at the right (very intense; see **Figure 1**).

#### *Corrugator electromyography (EMG)*

Corrugator activity has been shown to be sensitive to stimulus valence, with greater activity being associated with higher levels of stimulus unpleasantness (Bradley and Lang, 2007). Two 4-mm Ag/AgCl electrodes were placed in bipolar configuration over the right eye per Fridlund and Cacioppo (1986). One ground was placed on the forehead. The data were sampled at 1000 Hz and

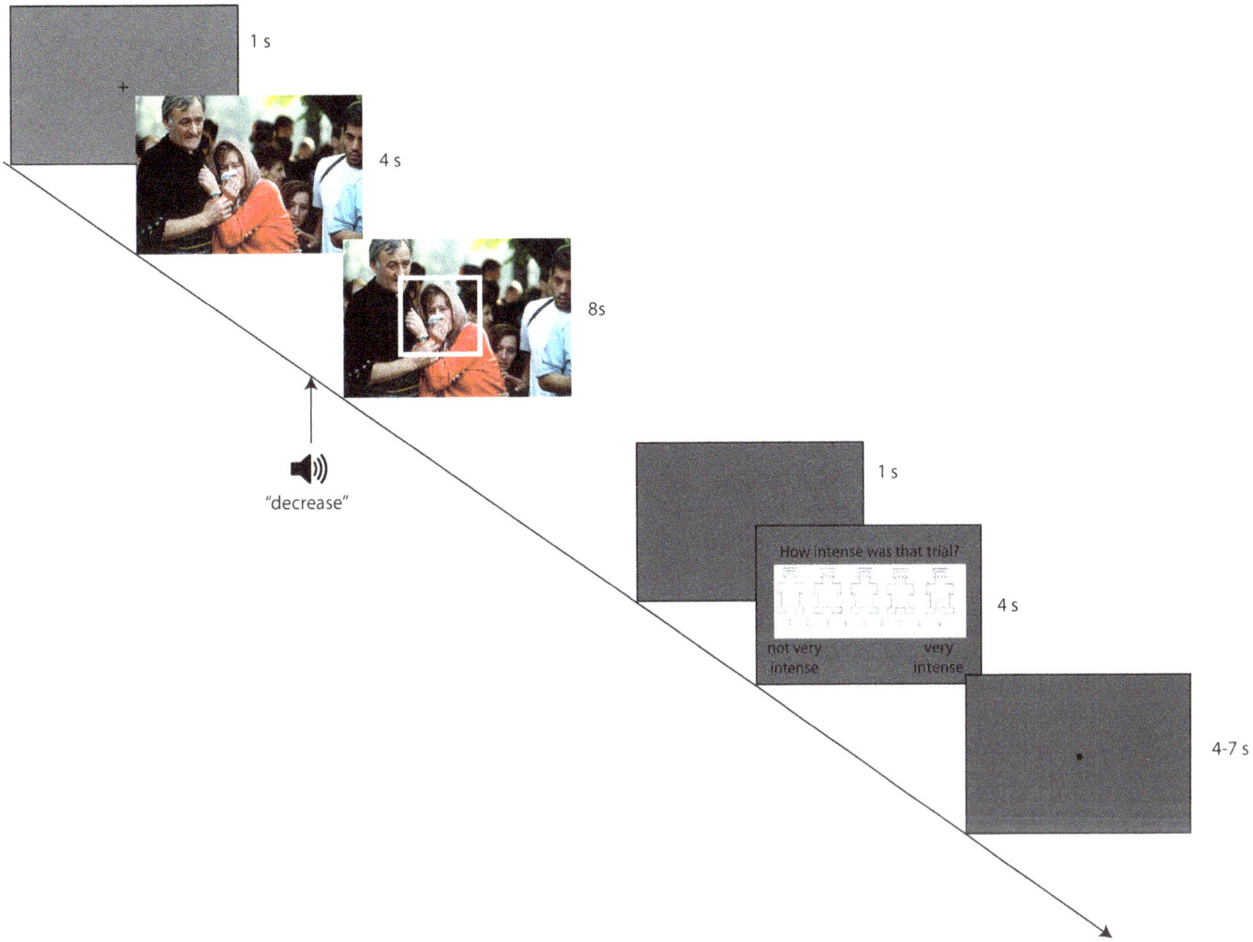


**FIGURE 1 | Trial structure.** Participants first saw a fixation cross for 1 s, followed by a picture for a total of 12 s. Three seconds after picture onset, participants heard the cognitive reappraisal (CR) instruction for that trial, if applicable (in this case, "decrease"). One second thereafter, a box directed them to look in an arousing or nonarousing area of the picture, if applicable (in this case, the box is directing gaze to an arousing area). After the 8-s regulatory period during which they followed the CR and gaze direction instructions, participants briefly saw a gray screen (1 s). This was followed by a 9-point intensity rating screen which was available for up to 4 s. After the rating screen, a gray screen with a black dot signaled a break between trials, which varied from 4 to 7 s. Photo of mourning family from Evstafiev (1992). Used with permission of the photographer.

bandpass filtered online (5 Hz to 3 kHz; 60-Hz notch filter on). Offline, data were resampled to 400 Hz, rectified, filtered (16 Hz low-pass), decimated to 4 Hz, and smoothed (1-s prior moving average).

#### *Electrocardiography*

Electrocardiography was used to measure HR, which is dually innervated by the sympathetic and parasympathetic branches of the autonomic nervous system. In event-related paradigms involving passive viewing of negative pictures, HR is sensitive to stimulus valence and often exhibits an initial, parasympathetically mediated deceleration (Bradley and Lang, 2007). Two disposable Ag/AgCl electrodes pregelled with 7% chloride gel (1 cm circular contact area) were placed under the left and right collarbones on the chest after swabbing with an alcohol or an electrode prep pad. ECG was acquired continuously at 1000 Hz. Offline, the ECG signal was downsampled to 400 Hz and bandpass-filtered from 0.5 to 40 Hz.

Interbeat interval series were created by identifying R-spikes using automated ANSLAB algorithms. R-spikes that were not detected automatically, thus leading to an erroneously long period between successive R-spikes, were marked for inclusion by hand. Similarly, R-spikes that were identified incorrectly, thus leading to an erroneously short period between successive R-spikes, were removed by hand. Following such artifact correction, the interbeat interval series was converted to HR in beats per minute. HR data were decimated to 10 Hz and then smoothed with a 1-s prior moving average filter.

#### *Electrodermal activity*

EDA was selected as a pure measure of sympathetic activation of the autonomic nervous system. Two disposable Ag/AgCl electrodes pregelled with 0.5% chloride isotonic gel (1 cm circular contact area) were attached to the distal phalanges of the index and middle fingers on the left hand. EDA level was recorded with DC coupling and constant voltage electrode excitation at 31.25 Hz (sensitivity = 0.7 nS). Offline, EDA was smoothed with a 1-Hz, low-pass filter, decimated to 10 Hz, and linearly detrended on a trial-by-trial basis. One ground electrode for all physiological channels was placed on the forehead.

### PROCEDURES

After providing informed consent, participants completed the BD, CD, DS, and VC subtests of the WAIS-IV in the order described above. Participants were then prepared for physiological recording and completed the training procedure for the CR task. Immediately following this training, participants completed the CR task. At various points in the session, participants completed additional questionnaires and a second set of WAIS-IV subtests. These additional procedures were not the focus of this report and some were subject to an unrelated manipulation thus the data are not reported here[1].

### DATA REDUCTION, RETENTION, AND ANALYSIS

For the continuous peripheral physiological measures, we summarized raw activity for two periods of interest in each trial, pre-instruction activity (reactivity period; mean of activity occurring 4 s after picture onset) and post-instruction activity (regulation period; mean of activity occurring 8 s after both ER manipulations). To prevent leveraging of condition estimates by outlying values in the dependent variables, trials for which the estimate of Mahalanobis Distance within each measure was too large ($p <$ 0.001) were set to missing (see Fidell and Tabachnick, 2003). An average of 95.4% ($SD = 0.789$; minimum = 94.2%, maximum = 96.0%) of all observations were available for analysis.

Multilevel analyses with two levels, some incorporating latent variables (see Hox, 2002; Kline, 2010), were conducted using Mplus v. 7.11 (Muthén and Muthén, 1998–2013). Continuous predictors were grand-mean centered. Estimates were generated (and missing values handled) using full information maximum likelihood estimation with robust standard errors. Although multilevel analyses are reported less often than traditional repeated measures analyses, they have three key advantages. First, this approach allows us to model emotional responding as a latent construct with experiential (self-reported intensity), expressive (corrugator activity), and autonomic physiological (HR, EDA) components. Traditional analyses compel one to analyze each measure as if they were independent. Second, this approach allows us to model trial-related variation in the dependent variable within each condition. Traditional analyses compel one to average across trials within each condition with the perhaps unfounded assumption that there is no trial-related variation. Third, this approach provides estimates using all available data. Traditional analyses compel listwise deletion of cases with missing observations.

[1] Before and after the WAIS-IV subtests reported here, participants completed items assessing appraisals of threat and challenge and current emotional state. Immediately after the CR task, participants provided open-ended reports of strategies used, and items assessing satisfaction with life, state and trait anxiety, ER, perceived stress, health, quality of life, and socioeconomic status. Participants then received information related to a between-subjects stereotype threat manipulation and completed the second set of WAIS-IV subtests (matrix reasoning, letter-number sequencing, symbol search, and the second, difficulty-matched VC subtest). Before and after the second set of WAIS-IV subtests, participants again completed items assessing appraisals of threat and challenge and current emotional state. At the end of the session, participants completed items assessing test anxiety, beliefs about the malleability of intelligence and emotions, age-related stereotypes of cognitive performance, and thoughts about what the experiment was about.

## RESULTS

Results are presented below in four sections. We first present preliminary analyses undertaken to determine (1) whether there are individual differences in pre-instruction emotion reactivity, and (2) whether there are main and/or interactive effects of our CR and gaze direction manipulations. Then, in pursuit of our primary goal, we present analyses germane to determining whether cognitive ability predicts successful CR. Next, in pursuit of our secondary goal, we present analyses germane to determining whether there are age differences in CR success. Finally, we report supplemental analyses that provide estimates of emotional responding as a function of age group, CR, and gaze direction during the regulation period on a measure-by-measure basis.

### PRELIMINARY ANALYSES

#### *Individual differences in pre-instruction emotion reactivity*

Using a two-level structural equation model, we examined whether there were individual differences in pre-instruction reactivity to the stimuli as a function of between-subjects variables of primary and secondary interest in this research (fluid cognitive ability, crystallized cognitive ability, age group). We also examined education level and marital status, both of which varied as a function of age group and thus represent control variables of interest.

On the first (within-subjects) level, activity during the reactivity period was regressed on baseline activity (mean of activity occurring 1 s prior to picture onset) for each of the three physiological measures.

On the second (between-subjects) level, activity during the reactivity period for each measure (self-reported intensity corrugator activity, HR, and EDA) was regressed on five between-subjects predictors as follows: fluid cognitive ability, crystallized cognitive ability, age group (older = 1, younger = 0), ever married (1 = yes, 0 = no), and education level. Fluid cognitive ability was modeled as a latent predictor variable with three manifest indicators, BD, CD, DS; variance was constrained at 1. Crystallized cognitive ability was modeled as the stand-alone manifest indicator, VC.

Participants exhibited significant, nonzero values for all four criterion variables (self-reported intensity $B = 4.26$, $SE = 0.353$; corrugator activity $B = 7.15$, $SE = 0.459$; HR $B = 72.1$ $SE = 0.876$; and EDA $B = 11.57$, $SE = 0.014$, all $ps < 0.001$). Factor loadings for the fluid cognitive ability latent predictor variable were positive and significant ($p = 0.001$ for BD and CD; $p = 0.002$ for DS). Finally, there were some significant individual differences in the criterion variables as follows: Higher fluid cognitive ability and lower crystallized cognitive ability were associated with lower EDA ($B = -0.02$, $SE = 0.009$, $p = 0.031$ and $B = 0.002$, $SE = 0.001$, $p = 0.031$, respectively) but not self-reported intensity, corrugator activity, or HR (all $ps > 0.20$). Older age was associated with lower corrugator activity ($B = -1.63$, $SE = 0.782$, $p = 0.037$) but not self-reported intensity, HR, or EDA (all *ps* $> 0.70$). Ever having been married was associated with higher corrugator activity ($B = 1.37$, $SE = 0.451$, $p = 0.002$), lower HR ($B = -3.28$, $SE = 1.557$, $p = 0.035$), and lower EDA ($B = -0.06$, $SE = 0.027$, $p = 0.026$) but not self-reported intensity ($p = 0.763$). Education level was not associated with any of the criterion variables (all *ps* $> 0.17$). We do not consider these isolated and non-predicted findings further.

### *Main and interactive effects of CR and gaze direction*

In a second two-level structural equation model, we tested the main and interactive effects of the CR and gaze direction manipulations on within-subjects (trial-by-trial) variation in emotional responding. The first column of **Table 2** summarizes the criterion and predictor variables in this preliminary analysis.

On the first level, activity during the regulation period was regressed on activity during the reactivity period for each physiological measure in order to isolate CR- and gaze direction-related variation in emotional responding. Emotional responding was then modeled as one latent dependent variable with variance constrained at 1. Emotional responding had four manifest indicators, namely self-reported emotional intensity and corrugator activity, HR, and EDA during the regulation period.

The emotional responding latent dependent variable was regressed on three CR condition contrasts [increase (1) vs. view (−1), decrease (1) vs. view (−1), and no CR (1) vs. view (−1)] to estimate the effects of CR, and two gaze direction condition contrasts [arousing (1) vs. not directed (−1) and non-arousing (1) vs. not directed (−1)] to estimate the effects of gaze direction. The latent variable was also regressed on six contrasts reflecting the products of each of the CR condition contrasts with each of the gaze direction condition contrasts to estimate the interaction between CR and gaze direction.

On the second level, random slopes were estimated for the decrease and increase CR predictors and the arousing and non-arousing gaze direction predictors from the first level. Random slopes were not estimated for the no CR predictor, which was a covariate of no interest, or for the six interaction contrasts by convention (Hoffman and Rovine, 2007).

As shown in the second column of **Table 2**, this analysis revealed that two of four manifest indicators, self-reported intensity and corrugator activity, loaded positively and significantly on the latent emotional response dependent variable on the first level (both $p = 0.001$); a third, skin conductance, exhibited a trend in the same direction ($p = 0.083$). In addition, the CR manipulation impacted emotional responding as expected. Participants responded with greater emotion in the increase condition vs. the view condition ($B = 1.00$, $p < 0.001$), lower emotion in the decrease condition vs. the view condition ($B = -0.64$, $p < 0.001$), and lower emotion in the no CR condition vs. the view condition ($B = -0.18$, $p = 0.006$).

The gaze direction manipulation also impacted emotional responding. Participants responded with greater emotion when gaze was directed to an arousing area vs. when gaze was not directed ($B = 0.07$, $p = 0.086$, a nonsignificant trend), and lower emotion when gaze was directed to a non-arousing area vs. when gaze was not directed ($B = -0.17$, $p = 0.016$). Importantly, gaze direction moderated the decrease CR effect, significantly for the non-arousing gaze direction contrast ($B = 0.20$, $p = 0.013$) but not significantly for the arousing gaze direction contrast ($B = -0.11$, $p = 0.108$). Neither gaze direction contrast moderated the increase CR effect (both $p > 0.40$).

In light of the significant interaction above, we conducted a set of follow-up analyses in which we estimated the three CR effects separately for each of the three gaze direction conditions. In these analyses, a random slope was estimated at the between-subjects level for the decrease CR contrast. When gaze was not directed, participants responded with lower emotion in the decrease condition vs. the view condition ($B = -0.42$, $p = 0.009$). When gaze was directed to an arousing area, this decrease CR effect was even stronger ($B = -0.98$, $p < 0.001$). However, when gaze was directed to a non-arousing area, the decrease CR effect narrowly reached significance in the opposite direction ($B = 0.35$, $p = 0.048$).

These results suggest that CR generally impacts emotional responding in expected ways. However, using CR to decrease emotional responding was effective only when participants were directing attention to emotional information in the pictures, either on their own or as cued by us. Because gaze direction moderated some CR effects, subsequent hypothesis testing analyses retained gaze direction contrasts and their interaction terms as fixed effects within subjects.

**Table 2 | Parameter estimates from preliminary analysis examining cognitive reappraisal and gaze direction effects on emotional responding.**

| Emotion response latent criterion variable | *B* (*SE*) |
|---|---|
| **Indicators** | **Factor loadings** |
| Self-reported intensity | 0.961 (0.279)* |
| Corrugator activity | 0.508 (0.085)** |
| Heart rate | 0.077 (0.1) |
| Skin conductance | 0.003 (0.001)+ |
| **Within-subjects predictors** | ***B* (*SE*)** |
| **CR CONTRASTS** | |
| Decrease—view[a] | −0.637 (0.171)** |
| Increase—view[a] | 0.997 (0.237)** |
| No CR—view | −0.176 (0.063)* |
| **GAZE DIRECTION CONTRASTS** | |
| Arousing—not directed[a] | 0.07 (0.04)+ |
| Non-arousing—not directed[a] | −0.166 (0.069)* |
| **CR × GAZE DIRECTION INTERACTION CONTRASTS** | |
| (Decrease—view) × (Arousing—not directed) | −0.112 (0.07) |
| (Increase—view) × (Arousing—not directed) | 0.051 (0.066) |
| (No CR—view) × (Arousing—not directed) | −0.021 (0.062) |
| (Decrease—view) × (Non-arousing—not directed) | 0.197 (0.079)* |
| (Increase—view) × (Non-arousing—not directed) | −0.045 (0.061) |
| (No CR—view) × (Non-arousing—not directed) | −0.037 (0.06) |

*CR, cognitive reappraisal. Pre-instruction activity was a positive, significant predictor of post-instruction activity for all three physiological measures; these estimates are not reported for the sake of brevity.*

*[a] Slope was estimated as a random effect.*

*$^{**}p < 0.001$, $^{*}p < 0.05$, $^{+}p < 0.10$.*

**PRIMARY ANALYSES**

To test our hypothesis that higher cognitive ability would predict more successful CR, we evaluated a two-level structural equation model (referred to as the Cognitive Ability Model in **Table 3**).

On the first level, the predictor and criterion variables were the same as noted for the preliminary analysis that tested the main and interactive effects of CR and gaze direction[2].

On the second level, the slopes estimated from the decrease and increase CR predictors on the first level were treated as criterion variables that were regressed on two between-subjects predictors, fluid cognitive ability and crystallized cognitive ability. Fluid cognitive ability was modeled as a latent predictor variable with three manifest indicators, BD, CD, DS; variance was constrained at 1. Crystallized cognitive ability was modeled as the stand-alone manifest indicator, VC.

As shown in **Table 3**, factor loadings for the fluid cognitive ability latent predictor variable were positive and significant or nearly so ($p = 0.001$ for BD and CD; $p = 0.070$ for DS). Note that negative estimates of the association between cognitive ability and CR success are expected for the decrease effect since the contrast was calculated as decrease minus view. Positive estimates are expected for the increase effect since the contrast was calculated as increase minus view. Consistent with our hypothesis, this analysis revealed that higher fluid cognitive ability was associated with greater success at decreasing ($B = -0.37, p < 0.001$) and increasing ($B = 0.42, p = 0.001$) emotional responding. Crystallized cognitive ability as indexed by VC was not associated with the decrease or increase CR effect (both $p > 0.30$).

[2]The no CR vs. view contrast is retained in all models. We focus in text on comparisons between the increase and decrease conditions vs. the view condition. We do so because the view condition is a better control than the no CR condition because the view, increase, and decrease conditions all include an auditory instruction on each trial whereas the no CR condition does not.

In follow-up analyses, we repeated the analyses above, but this time specified the fluid cognitive ability latent predictor variable with just one indicator, setting its residual variance and the slopes for the remaining two indicators to 0. In these analyses, higher levels of CD on its own were associated with greater success at decreasing ($B = -0.19, p = 0.023$) and increasing ($B = 0.24, p = 0.058$, a trend) emotional responding. Similarly, higher levels of BD on its own were associated with greater success at decreasing ($B = -0.80, p = 0.081$, a trend) and increasing ($B = 0.07, p = 0.033$) emotional responding. Neither of these associations was significant when considering DS on its own (both $ps > 0.10$). In another follow-up analysis, we dropped the latent fluid cognitive ability predictor variable and instead estimated a random effect for each of the four indicators of cognitive ability simultaneously. In this analysis, none of the four indicators was uniquely associated with CR success. Together, these results suggest that it is variance shared primarily between perceptual reasoning (BD) and PS (CD)—putatively fluid cognitive ability—that predicts successful CR.

**SECONDARY ANALYSES**

In pursuit of our secondary goal, we next present analyses that examine whether there are age differences in cognitive ability and CR success.

***Age differences in cognitive ability***

To examine whether the older and YA in this sample exhibited differences in fluid and/or crystallized cognitive ability as in previous studies, we conducted a between-subjects structural equation model. Fluid cognitive ability was estimated as a latent variable with BD, CD, and DS as manifest indicators; crystallized cognitive ability was estimated as the manifest indicator, VC. Both were regressed on age group (1 = older, 0 = younger). This structural equation model fit the data well, $\chi^2(4, N = 60) = 1.40$,

**Table 3 | Parameter estimates from hypothesis tests examining cognitive ability or age group as predictors of cognitive reappraisal success.**

| Fluid cognitive ability latent variable | Cognitive ability model | | Age group model | | Expanded model | |
|---|---|---|---|---|---|---|
| | ***B* (*SE*)** | | ***B* (*SE*)** | | ***B* (*SE*)** | |
| Indicators | Factor loadings | | | | Factor loadings | |
| BD | 7.811 (2.305)* | | – | | 10.607 (1.274)** | |
| CD | 11.039 (3.317)* | | – | | 12.688 (2.22)** | |
| DS | 1.63 (0.899)+ | | – | | 2.31 (0.767)* | |
| **Between-subjects predictors** | **Decrease–view criterion** | **Decrease–view criterion** | **Decrease–view criterion** | **Increase–view criterion** | **Decrease–view criterion** | **Increase–view criterion** |
| Fluid cognitive ability | −0.367 (0.08)** | 0.431 (0.128)* | – | – | −0.423 (0.107)** | 0.479 (0.152)* |
| Crystallized cognitive ability (VC) | 0.007 (0.007) | −0.004 (0.01) | – | – | 0.006 (0.008) | −0.002 (0.011) |
| Age group (older = 1, younger = 0) | – | – | 0.207 (0.13) | −0.226 (0.18) | 0.102 (0.197) | −0.388 (0.239) |
| Ever married (yes = 1, 0 = no) | – | – | – | – | −0.558 (0.159)** | 0.909 (0.217)** |
| Education level (higher values = more educated) | – | – | – | – | −0.012 (0.079) | 0.062 (0.096) |

*Within-subjects effects recapitulate effects reported in **Table 2** and thus are not reported here. BD, Block Design; CD, Coding; DS, Digit Span.*

*$^{**}p < 0.001$, $^{*}p < 0.05$, $^{+}p < 0.10$.*

$p = 0.844$, RMSEA $= 0.00$, 90% CI [0.00, 0.10], CFI $= 1.00$, SRMR $= 0.019$.

Results confirmed significant positive factor loadings for all three manifest indicators of the fluid cognitive ability latent variable (all $p < 0.01$). In addition, higher fluid cognitive ability was associated with higher crystallized cognitive ability ($\beta = 0.51$, $p = 0.002$). Importantly, although older age was not significantly associated with crystallized cognitive ability ($\beta = -0.08$, $p = 0.525$), older age was significantly associated with lower fluid cognitive ability ($\beta = -0.89$, $p < 0.001$).

### *Age differences in CR success*

In light of the preceding analysis indicating a high degree of shared variance between age group and fluid cognitive ability, we first treated older age as the sole between-subjects predictor of emotional responding in a two-level model (referred to as the Age Group Model in **Table 3**).

On the first level, the predictor and criterion variables were the same as noted for the preliminary analysis that tested the main and interactive effects of CR and gaze direction.

On the second level, the slopes estimated from the decrease and increase CR predictors on the first level were treated as criterion variables that were regressed on one between-subjects predictor, age group (older = 1, younger = 0).

Relative to the moderating effect of fluid cognitive ability, the moderating effect of age group on using CR to decrease ($B = 0.21$, $p = 0.112$) and increase ($B = -0.23$, $p = 0.209$) emotional responding relative to the view condition were modest in magnitude—roughly half the magnitude of the effects reported for fluid cognitive ability. The directions of these effects are consistent with older age predicting reduced CR success (see **Figure 2**) but they were not statistically significant. Follow-up analyses assessing the age difference within each gaze direction condition revealed effects that also were not statistically significant (results not shown; all $ps > 0.10$).

### *Age differences in CR success: expanded model*

It was possible that age differences in CR success were being obscured by individual differences in variables that covaried with age group (fluid cognitive ability, marital status, and education level). Thus, next we examined several simultaneous between-subjects predictors of emotional responding in a two-level structural equation model (referred to as the Expanded Model in **Table 3**)[3].

On the first level, the predictor and criterion variables were the same as noted previously.

On the second level, the slopes estimated from the decrease and increase CR predictors on the first level were treated as criterion variables. This time, they were regressed on five between-subjects predictors as follows: fluid cognitive ability, crystallized cognitive ability, age group (older = 1, younger = 0), ever married (1 = yes, 0 = no), and education level.

[3]Because of shared variance between predictors, estimates of the association between each predictor and the criterion variables should be interpreted with caution. In addition, although we attempted to test the interaction between age group and cognitive ability, this model would not converge, even when orthogonalizing cognitive ability with respect to age group.

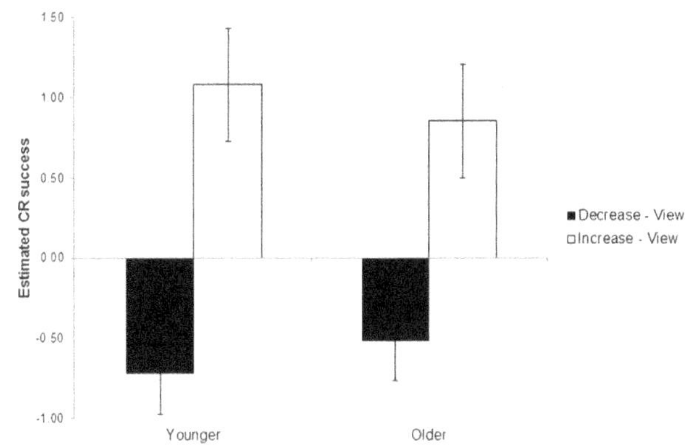


**FIGURE 2 | This figure depicts success using cognitive reappraisal to decrease (black bars) and increase (white bars) emotional responding as a function of age group in the Age Group Model (see Table 3).** Note that larger negative parameter estimates signal greater success for decrease vs. view whereas larger positive parameter estimates signal greater success for increase vs. view. Success scores were modestly lower in magnitude for older adults (right) than younger adults (left) but neither age difference was statistically significant. Error bars reflect the 95% confidence interval around the estimate of the age difference in cognitive reappraisal (CR) success.

In this analysis, higher fluid cognitive ability continued to be associated with greater success at decreasing ($B = -0.42$, $p < 0.001$) and increasing ($B = 0.48$, $p = 0.002$) emotional responding. There remained no significant effect of age group on using CR to decrease ($B = 0.10$, $p = 0.606$) or increase ($B = -0.39$, $p = 0.105$) emotional responding relative to the view condition. Notably, relative to when age group was modeled on its own, the magnitude of the effect of age group on using CR to decrease emotional responding was smaller by about one-half; the magnitude of the effect of age group on using CR to increase emotional responding was bigger by about one-half (and just barely approached marginal significance). Interestingly, ever having been married was associated with greater success using CR to decrease ($B = -0.56$, $p < 0.001$) and increase ($B = 0.91$, $p < 0.001$) emotional responding. Neither crystallized cognitive ability nor education level predicted success at decreasing or increasing emotional responding (see **Table 3**).

### *Estimates of emotional responding during the regulation period on a measure-by-measure basis*

The primary and secondary analyses reported above focused on variation in emotional responding during the regulation period modeled as a latent variable with four indicators. Some readers may be interested to examine estimates for each indicator individually as a function of age group, CR instruction, and gaze direction. To produce these estimates, we computed a series of 24 two-level models.

On the first level, there were four criterion variables (self-reported emotional intensity, corrugator activity, HR, EDA during the regulation period). These criterion variables were regressed on three within-subjects, dummy-coded CR instruction predictors. The physiological criterion variables were each additionally regressed on activity during the reactivity period.

On the second level, there were no explicit between-subjects predictors.

In **Table 4**, we report the B and SE for the intercept, which represents the mean value for the one CR instruction that was not included as a predictor in each model.

## DISCUSSION

The SOC-ER framework suggests that people might be most successful regulating their emotions when they use strategies for which they have the prerequisite resources in a given situation (Urry and Gross, 2010; Opitz et al., 2012b). In this study, we assessed the role of one class of resources, cognitive ability, in the success of one ER process, CR. Specifically, we examined whether higher levels of cognitive ability would predict greater CR success.

Three important observations emerged from this effort. First, higher levels of fluid cognitive ability predicted greater success at using CR to regulate emotional responses to sad stimuli. Second, fluid cognitive ability predicted greater success at using CR irrespective of whether the regulatory goal was to increase or decrease the emotional response. Finally, despite age differences in cognitive ability in this sample, older age was not associated with variation in success at using CR. We discuss these results in turn below. We then consider broader implications of this work, limitations, and future directions.

### COGNITIVE ABILITY PREDICTS SUCCESSFUL CR

Based on existing neuroimaging studies (see Buhle et al., 2013, for a meta-analysis) and the recent work of Schmeichel et al. (2008), McRae et al. (2012), and Malooly et al. (2013), we tested the prediction that cognitive abilities would predict CR success. Although correlational data preclude causal inference, the present findings are consistent with the idea that fluid cognitive abilities are resources for successful CR. Our results thus support a key tenet of the SOC-ER framework, namely that ER strategies draw on resources—internal abilities and/or environmental affordances that promote the use of a given ER strategy.

Not all previous studies have supported the idea that cognitive abilities should be associated with ER. For example, Farrelly and Austin (2007) failed to observe associations between cognitive ability and "managing emotions" as measured by the Mayer-Salovey-Caruso Emotional Intelligence Test (MSCEIT), the subscale most closely aligned with ER as conceptualized herein. In addition, Gross and John (2003) did not observe correlations between typical use of CR, as measured using the self-report Emotion Regulation Questionnaire (ERQ) and tests of scholastic performance and intelligence. Why, then, did we observe associations between fluid cognitive ability and CR success in this study?

One explanation pertains to the conceptualization and measurement of ER. While the MSCEIT and ERQ tap important aspects of ER, neither assesses success in modulating evoked emotional responses in accord with the emotion-regulatory goal. This is important because generally knowing the best emotion-regulating action to use in a particular context (which is assessed by the MSCEIT) or typically choosing to use CR (which is assessed by the ERQ) may be independent of how well one actually changes their emotional response in the midst of an emotion-triggering situation. Fluid cognitive abilities may be particularly relevant to how well one actually changes one's emotional response in accordance with the regulatory goal in an emotion-triggering situation, particularly in the face of a time limit and complex visual information to appreciate as was the case in this study.

**Table 4 | Estimates of emotional responding for each measure as a function of Cognitive Reappraisal (CR) instruction, gaze direction, and age group.**

| | Younger adults | | | | Older adults | | | |
|---|---|---|---|---|---|---|---|---|
| | Decrease | View | Increase | No CR | Decrease | View | Increase | No CR |
| **CORRUGATOR ACTIVITY** | | | | | | | | |
| Arousing | 1.267 (0.462) | 1.809 (0.517) | 2.047 (0.504) | 1.956 (0.598) | 1.736 (0.47) | 2.431 (0.636) | 2.984 (0.612) | 2.054 (0.453) |
| Not directed | 1.479 (0.539) | 2.247 (0.613) | 2.37 (0.594) | 2.362 (0.667) | 1.199 (0.479) | 1.8 (0.755) | 1.839 (0.542) | 1.603 (0.554) |
| Non-arousing | 1.11 (0.34) | 1.339 (0.334) | 2.018 (0.478) | 1.536 (0.37) | 1.188 (0.543) | 1.404 (0.558) | 1.245 (0.457) | 1.344 (0.486) |
| **HEART RATE** | | | | | | | | |
| Arousing | 35.424 (3.181) | 35.467 (3.048) | 35.992 (3.139) | 35.636 (3.171) | 29.447 (3.494) | 29.534 (3.442) | 29.62 (3.443) | 29.471 (3.449) |
| Not directed | 33.499 (3.807) | 33.685 (3.886) | 33.728 (3.794) | 33.476 (3.847) | 32.764 (3.079) | 32.866 (3.026) | 32.908 (3.001) | 32.849 (3.021) |
| Non-arousing | 36.299 (2.659) | 36.512 (2.666) | 37.335 (2.576) | 36.46 (2.541) | 29.457 (3.497) | 29.482 (3.475) | 29.506 (3.469) | 29.485 (3.48) |
| **ELECTRODERMAL ACTIVITY** | | | | | | | | |
| Arousing | −0.015 (0.012) | −0.026 (0.018) | 0.002 (0.01) | −0.003 (0.012) | 0.004 (0.007) | 0.003 (0.006) | −0.003 (0.005) | 0 (0.003) |
| Not directed | −0.007 (0.011) | −0.015 (0.009) | 0.002 (0.015) | 0.007 (0.012) | 0.007 (0.003) | 0.007 (0.005) | 0.007 (0.003) | 0.004 (0.003) |
| Non-arousing | 0.018 (0.01) | −0.001 (0.007) | 0.019 (0.011) | 0.015 (0.01) | 0.001 (0.005) | −0.004 (0.004) | 0.003 (0.004) | −0.002 (0.004) |
| **INTENSITY RATING** | | | | | | | | |
| Arousing | 3.658 (0.204) | 4.293 (0.238) | 5.412 (0.243) | 3.967 (0.249) | 4.111 (0.28) | 4.6 (0.246) | 5.771 (0.296) | 4.753 (0.282) |
| Not directed | 3.481 (0.203) | 4.104 (0.271) | 5.491 (0.226) | 4.208 (0.236) | 4.359 (0.277) | 4.655 (0.274) | 5.701 (0.273) | 4.646 (0.249) |
| Non-arousing | 3.562 (0.206) | 3.728 (0.224) | 5.136 (0.261) | 3.745 (0.235) | 4.343 (0.244) | 4.371 (0.268) | 5.548 (0.3) | 4.523 (0.272) |

*Estimates were determined via a series of two-level multilevel models, one for each age group, gaze direction, and CR instruction as described in text. Reported here is the intercept B(SE) from each model, which represents the mean value for the one CR instruction in each model that was not included as a predictor.*

### COGNITIVE ABILITY PREDICTS SUCCESSFUL CR, NO MATTER THE GOAL

Much ER research has focused on the down-regulation of negative emotions. This approach is motivated by the idea that prohedonic regulatory goals (e.g., "decrease negative") are commonly pursued in daily life (Gross et al., 2006; Riediger et al., 2011), and may have important clinical implications (Goldin et al., 2012; Gross, 2013). However, research focusing on the up-regulation of negative emotions is also warranted for two reasons. First, people also pursue contrahedonic regulatory (e.g., "increase negative") goals (Riediger et al., 2009, 2011; Tamir et al., 2013). Second, manipulating both pro- and contrahedonic ER in the same study helps to disambiguate the cognitive effort required to reappraise from changes in emotional arousal (see, e.g., Urry et al., 2009).

Examining both pro- and contra-hedonic goals in the present study gave us the opportunity to determine whether success in achieving these two ER goals is differentially predicted by cognitive ability. The existing literature provides mixed suggestions about these potentially differential relationships. On the one hand, prior work suggested that prohedonic ER goals may be more difficult to achieve than contrahedonic ER goals (Ochsner et al., 2004). This implies that fluid cognitive ability should be more useful when decreasing negative emotion than when increasing negative emotion. On the other hand, evidence also suggests that the association between working memory—one cognitive resource—and preferences for contrahedonic emotions is stronger than the association between working memory and preferences for prohedonic emotions (Riediger et al., 2011). This implies that fluid cognitive ability should be *less* useful when decreasing negative emotion than when increasing negative emotion.

Contrary to both possibilities, we found no difference in the extent to which higher levels of fluid cognitive ability predicted successful CR in pursuit of contrahedonic vs. prohedonic goals. Of course, it is possible that features of our design facilitated this outcome. For example, the use of mildly intense sad stimuli and a pseudo-block design may have reduced the typical disparity in difficulty. Future studies will be needed to understand the conditions that moderate how resources like fluid cognitive ability contribute to differential success of ER strategies as a function of contrahedonic or prohedonic aims.

### AGE DIFFERENCES IN COGNITIVE ABILITY BUT NOT CR SUCCESS

Theoretical models suggest that we might expect age differences in emotion and/or its regulation, at least in some contexts (e.g., Socioemotional Selectivity Theory Carstensen et al., 1999, Strength and Vulnerability Integration Charles, 2010). Indeed, consistent with that expectation, Opitz et al. (2012a) previously demonstrated that OA were less successful than YA at using CR to decrease negative emotions, but more successful at using CR to increase negative emotions. OA in that study also exhibited reduced CR-related activation in brain regions implicated in cognitive control processes like information selection and conflict monitoring compared to YA. The authors concluded that OA may lack the cognitive resources to reduce negative emotion using the particular form of CR that was studied. However, it is important to acknowledge that some of the stimuli used in that study may have been less relevant to OA. Moreover, participants had to frequently switch between ER goals and the regulation period was very brief. That particular design may therefore have put OA at a disadvantage in applying CR.

In the current study, we used only sad, moderately intense pictures which had face-valid relevance to both younger and OA. Additionally, participants had more time to use CR and only had to switch between one active CR condition and the view and no CR control conditions within each block. These changes likely reduced the degree to which OA would be at a disadvantage relative to YA in being able to successfully apply CR. With these changes in place, we observed significant associations between fluid cognitive ability and CR success but not between age group and CR success. Of course, this may in part be because of insufficient power to detect small effects in the present study. However, alternatively or in addition, the age differences in CR success observed by Opitz et al. (2012a) based on fewer participants may have been due to age-related variation in cognitive ability as well as age-related inequality in opportunity for success. Together, these two studies are consistent with the idea that age differences in affective responding are apt to be observed only in "highly resource-demanding situations that overtax OA capacities" (Wrzus et al., 2013, p. 386).

It is important to note that our ability to examine age differences in CR success in this study was hampered for at least two reasons. For one, the age range in the older and younger samples differed (16-year span vs. 4-year span, respectively). The larger age range in the older adult group may introduce greater within-group variation, thus reducing sensitivity to between-group differences. In addition, the two age groups differed not just in terms of age but also in terms of education, marital status, and fluid cognitive ability; OA had more education, were more likely to have been married, and had lower fluid cognitive ability than YA. Thus, even if we had identified age differences in CR success, it would ultimately be unclear whether age itself or one or more of these other variables represents the source of those differences. Importantly, when we modeled all of these as simultaneous predictors in one model, we did not observe any statistically significant effects of age group; instead, ever having been married was associated with greater CR success. Although intriguing, we are reluctant to make inferences about these marital status effects (and the absence of age effects) because none of the YA had ever been married and only three of the OA had never been married; as such, marital status is confounded with older age in this sample. It remains for future research to determine whether ever having been married really does relate to greater CR success, as potentially suggested by our results.

We did not have *a priori* predictions about age differences in the relation between cognitive ability and CR success. Even if we did, as noted above, age was significantly associated with fluid cognitive ability, marital status, and education level in the present sample, which hampers our ability to isolate unique effects. Thus, we suggest that fluid cognitive ability was perhaps a resource for successful CR across the whole sample. We also speculate that the inclusion of older and YA in our sample increased the range of meaningful variation in fluid cognitive ability; this may have enhanced sensitivity to the association between fluid cognitive ability and CR success.

## LIMITATIONS AND DIRECTIONS FOR FUTURE RESEARCH

While this study had numerous strengths, including the multi-method approach to measuring emotional responding, inclusion of both younger and older adult participants, and use of multi-level structural equation modeling to test our hypothesis, we acknowledge that this study has some important limitations to be addressed in future research. First, we concentrated on CR, which is just one of five families of ER processes. While individual differences in fluid cognitive ability predict the success of CR, this should not be taken to indicate that fluid cognitive ability would similarly predict the success of other ER strategies. This should also not be taken to indicate that fluid cognitive ability, as indexed by perceptual reasoning, PS, and working memory, are the only resources for CR. By the same token, the present study used only sad picture stimuli. It is unclear whether the current results will generalize to other specific emotions, like fear, disgust, or anger, or to positive emotions like happiness. It will be important in future studies to determine whether the cognitive abilities studied here serve as resources for other families of ER, to identify other resources that support successful CR, and to determine whether these resources play similar roles in the regulation of emotions other than sadness.

Second, cognitive ability is largely internal to an individual. Other resources that might be involved in CR might include resources that are largely *external*. Previous work has proposed, for example, that having access to people who help one generate new meanings for emotion-triggering situations may be a resource for CR (Urry and Gross, 2010). The elegant work of Coan et al. (2006) has demonstrated that stress-sensitive brain regions responded less in women who held someone's hand while undergoing threat of shock compared to women who did not hold someone's hand. While that example is not specific to CR, it suggests that social support in the form of hand-holding may be an external resource that facilitates ER. Assessing external resources for ER is an important direction for future research.

Third, our sample was mostly Caucasian and there were not enough participants to assess potential gender differences in the relations we have reported. In addition, these are cross-sectional, correlational data, which preclude drawing inferences about the putative causal direction on which we have focused here—namely that resources contribute to regulatory success. In order to determine the generalizability of these findings, it will be important to introduce heterogeneity with respect to the types of participants who are recruited for future studies. In addition, to facilitate causal inference, it will be important to (1) measure resources and regulatory success at multiple time points to examine whether a change in resources precedes a change in regulatory success and/or (2) manipulate the resources to see whether a change in resources effects a change in regulatory success.

## CONCLUSION

In this paper, we provide evidence that higher levels of fluid cognitive ability predict greater success at using CR to increase and decrease sad emotion. This finding supports a basic tenet of the SOC-ER framework (Urry and Gross, 2010), which proposes that higher levels of relevant resources contribute to greater ER success. Importantly, the relation between cognitive ability and successful CR was invariant with respect to whether the goal of CR was contrahedonic or prohedonic. This paper sets the stage for research that seeks to understand variation in successful ER in the context of fluctuating resources. Of key interest from the perspective of SOC-ER is determining the ways in which we compensate for lost resources by (a) selecting different strategies that do not require lost resources and/or (b) optimizing our skill at using strategies for which resources have been compromised. We believe this is an important set of steps to take to further our basic understanding of emotion and its regulation and to further applied goals vis-à-vis augmenting well-being.

## AUTHOR CONTRIBUTIONS

Philipp C. Opitz and Heather L. Urry conceived and designed the study, with significant input from James J. Gross. Philipp C. Opitz collected most of the data. Philipp C. Opitz, Ihno A. Lee, and Heather L. Urry analyzed the data. Philipp C. Opitz, Ihno A. Lee, James J. Gross, and Heather L. Urry wrote the manuscript.

## ACKNOWLEDGMENTS

We are grateful to Tufts University for their assistance in funding this work via a Graduate Student Research Award to Philipp C. Opitz. We also thank the following individuals: E. Brown and D. Millstein for assistance with data collection and processing, J. L. Birk, S. R. Cavanagh, and J. A. DiCorcia for many valuable discussions, and F. Wilhelm and P. Peyk for making ANSLAB, a suite of open source Matlab routines used to process physiological data, available as freeware in the Society for Psychophysiological Research Software Repository (http://www.sprweb.org/repository).

## REFERENCES

Appleton, A. A., Buka, S. L., Loucks, E. B., Gilman, S. E., and Kubzansky, L. D. (2013). Divergent associations of adaptive and maladaptive emotion regulation strategies with inflammation. *Health Psychol.* 32, 748–756. doi: 10.1037/a0030068

Arditi, A. (2005). Improving the design of the letter contrast sensitivity test. *Invest. Ophthalmol. Vis. Sci.* 46, 2225–2229. doi: 10.1167/iovs.04-1198

Bradley, M. M., and Lang, P. J. (2007). "Emotion and motivation," in *Handbook of Psychophysiology.* 3rd Edn., eds J. T. Cacioppo, L. G. Tassinary, and G. G. Berntson (Cambridge: Cambridge University Press), 581–607.

Buhle, J. T., Silvers, J. A., Wager, T. D., Lopez, R., Onyemekwu, C., Kober, H., et al. (2013). Cognitive reappraisal of emotion: A meta-analysis of human neuroimaging studies. *Cereb. Cortex.* doi: 10.1093/cercor/bht154. [Epub ahead of print].

Carstensen, L. L., Isaacowitz, D. M., and Charles, S. T. (1999). Taking time seriously: a theory of socioemotional selectivity. *Am. Psychol.* 54, 165.

Charles, S. T. (2010). Strength and vulnerability integration: a model of emotional well-being across adulthood. *Psychol. Bull.* 136, 1068. doi: 10.1037/a0021232

Coan, J. A., Schaefer, H. S., and Davidson, R. J. (2006). Lending a hand: social regulation of the neural response to threat. *Psychol. Sci.* 17, 1032–1039. doi: 10.1111/j.1467-9280.2006.01832.x

Dougherty, B., Flom, R., and Bullimore, M. (2005). An evaluation of the mars letter contrast sensitivity test. *Optom. Vis. Sci.* 82, 970–975. doi: 10.1097/01.opx.0000187844.27025.ea

Evstafiev, M. (1992). *A Family Mourns During a Funeral at the Lion's Cemetery in Sarajevo, 1992 [Photo].* Available online at: http://commons.wikimedia.org/wiki/File:Evstafiev-bosnia-sarajevo-funeral-reaction.jpg

Farrelly, D., and Austin, E. J. (2007). Ability EI as an intelligence? Associations of the MSCEIT with performance on emotion processing and social tasks and with cognitive ability. *Cogn. Emot.* 21, 1043–1063. doi: 10.1080/02699930601069404

Fidell, L. S., Tabachnick, B. G. (2003). "Research methods in psychology," in *Handbook of Psychology*. Vol. 2., eds J. A. Schinka, and W. F. Velicer (Hoboken, NJ: John Wiley & Sons Inc. xxiii, 115–141, 711.

Ford, B. Q., and Tamir, M. (2012). When getting angry is smart: emotional preferences and emotional intelligence. *Emotion* 12, 685–689. doi: 10.1037/a0027149

Fridlund, A., and Cacioppo, J. (1986). Guidelines for human electromyographic research. *Psychophysiology* 23, 567–589.

Goldin, P. R., Ziv, M., Jazaieri, H., Werner, K., Kraemer, H., Heimberg, R. G., et al. (2012). Cognitive reappraisal self-efficacy mediates the effects of individual cognitive-behavioral therapy for social anxiety disorder. *J. Consul. Clin. Psychol.* 80, 1034–1040. doi: 10.1037/a0028555

Gross, J. J. (2013). Emotion regulation: taking stock and moving forward. *Emotion* 13, 359–365. doi: 10.1037/a0032135

Gross, J. J. (ed.). (2014). *Handbook of Emotion Regulation.* 2nd Edn. New York, NY: Guilford.

Gross, J. J. (1998). The emerging field of emotion regulation: an integrative review. *Rev. Gen. Psychol.* 2, 271–299.

Gross, J. J., Richards, J. M., and John, O. P. (2006). "Emotion regulation in everyday life," in *Emotion Regulation in Couples and Families: Pathways to Dysfunction and Health,* eds D. K. Snyder, J. A. Simpson, and J. N. Hughes (Washington, DC: American Psychological Association), 13–35.

Gross, J. J., and John, O. P. (2003). Individual differences in two emotion regulation processes: implications for affect, relationships, and well-being. *J. Pers. Soc. Psychol.* 85, 348–362. doi: 10.1037/0022-3514.85.2.348

Hedden, T., and Gabrieli, J. D. E. (2004). Insights into the ageing mind: a view from cognitive neuroscience. *Nat. Rev. Neurosci.* 5, 87–96. doi: 10.1038/nrn1323

Hoffman, L., and Rovine, M. J. (2007). Multilevel models for the experimental psychologist: foundations and illustrative examples. *Behav. Res. Methods* 39, 101–117. doi: 10.3758/BF03192848

Hox, J. (2002). *Multilevel Analysis: Techniques and Applications.* Manwah, NJ: Lawrence Erlbaum.

Isaacowitz, D. M., Toner, K., Goren, D., and Wilson, H. R. (2008). Looking while unhappy: mood-congruent gaze in young adults, positive gaze in older adults. *Psychol. Sci.* 19, 848–853. doi: 10.1111/j.1467-9280.2008.02167.x

Isaacowitz, D. M., Toner, K., and Neupert, S. D. (2009). Use of gaze for real-time mood regulation: effects of age and attentional functioning. *Psychol. Aging* 24, 989–994. doi: 10.1037/a0017706

Kline, R. B. (2010). *Principles and Practice of Structural Equation Modeling.* 3rd Edn. New York, NY: Guildford.

Lang, P. J., Bradley, M. M., and Cuthbert, B. N. (2008). "International affective picture system (IAPS): affective ratings of pictures and instruction manual," in *Technical Report A-8,* (Gainesville, FL: University of Florida).

Lohani, M., and Isaacowitz, D. M. (2013). Age differences in managing response to sadness elicitors using attentional deployment, positive reappraisal and suppression. *Cogn. Emot.* 28, 678–697. doi: 10.1080/02699931.2013.853648

Malooly, A. M., Genet, J., and Siemer, M. (2013). Individual differences in reappraisal effectiveness: the role of affective flexibility. *Emotion* 13, 302–313. doi: 10.1037/a0029980

Mauss, I. B., Levenson, R. W., Mccarter, L., Wilhelm, F. H., and Gross, J. J. (2005). The tie that binds? Coherence among emotion experience, behavior, and physiology. *Emotion* 5, 175–190. doi: 10.1037/1528-3542.5.2.175

McRae, K., Hughes, B., Chopra, S., Gabrieli, J. D. E., Gross, J. J. and Ochsner, K. N. (2010). The neural bases of distraction and reappraisal. *J. Cogn. Neurosci.* 22, 248–262. doi: 10.1162/jocn.2009.21243

McRae, K., Jacobs, S. E., Ray, R. D., John, O. P., and Gross, J. J. (2012). Individual differences in reappraisal ability: Links to reappraisal frequency, well-being, and cognitive control. *J. Res. Pers.* 46, 2–7. doi: 10.1016/j.jrp.2011.10.003

Mikels, J., Fredrickson, B., Larkin, G., Lindberg, C., Maglio, S., and Reuter-Lorenz, P. (2005). Emotional category data on images from the International affective picture system. *Behav. Res. Methods* 37, 626–630. doi: 10.3758/BF03192732

Muthén, L. K., and Muthén, B. O. (1998–2013). *Mplus User's Guide.* 7th Edn. Los Angeles, CA: Muthén & Muthén.

Ochsner, K. N., Bunge, S. A., Gross, J. J., and Gabrieli, J. D. E. (2002). Rethinking feelings: an FMRI study of the cognitive regulation of emotion. *J. Cogn. Neurosci.* 14, 1215–1229. doi: 10.1162/089892902760807212

Ochsner, K. N., Day, R. D., Cooper, J. C., Robertson, E. R., Chopra, S., Gabrieli, J. D. E., et al. (2004). For better or for worse: neural systems supporting the cognitive down- and up-regulation of negative emotion. *Neuroimage* 23, 483–499. doi: 10.1016/j.neuroimage.2004.06.030

Opitz, P. C., Gross, J. J., and Urry, H. L. (2012b). Selection, optimization, and compensation in the domain of emotion regulation: applications to adolescence, older age, and major depressive disorder. *Soc. Pers. Psychol. Compass* 6, 142–155. doi: 10.1111/j.1751-9004.2011.00413.x

Opitz, P. C., Rauch, L. C., Terry, D. P., and Urry, H. L. (2012a). Prefrontal mediation of age differences in cognitive reappraisal. *Neurobiol. Aging,* 33, 645–655. doi: 10.1016/j.neurobiolaging.2010.06.004

Riediger, M., Schmiedek, F., Wagner, G. G., and Lindenberger, U. (2009). Seeking pleasure and seeking pain: differences in prohedonic and contra-hedonic motivation from adolescence to old age. *Psychol. Sci.* 20, 1529–1535. doi: 10.1111/j.1467-9280.2009.02473.x

Riediger, M., Wrzus, C., Schmiedek, F., Wagner, G. G., and Lindenberger, U. (2011). Is seeking bad mood cognitively demanding? Contra-hedonic orientation and working-memory capacity in everyday life. *Emotion* 11, 656–665. doi: 10.1037/a0022756

Salthouse, T. A., Atkinson, T. M., and Berish, D. E. (2003). Executive functioning as a potential mediator of age-related cognitive decline in normal adults. *J. Exp. Psychol.* 132, 566–594. doi: 10.1037/0096-3445.132.4.566

Sheppes, G., and Meiran, N. (2007). Better late than never? On the dynamics of online regulation of sadness using distraction and cognitive reappraisal. *Pers. Soc. Psychol. Bull.* 33, 1518–1532. doi: 10.1177/0146167207305537

Shiota, M. N., and Levenson, R. W. (2009). Effects of aging on experimentally instructed detached reappraisal, positive reappraisal, and emotional behavior suppression. *Psychol. Aging* 24, 890–900. doi: 10.1037/a0017896

Schmeichel, B. J., Volokhov, R. N., and Demaree, H. A. (2008). Working memory capacity and the self-regulation of emotional expression and experience. *J. Pers. Soc. Psychol.* 95, 1526–1540. doi: 10.1037/a0013345

Tamir, M., and Ford, B. Q. (2012). Should people pursue feelings that feel good or feelings that do good? Emotional preferences and well-being. *Emotion* 12, 1061–1070. doi: 10.1037/a0027223

Tamir, M., Ford, B. Q., and Gilliam, M. (2013). Evidence for utilitarian motives in emotion regulation. *Cogn. Emot.* 27, 483–491. doi: 10.1080/02699931.2012.715079

Urry, H. L. (2010). Seeing, thinking, and feeling: emotion-regulating effects of gaze-directed cognitive reappraisal. *Emotion* 10, 125. doi: 10.1037/a0017434

Urry, H. L., and Gross, J. J. (2010). Emotion regulation in older age. *Curr. Dir. Psychol. Sci.* 19, 352. doi: 10.1177/0963721410388395

Urry, H. L., van Reekum, C. M., Johnstone, T., and Davidson, R. J. (2009). Individual differences in some (but not all) medial prefrontal regions reflect cognitive demand while regulating unpleasant emotion. *Neuroimage* 47, 852–863. doi: 10.1016/j.neuroimage.2009.05.069

Wilhelm, F. H., and Peyk, P. (2005). *ANSLAB: Autonomic Nervous System Laboratory (Version 4.0).* Available online at the SPR Software Respository: http://www.sprweb.org

Wrzus, C., Müller, V., Wagner, G. G., Lindenberger, U., and Riediger, M. (2013). Affective and cardiovascular responding to unpleasant events from adolescence to old age: complexity of events matters. *Dev. Psychol.* 49, 384–397. doi: 10.1037/a0028325

9

# The ties to unbind: age-related differences in feature (un)binding in working memory for emotional faces

**_Didem Pehlivanoglu*, Shivangi Jain, Robert Ariel and Paul Verhaeghen_**

*School of Psychology, Georgia Institute of Technology, Atlanta, GA, USA*

***Edited by:***
*Natalie Ebner, University of Florida, USA*

***Reviewed by:***
*Natalie Ebner, University of Florida, USA*
*Carla Marie Strickland-Hughes, University of Florida, USA*
*Christina M. Leclerc, State University of New York at Oswego, USA*
*Lixia Yang, Ryerson University, Canada*

***Correspondence:***
*Didem Pehlivanoglu, School of Psychology, Georgia Institute of Technology, J. S. Coon Building, 654 Cherry Street, Atlanta, GA 30332, USA*
*e-mail: dpehlivanoglu3@gatech.edu*

In the present study, we investigated age-related differences in the processing of emotional stimuli. Specifically, we were interested in whether older adults would show deficits in unbinding emotional expression (i.e., either no emotion, happiness, anger, or disgust) from bound stimuli (i.e., photographs of faces expressing these emotions), as a hyper-binding account of age-related differences in working memory would predict. Younger and older adults completed different *N*-Back tasks (side-by-side 0-Back, 1-Back, 2-Back) under three conditions: match/mismatch judgments based on either the identity of the face (identity condition), the face's emotional expression (expression condition), or both identity and expression of the face (both condition). The two age groups performed more slowly and with lower accuracy in the expression condition than in the both condition, indicating the presence of an unbinding process. This unbinding effect was more pronounced in older adults than in younger adults, but only in the 2-Back task. Thus, older adults seemed to have a specific deficit in unbinding in working memory. Additionally, no age-related differences were found in accuracy in the 0-Back task, but such differences emerged in the 1-Back task, and were further magnified in the 2-Back task, indicating independent age-related differences in attention/STM and working memory. Pupil dilation data confirmed that the attention/STM version of the task (1-Back) is more effortful for older adults than younger adults.

**Keywords: hyper-binding, memory binding, working memory, aging, pupillary response, emotion**

## INTRODUCTION

Working memory is the workspace of the mind, where passive storage and active manipulation/transformation of information engage in dynamic interplay (Baddeley and Hitch, 1974; Miyake and Shah, 1999; Kane et al., 2001). An effective working memory system is crucial for high-level performance in a multitude of cognitive tasks, perhaps because an effective working memory system depends on the efficient implementation of a host of basic cognitive control operations that are likely involved in most, if not all aspects of the cognitive system. For instance, significant relations have been demonstrated between fluid intelligence and working memory capacity, and between spatial and language abilities and working memory (e.g., Kyllonen, 1996; Engle et al., 1999; Conway et al., 2002; Kemper et al., 2003).

Given the centrality of the working memory construct, it is not surprising that there is a growing literature on the effects of aging on its capacity and dynamics. The brunt of the research shows that working memory capacity declines with advancing adult age. Small age differences are already found in the performance of short-term memory (STM) tasks that do not require much cognitive control or attentional resources, such as digit span tasks, but age-related deficits in working memory, as measured by tasks such as reading span, listening span, or operation span, are demonstrably larger. In a meta-analysis compiling a total of 123 studies from 104 papers, Bopp and Verhaeghen (2007) found that older adults' capacity in simple STM span tasks was 92% that of the capacity of younger adults; their capacity on true working memory tasks, however, was only 74% that of younger adults. This decline in working memory capacity has consequences for complex aspects of cognition: on average, working memory capacity explains 52% of the age-related variance in episodic memory performance, 63% of the age-related variance in spatial abilities, and 72% of the age-related variance in reasoning abilities; STM, in contrast, explains 9% or less of the age-related variance (Verhaeghen, 2014).

One particular determinant of working memory capacity that has consistently been found to be age-sensitive is the availability of information that has left focus of attention and needs to be retrieved after a bout of intermittent processing. Our lab and others have studied this topic using variations on the *N*-Back task – the task we will also use here (e.g., Oberauer, 2002; Verhaeghen and Basak, 2005; Chen and Li, 2007; Vaughan et al., 2008; Verhaeghen, 2012; Zhang et al., 2012). In an *N*-Back task, subjects indicate whether the stimulus currently on the screen matches the stimulus presented *N* positions back. The typical finding in our experiments (but see Kirchner, 1958; Dobbs and Rule, 1989) is that older and younger adults are equally (and highly) accurate in the 1-Back version of the task, but that age differences in accuracy consistently emerge when $N > 1$. We would argue that 1-Back tasks primarily reflect the workings of attention, with a possible STM component as well (i.e., subjects have to retain information passively over a very brief duration – 2 s in our experiment). A 2-Back version adds a true working memory component to the task, in the form of intervening items that need to be processed.

The finding then echoes other reports (e.g., Bopp and Verhaeghen, 2007) that older adults show small or not deficits in STM tasks, but substantial deficits in working memory tasks. Additionally, in the present study, we will include a 0-Back condition where two stimuli are shown side-by-side, to test and/or control for perceptual deficiencies in older adults.

The finding of an age-related deficit in the working memory component, but not the attentional/STM component of working memory leads to an obvious question: can this result be reduced to a deeper deficit in a known process, or is this aspect of working memory – retrieval of items stored outside immediate attention – a cognitive primitive that is especially age-sensitive? This is the research question we will address in the present paper. To foreshadow: the cognitive primitive we will investigate is association, more precisely, the binding of features into objects and the concomitant unbinding of objects into features; the objects we will use, for reasons explained below, are faces displaying emotional expressions (presenting emotion and identity into a compound percept). Additionally, we will use a physiological measure (pupil dilation) to independently verify the commitment of attentional resources throughout the task. As a side effect, the use of emotional stimuli will allow us to investigate the claims of an age-related positivity effect in a domain where such effects have rarely been investigated, namely that of working memory.

One popular hypothesis to explain age-related differences in working memory functioning is the hypothesis of an age-related associative deficit. The claim is that older adults fail to efficiently and/or effectively link individual features of a learning episode together; one consequence is a particular difficulty in forming or retrieving the associations or bindings between the features of objects, compared to maintaining the single features in memory (Chalfonte and Johnson, 1996; Naveh-Benjamin et al., 2004; Cowan et al., 2006). The associative-binding theory has fared extremely well in the domain of episodic memory (e.g., Old and Naveh-Benjamin, 2008), but evidence from the domain of working memory have been decidedly mixed.

In support of the associative-deficit hypothesis, Cowan et al. (2006), in a delayed match-to-sample task, did indeed find evidence that older adults were especially poor at detecting binding changes. Importantly, this deficit was not due to age-related differences in attentional resources per se, because the decline was evident even when the set size of the array was reduced to be well below capacity limits. Other researchers, in contrast, have failed to discover evidence for an associative deficit in working memory, concluding instead that aging is governed by a rather general deficit in working memory functioning. For instance, in three change-detection experiments, Brockmole et al. (2008) found overall lower working memory performance in older adults, but no specific age-related deficit emerged in a feature-binding condition. Importantly, in this study, older adults were more affected by increases in set size than younger adults were, suggesting that the age-related decline in working memory performance is tied to a fundamental change in capacity rather than to associative deficits. With a very different task – a repetition-detection paradigm – Bopp and Verhaeghen (2009) found, in line with the Brockmole et al. (2008) findings, that the necessity to bind content to context decreased performance in both age groups to the same degree.

In the present paper, we approach the binding problem from a different angle, inspired by a recent study that found evidence – in episodic memory – of the existence of the third possible empirical outcome, namely that older adults are better at associative binding than younger adults. That is, Campbell et al. (2010) found that when to-be-remembered stimuli (in this case: line drawings) were paired with stimuli explicitly labeled as irrelevant (in this case: words) older participants showed better memory for the drawing–word conjunction than younger adults did. The authors labeled this phenomenon hyper-binding, and see it as predicated on deficient inhibitory functioning. Under this hypothesis, older adults are unable to inhibit the irrelevant information, which therefore gets encoded (and maintained) along with the relevant information. The net result is a functional shrinkage in the capacity of working memory.

So far, age-related hyper-binding has not been demonstrated in working memory. Clearly, the three papers cited above report either no evidence for a binding deficit in old age, or the opposite of hyper-binding, that is, a binding deficit. It is also clear, however, that the standard set-up of experiments into the associative deficit hypothesis might not be easily conducive to elicit the phenomenon of age-related hyper-binding. One potential issue is that in classical association experiments (which often use artificial compound stimuli composed of random combinations of abstract features, e.g., Wheeler and Treisman, 2002) feature binding typically comes at a cost: remembering the compound object is more difficult than remembering the individual features. Working memory experiments reporting age-related binding deficits as evidenced by age by condition interactions could then simply be instantiations of a complexity or difficulty effect: age differences are "naturally" larger in tasks yielding lower performance, that is, in this case, the both condition (e.g., Cerella, 1985).

In the present study, we reversed this situation by using naturally occurring and ecologically valid compound objects that, by all accounts, are easier to remember than at least some of their constituent features. More specifically, we capitalized on an interesting finding in the face recognition literature, namely that when participants are confronted with a face showing a natural emotion, recognition of facial identity (i.e., who is this person?) typically occurs faster and with higher accuracy than recognition of the emotional expression (e.g., Ganel and Goshen-Gottstein, 2004; Martens et al., 2010). At the same time, matching on both identity and emotional expression typically occurs no faster or more accurately than matching on identity alone (e.g., Soto and Wasserman, 2011). These findings suggest that identity of faces is processed easily, maybe even automatically, whereas extraction of emotional expression is a much slower, potentially effortful process. (Note that there is some controversy over whether these two types of judgments – identity or emotional expression – are independent; Bruce and Young, 1986; or interrelated; e.g., Ganel and Goshen-Gottstein, 2004. This question, however, is irrelevant to our current study, which concerns only the relative efficiency of these processes.) This particular quirk of the cognitive system makes emotional face recognition particularly well suited to investigate the hyper-binding hypothesis. If older adults indeed encode more of the stimulus than strictly needed for the task, the age-related deficit in performance would be larger in conditions in which only the emotional expression (a single feature) needs to be remembered compared to memory for the whole stimulus (i.e., identity bound with emotional expression), because older adults would be less inclined or less capable to extract and remember only the relevant feature. (Note that the age-related deficit for memory for facial identity (another single feature) should likely match that for memory of the whole stimulus, given that identity extraction typically comes at no cost.)

One added advantage of these stimuli lies in their emotional nature: it has often been claimed that the valence of emotions inherent in experimental stimuli moderates age-related differences in cognition. Our study allows us to investigate some of these claims explicitly, in a domain where these have been rarely researched. For instance, socioemotional selectivity theory (Carstensen et al., 1999) states that a shrinking time perspective leads older adults to focus on positive information rather than negative information – the so-called positivity bias. There are only a few studies that investigated the impact of emotional stimuli on working memory performance, but their usefulness for the present questions is limited: these studies included either only younger adults or negative stimuli (Kensinger and Corkin, 2003) or examined the effect of arousal but not emotion (Wurm et al., 2004). The literature on attention and the positivity bias suggests that the pattern may be complicated. For instance, Allard and Isaacowitz (2008) found that older adults fixated their gaze more on positive and neutral images compared to negative images, regardless of whether the images were presented in full or divided attention conditions; additionally, older adults' secondary task performance was as good as that of younger adults. This finding strongly suggests that processing positive emotional material does not require full attention. Other studies, however, have found that the presence of a distractor task leads older adults to remember proportionally more negative images than positive images (Mather and Knight, 2005) and to exhibit an attentional preference for negative images relative to positive images (Knight et al., 2007). This set of findings then indicates that processing positive emotional material does require attention, and that the age-related positivity bias may disappear or reverse under conditions of high cognitive load. Our study could shed further light on this controversy. That is, if the cognitive or memory load explanation has any validity, we would expect an age-related positivity effect for the *N*-Back conditions with low cognitive load (i.e., 0-Back or 1-Back), but a reversal of the effect for the 2-Back version, which has an added memory component which has been shown to increase response time (RT) and decrease accuracy (e.g., Verhaeghen and Basak, 2005).

We additionally recorded changes in participants' pupil diameter during stimulus processing. The aim was to investigate how this response changes with age and/or as a function of processing demands and emotional content of the stimuli. Pupil dilations have long been thought to reflect a brain activity during perceptual and cognitive processing (Kahneman and Beatty, 1966). Task-evoked pupillary responses occur during the processing of stimuli and have been interpreted as indicators of cognitive effort and emotional arousal (for a review, see Beatty, 1982; Goldinger and Papesh, 2012). In line with this reasoning, pupil diameter typically increases as task demand increases (e.g., Karatekin et al., 2007; Van Gerven et al., 2004; Heitz et al., 2008) and as task/response interference increases (e.g., Porter et al., 2007; Laeng et al., 2011). Pupils also dilate during emotional processing, with larger pupil dilations occurring in response to positively valenced images (Hess, 1965), sexually arousing stimuli (Hicks et al., 1967), and positively and negatively arousing sounds (Partala and Surakka, 2003).

Surprisingly, few studies have investigated the joint influence of processing demands and emotional content on task-evoked pupillary responses. One exception is Stanners et al. (1979) who manipulated both processing demands (difficulty level of an arithmetic task) and arousal (threat of shock) or only arousal without processing demands. They found that pupillary responses increased with the difficulty of the arithmetic problems regardless of threat of shock, suggesting that pupillary responses are influenced mainly by cognitive demands of the task regardless of emotional arousal. In the low-difficulty task, however, arousal did influence pupil dilations. The two results combined suggest that arousal influences pupillary responses in low-demand situations, but that high cognitive demand may override the arousal-related response.

Based on this literature, we propose that pupil dilation during stimulus processing (relative to a baseline pupil measurement) could provide an independent, physiological indication of age-related differences in the effects of working memory demands (by comparing responses in the 2-Back task with responses in the 0-Back and 1-Back tasks) and potentially also of age-related differences in phasic changes due to emotion-specific arousal; the latter effect will likely only be observable in the low-demand conditions (i.e., 0-Back and 1-Back), as observed by Stanners et al. (1979).

To summarize, in the present study, we investigate one potential source of the oft-noted age-related differences in working memory performance, namely the possibility that older adults are less flexible than younger adults in unbinding information in working memory when representing the bound object is unnecessary – the so-called hyper-binding hypothesis. To maximize the chances of hyper-binding, we used emotional faces as stimuli; it has been shown that extracting the emotion content from such faces is an effortful process. The task is a subject-paced *N*-Back task. In its side-by-side 0-Back form, this task measures perceptual discrimination; its 1-Back version adds an attentional/STM requirement; the 2-Back version adds a working memory component. If older adults do hyper-bind, they would need more time and/or be less accurate in unbinding a stimulus into its features. As a consequence, we would expect larger age differences in the condition in which subjects respond only to the emotional expression. Additionally, we investigated the role of emotional valence on age differences in perception, attention, and memory, expecting, from the one extant study (Knight et al., 2007), a positivity bias in perception and attention (i.e., in 0-Back and 1-Back) and a negativity bias in working memory (i.e., in 2-Back), possibly (Knight et al., 2007) modulated by task difficulty such that the positivity bias would only show in the simpler tasks (i.e., 0-Back or 1-Back). Pupil dilation data will provide information as to the resource investment in each of the conditions. Given previous reports of age differences in performance in *N*-Back tasks, we expect that older adults would show a higher investment of resources in this task than younger adults.

The present work breaks modest new ground in at least two aspects. First, as far as we know, although emotional faces have been used extensively in perceptual paradigms such as stimulus discrimination or classification, there are fewer data on how working memory handles this class of stimuli (for one exception, see Kensinger and Corkin, 2003), and none in the field of aging. Second, as far as we know, we are the first research team to employ a physiological measure, pupil dilation, as independent verification of adult age-related differences in the task difficulty presumably involved in working memory encoding and/or retrieval and in the processing of emotional content.

## MATERIALS AND METHODS

### PARTICIPANTS

Twenty-one younger (67% female) and 21 older (71% female) adults participated in this experiment. Older participants were recruited from the community; they received cash payment ($10/hour) as compensation for participation. Younger adults were students at Georgia Institute of Technology; they were given either course credit or cash payment ($10/hour) for participation.

One older adult whose data could not be recorded due to technical problems was excluded from the analyses. The mean age of the remaining 20 older adults was 70.55 ($SD = 4.3$); mean age of younger adults was 20.33 ($SD = 1.62$). Older adults ($M = 16.7$, $SD = 3.16$) had completed more years of education than younger adults ($M = 14.21$, $SD = 1.49$), $t(39) = 3.25$, $p = 0.002$. Younger adults ($M = 62.9$, $SD = 8.04$) performed significantly better than older adults ($M = 45.65$, $SD = 8.57$) on a symbol digit test, $t(39) = 6.65$, $p < 0.001$. On the other hand, older adults' performance ($M = 34.1$, $SD = 4.51$) on the Shipley Vocabulary test was significantly higher than performance of younger adults ($M = 31.33$, $SD = 3.61$), $t(39) = 2.18$, $p = 0.04$.

### MATERIALS

#### *Faces*

Forty-eight faces were selected from the FACES database (Ebner et al., 2010), with 12 different young-female actors portraying either angry, happy, neutral, or disgusted expressions. One of the faces, showing all these emotions is presented in **Figure 1A**. To keep the number of to-be-analyzed variables manageable we included only young and female faces in the study. Previous research has shown effects of age (young vs. old) and sex (female vs. male) of face stimuli on attention and memory performance of younger and older adults (for a meta-analytic review, see Rhodes and Anastasi, 2012); however, investigation of the effect of these variables is out of the scope of the current study.

Our choice of emotional expressions was guided by previous findings concerning age-related differences in emotion processing; the aim was to bias the results toward observing age by condition interactions. We included happy and angry faces specifically because older adults have been shown to show high recognition accuracy for happy stimuli (e.g., Carstensen et al., 1999) while younger adults tend to show a memory bias for angry faces (Mikels et al., 2005). Additionally, we included disgust to see whether recognition of disgust appears to be relatively preserved in old age as shown in a couple of studies (e.g., Calder et al., 2003).

We selected a subset of 12 young-female faces with happy, angry, neutral, and disgusted expressions from the FACES database based on correct identification of these facial expressions by younger-female, younger-male, older-female, and older-male raters in the norming study (Ebner et al., 2010)[1]. Given that we were interested in the effects of emotion alone, arousal level of the stimuli is a potential confound. Since arousal ratings are not available in FACES database, we conducted a separate study including 42 young adults (55% female) recruited from the Georgia Institute of Technology (mean age 19.81, $SD = 2.12$). Participants provided arousal ratings for each face on a 9-point Likert scale (1 – *not arousing at all*, 9 – *highly arousing*) using the Self-Assessment Manikin (Bradley and Lang, 1994). As expected, participants rated neutral faces ($M = 3.13$, $SD = 1.42$) as less arousing than happy ($M = 5.26$, $SD = 1.56$), disgusted ($M = 6.00$, $SD = 1.73$), or angry faces ($M = 5.56$, $SD = 1.53$), all $ts(41) > 6.35$, $ps < 0.001$. Although the perceived arousal level of individual face pictures in each emotion category varied, disgusted and angry faces were on average not more arousing than happy faces. The only significant difference was between angry and disgusted faces, $t(41) = 4.41$, $p < 0.001$.

#### *Apparatus*

Pupil data were recorded binocularly using a head-mounted SR Inc. Eyelink II eyetracker with a 500-Hz sample rate. To obtain baseline pupil estimates, an 8,000 ms fixation cross was presented at the beginning of each block. For each block, the average pupil size recorded during this 8,000 ms period served as the baseline pupil estimate for that block. Peak pupil sizes were recorded during presentation of the face photos and during the interstimulus interval. For the analyses, the peak pupil size value during stimulus presentation and the interstimulus interval for each trial was determined. The percentage change was calculated as max pupil size at each trial minus the baseline pupil value divided by the baseline, thus scaling responses as a function of each individual subject's baseline (e.g., Iqbal et al., 2004).

All tasks were prepared and presented by E-Prime 2.2. Stimuli were presented on a 14-inch computer screen (resolution 1024 × 768 pixel) over a gray background (RGB: 150, 150, 150) as bitmap images (231 × 185 pixels). The face stimuli subtended

[1]In the norm study (Ebner et al., 2010), for our subset of the stimuli, the mean accuracy of emotional expression identification by younger women was 93.15 ($SD = 11.31$), by younger men was 90.56 ($SD = 10.91$), by older women was 86.42 ($SD = 15.17$), and by older men was 83.67 ($SD = 16.42$).

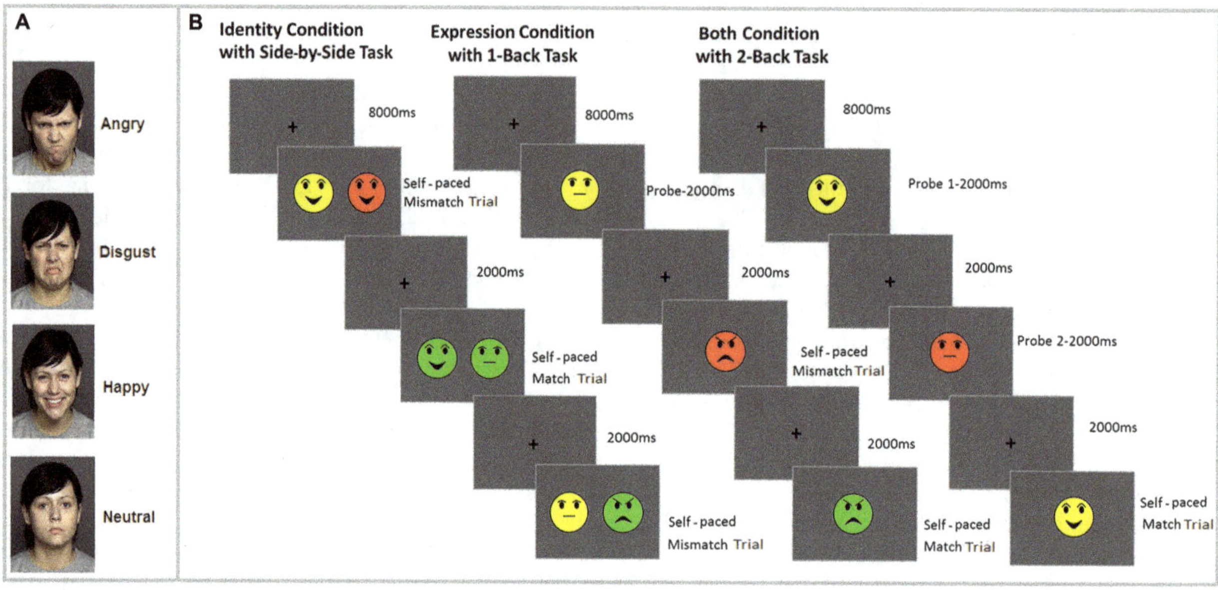


**FIGURE 1 | Illustration of the one of the faces with all emotional expressions (angry, disgust, happy, neutral) used in the study (A) and the experimental procedure, with a sample *N*-Back task for each of the three conditions: identity (side-by-side 0-Back task), expression (1-Back task) and both (2-Back task) (B).** Note that different colors represent different individual faces.

a horizontal visual angle of 7.5° and a vertical visual angle of 6.6°.

### *Task design*

The experiment consisted of identity, expression, and both conditions with three *N*-Back tasks (side-by-side 0-Back, 1-Back, and 2-Back). The task design for each condition is illustrated in **Figure 1B**[2]. Each condition involved making match/mismatch judgments based on either the identity of the face (identity condition), the face's emotional expression (expression condition), or joint identity and expression of the faces (both condition). Each condition consisted of two blocks of 48 trials of each *N*-Back task. Since we had three different *N*-Back tasks, there were a total of 288 trials in each of the three conditions (identity, expression, both). The number of match and mismatch trials was equally distributed across the 48 trials within each block. Furthermore, different trials included equal number of difficult and easy lures in each *N*-Back tasks. For instance, when participants were shown the face of person "A" with happy facial expression in the identity condition, the face of person "B" with happy facial expression was considered a difficult lure, whereas the face of person "B" with angry facial expression was an easy lure. Within each condition and task, the same set of face stimuli were used. This was done to ensure that performance differences between the different tasks and conditions could not be attributable to the stimuli. Emotional expressions and facial identity were pseudo-randomized so that each face and emotional expression was presented an equal number of times within each *N*-Back task. Conditions were blocked.

[2]Since the FACES database agreement provides only one young-female face to use in scientific publications, it was not possible to demonstrate the tasks we used in this study using the real stimuli. Thus, for the purposes of task design illustration, we used emoticons in **Figure 1B**.

The order of presentation of *N*-Back tasks and conditions was counterbalanced using a Latin square design. There was no effect of counterbalancing on performance.

#### *Side-by-side 0-Back task*

For the side-by-side 0-Back task, two face pictures were presented side-by-side on the screen and participants decided whether the two pictures were identical or not in terms of either identity or emotional expression, or of both identity and emotional expression, depending on condition. The purpose of the side-by-side task was to evaluate potential age differences in perceptual discrimination of facial identity, emotional expression, and their conjunction. Note that this side-by-side comparison likely involves saccadic eye movements, making it likely that the RTs for the 0-Back task will be larger than those of the 1-Back and 2-Back tasks.

#### *1-Back and 2-Back tasks*

In these tasks, participants were asked to compare either identity, emotional expression, or joint identity and emotional expression of a face with the face presented one position back (1-Back) or two positions back (2-Back task).

### PROCEDURE

Participants were tested individually. Before the experiment, each participant signed a consent form. Each condition began with 12 practice trials. During the study, the eye tracker was calibrated before each block in each condition to establish a map between each participant's gaze position and the eye tracker. Each block began with an 8,000 ms presentation of a fixation cross that served to collect the baseline pupil measurement. Next, participants were presented with a probe face (1-Back) or two probe faces (2-Back) for 2,000 ms each, or no probe (side-by-side 0-Back task). Following probe trials, participants completed 48 self-paced trials. In each trial, a single face (1-Back and 2-Back conditions) or two side-by-side faces (0-Back condition) were presented; subjects indicated whether the relevant feature(s) of the presented face matched the relevant feature(s) of the face presented one face back (1-Back condition), two faces back (2-Back condition), or whether the relevant feature(s) of the two side-by-side faces matched (0-Back). Because face trials were self-paced and peak pupil dilation typically occurs 1,800–2,000 ms post-stimulus onset (Beatty, 1982), each face trial was followed by a 2,000 ms interstimulus interval to allow sufficient time for the pupil to reach peak dilation. After 48 trials, a new block began. Pupil dilation was continuously recorded throughout the task. The total duration of the experiment was approximately 120 min.

## RESULTS

### CORRECTED RECOGNITION RATES

Corrected recognition rates (proportion of hit rates minus false alarm rates) were calculated for each participant and entered in a three-way mixed analysis of variance (ANOVA): 2 (Age: young, old) × 3 (Condition: identity, expression, both) × 3 (*N*-Back: side-by-side 0-Back, 1-Back, 2-Back). The data for younger and older adults are presented in **Figures 2A,B**, respectively. Younger adults ($M = 0.87$, $SD = 0.08$) performed significantly better than older participants ($M = 0.77$, $SD = 0.08$), $F(1,39) = 18.74$, $MSE = 0.05$, $p < 0.001$, $\eta_p^2 = 0.33$. There was a main effect of condition [$F(2,78) = 9.87$, $MSE = 0.02$, $p < 0.001$, $\eta_p^2 = 0.2$] showing that participants performed better in the both ($M = 0.86$, $SD = 0.11$) than in the expression condition ($M = 0.79$, $SD = 0.10$), $t(40) = 4.44$, $p < 0.001$. Performance in the identity condition ($M = 0.82$, $SD = 0.12$) was not significantly different from performance in the expression and both conditions (all $ps > 0.10$). The main effect of *N*-Back task [$F(2,78) = 134.58$, $MSE = 0.01$, $p < 0.001$, $\eta_p^2 = 0.78$] revealed that participants had higher corrected recognition responses in the side-by-side 0-Back task ($M = 0.89$, $SD = 0.07$) than in the 1-Back task ($M = 0.86$, $SD = 0.09$), $t(40) = 2.9$, $p = 0.006$, and 2-Back task ($M = 0.71$, $SD = 0.15$), $t(40) = 9.22$, $p < 0.001$. Performance was higher in the 1-Back task than 2-Back task, $t(40) = 9.89$, $p < 0.001$.

Additionally, the ANOVA revealed a significant Age × *N*-Back interaction [$F(2,78) = 27.65$, $MSE = 0.01$, $p < 0.001$, $\eta_p^2 = 0.42$]. Follow-up analyses indicated that there was no age difference in the side-by-side task. Older adults performed significantly worse than younger adults in the 1-Back [$t(39) = 2.79$, $p = 0.008$] and 2-Back tasks [$t(39) = 5.89$, $p < 0.001$]. Moreover, while both age groups performed poorer in the 2-Back task than in the 1-Back and 0-Back versions, only older adults showed significantly poorer performance in the 1-Back compared to the 0-Back version [$t(19) = 3.02$, $p = 0.007$]. To examine the unbinding cost directly, a separate ANOVA: 2 (Age: young, old) × 2 (Condition: expression, both) × 3 (*N*-Back: side-by-side 0-Back, 1-Back, 2-Back) showed a significant Condition × *N*-Back × Age interaction [$F(2,78) = 4.34$, $MSE = 0.01$, $p = 0.016$, $\eta_p^2 = 0.10$][3]. In the side-by-side 0-Back task, there was no age difference in the expression and both conditions. With regard to 1-Back task, there was no age difference in the both condition, but older adults performed worse than younger adults in the expression condition [$t(39) = 2.59$, $p < 0.05$]. For 2-Back task, older adults performed worse than younger adults in the expression [$t(39) = 4.99$, $p < 0.001$] and both [$t(39) = 4.12$, $p < 0.001$] conditions. More importantly, within the 2-Back task, older adults' performance in the both condition exceeded that in the expression condition [$t(19) = 3.25$, $p = 0.004$]. However, younger adults did not show such difficulty in the expression condition compared to the both condition in the 2-Back task. For younger adults, the only difference between expression and both condition was within the side-by-side 0-Back task [$t(20) = 3.09$, $p = 0.006$]; their side-by-side 0-Back task performance was better in the both condition than the performance in the expression condition.

### RESPONSE TIMES

Any RTs 3 *SD* above or below the group mean values were excluded from the analyses. To eliminate the effect of age-related slowing in age by condition interaction analyses (Faust et al., 1999), a logarithmic transformation was applied on the RT data prior to analysis. Only hit trials were included in RT data analyses. The data for younger and older adults are presented in **Figures 2C,D**, respectively. A three-way mixed ANOVA on log transformed RTs showed that younger participants ($M = 787.37$, $SD = 172.69$) had faster reaction times than older participants ($M = 1359.93$, $SD = 348.34$), $F(1,39) = 114.79$, $MSE = 0.22$, $p < 0.001$, $\eta_p^2 = 0.75$. There was a main effect of task [$F(2,78) = 122.66$, $MSE = 0.03$, $p < 0.001$, $\eta_p^2 = 0.76$]. Participants had significantly longer RTs in side-by-side 0-Back task ($M = 1194.7$, $SD = 296.13$) than they had in 1-Back ($M = 884.02$, $SD = 219.95$), $t(40) = 15.86$, $p < 0.001$ and 2-Back tasks ($M = 1142.22$, $SD = 265.45$), $t(40) = 3.72$, $p = 0.001$. RTs were longer in 2-Back task than in 1-Back task [$t(40) = 11.76$, $p < 0.001$]. Longer RTs in the side-by-side task are consistent with participants' verbal reports that they looked for differences in fine details between the two pictures; it is also likely that this RT included saccadic eye movements. ANOVA revealed a significant main effect of condition, $F(2,78) = 17.58$, $MSE = 0.05$, $p < 0.001$, $\eta_p^2 = 0.31$. Participants had longer RTs in the expression ($M = 1176.93$, $SD = 250.89$) condition than in the identity [$M = 1022.43$, $SD = 237.28$; $t(40) > 6.26$, $p < 0.001$] and both conditions [$M = 1021.58$, $SD = 293.37$; $t(40) = 5.01$, $p < 0.001$].

### INFLUENCE OF EMOTION ON ACCURACY

The analysis of the effect of emotional expression was restricted to the 1-Back and 2-Back tasks (the side-by-side comparison in the 0-Back task makes it impossible to assess which of the emotional expressions influenced performance), and to the expression and both conditions (in the identity condition, participants were supposed to disregard emotional information, and therefore any calculation of accuracy for expression is not meaningful in this condition).

A four-way mixed ANOVA: 2 (Age: young, old) × 2 (Condition: expression, both) × 2 (*N*-Back: 1-Back, 2-Back) × 4

[3]When we conducted a separate ANOVA: 2 (Age: young, old) × 2 (Condition: identity, both) × 3 (*N*-Back: side-by-side 0-Back, 1-Back, 2-Back) to see whether age-related unbinding cost would occur for identity task, the Condition × *N*-Back × Age interaction was not significant, indicating no differential cost of unbinding for older adults in the identity condition.

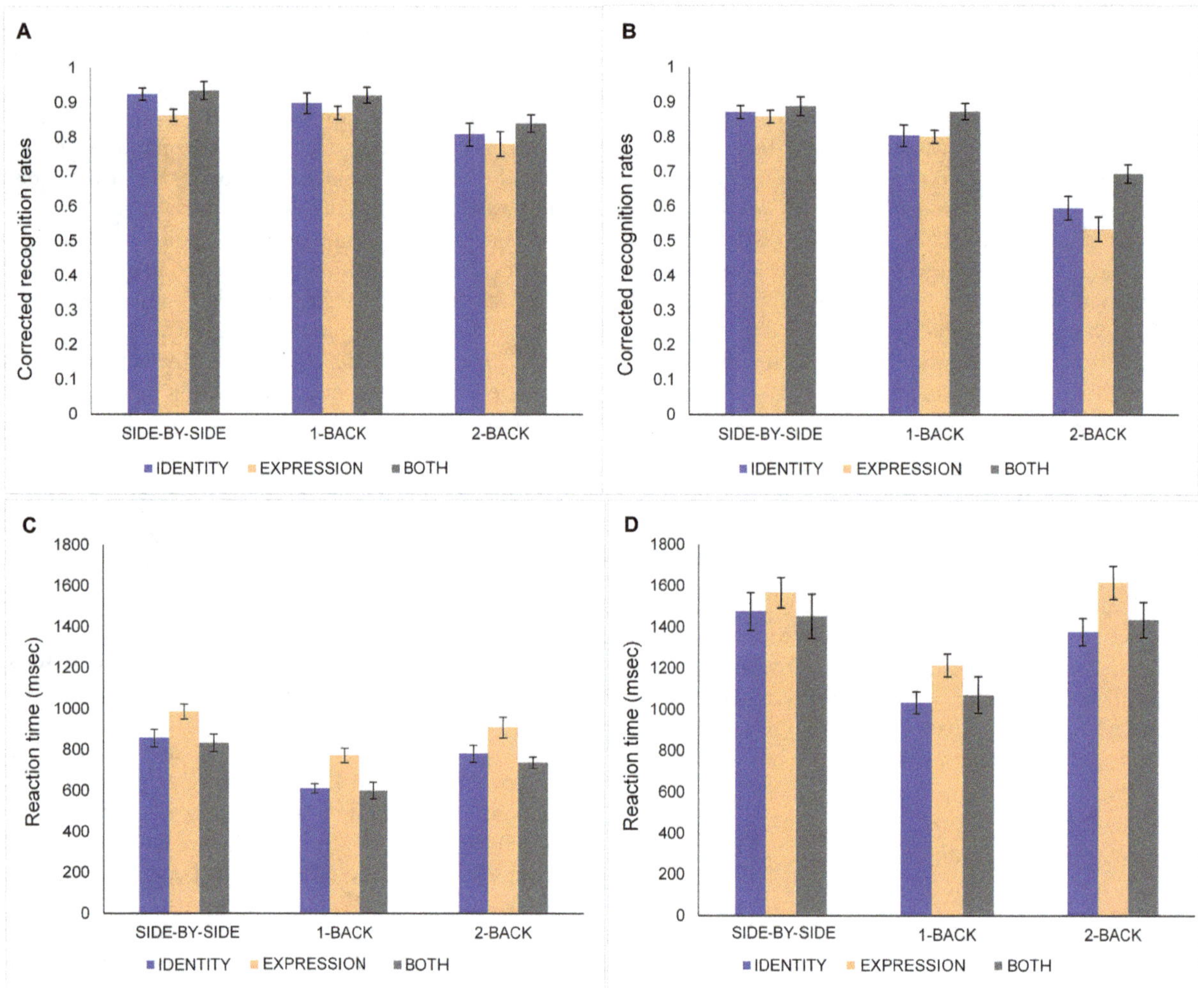

**FIGURE 2 | Corrected recognition rates (proportion of hits minus false alarms) and response times of younger (A,C) and older (B,D) adults in the identity, expression, and both conditions for side-by-side 0-Back, 1-Back, and 2-Back tasks.** Error bars denote standard error.

(Emotion: happy, angry, neutral, disgust) was performed on corrected recognition rates (proportion of hit minus false alarm rates) for each emotional expression. The data for younger and older adults are represented in **Figures 3A,B**, respectively. The main effect of emotion [$F(3,117) = 18.87$, $MSE = 0.02$, $p < 0.001$, $\eta_p^2 = 0.33$] showed that happy ($M = 0.83$, $SD = 0.09$) and neutral ($M = 0.81$, $SD = 0.12$) faces were recognized better than angry faces ($M = 0.73$, $SD = 0.11$) [happy vs. angry, $t(40) = 6.86$, $p < 0.001$; neutral vs. angry, $t(40) = 5.82$, $p < 0.001$]. Additionally, disgusted faces ($M = 0.76$, $SD = 0.13$) were recognized significantly worse than happy [$t(40) = 3.93$, $p < 0.001$], and neutral faces [$t(40) = 3.21$, $p = 0.003$]. There was no significant difference between angry and disgusted faces [$t(40) = 2.04$, $p = 0.048$] and between happy and neutral faces [$t(40) = 0.99$, $p > 0.10$]. Furthermore, the Condition by Emotion interaction [$F(3,117) = 17.85$, $MSE = 0.02$, $p < 0.001$, $\eta_p^2 = 0.32$] was significant. Follow-up analyses showed that in the expression condition, happy faces were recognized better than angry [$t(40) = 8.39$, $p < 0.001$], disgusted [$t(40) = 5.62$, $p < 0.001$] and, neutral faces [$t(40) = 3.21$, $p = 0.003$] while there was no difference in recognition of the faces in the both condition [all $ts(40) < 2.05$, $ps > 0.09$]. Additionally, participants performed better in the both condition than in the expression condition for angry [$t(40) = 6.3$, $p < 0.001$], and disgusted [$t(40) = 4.48$, $p < 0.001$] faces. There was no age-related recognition bias for the specific type of emotional stimuli shown, as indexed by a non-significant interaction between age and emotion [$F(3,117) = 1.83$, $MSE = 0.02$, $p > 0.10$, $\eta_p^2 = 0.05$].

### INFLUENCE OF EMOTION ON RESPONSE TIMES

The data for younger and older adults are shown in **Figures 3C,D**, respectively. The main effect of emotion was significant [$F(3,117) = 15.79$, $MSE = 0.09$, $p < 0.001$, $\eta_p^2 = 0.29$]. Participants' RTs were significantly faster for happy ($M = 937.87$, $SD = 55.67$) faces than for angry [$M = 1112.47$, $SD = 59.21$; $t(40) = 6.58$, $p < 0.001$], disgusted [$M = 1080.38$, $SD = 55.35$; $t(40) = 4.36$, $p < 0.001$], or neutral faces [$M = 1027.71$,

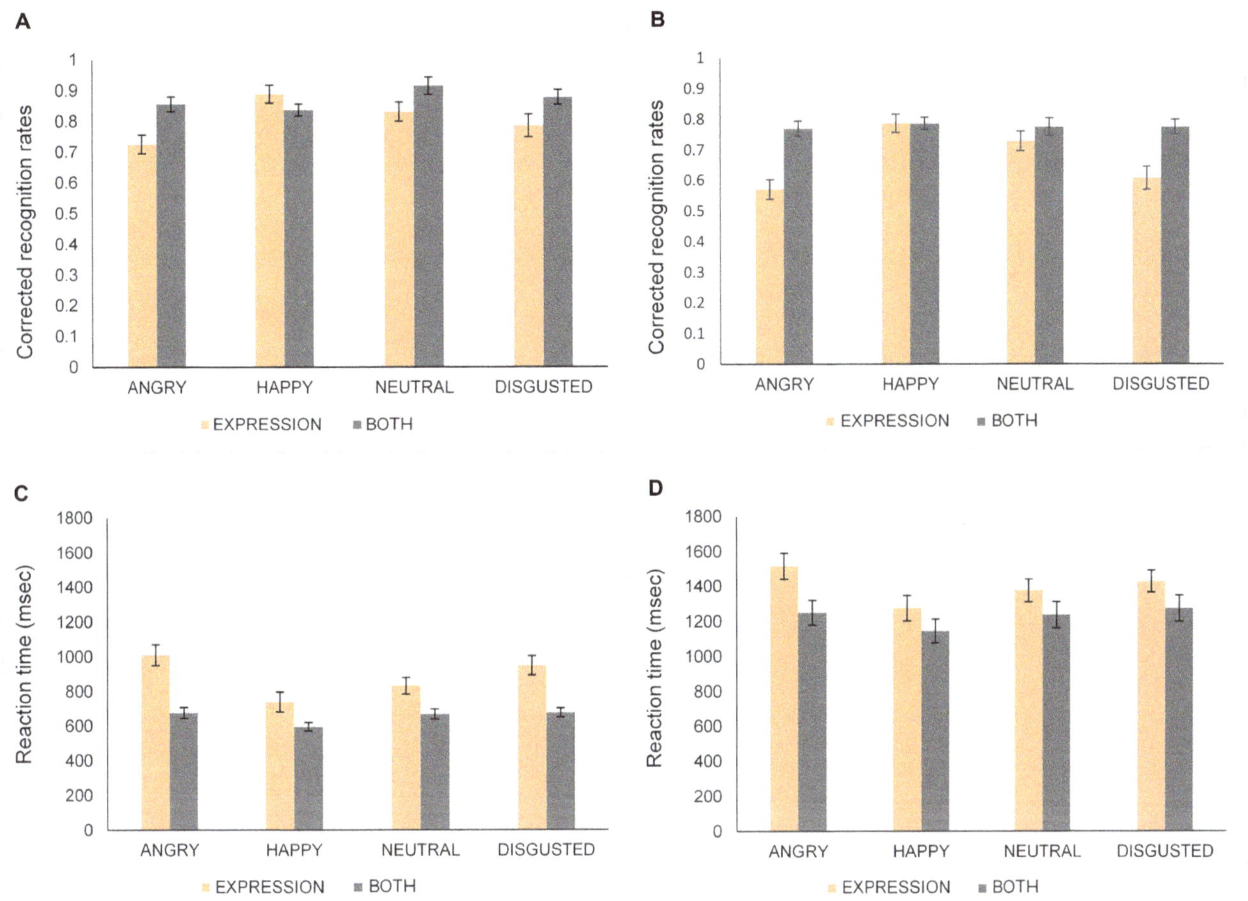


**FIGURE 3 | Corrected recognition rates (proportion of hits minus false alarms) and response times of younger (A,C) and older (B,D) adults for angry, happy, neutral, and disgusted faces in the identity, expression, and both conditions.** Error bars denote standard error.

*SD* = 54.6; $t(40) = 3.52$, $p = 0.001$]. In addition, neutral faces were detected faster than angry faces [$t(40) > 3.9$, $p < 0.001$]. Moreover, the Condition × Emotion interaction was significant [$F(3,117) = 3.72$, $MSE = 0.07$, $p = 0.01$, $\eta_p^2 = 0.09$]. Follow-up analyses showed that in the expression condition, happy faces were recognized faster than angry [$t(40) = 7.55$, $p < 0.001$], disgusted [$t(40) = 4.73$, $p < 0.001$], or neutral faces [$t(40) = 4.58$, $p < 0.001$]. Additionally, neutral faces were recognized faster than angry faces [$t(40) = 4.73$, $p < 0.001$]. For happy faces, there was no RT difference between conditions whereas the expression condition yielded slower RTs than the both condition for angry [$t(40) = 6.94$, $p < 0.001$], neutral [$t(40) = 3.46$, $p = 0.001$], and disgusted faces [$t(40) = 4.22$, $p < 0.001$]. Consistent with the accuracy data, a non-significant Age × Emotion interaction [$F(3,117) = 1.94$, $MSE = 0.09$, $p > 0.10$, $\eta_p^2 = 0.05$] reflects an absence of age-related speed bias for any type of emotional expression.

## INFLUENCE OF EMOTION AND COGNITIVE LOAD ON PUPIL RESPONSES

Prior to analysis, pupil data with missing observations due to eyeblinks or signal loss were discarded. Additionally, pupil values above 2.5 *SD* from the average of their 10 immediate neighbors were removed within each individual and replaced by linear interpolation, in accordance with guidelines by Goldinger et al. (2009). This procedure resulted in fewer than 4% corrected trials per participant. For the analyses, the max peak pupil size value during stimulus presentation and the inter-stimulus interval for each trial was determined. The percentage change was calculated as max pupil size at each trial minus the baseline pupil value divided by the baseline (e.g., Iqbal et al., 2004). Baseline pupil size was the average pupil size recorded during this 8,000 ms fixation cross presented at the beginning of each block. Only hit responses were included in the analyses.

To understand the joint effects of emotion and cognitive task on pupil size, average percentage change in pupil size was calculated for each emotional expression within the 1-Back and 2-Back versions of the task. As in the previous analyses focusing on emotion, side-by-side tasks in each condition and identity condition as a whole were not included. A four-way mixed ANOVA: 2 (Age: young, old) × 2 (Condition: expression, both) × 2 (*N*-Back: 1-Back, 2-Back) × 4 (Emotion: angry, happy, neutral, disgust) was performed on average percentage change in pupil size. Only hit trials were considered. The data for younger and older adults are presented in **Figures 4A,B**, respectively.

There was a main effect of emotion [$F(3,117) = 6.77$, $MSE = 0.00$, $p < 0.001$, $\eta_p^2 = 0.15$) with larger pupil dilation for disgusted and angry faces than neutral faces [disgusted vs. neutral faces, $t(40) = 3.46$, $p = 0.001$; angry vs. neutral faces $t(40) = 3.37$, $p = 0.001$]. More importantly, we obtained a significant N-Back × Emotion × Age interaction [$F(3,117) = 3.55$, $MSE = 0.00$, $p = 0.02$, $\eta_p^2 = 0.08$]. To follow-up, we ran separate ANOVAs on *N*-Back and Emotion within the groups of younger and older adults. Younger adults' pupil dilation was larger in 2-Back task than 1-Back task [$F(1,20) = 9.32$, $MSE = 0.00$, $p = 0.006$, $\eta_p^2 = 0.32$] while older adults did not show a significant main effect of *N*-Back task [$F(1,19) = 0.22$, $MSE = 0.00$, $p > 0.10$, $\eta_p^2 = 0.01$]. For younger adults, pupil dilation was larger for angry and disgusted faces than neutral and happy faces in 1-Back task [angry vs. neutral, $t(20) = 3.56$, $p = 0.002$; disgust vs. neutral, $t(20) = 3.33$, $p = 0.003$; disgust vs. happy, $t(20) = 3.28$, $p = 0.004$]. However, there was no differential effect of any emotion on pupil dilation in 2-Back task for younger adults. These findings indicated that the effect of emotion on pupil dilation was evident only under low cognitive demand condition (in 1-Back task) for younger adults. On the other hand, the *N*-Back × Emotion interaction was not significant for older adults, showing that older adults' pupil dilation was not different for the faces across *N*-Back tasks.

## DISCUSSION

Before we discuss the age-related effects in the data, we first turn to the general-psychological findings.

First, we indeed obtained the predicted difficulty effects for our *N*-Back tasks. Crucial for our main investigation, we found that the 1-Back task, which involves sequential comparisons between two stimuli, and is thus primarily a measure of attention and STM, is easier (i.e., it leads to higher accuracy and faster RT) than the 2-Back task, which involves retrieving a memory presentation stored outside the immediate focus of attention, and is thus primarily a measure of working memory performance. In older adults, the 0-Back task, which involves a side-by-side comparison and is thus primarily a measure of perceptual discrimination, was also easier (i.e., it led to higher accuracy) than the 1-Back task; younger adults showed statistically indistinguishable accuracy for the two tasks. Note that RT for the 0-Back task is much higher than for the other tasks. This is probably due to the peculiarity of our set-up: the two stimuli are presented side-by-side, likely prompting saccadic eye movements during the comparison process.

Second, our results concerning binding and unbinding of identity and emotion in the face stimuli are in line with expectations as well. Analysis of RTs showed that the identity condition (where only the identity of the face needed to be matched) and the both condition (where both identity and emotional expression needed to be matched) were statistically indistinguishable, and that they were performed on average about 150 ms faster than the expression condition (where only the emotional expression of the face needed to be matched). These results are in line with the literature on perceptual discrimination for emotional faces, where extraction of identity appears to happen relatively automatically, but extraction of emotional expression is an effortful, time-demanding process (e.g., Ganel and Goshen-Gottstein, 2004). The accuracy analyses added a subtle twist to these findings: subjects were more accurate in the both condition than in the expression condition, with the identity condition situated in between (and not significantly different from either). For younger adults (we will return to the older-adults data below), this effect is already present in the side-by-side 0-Back condition, and is simply carried over to the 1-Back and 2-Back versions of the task. This suggests that for younger adults the effect operates at the perceptual stage only – it is not further exacerbated by the attentional/STM requirement in the 1-Back, or the working memory requirement in the 2-Back task. In sum, the accuracy findings reaffirm that expression extraction is an added, effortful process, leading to lower accuracy, and suggest that identity extraction may come at a

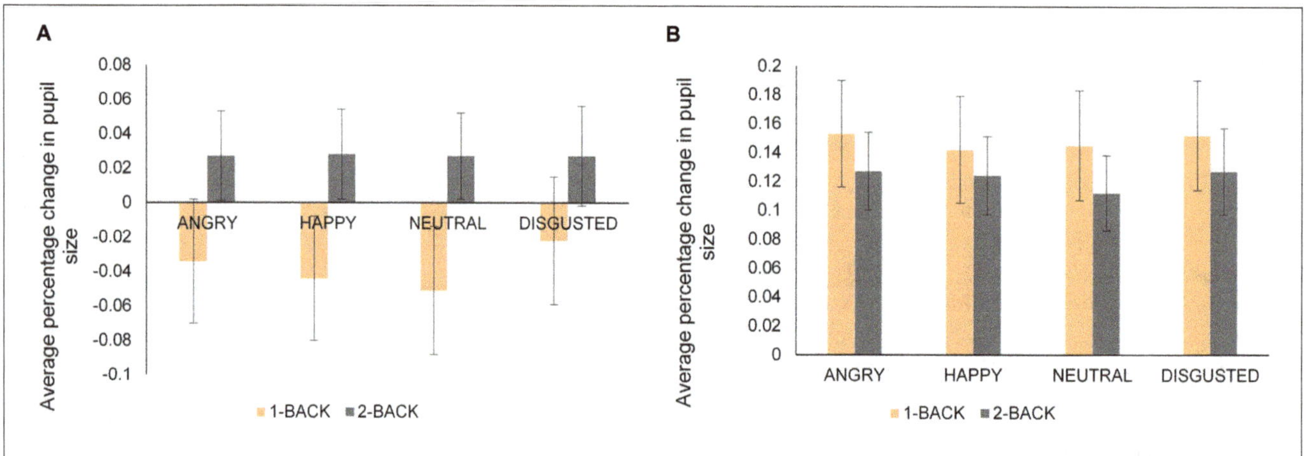


**FIGURE 4 | Average percentage change in pupil size from a fixation-cross baseline for younger (A) and older (B) adults for angry, happy, neutral, and disgusted faces in 1-Back and 2-Back tasks.** Error bars denote standard error. Note the different scale of the vertical axis for younger and older adults.

small (and, in the present study, not significant) cost in error rates.

The third set of findings concerns the effects of particular emotions on performance. This analysis was restricted to the 1-Back and 2-Back versions of the task (in mismatch stimuli in the 0-Back task, it is impossible to ascertain which of the two emotions displayed drives the effect); the analysis was also restricted to the two conditions were the emotional expressions were explicitly part of the decision process – the both condition and the expression condition. Overall, the evidence points at a positivity effect: happy and neutral faces yielded higher accuracy than angry and disgusted faces. This effect, however, only operated in the expression condition, not in the both condition, where no significant difference between accuracy for the different emotions was observed. RT data largely confirm this picture, with the exception of a less flat profile for the both condition, where happy faces were responded to faster than any other emotion. We note that the positivity effect in accuracy and RT may be due to the valence of the emotion, but it could also partially related to perceptual factors specific to happy faces, which tend to display more perceptually distinct features (i.e., open mouth, visible teeth) than negative and neutral faces. RTs in the both condition, with happy faces being the only stand-out (and being responded to fastest), lend some credence to the perceptual-distinctiveness hypothesis. Additionally, we showed that disgusted and angry emotions were more easily recognized in the both condition than in the expression condition. More accurate recognition of negative and potentially threatening emotions in the condition in which faces are processed as a whole may have its origin in the evolutionary survival value of swift action in the face of such emotions (e.g., Ackerman et al., 2006).

The final set of general findings pertains to pupil dilation. We highlight two results. First, for younger adults, we found evidence for a separation between the 1-Back task, which did not lead to larger pupil dilation compared to baseline, and the 2-Back task, which did. This finding is clearly in line with previous work showing that pupil dilation indexes cognitive resources (e.g., Granholm et al., 1996; Van Gerven et al., 2004; Goldinger and Papesh, 2012). Second, also for younger adults, but only for the 1-Back condition, we found a differential effect for emotion, with disgusted faces showing the highest amount of dilation, and angry the second highest. One observation here is that the emotions that yielded the lowest accuracy also elicit the largest pupil dilation, suggesting that higher effort (as evidenced by pupil dilation) is associated with more difficulties in maintaining attention across sequential presentation of stimuli. It also suggests that the recognition and reaction time advantage for happy faces is not due to attentional biases: one would expect that higher attentional effort would lead to better recognition and faster decisions, and therefore larger pupil dilation would be observed for happy faces. However, the opposite was true. We can solve this apparent puzzle if we assume that in the present case, pupil dilation does not index effort, but arousal (e.g., Stanners et al., 1979). In the separate study we conducted to assess arousal value of the stimuli (see Materials and Methods), the rank ordering of arousal values (from lowest to highest: neutral, happy, angry, disgusted) nicely tracks the pupil dilation date in the 1-Back condition for younger adults. We note that this differential effect of emotion disappeared in the 2-Back condition. The reason for this may be a functional ceiling in pupil dilation, in which the larger dilation associated with cognitive effort masks or trumps the arousal-related changes visible under conditions of low effort.

One goal of our study was to investigate age-related changes in the efficiency and/or efficacy of binding of information in working memory. Recall that binding emotional expressions to the identity of faces seems to be the default, and that abstracting emotional expressions from faces is effortful, as exemplified in higher accuracy and faster RTs for emotional faces than for the emotional expression on its own. Also recall that in younger adults, this effect operates at the perceptual stage, simply carrying over into the attentional/STM and working memory stages of processing (i.e., in the 1-Back and 2-Back task, respectively). The picture is different for older adults: age-related unbinding problems (operationalized as the difference between the expression condition and the both condition) become apparent in the 2-Back version of the task. Thus, older adults are as good (or as bad) as younger adults in unbinding the emotional feature from the compound stimulus in the perceptual and attentional/STM stages of the task; an added working memory component, however, widens the observed age difference. This suggests that older adults have a specific deficit, at least in this task, either with keeping unbound, feature-level information active and/or retrievable in memory, or with keeping the bound representation that is stored in working memory sufficiently detailed to easily abstract the emotional content from it. Further research is necessary to more precisely pinpoint the locus of or mechanism behind the effect. The result does not suggest a specific age-related problem of hyper-binding in the sense that older adults would keep the representation bound and younger adults do not: both age groups incur an unbinding cost in both accuracy and RT in the expression condition.

There is another possibility as well – an age-related deficit in flexible strategy use. Note that conditions were blocked, so that participants could freely apply strategic processing to the task, such as extraction of the relevant feature at the encoding stage rather than from a retrieved memory representation. If this strategy was used at all, the results suggest it was used more often, or with greater efficacy, by younger adults. In sum, the evidence points at the existence of hyper-binding in working memory in older adults, at least in this task, where the default modus operandi is to process stimuli in a bound state.

A second results concerns the emergence of age-related differences in the 1-Back task. In our previous work using the *N*-Back task (e.g., Verhaeghen et al., 2004; Vaughan et al., 2008), we consistently observed age-related differences in 2-Back tasks, but not in 1-Back tasks. The present experiment is the first where we do obtain age-related deficits in a 1-Back task. We can see at least two possible reasons for this difference. First, in our previous work, we used digits; the present study uses faces. Faces contain much more detail than digits, and so it is possible that this result signifies that older adults are less able to keep informational detail alive than younger adults do, even in the simple 1-Back task (for a related theoretical argument, see Myerson et al., 1990). The second possible reason is related to the brief interstimulus interval – 2,000 ms – built into the present, but not previous studies.

The interpretation would then be that older adults lose informational detail at a faster clip than younger adults do. We are not aware of relevant data in visual working memory, but decay rates in verbal working memory are indeed faster in older than younger adults – the half-life of older adults' STM representations is about 70% shorter than that of younger adults (Verhaeghen, 2014). Further research is necessary to assess to what degree each of those potential mechanisms operates to create the effect. We do know that this age-related deficit in attentional/STM processing cannot be due to perceptual deficits – younger and older adults performed equally well in the side-by-side comparison task.

Whatever the mechanism, it seems quite counterintuitive that age differences would appear with so minimal a cognitive load: all that is required of the subject in the 1-Back task is to retain an image of a face for 2 s, with no additional requirements. The pupil data confirm, however, that what one might consider a minimal load is far from minimal for older adults. First, older adults had elevated pupil dilations compared to younger adults in the 1-Back task, indicating that the 1-Back task is more effortful for older than for younger adults. Second, while we observed a clear separation between the 1-Back and the 2-Back version of the task in younger adults, older adults showed only nominally smaller pupil dilation for 1-Back that for 2-Back. This finding suggests that for older adults the cognitive load of passively maintaining a representation in the focus of attention is about as large as that for maintaining a representation in working memory while performing a concurrent task. One possible complication with the interpretation of this second finding is that there might be a functional ceiling for pupil dilation, and that statistical identity of 1-Back and 2-Back performance can therefore not directly equated with equal effort. Even under this interpretation, however, it is clear that the 1-Back task does not require attentional resources in younger adults, as testified by the lack of pupil dilation compared to baseline, whereas it clearly does in older adults.

A third age-related result concerns the differential effect of the emotion content of the stimuli. In general, and perhaps surprisingly, we observed a positivity effect, where happy and neutral faces were generally responded to faster and more accurately than angry and disgusted faces. Socioemotional selectivity theory (Carstensen et al., 1999) would predict this effect to be larger in older adults. One recent refinement of the theory (Mather and Knight, 2005) claimed that processing positive emotional material does require attention, and that the age-related positivity bias should then disappear or reverse under conditions of high cognitive load, as in our 2-Back task. We did not find any evidence for either hypothesis: no age by emotion interactions were observed in either accuracy or RTs, thus suggesting both an absence of an age-specific positivity effect and the absence of an effect of load on age-related difference in emotion-specific processing. Thus, the impact of the type of emotion was identical across age groups, regardless of processing stage (perceptual, attentional/STM, or memory) or cognitive load. This result runs counter socioemotional selectivity theory (including modifications of this theory that take cognitive load into account; e.g., Knight et al., 2007), but is in line with the one extant meta-analysis (Murphy and Isaacowitz, 2008) which found no significant difference in the preference for positive emotional stimuli of younger and older adults in either memory or attention studies.

Summarized, our results indicate that older adults do have more difficulty unbinding a bound stimulus than younger adults do, and that this difficulty is restricted to a working memory condition (2-Back); tasks primarily measuring perceptual clarity and attention/STM do not show age-related hyper-binding. Additionally, we found that, in general, older adults show deficits in attentional/STM processing (1-Back) as well as working memory processing; pupil dilation data suggest that attentional processing mobilizes and possibly requires more cognitive resources in older adults compared to younger adults. Finally, and importantly, our study adds to the body of literature suggesting a lack of age sensitivity in differential effects of different emotional stimuli on perception, attention, and working memory, counter the so-called positivity effect posited by socioemotional selectivity theory.

We note some important limitations of our study. One potential issue concerns the stimulus set: we used only young, female (and white) faces. Given the potential for own-age biases in attention and/or memory (Rhodes and Anastasi, 2012), it might be advisable to replicate this work using older-adult faces as well. We reiterative that same-age biases in face discrimination or face memory would influence mean levels of accuracy, but there is no reason to expect that that would influence interactions involving age.

Likewise, we obtained arousal data for these stimuli only from younger adults. Given that our study included both younger and older adults, arousal ratings from a sample of older adults would have been useful to ensure that older adults did not perceive the emotional faces differently than younger adults. Although some face databases (e.g., The Karolinska Directed Emotional Faces by Goeleven et al., 2008) measured perceived arousal level of the emotional face stimuli in the norming study, to our knowledge none of the databases included older adults as raters in their norming studies. When we look at non-face stimuli, Grühn and Scheibe (2008) investigated age-related differences in perceived levels of IAPS pictures and found that older adults perceived negative pictures as being more arousing and positive pictures as being less arousing than young adults did. If this result were to generalize to faces, we would expect larger pupil dilation for angry and disgusted faces in older adults compared to younger adults, and perhaps pupil contraction for happy faces. This is not what was found. We do note that this limitation is likely moot in the present study: only younger adults showed modulation of their pupil responses that could be interpreted as arousal-mediated, and then only in the 1-Back condition. Older adults, as well as younger adults in the more demanding condition (2-Back), showed elevated pupil dilation and no modulation by emotion, suggesting that the cognitive demands of the task wiped out any arousal-based effects on pupil dilation. Of course, it remains theoretically possible that older adults perceived all faces as much more arousing than younger adults did, thereby in effect attenuating all differential effects of emotion on pupil dilation.

A third limitation is that we scaled our pupillometry data as percentage of baseline; recent work (unknown to us when we were designing the experiment) has used a different approach, scaling pupil size as a function of maximum possible pupil change (Piquado et al., 2010). We cannot retroactively apply this metric to our data, but this rescaling would have been useful to see if older adults' asymptoting of pupil size in the 1-Back condition reflects a limit on the deployment of attentional/STM resources or a physiological limit on pupil size.

Many questions remain. For instance, it is not clear whether the unbinding deficit in old age is a specific deficit, or merely an instantiation of the complexity effect – age differences in perception and attention are magnified in memory tasks, with the larger age differences then observed in the more difficult task. Under most circumstances, binding would be more difficult (a finding in line with the results on associative deficits summarized in the Introduction), but in the present study, unbinding was more difficult, and hence we found evidence for hyper-binding in older adults. Likewise, it is unclear what exactly makes the 1-Back, attention-centered condition so hard and effortful for older adults: information detail, the 2-s delay, or some other mechanism. It would also be worthwhile to get neuroimaging data on the brain locus of this effect, and see whether it (as one would expect) originates in parts of the control network.

## ACKNOWLEDGMENT

This research was supported by the grant AG-16201 of National Institute of Health, USA.

## REFERENCES


Ackerman, J. M., Shapiro, J. R., Neuberg, S. L., Kenrick, D. T., Becker, D. V., Griskevicius, V., et al. (2006). They all look the same to me (unless they're angry): from out-group homogeneity to outgroup heterogeneity. *Psychol. Sci.* 17, 836–840. doi: 10.1111/j.1467-9280.2006.01790.x

Allard, E. S., and Isaacowitz, D. M. (2008). Are preferences in emotional processing affected by distraction? Examining the age-related positivity effect in visual fixation within a dual-task paradigm. *Aging Neuropsychol. Cogn.* 15, 725–743. doi: 10.1080/13825580802348562

Baddeley, A. D., and Hitch, G. J. (1974). "Working memory," in *The Psychology of Learning and Motivation*, eds G. H. Bower (New York: Academic Press), 47–89.

Beatty, J. (1982). Task-evoked pupillary responses, processing load, and the structure of processing resources. *Psychol. Bull.* 91, 276–292. doi: 10.1037/0033-2909.91.2.276

Bopp, K. L., and Verhaeghen, P. (2007). Age-related differences in control processes in verbal and visuo-spatial working memory: storage, transformation, supervision, and coordination. *J. Gerontol. B Psychol. Sci. Soc. Sci.* 62, 239–246. doi: 10.1093/geronb/62.5.P239

Bopp, K. L., and Verhaeghen, P. (2009). Working memory and aging: separating the effects of content and context. *Psychol. Aging* 24, 968–980. doi: 10.1037/a0017731

Bradley, M. M., and Lang, P. J. (1994). Measuring emotion: the self-assessment manikin and the semantic differential. *J. Behav. Ther. Exp. Psychiatry* 25, 49–59. doi: 10.1016/0005-7916(94)90063-9

Brockmole, J. R., Parra, M. A., Della Sala, S., and Logie, R. H. (2008). Do binding deficits account for age-related decline in visual working memory? *Psychon. Bull. Rev.* 15, 543–547. doi: 10.3758/PBR.15.3.543

Bruce, V., and Young, A. W. (1986). Understanding face recognition. *Br. J. Psychol.* 77, 305–327. doi: 10.1111/j.2044-8295.1986.tb02199.x

Calder, A. J., Keane, J., Manly, T., Sprengelmeyer, R., Scott, S., Nimmo-Smith, I., et al. (2003). Facial expression recognition across the adult life span. *Neuropsychologia* 41, 195–202. doi: 10.1016/S0028-3932(02)00149-5

Campbell, K. L., Hasher, L., and Thomas, R. C. (2010). Hyper-binding: a unique age effect. *Psychol. Sci.* 21, 399–405. doi: 10.1177/0956797609359910

Carstensen, L. L., Isaacowitz, D., and Charles, S. T. (1999). Taking time seriously: a theory of socioemotional selectivity. *Am. Psychol.* 54, 165–181. doi: 10.1037/0003-066X.54.3.165

Cerella, J. (1985). Information processing rates in the elderly. *Psychol. Bull.* 98, 67–83. doi: 10.1037/0033-2909.98.1.67

Chalfonte, B. L., and Johnson, M. K. (1996). Feature memory and binding in young and older adults. *Mem. Cogn.* 24, 403–416. doi: 10.3758/BF03200930

Chen, T., and Li, D. (2007). The roles of working memory updating and processing speed in mediating age-related differences in fluid intelligence. *Neuropsychol. Dev. Cogn. B Aging Neuropsychol. Cogn.* 14, 631–646. doi: 10.1080/13825580600987660

Conway, A. R. A., Cowan, N., Bunting, M. F., Therriault, D. J., and Minkoff, S. R. B. (2002). A latent variable analysis of working memory capacity, short-term memory capacity, processing speed, and general fluid intelligence. *Intelligence* 30, 163–183. doi: 10.1016/S0160-2896(01)00096-4

Cowan, N., Naveh-Benjamin, M., Kilb, A., and Saults, J. S. (2006). Life-span development of visual working memory: when is feature binding difficult? *Dev. Psychol.* 42, 1089–1102. doi: 10.1037/0012-1649.42.6.1089

Dobbs, A. R., and Rule, B. G. (1989). Adult age differences in working memory. *Psychol. Aging* 4, 500–503. doi: 10.1037/0882-7974.4.4.500

Ebner, N., Riediger, M., and Lindenberger, U. (2010). FACES – a database of facial expressions in young, middle-aged, and older women and men: development and validation. *Behav. Res. Methods* 42, 351–362. doi: 10.3758/BRM.42.1.351

Engle, R. W., Kane, M. J., and Tuholski, S. W. (1999). "Individual differences in working memory capacity and what they tell us about controlled attention, general fluid intelligence and functions of the prefrontal cortex," in *Models of Working Memory: Mechanisms of Active Maintenance and Executive Control*, eds A. Miyake and P. Shah (London: Cambridge University Press), 102–134.

Faust, M. E., Balota, D. A., Spieler, D. H., and Ferraro, F. R. (1999). Individual differences in information-processing rate and amount: implications for group differences in response latency. *Psychol. Bull.* 125, 777–799. doi: 10.1037/0033-2909.125.6.777

Ganel, T., and Goshen-Gottstein, Y. (2004). Effects of familiarity on the perceptual integrality of the identity and expression of faces: the parallel-route hypothesis revisited. *J. Exp. Psychol. Hum. Percept. Perform.* 30, 583–597. doi: 10.1037/0096-1523.30.3.583

Goeleven, E., Raedt, R., Leyman, L., and Verschuere, B. (2008). The Karolinska directed emotional faces: a validation study. *Cogn. Emot.* 22, 1094–1118. doi: 10.1080/02699930701626582

Goldinger, S. D., and Papesh, M. H. (2012). Pupil dilation reflects the creation and retrieval of memories. *Curr. Dir. Psychol. Sci.* 21, 90–95. doi: 10.1177/0963721412436811

Goldinger, S. D., He, Y., and Papesh, M. (2009). Deficits in cross-race face learning: insights from eye-movements and pupillometry. *J. Exp. Psychol. Learn. Mem. Cogn.* 35, 1105–1122. doi: 10.1037/a0016548

Granholm, E., Asarnow, R. F., Sarkin, A. J., and Dykes, K. L. (1996). Pupillary responses index cognitive resource limitations. *Psychophysiology* 33, 457–461. doi: 10.1111/j.1469-8986.1996.tb01071.x

Grühn, D., and Scheibe, S. (2008). Age-related differences in valence and arousal ratings of pictures from the International Affective Picture System (IAPS): do ratings become more extreme with age? *Behav. Res. Methods* 40, 512–521. doi: 10.3758/BRM.40.2.512

Heitz, R. P., Schrock, J. C., Payne, T. W., and Engle, R. W. (2008). Effect of incentive on working memory capacity: behavioral and pupillometric data. *Psychophysiology* 45, 119–129. doi: 10.1111/j.1469-8986.2007.00605.x

Hess, E. H. (1965). Attitude and pupil size. *Sci. Am.* 212, 46–54. doi: 10.1038/scientificamerican0465-46

Hicks, R. A., Reaney, T., and Hill, L. (1967). Effects of pupil size and facial angle on preference for photographs of a young woman. *Percept. Mot. Skills* 24, 388–390. doi: 10.2466/pms.1967.24.2.388

Iqbal, S. T., Zheng, X. S., and Bailey, B. P. (2004). "Task-evoked pupillary response to mental workload in human-computer interaction," in *Proceedings of the Conference on Human Factors in Computing Systems*, Vienna, Austria, 2004, 1477–1480. doi: 10.1145/985921.986094

Kahneman, D., and Beatty, J. (1966). Pupil diameter and load on memory. *Science* 154, 1583–1585. doi: 10.1126/science.154.3756.1583

Kane, M. J., Bleckley, M. K., Conway, A. R. A., and Engle, R. W. (2001). A controlled-attention view of working memory capacity: individual differences in memory span and the control of visual orienting. *J. Exp. Psychol. Gen.* 130, 169–183. doi: 10.1037/0096-3445.130.2.169

Karatekin, C., Marcus, D. J., and Couperus, J. W. (2007). Regulation of cognitive resources during sustained attention and working memory in 10-year-olds and adults. *Psychophysiology* 44, 128–144. doi: 10.1111/j.1469-8986.2006.00477.x

Kemper, S., Herman, R. E., and Lian, C. H. T. (2003). The costs of doing two things at once for young and older adults: talking while walking, finger tapping, and ignoring speech or noise. *Psychol. Aging* 18, 181–192. doi: 10.1037/0882-7974.18.2.181

Kensinger, E. A., and Corkin, S. (2003). Effects of negative emotional content on working memory and long-term memory. *Emotion* 3, 378–393. doi: 10.1037/1528-3542.3.4.378

Kirchner, W. K. (1958). Age differences in short-term retention of rapidly changing information. *J. Exp. Psychol.* 55, 352–358. doi: 10.1037/h0043688

Knight, M., Seymour, T. L., Gaunt, J. T., Baker, C., Nesmith, K., and Mather, M. (2007). Aging and goal directed emotional attention: distraction reverses emotional biases. *Emotion* 7, 705–714. doi: 10.1037/1528-3542.7.4.705

Kyllonen, P. C. (1996). "Is working memory capacity Spearman's g?," in *Human Abilities: Their Nature and Measurement*, eds I. Dennis and P. Tapsfield (Mahwah, NJ: Erlbaum), 49–75.

Laeng, B., Ørbo, M., Holmlund, T., and Miozzo, M. (2011). Pupillary Stroop effects. *Cogn. Process.* 12, 13–21. doi: 10.1007/s10339-010-0370-z

Martens, U., Leuthold, H., and Schweinberger, S. R. (2010). On the temporal organization of facial identity and expression analysis: inferences from event-related brain potentials. *Cogn. Affect. Behav. Neurosci.* 10, 505–522. doi: 10.3758/CABN.10.4.505

Mather, M., and Knight, M. (2005). Goal-directed memory: the role of cognitive control in older adults' emotional memory. *Psychol. Aging* 20, 554–570. doi: 10.1037/0882-7974.20.4.554

Mikels, J. A., Larkin, G. R., Reuter-Lorenz, P. A., and Cartensen, L. L. (2005). Divergent trajectories in the aging mind: changes in working memory for affective versus visual information with age. *Psychol. Aging.* 20, 542–553. doi: 10.1037/0882-7974.20.4.542

Miyake, A., and Shah, P. (1999). "Toward unified theories of working memory: emerging general consensus, unresolved theoretical issues, and future research directions," in *Models of Working Memory: Mechanisms of Active Maintenance and Executive Control*, eds A. Miyake and P. Shah (Cambridge: Cambridge University Press), 442–481. doi: 10.1017/CBO9781139174909

Murphy, N. A., and Isaacowitz, D. M. (2008). Preferences for emotional information in older adults: a meta-analysis of memory and attention studies. *Psychol. Aging* 23, 263–286. doi: 10.1037/0882-7974.23.2.263

Myerson, J., Hale, S., Wagstaff, D., Poon, L. W., and Smith, G. A. (1990). The information-loss model: A mathematical theory of age-related cognitive slowing. *Psychol. Rev.* 97, 475–487. doi: 10.1037/0033-295X.97.4.475

Naveh-Benjamin, M., Guez, J., Kilb, A., and Reedy, S. (2004). The associative deficit of older adults: further support using face-name associations. *Psychol. Aging* 19, 541–546. doi: 10.1037/0882-7974.19.3.541

Oberauer, K. (2002). Access to information in working memory: exploring the focus of attention. *J. Exp. Psychol. Learn. Mem. Cogn.* 28, 411–421. doi: 10.1037/0278-7393.28.3.411

Old, S., and Naveh-Benjamin, M. (2008). Differential effects of age on item and associative measures of memory: a meta-analysis. *Psychol. Aging* 23, 104–118. doi: 10.1037/0882-7974.23.1.104

Partala, T., and Surakka, V. (2003). Pupil size variation as an indication of affective processing. *Int. J. Hum. Comput. Stud.* 59, 185–198. doi: 10.1016/S1071-5819(03)00017.x

Piquado, T., Isaacowitz, D. M., and Wingfield, A. (2010). Pupillometry as a measure of cognitive effort in younger and older adults. *Psychophysiology* 47, 560–569. doi: 10.1111/j.1469-8986.2009.00947.x

Porter, G., Troscianko, T., and Gilchrist, I. D. (2007). Effort during visual search and counting: insights from pupillometry. *Q. J. Exp. Psychol.* 60, 211–229. doi: 10.1080/17470210600673818

Rhodes, M. G., and Anastasi, J. S. (2012). The own-age bias in face recognition: a meta-analytic and theoretical review. *Psychol. Bull.* 138, 146–174. doi; 10.1037/a0025750

Soto, F. A., and Wasserman, E. A. (2011). Asymmetrical interactions in the perception of face identity and emotional expression are not unique to the primate visual system. *J. Vis.* 11:24. doi: 10.1167/11.3.24

Stanners, R., Coulter, M., Sweet, A., and Murphy, P. (1979). The pupillary response as an indicator of arousal and cognition. *Motiv. Emot.* 3, 319–340. doi: 10.1007/BF00994048

Van Gerven, P. W. M., Paas, F., Van Merriënboer, J. J. G., and Schmidt, H. G. (2004). Memory load and the cognitive pupillary response in aging. *Psychophysiology* 167–174. doi: 10.1111/j.1469-8986.2003.00148.x

Vaughan, L., Basak, C., Hartman, M., and Verhaeghen, P. (2008). Aging and working memory inside and outside the focus of attention: dissociations of availability and accessibility. *Aging Neuropsychol. Cogn.* 15, 1–22. doi: 10.1080/13825580802061645

Verhaeghen, P. (2012). "Working memory still working: age-related differences in working memory and executive control," in *Memory and Aging*, eds N. Ohta and M. Naveh-Benjamin (New York: Psychology Press), 3–30.

Verhaeghen, P. (2014). *The Elements of Cognitive Aging: Meta-Analyses of Age-Related Differences in Processing Speed and Their Consequences.* New York, NY: Oxford University Press.

Verhaeghen, P., and Basak, C. (2005). Aging and switching of the focus of attention in working memory: results from a modified *N*-Back task. *Q. J. Exp. Psychol. A* 58, 134–154. doi: 10.1080/02724980443000241

Verhaeghen, P., Cerella, J., and Basak, C. (2004). A working memory workout: how to change to size of the focus of attention from one to four in ten hours or less. *J. Exp. Psychol. Learn. Mem. Cogn.* 30, 1322–1337. doi: 10.1037/0278-7393.30.6.1322

Wheeler, M. E., and Treisman, A. M. (2002). Binding in short-term visual memory. *J. Exp. Psychol. Gen.* 131, 48–64. doi: 10.1037/0096-3445.131.1.48

Wurm, L. H., Labouvie-Vief, G., Aycock, J., Rebucal, K. A., and Koch, H. E. (2004). Performance in auditory and visual emotional Stroop tasks: a comparison of older and younger adults. *Psychol. Aging* 19, 523–535. doi: 10.1037/0882-7974.19.3.523

Zhang, Y., Verhaeghen, P., and Cerella, J. (2012). Working memory at work: how the updating process alters the nature of memory encoding. *Acta Psychol.* 139, 77–83. doi: 10.1016/j.actpsy.2011.10.012

# 10

# Emotional aging: a discrete emotions perspective

**Ute Kunzmann[1]*, Cathleen Kappes[1] and Carsten Wrosch[2]**

[1] Institute of Psychology, University of Leipzig, Leipzig, Germany
[2] Department of Psychology, Concordia University, Montreal, QC, Canada

**Edited by:**
Natalie Ebner, University of Florida, USA

**Reviewed by:**
Natalie Ebner, University of Florida, USA
Manuel C. Voelkle, Max Planck Institute for Human Development, Germany
Andrew Mienaltowski, Western Kentucky University, USA

***Correspondence:**
Ute Kunzmann, Institute of Psychology, University of Leipzig, Seeburgstrasse 14-20, Leipzig 04103, Germany
e-mail: kunzmann@uni-leipzig.de

Perhaps the most important single finding in the field of emotional aging has been that the overall quality of affective experience steadily improves during adulthood and can be maintained into old age. Recent lifespan developmental theories have provided motivation- and experience-based explanations for this phenomenon. These theories suggest that, as individuals grow older, they become increasingly motivated and able to regulate their emotions, which could result in reduced negativity and enhanced positivity. The objective of this paper is to expand existing theories and empirical research on emotional aging by presenting a discrete emotions perspective. To illustrate the usefulness of this approach, we focus on a discussion of the literature examining age differences in anger and sadness. These two negative emotions have typically been subsumed under the singular concept of negative affect. From a discrete emotions perspective, however, they are highly distinct and show multidirectional age differences. We propose that such contrasting age differences in specific negative emotions have important implications for our understanding of long-term patterns of affective well-being across the adult lifespan.

**Keywords: emotional aging, adult lifespan, anger, sadness, affective well-being**

The single most important finding in the field of emotional aging is perhaps that affective well-being does not decline during most of the adult lifespan (e.g., Charles and Carstensen, 2007; Scheibe and Carstensen, 2010; Isaacowitz and Blanchard-Fields, 2012). Research based on the most prominent life-span theories of developmental regulation and emotional aging have provided different explanations for this phenomenon by examining broad dimensions of emotions (i.e., negative affect and positive affect; e.g., Baltes and Baltes, 1990; Brandtstädter and Greve, 1994; Heckhausen, 1997; Carstensen, 2006). Complementing these theories, we present a discrete emotions perspective, that considers specific positive and negative emotions. To illustrate the usefulness of this approach, we focus on a discussion of age differences in the experience of anger and sadness. These two negative emotions have typically been subsumed under the singular concept of negative affect. From a discrete emotions perspective, however, they are highly distinct and show multidirectional age differences. We propose that such contrasting age differences in specific emotions have important implications for understanding long-term patterns of affective well-being across the adult lifespan.

## LIFE-SPAN THEORIES OF DEVELOPMENTAL REGULATION AND EMOTIONAL AGING

Prominent theories of developmental regulation postulate that individuals can avoid the adverse emotional effects of life's challenges, threats, and losses if they engage in effective self-regulatory strategies (e.g., Baltes and Baltes, 1990; Brandtstädter and Renner, 1990; Heckhausen et al., 2010). Although the nature of strategies has been defined and labeled differently by different theories, the various strategies seem to cluster according to whether they refer to continued engagement in attaining goals or to disengagement from unattainable goals (Haase et al., 2013). Further, the extent to which these two higher-order categories of developmental regulation protect affective well-being is thought to differ as a function of an individual's place in the life-cycle, which can be considered a proxy for individual differences in control opportunities and constraints. Given that individuals' capacity to influence their environment is relatively high in young adulthood and often declines in old age, processes of goal engagement should be used more frequently and adaptive in young adulthood. Processes of goal disengagement, by contrast, should become increasingly salient and adaptive in older adulthood. A large number of longitudinal and intervention studies have supported these propositions (reviews: Wrosch et al., 2006; Heckhausen et al., 2010).

Socioemotional Selectivity Theory (SST; Carstensen, 2006; Scheibe and Carstensen, 2010; Reed and Carstensen, 2012), a prominent theory of emotional aging, explains the maintenance of affective well-being in old age by focusing on future-related expectations, particularly older individuals' estimations of their remaining life-time. According to SST, because advancing age is naturally associated with endings and a limited lifetime, older adults prioritize social and emotional goals related to the optimization of immediate affective well-being over longer-term knowledge-related goals aimed at optimizing future resources (Carstensen et al., 1999). In support of SST's main predictions, a large body of evidence suggests that, in comparison with their younger counterparts, older adults are more selective in their choice of social partners and make their social interactions more emotionally satisfying (reviews: Carstensen et al., 1999; Fingerman and Charles, 2010). There is also substantial evidence for systematic age differences in basic affective information processing. Older adults appear to be generally more sensitive to positive information and less sensitive to negative information than young adults, a phenomenon termed the "positivity effect" (Carstensen and Mikels, 2005). SST states that this positivity effect is the result of an age-related increase in the allocation of cognitive resources toward emotion regulation (reviews: Mather and Carstensen, 2005; Kryla-Lighthall and Mather, 2009; Mather, 2012).

Overall, life-span developmental theories have provided valuable insights into how older individuals can maintain or enhance their affective well-being despite age-related losses in many life domains. Independent of their specific explanatory processes, however, affective well-being has been considered in these theories from a broad and dimensional perspective. That is, research based on these theories typically examined whether processes of developmental regulation, socio-emotional selectivity, or biases in affective information processing are associated with a broader aggregate of emotional experiences such as positive affect or negative affect. Past theoretical work is thus well suited to explain age differences in broad affective dimensions, but it may fall short in explaining age-differences in the salience and functions of different discrete negative or positive emotions subsumed under positive or positive affect. As a consequence, a discrete emotions perspective may be needed to complement past theoretical work. Such an approach may help better understand multidirectional age differences in short-term affective reactions and longer-term affective well-being. In addition, it may raise awareness that emotions are not only consequences of cognitive or motivational processes, but also can cause effective cognitions and behaviors.

## A DISCRETE EMOTIONS PERSPECTIVE ON EMOTIONAL AGING

Functional emotion theories emphasize the adaptive value of discrete emotions and emotional dispositions (e.g., Frijda, 1986; Campos et al., 1989; Lazarus, 1991; Izard, 1993; Levenson, 1994; Ekman, 1999; Keltner and Gross, 1999). According to these theories, emotions provide important information to the self and others and help motivate our own and others' behavior. For example, some emotions push individuals away from certain thoughts, memories, or actions, whereas other emotions make certain thoughts, memories, or actions more likely. Functional approaches traditionally have focused on the adaptive value of negative emotions. From this perspective, the overall purpose of negative emotions is to eliminate a threat or an imbalance between the individual and his or her environment. More specifically, negative emotions are thought to prompt time-tested adaptive actions enabled and supported by specific action tendencies (Frijda, 1986), patterns of physiological activity (Levenson, 1994), configurations of facial expressions (Ekman, 1999), and subjective feelings (e.g., Izard, 1993). Functional approaches to emotion have emphasized that each discrete negative emotion serves a specific and distinct function (e.g., fear creates the urge to escape, disgust the urge to expel; e.g., Frijda, 1986; Levenson, 1992).

### AGE DIFFERENCES IN NEGATIVE AFFECT: THE SAMPLE CASE OF ANGER AND SADNESS

To explore the usefulness of a discrete emotion approach, we focus on the functions of two emotions, anger and sadness for two reasons. First, empirical studies examining age differences in discrete emotions have largely focused on these two emotions. Second, and more important, different from other discrete emotions, anger and sadness are closely and differentially associated with the two higher-order classes of developmental regulation, goal engagement and goal disengagement. As a consequence, a theoretical framework that addresses age differences in the salience and adaptivity of anger and sadness appears to be a reasonable starting point for developing a more comprehensive discrete emotions approach.

A central tenet of theories of life-span development has been that each stage in the life cycle is characterized by a specific configuration of environmental challenges as well as personal needs, beliefs, and future expectations (e.g., Heckhausen and Schulz, 1995). We build on this assumption and argue that age-specific configurations may increase or decrease the experience and adaptive value of specific emotions (see also Haase et al., 2012). This proposition provides a theoretically important extension of functional emotion theories as it suggests that not only the emotion itself but also characteristics of the individual and his or her immediate and broader social context, most of which substantially change across the adult life-span, determine the adaptive value of specific emotions.

To begin, young adulthood has been described as a phase of growth during which individuals have greater opportunities to develop their potentials than their older counterparts. Thus, processes of growth and optimization rather than maintenance or compensation should have priority in young adulthood (Baltes and Baltes, 1990; Freund and Baltes, 1998, 2002; Ebner et al., 2006). Consistent with this view, SST assumes that young, as compared with older adults' goals tend to be more future-oriented and focused on acquiring new resources such as knowledge or information (e.g., Carstensen et al., 1999). Moreover, life-span theories of developmental regulation (e.g., Brandtstädter and Greve, 1994; Heckhausen et al., 2010) have proposed that, in young adulthood, perceptions of high personal control and a tenacious pursuit of goals are not only highly prevalent, but also closely tied to well-being (Wrosch and Heckhausen, 1999; Rothermund and Brandtstädter, 2003; Lachman, 2006). Finally, there is evidence suggesting that individuals are most willing to engage in and reflect on social conflicts when they are young (Labouvie-Vief et al., 1989; Birditt and Fingerman, 2005; Blanchard-Fields et al., 2007).

Given that young adults typically pursue many future-related goals and have a strong need to accomplish them, the elicitor of anger, which is the appraisal that one's own goals are intentionally ignored or blocked by others, should be particularly frequent and salient in young adulthood. In addition, the situational control appraisals, action tendencies, and social motivations typical of anger are likely to be more readily accessible in young adulthood than in old age. In fact, according to discrete emotion theories, anger prototypically involves the belief in high situational control (Lazarus, 1991), triggers a reactant "moving against" state of action readiness (Frijda et al., 1989), and promotes goal persistence (Lench and Levine, 2008). In addition, anger facilitates efforts to bring others' behaviors back in line with one's own goals (Fischer and Roseman, 2007). Thus, relative to older adults, young adults should experience anger more intensively and more frequently. Moreover, because anger may at times help young adults to overcome obstacles in accomplishing age-normative tasks, it could be adaptive, at least in certain contexts, and benefit young adults' longer-term affective well-being (Haase et al., 2012).

In marked contrast to young adulthood, old age has been characterized as a phase of loss and decline (Lindenberger and Baltes, 1997; Smith and Baltes, 1997; Baltes and Mayer, 1999) during which social, cognitive, and physical resources become increasingly limited and processes of maintenance and compensation gain importance (Baltes and Baltes, 1990; Labouvie-Vief, 2003). Life-span theories have proposed that, given the limited resources in old age, perceptions of low personal control and goal adjustment processes become increasingly frequent and adaptive (e.g., Wrosch and Heckhausen, 1999; Rothermund and Brandtstädter, 2003; Lachman, 2006). In addition, according to SST, because perceived future life-time shrinks with increasing age, older adults' tend to be particularly present-oriented in their goal pursuits, focused on creating emotionally meaningful experiences, and likely to avoid social conflicts for the sake of maintaining social harmony in the current moment (Birditt and Fingerman, 2005; Carstensen, 2006; Blanchard-Fields, 2007).

Given that, relative to young adults, older adults increasingly face losses of fundamental resources and tend to adjust their goals accordingly, the elicitor of sadness, that is, the appraisal of a situation as an irreversible loss, should be particularly frequent and salient in old age. In addition, the situational control appraisals, action tendencies, and social motivations that are linked to sadness are likely to be more readily accessible in old age than in earlier life periods. In support of this assumption, discrete emotion theories suggest that sadness prototypically goes hand in hand with a perception of low situational control (Lazarus, 1991). In addition, it triggers processes of adaptive goal disengagement (Frijda et al., 1989; Nesse, 2000; Wrosch and Miller, 2009) and signals to others the need for closeness, sympathy, and support (Andrews and Thomson, 2009). As a consequence, relative to young adults, older adults should experience sadness more intensively and frequently. Moreover, because sadness is likely to help older adults deal with losses by facilitating disengagement from unattainable goals and enhancing social support, it could be adaptive, at least in certain contexts, and facilitate older adults' longer-term affective well-being (see also Kunzmann and Grühn, 2005; Haase et al., 2012).

### EMPIRICAL EVIDENCE

A small but growing body of evidence is consistent with the notion that sadness and anger follow contrasting trajectories across the adult life-span. For example, research has shown that older adults report less anger and anger-related regulatory strategies during interpersonal conflicts than their younger counterparts (Blanchard-Fields and Coats, 2008). An age-related reduction in the intensity of anger reactivity was also found when young and older adults were confronted with film clips of an old woman talking about problems in a nursing home (Charles et al., 2001) or audio-taped conversations, in which two individuals were ostensibly making disparaging remarks about a third person (Charles and Carstensen, 2008). Age differences in sadness-reactions, by contrast, have been shown to be reversed (i.e., higher among older adults) or non-significant (Charles et al., 2001; Charles and Carstensen, 2008). Other studies have investigated age differences in emotional reactions to stimuli specifically designed to elicit either anger or sadness. In this line of work, older, as compared with younger, adults reported less anger in response to anger-eliciting stimuli, but equal or higher sadness in response to sadness-eliciting stimuli (Tsai et al., 2000; Labouvie-Vief et al., 2003; Kunzmann and Grühn, 2005; Kunzmann and Richter, 2009; Seider et al., 2011; Streubel and Kunzmann, 2011).

Age-related differences in the experience of anger and sadness have also been examined on the level of affect frequency in a longitudinal field study with a national sample of German adults covering most of the adult lifespan (Kunzmann et al., 2013). More specifically, cross-sectional and longitudinal findings from this study consistently suggest that the frequency of anger increases from late adolescence into young adulthood, but shows a steady decrease from midlife to old age. By contrast, the frequency of sadness remained stable over most of adulthood and increased in old age (Kunzmann et al., 2013). Extending this work, a recent study explored age differences in anger and sadness by focusing on the intensity and frequency of emotional experiences on a typical day and their implicit associations with participants' self (Kunzmann and Thomas, 2014). Consistent with a discrete emotions perspective, older adults experienced anger less frequently and less intensively than young adults, but there were no age differences in the experience of sadness. Furthermore, this study provided initial evidence for the idea that anger, but not sadness, becomes less self-descriptive with age (Kunzmann and Thomas, 2014).

Finally, there is preliminary evidence indicating that the effects of anger and sadness on affective well-being are age-differential as well (Haase et al., 2012). In this laboratory study, anger experiences in response to neutral film clips with ambiguous contents were associated with high affective well-being in middle-aged adults but not in young or older adults. Sadness reactions, by contrast, were associated with high affective well-being in older adults, but not in younger or middle-aged adults (Haase et al., 2012). These findings lend support to our previous predictions, although according to our framework, anger should be adaptive in young adulthood as well.

## CONCLUSIONS AND OUTLOOK

Life-span theories' current focus on the explanation of age-related changes in the overall quality of affective experience does not account well for multidirectional and multifunctional age differences in specific emotions. A discrete emotions perspective on aging therefore complements life-span theories as it allows more differentiated predictions. According to this view, all emotions—positive and negative—are adaptive in particular contexts. Thus, although most individuals value high emotional well-being (Tsai et al., 2006), and report pro-hedonic emotion regulatory goals more frequently than contra-hedonic goals (Riediger et al., 2009), from a functionalist view, a life without negative emotions would be impoverished, unhealthy, and short. Instead, it assumes that negative emotions are useful experiences. They serve specific functions and may be adaptive if they enable individuals to manage critical life circumstances.

Our approach and review is consistent with this view by documenting the usefulness and importance of a discrete emotions approach. It demonstrates multidirectional age differences in the experience of anger and sadness by indicating that the salience of anger decreases across the life-span, particularly during middle adulthood and old age, whereas the intensity and frequency of sadness remains stable or increases in old age. In addition, it provides preliminary evidence suggesting such age differences in emotional reactions may contribute to individuals' general affective well-being.

To further clarify the roles of specific negative emotions, future research should determine the conditions that give rise to adaptive consequences of anger reactions (in young adulthood) and sadness reactions (in old age). Certainly, chronic or unwarranted anger and sadness are unlikely to contribute to high affective well-being at any age. Instead, it may be the match between situational circumstances and emotional reactions that could determine the adaptive value of age-related experiences of anger and sadness. To examine such situation by emotion interactions, future research should also incorporate time windows of different lengths because specific negative emotions may not be strongly associated with high levels of concurrent affective well-being. Rather, the experience of certain negative emotions could restore and optimize individuals' affective well-being over longer periods of time if they trigger and facilitate behavioral processes that over time help individuals to adjust successfully to age-related opportunities and constraints.

A second task for future work is to shed further light on the mechanisms that can explain age differences in anger and sadness. Our theoretical framework is motivational in nature in that we argue that each place in the life-cycle is characterized by a specific configuration of developmental conditions that make certain emotions more salient and adaptive. However, theoretical accounts of age differences in cognitive and physiological resources may provide additional insights (Labouvie-Vief, 2003; Cacioppo et al., 2011). For example, anger may involve greater physiological arousal and may require more cognitive resources than sadness, and this may imply that older adults have fewer resources to experience anger than sadness.

Finally, it will be interesting to extend our framework by considering additional distinct negative and positive emotions. For example, there is preliminary research suggesting age-related increases in fear and age-related declines in disgust (Kunzmann et al., 2005; Teachman and Gordon, 2009). Future research should clarify the mechanisms that underlie such age differences in a variety of distinct emotions. Research along these lines may also broaden the age range of inquiry by additionally examining children and adolescents and consider the influence of individual differences in available resources and types of goals. We think that future research from a discrete emotion perspective is warranted and has the potential to contribute to our understanding of successful development across the lifespan.

## AUTHOR NOTE

The completion of this manuscript was supported by grants from the German Research Foundation to Ute Kunzmann and by grants from Social Sciences and Humanities Research Council of Canada and Canadian Institutes of Health Research to Carsten Wrosch.

## REFERENCES

Andrews, P. W., and Thomson, J. A. Jr. (2009). The bright side of being blue: depression as an adaptation for analyzing complex problems. *Psychol. Rev.* 116, 620–654. doi: 10.1037/a0016242

Baltes, P. B., and Baltes, M. M. (1990). *Successful Aging: Perspectives From the Behavioral Sciences.* New York, NY: Cambridge University Press.

Baltes, P. B., and Mayer, K. U. (1999). *The Berlin Aging Study: Aging from 70 to 100.* New York, NY: Cambridge University Press.

Birditt, K. S., and Fingerman, K. L. (2005). Do we get better at picking our battles? Age group differences in descriptions of behavioral reactions to interpersonal tensions. *J. Gerontol. B Psychol. Sci. Soc. Sci.* 60B, P121–P128. doi: 10.1093/geronb/60.3.P121

Blanchard-Fields, F. (2007). Everyday problem solving and emotion: an adult developmental perspective. *Curr. Dir. Psychol. Sci.* 16, 26–31. doi: 10.1111/j.1467-8721.2007.00469.x

Blanchard-Fields, F., and Coats, A. H. (2008). The experience of anger and sadness in everyday problems impacts age differences in emotion regulation. *Dev. Psychol.* 44, 1547–1556. doi: 10.1037/a0013915

Blanchard-Fields, F., Mienaltowski, A., and Seay, R. B. (2007). Age differences in everyday problem-solving effectiveness: older adults select more effective strategies for interpersonal problems. *J. Gerontol. B Psychol. Sci. Soc. Sci.* 62B, P61–P64. doi: 10.1093/geronb/62.1.P61

Brandtstädter, J., and Greve, W. (1994). The aging self: stabilizing and protective processes. *Dev. Rev.* 14, 52–80.

Brandtstädter, J., and Renner, G. (1990). Tenacious goal pursuit and flexible goal adjustment: explication and age-related analysis of assimilative and accommodative strategies of coping. *Psychol. Aging* 5, 58–67. doi: 10.1037/0882-7974.5.1.58

Cacioppo, J. T., Berntson, G. G., Bechara, A., Tranel, D., and Hawkley, L. C. (2011). "Could an aging brain contribute to subjective well-being? The value added by a social neuroscience perspective," in *Social Neuroscience: Toward Understanding the Underpinnings of the Social Mind,* eds A. Todorov, S. T. Fiske and D. A. Prentice (New York, NY: Oxford University Press), 249–262.

Campos, J. J., Campos, R. G., and Barrett, K. C. (1989). Emergent themes in the study of emotional development and emotion regulation. *Dev. Psychol.* 25, 394–402. doi: 10.1037/0012-1649.25.3.394

Carstensen, L. L. (2006). The influence of a sense of time on human development. *Science* 312, 1913–1915. doi: 10.1126/science.1127488

Carstensen, L. L., Isaacowitz, D. M., and Charles, S. T. (1999). Taking time seriously: a theory of socioemotional selectivity. *Am. Psychol.* 54, 165–181. doi: 10.1037/0003-066x.54.3.165

Carstensen, L. L., and Mikels, J. A. (2005). At the intersection of emotion and cognition: aging and the positivity effect. *Curr. Dir. Psychol. Sci.* 14, 117–121. doi: 10.1111/j.0963-7214.2005.00348.x

Charles, S. T., and Carstensen, L. L. (2007). "Emotion regulation and aging," in *Handbook of Emotion Regulation,* ed J. J. Gross (New York, NY: Guilford Press), 307–327.

Charles, S. T., and Carstensen, L. L. (2008). Unpleasant situations elicit different emotional responses in younger and older adults. *Psychol. Aging* 23, 495–504. doi: 10.1037/a0013284

Charles, S. T., Carstensen, L. L., and Mcfall, R. M. (2001). Problem-solving in the nursing home environment: age and experience differences in emotional reactions and responses. *J. Clin. Geropsychol.* 7, 319–330. doi: 10.1023/a:1011352326374

Ebner, N. C., Freund, A. M., and Baltes, P. B. (2006). Developmental changes in personal goal orientation from young to late adulthood: from striving for gains to maintenance and prevention of losses. *Psychol. Aging* 21, 664–678. doi: 10.1037/0882-7974.21.4.664

Ekman, P. (1999). "Basic emotions," in *Handbook of Cognition and Emotion,* eds T. Dalgleish and M. J. Power (New York, NY: John Wiley & Sons Ltd), 45–60.

Fingerman, K. L., and Charles, S. T. (2010). It takes two to tango: why older people have the best relationships. *Curr. Dir. Psychol. Sci.* 19, 172–176. doi: 10.1177/0963721410370297

Fischer, A. H., and Roseman, I. J. (2007). Beat them or ban them: the characteristics and social functions of anger and contempt. *J. Pers. Soc. Psychol.* 93, 103–115. doi: 10.1037/0022-3514.93.1.103

Freund, A. M., and Baltes, P. B. (1998). Selection, optimization, and compensation as strategies of life management: correlations with subjective indicators of successful aging. *Psychol. Aging* 13, 531–543. doi: 10.1037/0882-7974.13.4.531

Freund, A. M., and Baltes, P. B. (2002). Life-management strategies of selection, optimization and compensation: measurement by self-report and construct validity. *J. Pers. Soc. Psychol.* 82, 642–662. doi: 10.1037/0022-3514.82.4.642

Frijda, N. H. (1986). *The Emotions.* New York; Paris: Cambridge University Press Editions de la Maison des Sciences de l'Homme.

Frijda, N. H., Kuipers, P., and Ter Schure, E. (1989). Relations among emotion, appraisal, and emotional action readiness. *J. Pers. Soc. Psychol.* 57, 212–228. doi: 10.1037/0022-3514.57.2.212

Haase, C. M., Heckhausen, J., and Wrosch, C. (2013). Developmental regulation across the life span: toward a new synthesis. *Dev. Psychol.* 49, 964–972. doi: 10.1037/a002923110.1037/a0029231

Haase, C. M., Seider, B. H., Shiota, M. N., and Levenson, R. W. (2012). Anger and sadness in response to an emotionally neutral film: evidence for age-specific associations with well-being. *Psychol. Aging* 27, 305–317. doi: 10.1037/a0024959

Heckhausen, J. (1997). Developmental regulation across adulthood: primary and secondary control of age-related challenges. *Dev. Psychol.* 33, 176–187. doi: 10.1037/0012-1649.33.1.176

Heckhausen, J., and Schulz, R. (1995). A life-span theory of control. *Psychol. Rev.* 102, 284–304. doi: 10.1037/0033-295x.102.2.284

Heckhausen, J., Wrosch, C., and Schulz, R. (2010). A motivational theory of life-span development. *Psychol. Rev.* 117, 32–60. doi: 10.1037/a0017668

Isaacowitz, D. M., and Blanchard-Fields, F. (2012). Linking process and outcome in the study of emotion and aging. *Perspect. Psychol. Sci.* 7, 3–17. doi: 10.1177/1745691611424750

Izard, C. E. (1993). Four systems for emotion activation: cognitive and noncognitive processes. *Psychol. Rev.* 100, 68–90. doi: 10.1037/0033-295x.100.1.68

Keltner, D., and Gross, J. J. (1999). Functional accounts of emotions. *Cogn. Emot.* 13, 467–480.

Kryla-Lighthall, N., and Mather, M. (2009). "The role of cognitive control in older adults' emotional well-being," in *Handbook of Theories of Aging, 2nd Edh.* eds V. L. Bengston, D. Gans, N. M. Pulney, and M. Silverstein (New York, NY: Springer Publishing Co), 323–344.

Kunzmann, U., and Grühn, D. (2005). Age differences in emotional reactivity: the sample case of sadness. *Psychol. Aging* 20, 47–59. doi: 10.1037/0882-7974.20.1.47

Kunzmann, U., Kupperbusch, C. S., and Levenson, R. W. (2005). Behavioral inhibition and amplification during emotional arousal: a comparison of two age groups. *Psychol. Aging* 20, 144–158. doi: 10.1037/0882-7974.20.1.144

Kunzmann, U., and Richter, D. (2009). Emotional reactivity across the adult life span: the cognitive pragmatics make a difference. *Psychol. Aging* 24, 879–889. doi: 10.1037/a0017347

Kunzmann, U., Richter, D., and Schmukle, S. C. (2013). Stability and change in affective experience across the adult life span: analyses with a national sample from Germany. *Emotion* 13, 1086–1095. doi: 10.1037/a0033572

Kunzmann, U., and Thomas, S. (2014). Multidirectional age differences in anger and sadness. *Psychol. Aging* 29, 16–27. doi: 10.1037/a0035751

Labouvie-Vief, G. (2003). Dynamic integration: affect, cognition, and the self in adulthood. *Curr. Dir. Psychol. Sci.* 12, 201–206. doi: 10.1046/j.0963-7214.2003.01262.x

Labouvie-Vief, G., Devoe, M., and Bulka, D. (1989). Speaking about feelings: conceptions of emotion across the life span. *Psychol. Aging* 4, 425–437. doi: 10.1037/0882-7974.4.4.425

Labouvie-Vief, G., Lumley, M. A., Jain, E., and Heinze, H. (2003). Age and gender differences in cardiac reactivity and subjective emotion responses to emotional autobiographical memories. *Emotion* 3, 115–126. doi: 10.1037/1528-3542.3.2.115

Lachman, M. E. (2006). Perceived control over aging-related declines: adaptive beliefs and behaviors. *Curr. Dir. Psychol. Sci.* 15, 282–286. doi: 10.1111/j.1467-8721.2006.00453.x

Lazarus, R. S. (1991). Cognition and motivation in emotion. *Am. Psychol.* 46, 352–367. doi: 10.1037/0003-066x.46.4.352

Lench, H. C., and Levine, L. J. (2008). Goals and responses to failure: knowing when to hold them and when to fold them. *Motiv. Emot.* 32, 127–140. doi: 10.1007/s11031-008-9085-1

Levenson, R. W. (1992). Autonomic nervous system differences among emotions. *Psychol. Sci.* 3, 23–27. doi: 10.1111/j.1467-9280.1992.tb00251.x

Levenson, R. W. (1994). "Human emotion: a functional view," in *The Nature of Emotion. Fundamental Questions*, eds P. Ekman and R. Davidson (New York, NY: Oxford University Press), 123–126.

Lindenberger, U., and Baltes, P. B. (1997). Intellectual functioning in old and very old age: cross-sectional results from the Berlin Aging Study. *Psychol. Aging* 12, 410–432. doi: 10.1037/0882-7974.12.3.410

Mather, M. (2012). The emotion paradox in the aging brain. *Ann. N.Y. Acad. Sci.* 1251, 33–49. doi: 10.1111/j.1749-6632.2012.06471.x

Mather, M., and Carstensen, L. L. (2005). Aging and motivated cognition: the positivity effect in attention and memory. *Trends Cogn. Sci.* 9, 496–502. doi: 10.1016/j.tics.2005.08.005

Nesse, R. M. (2000). Is depression an adaptation? *Arch. Gen. Psychiatry* 57, 14–20. doi: 10.1001/archpsyc.57.1.14

Reed, A. E., and Carstensen, L. L. (2012). The theory behind the age-related positivity effect. *Front. Psychol.* 3:339. doi: 10.3389/fpsyg.2012.00339

Riediger, M., Schmiedek, F., Wagner, G. G., and Lindenberger, U. (2009). Seeking pleasure and seeking pain: differences in prohedonic and contra-hedonic motivation from adolescence to old age. *Psychol. Sci.* 20, 1529–1535. doi: 10.1111/j.1467-9280.2009.02473.x

Rothermund, K., and Brandtstädter, J. (2003). Depression in later life: cross-sequential patterns and possible determinants. *Psychol. Aging* 18, 80–90. doi: 10.1037/0882-7974.18.1.80

Scheibe, S., and Carstensen, L. L. (2010). Emotional aging: recent findings and future trends. *J. Gerontol. B Psychol. Sci. Soc. Sci.* 65B, 135–144. doi: 10.1093/geronb/gbp132

Seider, B. H., Shiota, M. N., Whalen, P., and Levenson, R. W. (2011). Greater sadness reactivity in late life. *Soc. Cogn. Affect. Neurosci.* 6, 186–194. doi: 10.1093/scan/nsq069

Smith, J., and Baltes, P. B. (1997). Profiles of psychological functioning in the old and oldest old. *Psychol. Aging* 12, 458–472. doi: 10.1037/0882-7974.12.3.458

Streubel, B., and Kunzmann, U. (2011). Age differences in emotional reactions: arousal and age-relevance count. *Psychol. Aging* 26, 966–978. doi: 10.1037/a0023424

Teachman, B. A., and Gordon, T. (2009). Age differences in anxious responding: older and calmer, unless the trigger is physical. *Psychol. Aging* 24, 703–714. doi: 10.1037/a0016813

Tsai, J. L., Knutson, B., and Fung, H. H. (2006). Cultural variation in affect valuation. *J. Pers. Soc. Psychol.* 90, 288–307. doi: 10.1037/0022-3514.90.2.288

Tsai, J. L., Levenson, R. W., and Carstensen, L. L. (2000). Autonomic, subjective, and expressive responses to emotional films in older and younger Chinese Americans and European Americans. *Psychol. Aging* 15, 684–693. doi: 10.1037/0882-7974.15.4.684

Wrosch, C., Dunne, E., Scheier, M. F., and Schulz, R. (2006). Self-regulation of common age-related challenges: benefits for older adults' psychological and physical health. *J. Behav. Med.* 29, 299–306. doi: 10.1007/s10865-006-9051-x

Wrosch, C., and Heckhausen, J. (1999). Control processes before and after passing a developmental deadline: activation and deactivation of intimate relationship goals. *J. Pers. Soc. Psychol.* 77, 415–427. doi: 10.1037/0022-3514.77.2.415

Wrosch, C., and Miller, G. E. (2009). Depressive symptoms can be useful: self-regulatory and emotional benefits of dysphoric mood in adolescence. *J. Pers. Soc. Psychol.* 96, 1181–1190. doi: 10.1037/a0015172

11

# Adult age-differences in subjective impression of emotional faces are reflected in emotion-related attention and memory tasks

**Joakim Svärd[1]*, Håkan Fischer[1,2] and Daniel Lundqvist[3]**

[1] Aging Research Center, Karolinska Institutet and Stockholm University, Stockholm, Sweden
[2] Department of Psychology, Stockholm University, Stockholm, Sweden
[3] Department of Clinical Neuroscience, Karolinska Institutet, Stockholm, Sweden

**Edited by:**
Natalie Ebner, University of Florida, USA

**Reviewed by:**
Natalie Ebner, University of Florida, USA
Phoebe E. Bailey, University of Western Sydney, Australia
Katja Werheid, Humboldt Universität zu Berlin, Germany

***Correspondence:**
Joakim Svärd, Aging Research Center, Karolinska Institutet, Stockholm University, Gävlegatan 16, 113 30 Stockholm, Sweden
e-mail: joakim.svard@ki.se

Although younger and older adults appear to attend to and remember emotional faces differently, less is known about age-related differences in the subjective emotional impression (arousal, potency, and valence) of emotional faces and how these differences, in turn, are reflected in age differences in various emotional tasks. In the current study, we used the same facial emotional stimuli (angry and happy faces) in four tasks: emotional rating, attention, categorical perception, and visual short-term memory (VSTM). The aim of this study was to investigate effects of age on the subjective emotional impression of angry and happy faces and to examine whether any age differences were mirrored in measures of emotional behavior (attention, categorical perception, and memory). In addition, regression analyses were used to further study impression-behavior associations. Forty younger adults (range 20–30 years) and thirty-nine older adults (range 65–75 years) participated in the experiment. The emotional rating task showed that older adults perceived less arousal, potency, and valence than younger adults and that the difference was more pronounced for angry than happy faces. Similarly, the results of the attention and memory tasks demonstrated interaction effects between emotion and age, and age differences on these measures were larger for angry than for happy faces. Regression analyses confirmed that in both age groups, higher potency ratings predicted both visual search and VSTM efficiency. Future studies should consider the possibility that age differences in the subjective emotional impression of facial emotional stimuli may explain age differences in attention to and memory of such stimuli.

**Keywords: emotion, faces, arousal, aging, subjective rating, attention, categorical perception, memory**

## INTRODUCTION

The effects of age on the processing of emotional facial expression have been investigated in a broad range of emotion-cognition domains, such as attention (e.g., Isaacowitz et al., 2006), memory (e.g., Mather and Carstensen, 2003), and categorical perception (Kiffel et al., 2005). However, age differences in the subjective emotional experience of facial expressions have been less extensively investigated. For example, studies of age differences in ratings of valence (pleasantness/unpleasantness), arousal (active/passive), and potency (weak/strong) (see e.g., Osgood, 1966; Russell, 2003) of such stimuli are rare. Consequently, little is known about whether age-related differences in the subjective emotional impression—that is, the valence, arousal, and potency rating—of emotional stimuli is associated with emotional behavior (e.g., memory, attention).

### AGE AND EMOTIONAL PROCESSING OF FACIAL EXPRESSION

Studies on the processing of emotional facial expression, including studies on recognition, attention, and memory, have revealed that aging is associated with less efficient processing of negative than positive faces. More specifically, older adults have repeatedly demonstrated poorer recognition than younger adults of expressions that are fearful (e.g., McDowell et al., 1994; Calder et al., 2003; Keightley et al., 2006; Horning et al., 2012; Svärd et al., 2012; Suzuki and Akiyama, 2013), angry (McDowell et al., 1994; Calder et al., 2003; Ebner and Johnson, 2009; Suzuki and Akiyama, 2013), and sad (McDowell et al., 1994; Calder et al., 2003; Keightley et al., 2006; Horning et al., 2012; Suzuki and Akiyama, 2013). However, they have a preserved or even increased ability to recognize facial expressions that are happy (e.g., McDowell et al., 1994; Calder et al., 2003; Svärd et al., 2012, but see also Horning et al., 2012; Suzuki and Akiyama, 2013) and disgusted (Calder et al., 2003; Horning et al., 2012; Suzuki and Akiyama, 2013). This pattern of results from individual studies has been confirmed in a meta-analysis by Ruffman et al. (2008), who found that the largest age-related decrease occurred in the recognition of angry, fearful, and sad faces and that less of a decrease occurred in the recognition of happy and surprised faces.

A similar age-by-emotion interaction has been demonstrated in memory for emotional faces. For instance, Mather and

Carstensen (2003) have demonstrated that although older adults remembered more positive than negative faces, there was no such difference among younger adults. Similarly, Ebner and Johnson (2009) have reported that older adults' memory for angry faces was poorer than their memory for happy and neutral faces. Enhanced memory for negative faces has also been reported among younger but not older adults (Grady et al., 2007; but see also D'Argembeau and van der Linden, 2004; Fischer et al., 2010). Studies of the effects of age on VSTM for emotional material have shown either a general decrease with age (Borg et al., 2011) or age-by-emotion interactions, findings that are consistent with the above-mentioned pattern of effects. For example, Mikels et al. (2005) found that younger adults were able to maintain intensity judgments of negative emotional pictures to a larger extent than of positive emotional pictures, but the opposite was true for older adults. A similar finding was reported in a study by Langeslag and van Strien (2009) in which younger adults exhibited enhanced VSTM performance for unpleasant but not pleasant stimuli, and older adults exhibited similar VSTM for both types of stimuli. However, to the best of our knowledge, no studies have investigated the effects of age on VSTM of emotional faces.

The attention literature shows that older adults preferentially focus on happy rather than sad faces, whereas younger adults do not (Isaacowitz et al., 2006). Moreover, older adults focus away from negative faces in negative-neutral face-pairs, but younger adults do not (Mather and Carstensen, 2003). However, when the task requires detection of negative (angry) schematic faces, these positivity preferences in older adults diminish (Hahn et al., 2006; Mather and Knight, 2006; Ruffman et al., 2009; Lundqvist et al., 2013a).

The findings from recognition, attention, and memory studies all show that the processing of negative but not positive facial expressions decreases with increasing age. This age-by-emotion interaction is often discussed in the theoretical framework of the *socio-emotional selectivity theory* (SST; Carstensen et al., 1999), which proposes motivational shifts away from negative and toward positive stimuli in the processing of emotional material as a function of limited time perspectives (see e.g., Carstensen, 2006). However, the contribution of subjective emotional impression to emotional processing remains relatively unexplored in the literature on age and emotion. This is intriguing because, as described in the next section, a growing body of research on younger adults shows that subjective emotional impression affect emotional processing.

### EFFECTS OF AROUSAL ON EMOTIONAL PROCESSING

Several reviews of studies on the attention-emotion domain in younger adults show that a stimulus' score on emotional arousal measures is more important for processing efficiency than the valence of the stimulus (in particular, see Lundqvist et al., 2013b; also c.f. Phelps and LeDoux, 2005; Lang and Bradley, 2010; Mather and Sutherland, 2011; Harmon-Jones et al., 2012). Recent results support the idea that emotional arousal is also important in older adults; they suggest that arousal may be the main emotional impression factor involved in age-related flattening of affect (Lundqvist et al., 2013a). More specifically, these results showed a significant age-related reduction in minimum and maximum ratings on emotional arousal and potency measures in response to facial stimuli. The results also showed a relationship between arousal ratings, potency ratings, and attention measures for angry (but not for happy) faces, such that higher ratings on those scales were associated with shorter reaction times (RTs) in a visual search task. A growing body of research on younger adults also points to emotional arousal as an important factor in VSTM performance. More specifically, both maintenance (Langeslag et al., 2009; Lindström and Bohlin, 2011) and immediate recall and recognition performance seem to be boosted by emotionally arousing content (Jackson et al., 2009; Langeslag et al., 2009).

A potential mechanisms through which arousal may impact task performance in the reported tasks is by means of activation in core affective arousal-related brain regions such as the amygdala, PAG and orbitofrontal cortex, which, in turn, influence activity in cortical regions and visual cortex to facilitate both higher cognitive processing and more basic visual perception (see e.g., Phelps and LeDoux, 2005).

In summary, studies in younger adults show an association between emotional arousal and efficiency in processing emotional information in both the attention and memory domains. With the exception of one study that found that the association between arousal and attention is preserved in older age (Lundqvist et al., 2013a), the effect of arousal on emotional processing in other emotion-cognition domains remains largely unexplored in the literature on aging.

### A THREE DIMENSION APPROACH TO THE STUDY OF EMOTION

In the cognition-emotion literature, the dimension of valence has historically been the emotional dimension of largest interest (see e.g., Lundqvist et al., 2013b), whereas the dimensions of arousal and potency have been investigated to a much lesser degree. All three dimensions reoccur in the literature (since the mid-fifties) as the three main underlying dimensions of affective/emotional responses to a wide array of emotional stimuli (e.g., Osgood and Suci, 1955; Lundqvist et al., 1999). The steady reoccurrence demonstrates the importance of these dimensions in socio-emotional interactions, and makes it meaningful and motivated to include all three dimensions in studies of emotion-cognition relationships.

### IMPLICATIONS FOR THE STUDY OF EFFECTS OF AGE ON EMOTIONAL PROCESSING

The findings of an effect of emotional impression on behavior point to the importance of stimulus selection in studies of emotional behavior in younger and older adults. If emotional faces convey different impression to younger and older adults, this may in turn affect attention and memory processing. Given that both memory literature (which indicates that participants remember material and events of emotional character better than those that are neutral; see e.g., Buchanan, 2007, for a review) and recent attention literature, which has found that arousal affects attention processing (e.g., Lundqvist et al., 2013b), a decrease in emotional impression might thus dampen the effect of emotion on memory performance and attention processing. By assuming that younger and older adults perceive emotional material equally in terms of the key dimensions of emotional impression, researchers risk misattributing age effects in emotional behavior.

### EXTENSION TO ANOTHER EMOTION-COGNITION DOMAIN

Categorical perception is another emotion-cognition domain that remains relatively unexplored, both in terms of age and arousal effects. The phenomenon of categorical perception refers to the occurrence of perceived categories along a linear continuum of physically changing stimulus (see e.g., Bornstein and Korda, 1984 for a more detailed description). Such phenomena have been shown in studies of color perception (e.g., Bornstein and Korda, 1984), speech perception (Liberman et al., 1957), and facial expression recognition (Etcoff and Magee, 1992). Although the physical differences between pairs of emotional faces in the Etcoff and Magee study (1992) were held constant, discrete perceived boundaries occurred for a variety of the emotion-emotion and emotion-neutral face pairs. Even though this finding of categorical perception of emotional facial expressions has been replicated in numerous studies of younger adults (e.g., Calder et al., 1996; Young et al., 1997; Campanella et al., 2002), less is known about how this type of categorical perception might vary as a function of age. To the best of our knowledge, only one study has investigated the effects of age on categorical perception of emotional facial expressions. That study showed that although categorical perception of identity was affected by age, categorical perception of emotional expressions seemed to remain intact (Kiffel et al., 2005).

### THE AIM AND HYPOTHESIS OF THE STUDY

The overall aim of this study was to extend earlier studies on subjective emotional impression and attention in older people. The study had three specific aims. The first was to investigate differences between older and younger adults in subjective emotional impressions. The second was to explore whether any such differences were mirrored in the emotional-cognitive tasks of attention, categorical perception, and VSTM. The third was to analyze whether any differences in the impression were associated with differences in task performance.

The literature on emotion indicates that the emotional properties of stimuli influence stimulus processing in many different domains, from perception to visual attention and memory (see e.g., Phelps and LeDoux, 2005). In this study, these different domains were represented by our categorical perception task (perception), visual search task (attention), and VSTM task (memory). Because of our previous results (Lundqvist et al., 2013a) and the above-mentioned reviews, we expected to replicate our earlier findings, which showed lower ratings in emotional impression of facial expression in older adults and an age-independent association between arousal ratings and visual search performance. We further expected to find performance differences across the perception, attention, and VSTM tasks, in keeping with the idea that high arousal scores are associated with high performance on tasks, and vice versa. This predicted decline in categorical perception would contrast with the Kiffel et al. (2005) finding that categorical perception of emotional expressions seems to remain intact with age. However, their study did not include angry faces, and it is angry faces that we predict will garner lower emotional ratings in older but not younger adults. Because of our previous results (Lundqvist et al., 2013a) and the above-mentioned reviews, we expect arousal to be the dimension that most strongly predicts task performance. However, because of our previous findings (Lundqvist et al., 2013a) and suggestions that at least a third emotional dimension should be incorporated in the study of emotions (Russell and Mehrabian, 1977; Fontaine et al., 2007), we also expected emotional potency to be involved in task performance.

Specifically, we expected: (1) to find lower ratings (i.e., arousal, potency) of emotional stimuli in older than younger adults, (2) to demonstrate that such lower ratings (i.e., arousal, potency) are associated with response latencies on the visual search task, and (3) that subjective emotional impression of facial expressions would be associated with performance on VSTM and categorical perception tasks. We did not have any predictions whether these associations are restricted only to angry faces, because previous results have showed that high arousal ratings of both angry and happy faces visual are associated with increased search efficiency (Lundqvist et al., 2013b).

## METHODS

### PARTICIPANTS

**Table 1** shows the characteristics of the participants in this study. Although younger adults scored higher than older adults on the anxiety items on the Hospital Anxiety and Depression Scale (HADS), this difference most likely did not affect behavioral results because no age-related differences in either trait anxiety (STAI-T) or state anxiety (STAI-S) were measured at test. All participants had normal or corrected-to-normal vision. Written informed consent was collected prior the tests and participants received two movie vouchers for their participation. The same participants were enrolled in all four tasks. The study was approved by the local ethics committee.

### MATERIALS

#### *Rating and visual search tasks*

Faces from the Averaged Karolinska Directed Emotional Faces set (AKDEF; Lundqvist and Litton, 1998) were used in the study. The AKDEF faces consist of an averaged female and an averaged male face, each composed of 35 individuals (see **Figure 1**). In the emotional rating task and in the visual search task, angry, happy, and neutral expressions from both the averaged female face and the averaged male face were used as stimuli. Ratings of and visual search performance for fear, disgust, sadness, and surprise were also collected but not analyzed in the current study.

#### *Categorical perception and visual short-term memory tasks*

The stimuli shown in **Figure 1** were also the basis of the stimuli in the categorical perception and VSTM tasks. However, to enable investigation of categorical boundaries and VSTM performance on a continuum from a neutral to an emotional facial expression, the faces were modified to show emotional expressions at various intensities between 0 and 100%. The modification of the faces was performed using SqirlsMorph 2.1

**Table 1 | Participant characteristics by age group.**

| | Younger | Older | *p*-value | *d* |
|---|---|---|---|---|
| | M | M | | |
| Age in years (*SD*) | 25.2 (10.5) | 70.5 (2.8) | <0.001 | 13.127 |
| Sex | 21 F, 19 M | 24 F, 15 M | | |
| Education in years (*SD*) | 14.6 (2.9) | 14.5 (2.9) | 0.831 | 0.049 |
| MMSE (*SD*; range) | 29 (0.9; 26–30) | 28.7 (1.4; 24–30) | 0.295 | 0.237 |
| HADS[a] (*SD*; range) | 5 (3.5; 0–13) | 3.4 (3.0; 0–15) | 0.028 | 0.509 |
| HADS[d] (*SD*; range) | 3.1 (2.3; 0–12) | 2.9 (2.2; 0–10) | 0.653 | 0.102 |
| STAI-T (*SD*) | 47.7 (4.8; 27–59) | 47 (3.1; 42–56) | 0.390 | 0.196 |
| STAI-S (*SD*) | 30.1 (5.8; 20–42) | 29 (5.2; 20–40) | 0.381 | 0.201 |

*MMSE, mini mental state examination (Folstein et al., 1975); HADS, hospital anxiety and depression scale (Zigmond and Snaith, 1983); STAI, state-trait anxiety inventory (Spielberger et al., 1988); -T, Trait; -S, State; [a]anxiety items; [d]depression items; F, female; M, male; *$p < 0.05$.*

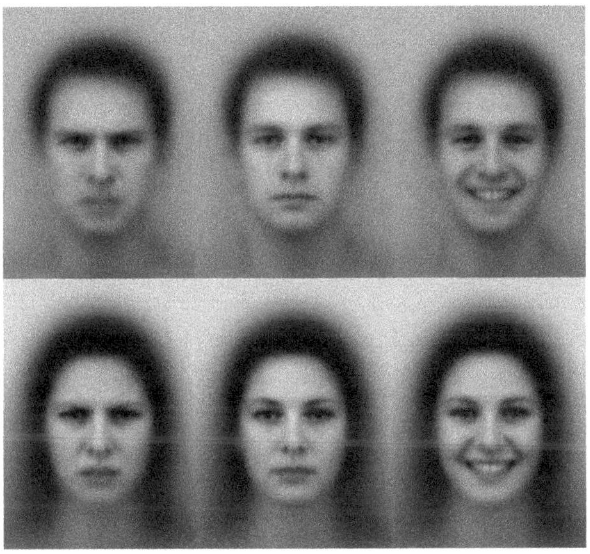

**FIGURE 1 | Examples of the face stimuli used in all four tasks.** Note: Faces from the Averaged Karolinska Directed Emotional Faces set (Lundqvist and Litton, 1998).

(http://www.xiberpix.net/), and key points were used to guide the morph between facial features (e.g., lips, mouth shape, eyes, nose wrinkles, facial outline). For the categorical perception task, 9 face pairs differing 20% in intensity (i.e., 20 steps apart along the 100-step morph) were created in the neutral-to-angry and neutral-to-happy continua for the female and male averaged faces respectively (see **Figure 2**). The size of each face was 7.5 × 10.5 cm.

## PROCEDURE

To minimize the risk of initiating any potential biases caused by elaborative processing, the rating task was performed last in the sequence. Although the order in which the tasks were conducted was visual search, categorical perception, visual short-term memory, and rating, to facilitate reading and interpretation of the manuscript, the rating experiment is presented first. The order of the tasks was the same for all participants. At study, participants sat on a chair in front of a computer screen (HP Compaq LA2405wg) at a distance of approximately 0.5 m. Behavioral responses were collected by key presses on an external keyboard. The experiment was programmed using Macromedia Director MX 2004 software (Macromedia Inc.). Total duration of the experiment was approximately 75 min. The visual search task took 30 min, and the rating, VSTM, and categorical perception tasks each took 15 min. Short breaks were given between the tasks to prevent fatigue.

### *Emotional rating task*

During the rating task, facial stimuli (**Figure 1**) with full emotional expressions (100% intensity) were presented one at a time on the computer screen. Participants used a visual analog scale (VAS) to rate the three key emotional dimensions arousal (active-inactive), valence (pleasant-unpleasant), and potency (weak-strong) of seven expressions on male faces and seven on female faces (a total of 42 faces). Cursors on three separated horizontal lines were used for the ratings. The scales ranged from −1 to 1 (actual values were not visible to the participants).

The three VAS scales were presented below the face and maneuvered with the right and left arrow keys. Participants were informed that the task was self-paced. However, they were encouraged to base their rating on the first impression of a face and not spend exaggerated time thinking. Once ratings on the three scales were completed, participants pressed the spacebar to continue to the next trial. The order and polarity of scales were randomized between trials.

### *Visual search task*

During the visual search task, circular displays of 6 faces were presented to the participants. In half of the trials (so-called target-absent trials), all faces in the array had the same emotional expression, while in the other half (so-called target-present trials), one of the faces was different from the other (e.g., an angry face among neutral faces).

Participants were instructed to determine whether each array consisted of faces that were all the same (in which case they were to press a button marked "all same" with their left index finger), or whether one of the faces was different from the others (in which

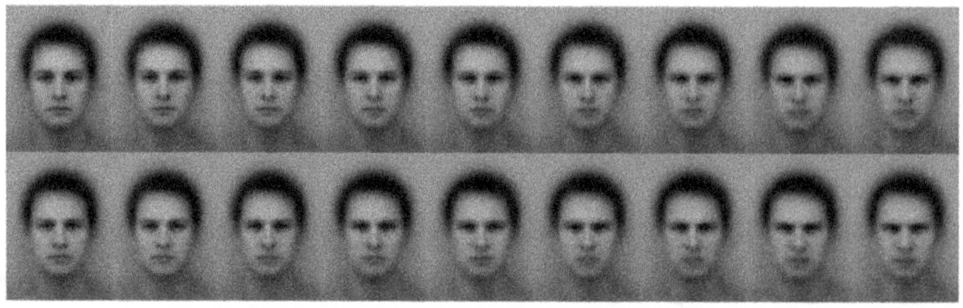


**FIGURE 2 | Examples of face pairs used in the categorical perception task (presented vertically).** At study, the faces in each pair were presented side by side.

case they were to press a button marked "one deviant" with their right index finger). They were instructed to respond as quickly and accurately as possible. A fixation cross initiated each trial. During target-absent conditions, all faces were afraid, angry, disgusted, happy, neutral, sad, or surprised. During target-present conditions, the background would either be *neutral*, with afraid, angry, disgusted, happy, sad, or surprised faces as the deviating target, or *emotional* (afraid, angry, disgusted, happy, sad, or surprised faces), with neutral as the deviating target. The target face was presented once at each position in the array. The presentation of trials was blocked by condition (emotional background or neutral background) and sex of faces (female or male). Thus, four blocks that included a total 288 faces (2 sexes, 6 expressions, 6 positions, 4 blocks) were used. As soon as a key was pressed ("all similar" or "one deviant"), the trial was terminated and the next trial was initiated. This article only includes information about the analyses of angry and happy emotional faces to make the effects of emotional stimuli (angry, happy) congruent with the stimuli used in the other tasks in the study. The order of blocks was randomized for each participant.

#### Categorical perception task

During the categorical perception task, pairs of faces were presented side by side on the screen. The physical difference between the faces in each pair was always 20%. Thus, a face showing 0% emotionality (i.e., a neutral face) was always paired with a face showing 20% emotionality, a face 10% emotionality was always paired with a face showing 30% emotionality, and so on (see **Figure 2**). Each pair was shown twice in a randomized order. Presentation of stimuli was however blocked for emotional expression and for the sex of the depicted face. Thus, each of the four blocked conditions (male, neutral to angry; male neural to happy; female, neutral to angry; and female, neutral to happy) contained 2*9 pairs, or a total of 72 pair of faces. The order of blocks was balanced over participants.

Participants were instructed to decide whether the two faces in each pair showed the same facial expression or not. Participants gave their answers by pressing keys labeled "same" or "different." Thus, a shift in Categorical perception from neutral to an emotional expression was investigated. Because pilot tests before start of the study showed that some participants tended to respond "different" on trials where the intensity rather than expression differed, it was emphasized that the task was to judge the facial expression of the face and not whether the expression showed the same intensity or not. The faces stayed on the screen until participants gave their response, which terminated the trial and initiated the next trial.

#### Visual short-term memory task

In the VSTM task, an emotional face (angry or happy) that varied in expressed emotional intensity in 10% intervals ranging from 10 to 90% was displayed on the screen for three seconds before it disappeared. After a one second interval, a face again appeared on the screen, but at a different (random) intensity level. Participants were instructed to remember the first face and upon display of the second (random) face, adjust the face's intensity level until it matched that of the first face. Intensity adjustments were made with the right and left arrow keys. After completing the adjustments, participants pressed the enter key, and a new trial was initiated. Each intensity interval was shown twice in a randomized order. The presentations were however blocked for emotional expression and for the sex of the depicted face. Thus, each of the four blocked conditions (male, neutral to angry; male neural to happy; female, neutral to angry; and female, neutral to happy) contained 2*9 faces, or a total of 72 presented faces. The order of blocks was balanced over participants.

### DATA PREPARATION AND STATISTICAL ANALYSIS

#### Rating task

Average ratings for the female and male faces were calculated separately for the emotional dimensions valence, arousal, and potency before statistical analyses were run.

#### Visual search task

Separate ANOVAs were run for reaction times (RTs) and accuracy. Correct responses were included in the analysis of RTs. Before analysis, raw RT data was log10-transformed to achieve normal distribution of data. Furthermore, individual outliers ($M >< \pm 3 * SD$) were replaced by ($M \pm 3 * SD$). However, to facilitate interpretation of the results, raw values are presented in the text and figures.

#### Categorical perception task

To analyze categorical perception data, a peak intensity interval (e.g., 30–50) was identified for each participant (separately for each of the two emotions). Within each emotion, data for the two AKDEF stimuli genders were collapsed before identifying the peak. Since there were clear differences in how many responses of "different" a participant tended to give (across intervals), the peak was identified by first identifying the interval with the most responses of "different" for that participant and that emotion (e.g., neutral to angry). If there were several responses with the same frequency across a span of intervals (e.g., 20–40; 30–50; 40–60) an average interval was calculated (here 30–50). The most frequent reported "different" pair was thus assumed to be the peak at which categorical perception occurred (Beale and Keil, 1995). The category border itself was assumed to be in the middle of the peak interval (e.g., at 40% if the peak was identified in a 30–50% pair). Thus, peaks were identified for angry and happy faces separately for each individual participant.

### *Visual short-term memory task*

To investigate VSTM performance, the intensity level of the face during encoding was subtracted from the intensity levels reported by the participant. That is, if the face showed 20% intensity at encoding and the participants adjusted the face to show 28% intensity at retrieval, the error score was 8%. Further, to transform all error scores to a positive value, all answers were square root transformed [$\sqrt{}$ (answer∗answer)] at the level of individual responses. The transformation was made after initial analyses where it was discovered that un-transformed errors made in both directions (e.g., −20 and +20% for two trials within one emotion) led to the false impression that this condition was reported with perfect accuracy ($M = 0\%$). Thus, to study effects of age and emotional impression on VSTM performance, transformed data were used in analyses.

## RESULTS

To investigate age effects on specific emotion-cognition domains separated ANOVAs were planned for the rating, visual search, VSTM, and categorical perception tasks. Regression analyses were carried out on each of the three behavior tasks to study the effects of emotional impression on emotional behavior. Because of the exploratory nature of this first study on emotional impression and its relation to different emotional behaviors, we decided that the risk of making a type I error was less important than the risk missing important findings. Therefore, corrections for multiple comparisons were not performed.

For all analyses, regular degrees of freedom are reported together with observed significance levels after Greenhouse-Geisser correction. Results were considered significant at $p \leq 0.05$.

### ANOVAs

A multivariate analysis revealed a significant effect of age on the combined task performance, $F_{(4, 63)} = 24.62$, $p < 0.001$, $\eta^2 = 0.610$. Analysis of each tasks confirmed the effect of age on rating, $F_{(1, 66)} = 13.22$, $p = 0.001$, $\eta^2 = 0.167$, visual search, $F_{(1, 66)} = 65.60$, $p < 0.001$, $\eta^2 = 0.498$, categorical perception, $F_{(1, 66)} = 12.92$, $p = 0.001$, $\eta^2 = 0.164$, and VSTM, $F_{(1, 66)} = 23.15$, $p < 0.001$, $\eta^2 = 0.260$, performance. Separated repeated ANOVAs were carried out to study effects of age and emotion on each of the tasks.

### *Rating task*

Separate ANOVAs were carried out for the emotional dimensions of valence, arousal, and potency. In the ANOVAs, age (young, old) was used as the between-subject variable and emotion (angry, happy) was used as within-subject variables. Planned $t$-tests were conducted to study the effect of age on each dimension of emotion. These tests were conducted separately for angry and happy faces. The results are presented in **Figure 3A**.

***Valence.*** The main effect of Emotion $F_{(1, 77)} = 133.73$, $p < 0.001$, $\eta^2 = 0.635$, showed overall higher ratings for Happy ($M = 0.51$, $SD = 0.43$) compared to Angry ($M = -0.35$, $SD = 0.35$)

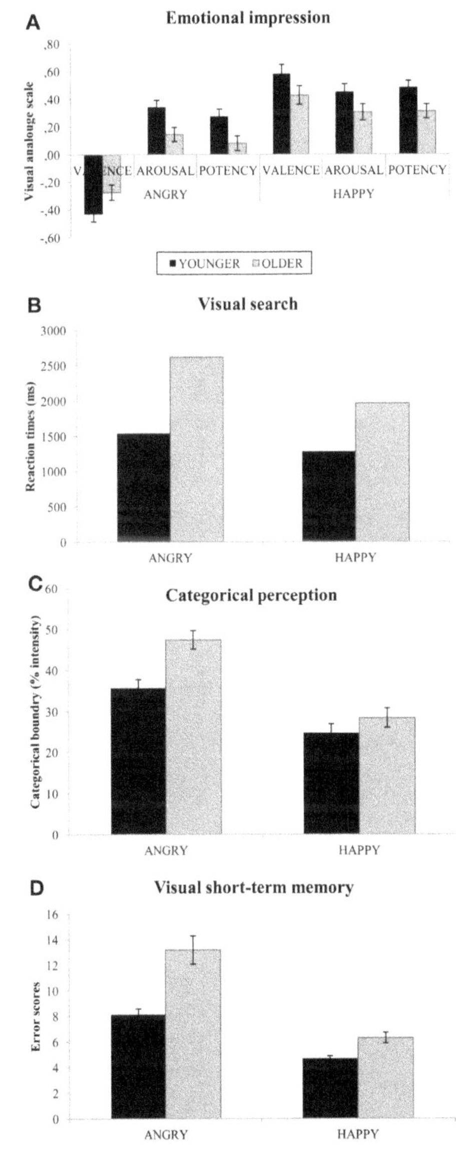


**FIGURE 3 | Mean (SE) performance in the rating task (A), visual search task (B), categorical perception task, (C) and visual short-term memory task (D) separately for expression and age.** Note. Error bars represent standard error. Results of the ANOVAs and $t$-tests for age differences are presented in the result section.

faces. There was also an interaction effect between Age and Emotion $F_{(1, 77)} = 4.35$, $p = 0.04$, $\eta^2 = 0.053$, that showed that the largest decrease in responsiveness among Older adults was for Angry faces. Follow up *t*-tests for the interaction revealed that Older adults ratings ($M = -0.28$, $SD = 0.38$) were lower than those of Younger adults ($M = -0.31$, $SD = 0.31$) for Angry faces, $t_{(77)} = 1.99$, $p = 0.05$, $d = 0.087$. For happy faces, there was no difference, $p = 0.11$.

***Arousal.*** The ANOVA on arousal revealed a main effect of Emotion, $F_{(1, 77)} = 7.80$, $p = 0.007$, $\eta^2 = 0.092$, that showed higher ratings for Happy ($M = 0.38$, $SD = 0.37$) compared to Angry ($M = 0.25$, $SD = 0.33$) faces. The main effect of Age, $F_{(1, 77)} = 7.96$, $p = 0.006$, $\eta^2 = 0.094$, showed that Older adults ($M = 0.22$, $SD = 0.23$) gave lower ratings than Younger adults ($M = 0.40$, $SD = 0.30$). The planned *t*-tests revealed that Older adults ratings ($M = 0.15$, $SD = 0.27$) were lower than those of Younger adults ($M = 0.34$, $SD = 0.36$) for Angry faces, $t_{(1, 77)} = 2.74$, $p = 0.008$, $d = 0.597$. For Happy faces, Older adults tended to give lower ratings ($M = 0.30$, $SD = 0.38$) than Younger adults ($M = 0.45$, $SD = 0.35$), which resulted in a trend toward an age difference, $t_{(1, 77)} = 1.78$, $p = 0.078$, $d = 0.411$.

***Potency.*** The main effect of Emotion, $F_{(1, 77)} = 16.95$, $p < 0.001$, $\eta^2 = 0.180$, showed higher ratings for Happy ($M = 0.40$, $SD = 0.33$) than for Angry ($M = 0.18$, $SD = 0.34$) faces. The effect of Age, $F_{(1, 77)} = 12.91$, $p = 001$, $\eta^2 = 0.144$, showed that Older adults ($M = 0.20$, $SD = 0.19$) gave lower ratings than Younger adults ($M = 0.38$, $SD = 0.26$). The planned *t*-tests revealed that Older adults ratings ($M = 0.08$, $SD = 0.29$) were lower than those of Younger adults ($M = 0.27$, $SD = 0.38$) for Angry faces, $t_{(1, 77)} = 2.6$, $p = 0.011$, $d = 0.533$. For Happy faces, Older adults' ratings ($M = 0.31$, $SD = 0.33$) were lower than those of Younger adults, ($M = 0.48$, $SD = 0.31$), $t_{(1, 77)} = 2.38$, $p = 0.020$, $d = 0.531$.

### Visual search task

***Accuracy (%).*** The ANOVA on Accuracy revealed a main effect of Emotion, $F_{(1, 77)} = 13.84$, $p < 0.001$, $\eta^2 = 0.152$, showing that across age Happy faces ($M = 96.10$, $SD = 0.07$) were detected with higher accuracy than Angry faces ($M = 90.71$, $SD = 0.14$). There was also a main effect of Age, $F_{(1, 77)} = 8.32$, $p = 0.005$, $\eta^2 = 0.098$, showing that across emotions, Older adults ($M = 96.20$, $SD = 0.01$) detected a deviant emotional face among neutral distractors more accurately than did Younger adults ($M = 90.70$, $SD = 0.10$).

***Reaction time (ms).*** The ANOVA on RTs revealed a main effect of Emotion, $F_{(1, 77)} = 118.23$, $p < 0.001$, $\eta^2 = 0.606$, showing that Happy faces ($M = 1618$, $SD = 525$) were detected faster than Angry faces ($M = 2071$, $SD = 925$). A main effect of Age, $F_{(1, 77)} = 76.30$, $p < 0.001$, $\eta^2 = 0.498$, showed that Older adults ($M = 2290$, $SD = 702$) were slower than Younger adults ($M = 1411$, $SD = 338$) in detecting a deviant face. There was also an interaction between Age and Emotion, $F_{(1, 77)} = 6.51$, $p = 0.013$, $\eta^2 = 0.078$, showing that although Older adults were slower than Younger adults in detecting both Angry and Happy faces, this effect was more pronounced for Angry faces (**Figure 3B**).

### Categorical perception task

Because of equipment failure, data from two older women were not collected. In addition, seven (3 younger and 4 older adults) non-responders (i.e., participants who did not report any different response at all) were excluded from the analysis (11.4% excluded in total). Thus, 37 (20 female) younger and 34 (20 female) older adults were included in this analysis.

The ANOVA on Categorical perception data demonstrated a main effect of Emotion, $F_{(1, 69)} = 44.72$, $p < 0.001$, $\eta^2 = 0.393$, showing that the shift in Categorical perception from neutral to an emotional expression occurred earlier for Happy ($M = 26.5$, $SD = 13.8$), than for Angry ($M = 41.3$, $SD = 14.2$) faces. The main effect of Age, $F_{(1, 69)} = 11.88$, $p < 0.001$, $\eta^2 = 0.147$, revealed that across emotions (Angry and Happy), Older adults categorical shift from a neutral to an emotional face occurred at a later stage ($M = 37.9$, $SD = 10.8$) along the continuum compared to Younger adults ($M = 30.2$, $SD = 8.2$). (**Figure 3C**). In addition, there was also an trend toward an Age by Emotion interaction, $F_{(1, 69)} = 3.22$, $p = 0.077$, $\eta^2 = 0.045$.

### Visual short-term memory task

Data inspection revealed two outliers (whose mean score was <> $\pm$ 3 *SD*), which were excluded from analyses together with one participant with missing data (3.8% excluded in total). Thus, analyses were computed for 40 younger (21 female) and 35 older (21 female) adults. The statistical design of the ANOVA on VSTM was a 2 (Emotion: Angry, Happy) by 9 (Intensity levels: 10–90%) design with Age (Young, Old) as a between-group variable.

The results revealed a main effect of Emotion, $F_{(1, 73)} = 104.23$, $p < 0.001$, $\eta^2 = 0.588$. Across intensity levels, both Younger and Older adults performed better (fewer errors) for Happy ($M = 5.32$, $SD = 1.90$) than for Angry ($M = 10.18$, $SD = 4.80$) faces. There was also a main effect of Age, $F_{(1, 73)} = 26.83$, $p < 0.001$, $\eta^2 = 0.269$: Older adults ($M = 9.32$, $SD = 3.13$) made more errors than Younger adults ($M = 6.38$, $SD = 1.67$). In addition, there was an interaction between Age and Emotion, $F_{(1, 73)} = 9.99$, $p = 0.002$, $\eta^2 = 0.120$: although Older adults performed worse than Younger adults for both emotions, the poorer performance of Older adults was more pronounced for Angry faces (**Figure 3D**). There was also a main effect of Intensity, $F_{(8, 584)} = 2.33$, $p = 0.029$, $\eta^2 = 0.031$. Contrast tests showed that in both age groups and for both emotions, participants made significantly more errors at the 90% intensity level than at any other level, $ps < 0.05$.

## REGRESSION ANALYSES

A multivariate multiple regression analysis revealed an association between emotional impression (all dimensions) and the combined task performance, $F_{(3, 64)} = 3.10$, $p = 0.033$, $\eta^2 = 0.127$. Analysis of each tasks confirmed the association between emotional impression and visual search, $F_{(1, 66)} = 6.92$, $p = 0.011$, $\eta^2 = 0.095$, VSTM, $F_{(1, 66)} = 6.79$, $p = 0.011$, $\eta^2 = 0.093$, but not categorical perception, $F_{(1, 66)} = 0.85$, $p = 0.361$, $\eta^2 = 0.013$, performance. Separated regressions were carried out to study associations between specific dimensions and tasks.

Regression analyses were conducted for each of the behavior tasks (for angry and happy faces separately). In these analyses, three models were used to explore the relationship between emotional impression and behavior. Model one was univariate; each emotional rating scale was tested alone as the predictor. Model 2 was multivariate; all three scales were included as predictors. Thus, in Model 2, any effects were adjusted for the influences of the other scales. Finally, in Model 3, age was included as a predictor, which means that any effect in this model holds even after controlling for age effects. Models 2 and 3 were performed using the enter method.

The univariate analyses for Angry faces revealed that both Arousal and Potency ratings were associated with Visual search performance ($ps < 0.05$). In addition, Potency ratings were also associated with VSTM performance ($p < 0.05$). The association between Arousal ratings and emotional behavior vanished when the analyses were adjusted for the influences of the other scales (Model 2) and the influences of the other scales and age (Model 3). However, the association between Potency ratings and Visual search and VSTM performance remained significant even after these adjustments ($ps < 0.05$). These age-independent relationships can be seen in **Figure 4** in the different location of younger (middle to top left area) and older adults' (middle to bottom right area) scores along the regression line. For Happy faces, there were no associations between any of the emotional rating scales and emotional behavior tasks ($ps > 0.05$). **Table 2** gives information regarding the predictor variables used in the different models.

## DISCUSSION

The emotional rating task revealed that older adults rated facial expressions as less emotional than younger adults, and these age differences were more pronounced for angry than happy faces. This age-by-emotion interaction was also evident in visual search and visual short-term memory performance. Regression analyses confirmed that in both age groups, higher potency ratings were the foremost predictor of both visual search and VSTM efficiency for angry faces but not for happy ones. We will briefly discuss the results separately for each task as well as results regarding the associations between subjective emotional impressions and emotional behavior.

### SPECIFIC EMOTION-COGNITION DOMAINS

#### *Rating*

The results of the rating task revealed a weaker emotional impression of facial expressions in older than in younger adults, which was more pronounced for angry than happy faces (**Figure 3A**, left panel). Older adults rated the angry faces as significantly less unpleasant (valence), less active (arousal), and weaker (potency) than did younger adults. A similar pattern was found for happy faces, but only the difference in the potency measure was statistically significant (see **Figure 3A**, right panel). These results are in line with previous results from our group (Lundqvist et al., 2013a), which show that the emotional impression of faces diminishes with advancing age, and that this dampening is most pronounced for angry faces.

#### *Visual search*

An age-by-emotion interaction in RTs revealed that although older adults were generally slower than younger adults, this effect was more pronounced for the detection of angry faces. To the best of our knowledge, this article is the first to report an age-by-emotion interaction in visual search efficiency for emotional faces. It should be noted that our results (which used photographic stimuli) are in disagreement with the results of overall age and emotion effects from previous studies that used schematic (Hahn et al., 2006; Mather and Knight, 2006; Ruffman et al., 2009; Lundqvist et al., 2013a) and photographic (Ruffman et al., 2009) faces. Our finding of faster detection of happy than angry faces is also in disagreement with the findings of the above-mentioned studies. The finding of an angry superiority effect (ASE) in previous studies and a happy superiority effect (HSE; for an overview, see Lundqvist et al., 2013a). in the present study is linked to the emotional impression of the stimuli used and will be discussed below.

The pattern of results in the visual search tasks shows that the older participants generate markedly longer RTs. However, it also shows that this slowness is not without advantages, as the older group also responds with greater accuracy. Whether the high accuracy is a side-effect from the slow responses, or part of a strategy is difficult to say from the present data, since we do not assess or address response strategies.

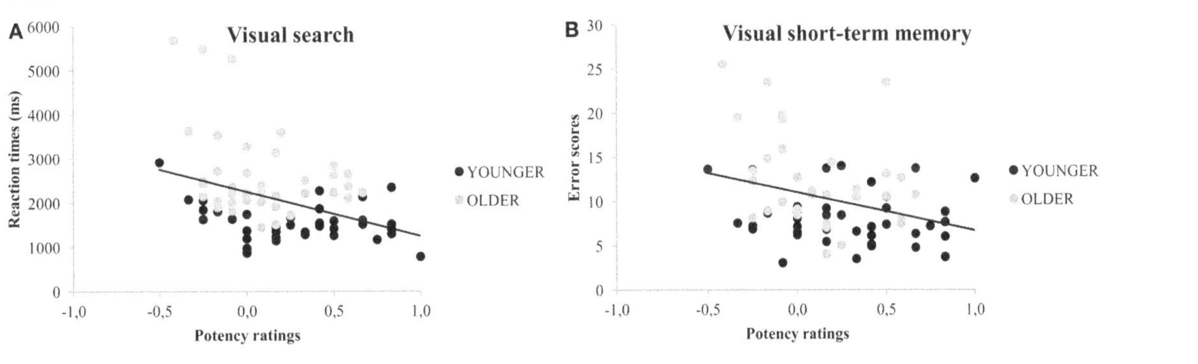


**FIGURE 4 | Scatterplots for potency ratings and emotional behavior tasks, separately for visual search (A) and visual short-term memory (B) performance for angry faces across age.** Note. Visual search: $r = -0.372$; Visual short-term memory: $r = -0.312$.

**Table 2 | β-coefficients (SE) and bivariate correlations for rating scores associated with emotional behavior.**

| Predictors | Angry | | | Happy | | |
|---|---|---|---|---|---|---|
| By task | Model 1[a] | Model 2[a] | Model 3[a] | Model 1[a] | Model 2[a] | Model 3[a] |
| **VISUAL SEARCH (RT)** | | | | | | |
| Arousal | −0.25 (0.06)* | −0.08 (0.06) | 0.03 (0.05) | −0.14 (0.04) | −0.15 (0.05) | −0.09 (0.04) |
| Potency | −0.36 (0.05)** | −0.31 (0.06)* | −0.21 (0.05)* | −0.11 (0.05) | −0.08 (0.05) | 0.07 (0.04) |
| Valence | 0.13 (0.05) | 0.01 (0.05) | −0.07 (0.04) | −0.03 (0.04) | 0.08 (0.04) | 0.11 (0.03) |
| **VISUAL SHORT-TERM MEMORY (ERROR SCORES)** | | | | | | |
| Arousal | −0.09 (1.68) | 0.12 (1.97) | 0.21 (1.78) | −0.10 (0.61) | −0.07 (0.73) | −0.04 (0.69) |
| Potency | −0.31 (1.53)* | −0.37 (1.86)* | −0.32 (1.67)* | −0.19 (0.66) | −0.20 (0.74) | −0.11 (0.72) |
| Valence | 0.11 (1.57) | 0.04 (1.62) | −0.04 (1.47) | −0.03 (0.52) | 0.09 (0.62) | 0.12 (0.59) |
| **CATEGORICAL PERCEPTION (PEAK)** | | | | | | |
| Arousal | −0.19 (5.05) | −0.17 (6.26) | −0.12 (5.82) | 0.10 (4.41) | 0.05 (5.14) | 0.07 (5.13) |
| Potency | −0.12 (4.97) | −0.03 (6.11) | 0.07 (5.78) | 0.04 (5.07) | −0.03 (5.66) | 0.00 (5.67) |
| Valence | 0.07 (5.03) | 0.00 (5.43) | −0.03 (5.05) | 0.15 (4.04) | 0.14 (4.84) | 0.16 (4.82) |
| **Correlations** | **Angry** | | | **Happy** | | |
| **Between predictors** | **Arousal** | **Potency** | **Valence** | **Arousal** | **Potency** | **Valence** |
| Arousal | – | 0.539** | −0.306* | – | 0.379** | 0.522** |
| Potency | | – | −0.288* | | – | 0.410** |

[a] *Model 1 was univariate; Model 2 was multivariate, adjusted for the other rating scales; and Model 3 was additionally adjusted for age.* $^{**}p \leq 0.01$; $^{*}0.01 < p \leq 0.05$.

### *Categorical perception*

The results of the categorical perception task show that both angry and happy faces were perceived categorically by both age groups. These results are in line with the results of several other studies on younger adults (e.g., Calder et al., 1996; Young et al., 1997; Campanella et al., 2002) and on older adults (Kiffel et al., 2005). The present study adds new information to the existing literature by showing that the perceptual category boundaries can vary as a function of both age and emotion. The current study used a neutral expression as a reference and paired it separately with an angry or a happy expression; the results showed reliable differences in the locus of boundaries for angry and happy faces. More specifically, our results showed that in both age groups, the locus of the boundary was further forward for angry than for happy faces, indicating that the angry faces were processed more ambiguously than the happy ones. In light of the results from the other tasks, the trend toward an interaction between age and emotion in this task is noteworthy. Although it did not reach a conventional statistical threshold, the relationship agrees with the general pattern of results in this article, which shows that older adults process angry faces less readily than younger adults.

### *Visual short-term memory*

The results of the VSTM task showed that the older adults performed less accurately than younger adults, and the difference in accuracy was greater for angry than for happy faces. Earlier studies have shown that older adults have a decreased ability to maintain unpleasant non-facial stimuli (Langeslag and van Strien, 2009) and negative intensity judgments (Mikels et al., 2005). Our results extend these previous findings into the domain of emotional expression by showing a relatively larger reduction in VSTM performance for angry than for happy facial expressions. The results agree on the general pattern of results in this article, which shows that older adults process angry faces less readily than younger adults.

## EMOTIONAL IMPRESSION-BEHAVIOR RELATIONSHIPS

A central aim of this study was to replicate and extend our previous findings (Lundqvist et al., 2013a) of an association between emotional impression and visual search efficiency to include new cognitive-emotion domains. As seen in **Table 2**, the emotional dimension of potency was associated with the results of two out of three emotional behavior tasks for angry faces.

The association between arousal and potency ratings and visual search efficiency replicates our previous findings of a similar relationship for schematic emotional faces (Lundqvist et al., 2013a). In that study, higher arousal and potency ratings were correlated with lower search times for angry but not happy faces. In accordance with the findings of the current study, this association was age-independent, which indicates that visual search performance in both younger and older adults is associated with potency measures. In the present analyses, this relationship can also be seen in **Figure 4A** in the differing location of younger (middle to top left area) and older adults' (middle to bottom right area) scores along the regression line. Both our previous findings (Lundqvist et al., 2013a) and our present results indicate that although older adults generally have lower visual search efficiency than younger adults, search efficiency is associated with the same underlying emotional dimensions (potency and arousal) regardless of age. This notion is also partially supported by the work of Leclerc and

Kensinger (2008, 2010), who found that when arousal levels of positive and negative stimuli were equated, all valence effects were absent. Importantly, the lack of interactions with age demonstrated an age-independent reliance on arousal in visual search performance.

Within the visual search literature, researchers usually report on whether their results show an ASE or a HSE (see Visual Search. above). In those terms, the present results demonstrate an HSE. A recent review article by Lundqvist et al. (2013b) concluded that when participants compared two facial expressions, the expression with the highest arousal ratings was detected most efficiently, regardless of whether that expression was happy or angry. The Lundqvist et al. (2013b) article may thus explain the disagreement between our findings of an HSE and previous studies' findings of an ASE. In accordance with the notion that the facial expression with the highest arousal rating is detected most efficiently, the current study showed a HSE in both arousal ratings and visual search performance. Thus, the current results help generalize the role played by arousal in visual attention to the later part of the adult life-span. In terms of behavior and related brain processes, the HSE effect is potentially associated with a more attention driven positivity bias associated with activity in the dorsolateral prefrontal cortex (Lindquist et al., 2012), a more elaborative cognitive bias associated with activity in the ventromedial prefrontal cortex (Ebner et al., 2012) and/or a more perceptually driven bias associated with activation in the occipital cortex (Lindquist et al., 2012). A recent review by Lundqvist et al. (2013b) however shows that both the HSE concept and its rivaling concept ASE may be confound by an uncontrolled influence from the arousal factor. The present data (showing overall lower scores on arousal for angry compared to happy faces indicates that the present HSE finding may well be explained by the arousal differences between the angry and happy stimuli.

Like attention processing, VSTM performance was associated with the potency ratings of stimuli, such that higher potency ratings were associated with fewer errors. This age-independent association can be seen in **Figure 4B** in the different location of younger (middle to top left area) and older adults' (middle to bottom right area) scores along the regression line. Like the emotion-attention relationship, this relationship indicate that although older adults generally have lower VSTM efficiency than younger adults, VSTM efficiency is associated with the same underlying emotional dimensions (potency and arousal) regardless of age. These findings of age-independent associations might contribute to the understanding of the preserved processing of the happy facial expression that is reported in recognition (e.g., Ruffman et al., 2008), attention (e.g., Isaacowitz et al., 2006), and memory (e.g., Mather and Carstensen, 2003). The age-related differences in emotional impression and the age-related differences in behavior were both less pronounced for happy than angry faces.

In summary, for angry faces, associations between subjective emotional impression and behavior were found in two out of three tasks. The lack of an association for happy faces are most likely due to a lower degree of variance in the processing of happy than angry faces.

### POTENCY AS A PREDICTOR OF EMOTIONAL BEHAVIOR

When analyzed as univariate predictors, both high arousal and high potency ratings were associated with an increase in visual search efficiency (i.e., lower RTs). However, after adjustments for arousal and valence in Model 2 and arousal, valance, age in Model 3, only high potency ratings predicted a reduction in RT for angry faces. A likely explanation of this might be the relatively high inter-correlation between the dimensions of arousal and potency ($r = 0.539$). Thus, although arousal may in itself have an effect on visual search performance, as indicated by the results of Model 1, this effect may have been masked by the statistically stronger effect of potency. Hence, although our prediction was of an association between arousal and behavior, our finding that potency is the stronger predictor is neither controversial nor in direct disagreement with our previous results. As mentioned in the introduction, the study of emotional dimensions beyond valence and arousal has been proposed previously (Russell and Mehrabian, 1977; Fontaine et al., 2007). Given that we have found associations between potency and search efficiency in the current study and in a previous one (Lundqvist et al., 2013a)—and an additional association between potency and VSTM performance in the current study—this dimension clearly deserves to be included and investigated in future studies in this field of research.

### LIMITATIONS

Using the same stimuli and the same study population across four tasks, we have consistently demonstrated a less accurate processing of angry faces in older than younger adults. Moreover, we found an association between emotional impression and emotional behavior, which indicates that subjective emotional impression influences behavior. However, some limitations are worth mentioning.

For example, the facial stimuli used all depicted younger adults. Although previous research on the recognition of facial expressions has demonstrated equal recognition processing of younger and older faces (Ebner and Johnson, 2009; Ebner et al., 2013), interactions between the age of poser and the age of participants might be present in other domains, such as those used in the present study. Thus, replication of the current study using both younger and older faces would increase the generalizability of our results.

A second potential limitation is the lack of an association between subjective emotional impression and categorical perception performance. A loss of almost 12% of the participants during the categorical perception task might have been sufficiently large to hinder the detection of such an association. The lack of an association might also be linked to nature of the task itself. Whereas the visual search task is related to response speed and the VSTM task is related to updating of information, the categorical perception task taps into categorical judgments or comparisons of two stimuli. Thus, this kind of more elaborative comparison ability might rely on a different behavior component than memory and attention processes, one that is hypothetically less affected by subjective emotional impression.

A third limitation is that because of the exploratory nature of this first study on emotional impression and behavior, we did not correct for multiple comparisons in the current

ANOVA or regression analyses. The current results must therefore be considered preliminary until they are replicated in future studies.

However, despite these potential shortcomings, our results uniquely and clearly demonstrate the importance of taking the emotional impression of the stimuli (including all three of the major emotional dimensions) into account in the study of emotional processing in general, and in aging research in particular.

### ADULT AGING RESEARCH AND PROCESSING OF EMOTIONAL STIMULI

The results of the current study point to the importance of stimulus selection in studies of emotional behavior in younger and older adults. As shown in the current study, emotional faces elicit different emotional impressions in younger and older adults, and this in turn affects attention and memory processing. The present results are in line both with the memory literature, which shows that people remember material and events of emotional character better than those that are neutral (e.g., see Buchanan, 2007 for a review) and recent attention literature, which has found that arousal affects attention processing (e.g., Lundqvist et al., 2013b). Thus, a decrease in emotional impression might dampen the effect of emotion on memory performance and attention processing. By assuming that younger and older adults perceive emotional material equally in terms of the key dimensions of emotional impression, we risk misattributing age effects in emotional behavior. As our results indicate, a decrease in subjective emotional impression of angry faces was associated with poorer performance on memory and attention processing tasks. An interesting topic for future research would be to more systematically manipulate emotional impression and study subsequent emotional behavior in younger and older adults.

## CONCLUSIONS

The results of all of the four tasks used in this study showed an age-related flattening of emotional impression of facial expressions that was more pronounced for angry than for happy faces. The lower level of emotional impression of angry faces in older adults was also mirrored in the two measures of emotional behavior (visual attention and VSTM) for the facial expressions. Regression analyses confirmed the association between emotional impression and behavior by showing that higher potency ratings predicted lower RTs in the visual search task and fewer errors in the VSTM task. These relationships were age-independent but statistically significant only for angry faces. The present findings of age differences in subjective emotional impression should be considered as a possible explanation of age differences in emotional effects on attention and memory in future studies.

## ACKNOWLEDGMENTS

This research was conducted at the Aging Research Center, Karolinska Institutet and Stockholm University, Stockholm, Sweden, and was supported by the Bank of Sweden Tercentenary Foundation awarded to Håkan Fischer. The authors wish to thank Elsa Larsson, Karin Calissendorf, and Therese Lindström for the data collection.

## REFERENCES

Beale, J. M., and Keil, F. C. (1995). Categorical effects in the perception of faces. *Cognition* 57, 217–239. doi: 10.1016/0010-0277(95)00669-X

Borg, C., Leroy, N., Favre, E., Laurent, B., and Thomas-Antérion, C. (2011). How emotional pictures influence visuospatial binding in short-term memory in ageing and Alzheimer's disease? *Brain Cogn.* 76, 20–25. doi:10.1016/j.bandc.2011.03.008

Bornstein, M. H., and Korda, N. O. (1984). Discrimination and matching within and between hues measured by reaction times: some implications for categorical perception and levels of information processing. *Psychol. Res.* 46, 207–222. doi: 10.1007/BF00308884

Buchanan, T. W. (2007). Retrieval of emotional memories. *Psychol. Bull.* 133, 761–779. doi: 10.1037/0033-2909.133.5.761

Calder, A. J., Keane, J., Manly, T., Sprengelmeyer, R., Scott, S., Nimmo-Smith, I., et al. (2003). Facial expression recognition across the adult life span. *Neuropsychologia* 41, 195–202. doi: 10.1016/S0028-3932(02)00149-5

Calder, A. J., Young, A. W., Perrett, D. I., Etcoff, N. L., and Rowland, D. (1996). Categorical perception of morphed facial expressions. *Vis. Cogn.* 3, 81–117. doi: 10.1080/713756735

Campanella, S., Quinet, P., Bruyer, R., Crommelinck, M., and Guerit, J.-M. (2002). Categorical perception of happiness and fear facial expressions: an ERP study. *J. Cogn. Neurosci.* 14, 210–227. doi:10.1162/089892902317236858

Carstensen, L. L. (2006). The influence of a sence of time on human development. *Science* 312, 1913–1915. doi: 10.1126/science.1127488

Carstensen, L. L., Isaacowitz, D. M., and Charles, S. T. (1999). Taking time seriously: a theory of socioemotional selectivity. *Am. Psychol.* 54, 165–181. doi: 10.1037/0003-066X.54.3.165

D'Argembeau, A., and van der Linden, M. (2004). Identity but not expression memory for unfamiliar faces is affected by ageing. *Memory* 12, 644–654. doi: 10.1080/09658210344000198

Ebner, N. C., and Johnson, M. K. (2009). Young and older emotional faces: are there age group differences in expression identification and memory? *Emotion* 9, 329–339. doi: 10.1037/a0015179

Ebner, N. C., Johnson, M. K., and Fischer, H. (2012). Neural mechanisms of reading facial emotions in young and older adults. *Front. Psychol.* 3:223. doi: 10.3389/fpsyg.2012.00223

Ebner, N. C., Johnson, M. R., Rieckmann, A., Durbin, K. A., Johnson, M. K., and Fischer, H. (2013). Processing own-age vs. other-age faces: neuro-behavioral correlates and effects of emotion. *Neuroimage* 78, 363–371. doi:10.1016/j.neuroimage.2013.04.029

Etcoff, N. L., and Magee, J. J. (1992). Categorical perception of facial expressions. *Cognition* 44, 227–240. doi: 10.1016/0010-0277(92)90002-Y

Folstein, M. F., Folstein, S. E., and McHugh, P. R. (1975). "Mini-mental state." A practical method for grading the cognitive state of patients for clinician. *J. Psychiatry Res.* 12, 189–198. doi: 10.1016/0022-3956(75)90026-6

Fischer, H., Nyberg, L., and Bäckman, L. (2010). Age-related differences in brain regions supporting successful encoding of emotional faces. *Cortex* 46, 490–497. doi: 10.1016/j.cortex.2009.05.011

Fontaine, J. R. J., Scherer, K. R., Roesch, E. B., and Ellsworth, P. C. (2007). The world of emotions is not two-dimensional. *Psychol. Sci.* 18, 1050–1057. doi: 10.1111/j.1467-9280.2007.02024.x

Grady, C. L., Hongwanishkul, D., Keightley, M., Lee, W., and Hasher, L. (2007). The effect of age on memory for emotional faces. *Neuropsychology* 21, 371–380. doi: 10.1037/0894-4105.21.3.371

Hahn, S., Carlson, C., Singer, S., and Gronlund, S. D. (2006). Aging and visual search: automatic and controlled attentional bias to threat faces. *Acta Psychol.* 123, 312–336. doi: 10.1016/j.actpsy.2006.01.008

Harmon-Jones, E., Gable, P., and Price, T. F. (2012). The influence of affective states varying in motivational intensity on cognitive scope. *Front. Integr. Neurosci.* 6:73. doi: 10.3389/fnint.2012.00073

Horning, S. M., Cornwell, R. E., and Davis, H. P. (2012). The recognition of facial expressions: an investigation of the influence of age and cognition. *Neuropsychol. Dev. Cogn. B Aging Neuropsychol. Cogn.* 19, 657–676. doi: 10.1080/13825585.2011.645011

Isaacowitz, D. M., Wadlinger, H. A., Goren, D., and Wilson, H. R. (2006). Is there an age-related positivity effect in visual attention? A comparison of two methodologies. *Emotion* 6, 511–516. doi: 10.1037/1528-3542.6.3.511

Jackson, M. C., Wu, C.-Y., Linden, D. E. J., and Raymond, J. E. (2009). Enhanced visual short-term memory for angry faces. *J. Exp. Psychol. Hum. Percept. Perform.* 35, 363–374. doi: 10.1037/a0013895

Keightley, M. L., Winocur, G., Burianova, H., Hongwanishkul, D., and Grady, C. L. (2006). Age effects on social cognition: faces tell a different story. *Psychol. Aging* 21, 558–572. doi: 10.1037/0882-7974.21.3.558

Kiffel, C., Campanella, S., and Bruyer, R. (2005). Categorical perception of faces and facial expressions: the age factor. *Exp. Aging Res.* 31, 119–147. doi: 10.1080/03610730590914985

Lang, P., and Bradley, M. (2010). Emotion and the motivational brain. *Biol. Psychol.* 84, 437–450. doi: 10.1016/j.biopsycho.2009.10.007

Langeslag, S. J. E., Morgan, H. M., Jackson, M. C., Linden, D. E. J., and Van Strien, J. W. (2009). Electrophysiological correlates of improved short-term memory for emotional faces. *Neuropsychologia* 47, 887–896. doi: 10.1016/j.neuropsychologia.2008.12.024

Langeslag, S. J. E., and van Strien, J. W. (2009). Aging and emotional memory: the co-occurrence of neurophysiological and behavioral positivity effects. *Emotion* 9, 369–377. doi: 10.1037/a0015356

Leclerc, C. M., and Kensinger, E. A. (2008). Effects of age on detection of emotional information. *Psychol. Aging* 23, 209–215. doi: 10.1037/0882-7974.23.1.209

Leclerc, C. M., and Kensinger, E. A. (2010). Age-related valence-based reversal in recruitment of medial prefrontal cortex on a visual search task. *Soc. Neurosci.* 5, 560–576. doi: 10.1080/17470910903512296

Liberman, A. M., Harris, K. S., Hoffman, H. S., and Griffith, B. C. (1957). The discrimination of speech sounds within and across phoneme boundaries. *J. Exp. Psychol.* 54, 358–368. doi: 10.1037/h0044417

Lindquist, K. A., Wager, T. D., Kober, H., Bliss-Moreau, E., and Barrett, L. F. (2012). The brain basis of emotion: a meta-analytic review. *Behav. Brain Sci.* 35, 121–202. doi: 10.1017/S0140525X11000446

Lindström, B. R., and Bohlin, G. (2011). Emotion processing facilitates working memory performance. *Cogn. Emot.* 25, 1196–1204. doi: 10.1080/02699931.2010.527703

Lundqvist, D., Esteves, F., and Öhman, A. (1999). The face of wrath: critical features for conveying facial threat. *Cogn. Emot.* 13, 691–711. doi: 10.1080/026999399379041

Lundqvist, D., Juth, P., and Öhman, A. (2013b). Using facial emotional stimuli in visual search experiments: the arousal factor explains contradictory results. *Cogn. Emot.* doi: 10.1080/02699931.2013.867479. [Epub ahead of print].

Lundqvist, D., and Litton, J. E. (1998). *The Averaged Karolinska Directed Emotional Faces – AKDEF.* Stockholm: CD ROM from Department of Clinical Neuroscience, Psychology section, Karolinska Institutet. ISBN: 91-630-7164-9.

Lundqvist, D., Svärd, J., and Fischer, H. (2013a). Age-related differences in sensitivity to emotional facial stimuli but age-independent association between arousal ratings and visual search efficiency. *Psychol. Topics* 22, 271–286.

Mather, M., and Carstensen, L. L. (2003). Aging and attentional biases for emotional faces. *Psychol. Sci.* 14, 409–415. doi: 10.1111/1467-9280.01455

Mather, M., and Knight, M. R. (2006). Angry faces get noticed quickly: threat detection is not impaired among older adults. *J. Gerontol. B Psychol. Sci. Soc. Sci.* 61, 54–57. doi: 10.1093/geronb/61.1.P54

Mather, M., and Sutherland, M. R. (2011). Arousal-biased competition in perception and memory. *Perspect. Psychol. Sci.* 6, 114–133. doi: 10.1177/1745691611400234

McDowell, C. L., Harrison, D. W., and Demaree, H. A. (1994). Is right hemisphere decline in the perception of emotion a function of aging? *Intern. J. Neurosci.* 79, 1–11.

Mikels, J. A., Larkin, G. R., Reuter-Lorenz, P. A., and Cartensen, L. L. (2005). Divergent trajectories in the aging mind: changes in working memory for affective versus visual information with age. *Psychol. Aging* 20, 542–553. doi: 10.1037/0882-7974.20.4.542

Osgood, C. E. (1966). Dimensionality of the semantic space for communication via facial expressions. *Scand. J. Psychol.* 7, 1–30. doi: 10.1111/j.1467-9450.1966.tb01334.x

Osgood, C. E., and Suci, G. J. (1955). Factor analysis of meaning. *J. Exp. Psychol.* 50, 325–338. doi: 10.1037/h0043965

Phelps, E. A., and LeDoux, J. E. (2005). Contributions of the amygdala to emotion processing: from animal models to human behavior. *Neuron* 48, 175–187. doi: 10.1016/j.neuron.2005.09.025

Ruffman, T., Henry, J. D., Livingstone, V., and Phillips, L. H. (2008). A meta-analytic review of emotion recognition and aging: implications for neuropsychological models of aging. *Neurosci. Biobehav. Rev.* 32, 863–881. doi: 10.1016/j.neubiorev.2008.01.001

Ruffman, T., Ng, M., and Jenkin, T. (2009). Older adults respond quickly to angry faces despite labeling difficulty. *J. Gerontol. B Psychol. Sci. Soc. Sci.* 64, 171–179. doi: 10.1093/geronb/gbn035

Russell, J. A. (2003). Core affect and the psychological construction of emotion. *Psychol. Rev.* 110, 145–172. doi: 10.1037/0033-295X.110.1.145

Russell, J. A., and Mehrabian, A. (1977). Evidence for a three-factor theory of emotions. *J. Res. Pers.* 11, 273–294. doi: 10.1016/0092-6566(77)90037-X *Front.*

Spielberger, C. D., Gorsuch, R. L., and Lushene, R. E. (1988). *STAI-Manual for the State Trait Anxiety Inventory, 3rd Edn.* Palo Alto, CA: Consulting Psychological Press.

Suzuki, A., and Akiyama, H. (2013). Cognitive aging explains age-related differences in face-based recognition of basic emotions except for anger and disgust. *Neuropsychol. Dev. Cogn. B Aging Neuropsychol. Cogn.* 20, 253–270. doi: 10.1080/13825585.2012.692761 *Acta*

Svärd, J., Wiens, S., and Fischer, H. (2012). Superior recognition performance for happy masked and unmasked faces in both younger and older adults. *Psychol.* 3:520. doi: 10.3389/fpsyg.2012.00520

Young, A. W., Rowland, D., Calder, A. J., Etcoff, N. L., Seth, A., and Perrett, D. I. (1997). Facial expression megamix: tests of dimensional and category accounts of emotion recognition. *Cognition* 63, 271–313. doi: 10.1016/S0010-0277(97)00003-6

Zigmond, A., and Snaith, R. (1983). The hospital anxiety depression scale. *Psychiatr. Scand.* 67, 361–370. doi: 10.1111/j.1600-0447.1983.tb09716.x

# 12

# Spatial navigational strategies correlate with gray matter in the hippocampus of healthy older adults tested in a virtual maze

***Kyoko Konishi and Véronique D. Bohbot****

*Department of Psychiatry, Douglas Institute, McGill University, Verdun, QC, Canada*

**Edited by:**
Thomas Wolbers, German Center for Neurodegenerative Diseases, Germany

**Reviewed by:**
Diego Ruano, University of Sevilla, Spain
Barbara Shukitt-Hale, United States Department of Agriculture, USA

***Correspondence:**
Véronique D. Bohbot, Department of Psychiatry, Faculty of Medicine, McGill University, Douglas Mental Health University Institute, FBC Building, 6875 boul. LaSalle, Verdun, QC H4H 1R3, Canada.
e-mail: veronique.bohbot@mcgill.ca

Healthy young adults use different strategies when navigating in a virtual maze. Spatial strategies involve using environmental landmarks while response strategies involve executing a series of movements from specific stimuli. Neuroimaging studies previously confirmed that people who use spatial strategies show increased activity and gray matter in the hippocampus, while those who use response strategies show increased activity and gray matter in caudate nucleus (Iaria et al., 2003; Bohbot et al., 2007). A growing number of studies report that cognitive decline that occurs with normal aging is correlated with a decrease in volume of the hippocampus. Here, we used voxel-based morphometry (VBM) to examine whether spatial strategies in aging are correlated with greater gray matter in the hippocampus, as found in our previous study with healthy young participants. Forty-five healthy older adults were tested on a virtual navigation task that allows spatial and response strategies. All participants learn the task to criterion after which a special "probe" trial that assesses spatial and response strategies is given. Results show that spontaneous spatial memory strategies, and not performance on the navigation task, positively correlate with gray matter in the hippocampus. Since numerous studies have shown that a decrease in the volume of the hippocampus correlates with cognitive deficits during normal aging and increases the risks of ensuing dementia, the current results suggest that older people who use their spatial memory strategies in their everyday lives may have increased gray matter in the hippocampus and enhance their probability of healthy and successful aging.

**Keywords: aging, radial maze, spatial memory, hippocampus, navigation**

## INTRODUCTION

Multiple studies have demonstrated that age impairs spatial memory in both humans and non-human species (Barnes et al., 1980; Marighetto et al., 1999; Driscoll et al., 2003; Wood and Dudchenko, 2003; Moffat et al., 2006; Antonova et al., 2009; Iaria et al., 2009). Older adults report to having more navigation problems with increasing age and admit to avoiding traveling unfamiliar routes (Burns, 1999). Furthermore, "getting lost" behavior and impairment in spatial memory are early symptoms of cognitive impairment and Alzheimer's disease (Klein et al., 1999; delpolyi et al., 2007; Hort et al., 2007).

When navigating in a virtual environment, studies showed that participants spontaneously use one of two navigational strategies (Packard and McGaugh, 1996; Iaria et al., 2003). Spatial memory, or the "spatial strategy," is one of two navigation strategies that can be used when going places (Packard et al., 1989; Packard and McGaugh, 1996; Iaria et al., 2003; Bohbot et al., 2007). It involves navigating within an environment by forming relationships between different landmarks in the environment and orientating oneself in relation to those landmarks. This process of forming associations between landmarks leads to the development of cognitive maps, i.e., mental representations of one's environment. Knowledge of the relationships between landmarks is characterized with flexibility, allowing, for example, one to derive a direct path to a target destination when navigating in a town (O'Keefe and Nadel, 1978). The spatial strategy is subserved by the hippocampus (O'Keefe and Nadel, 1978; Morris et al., 1982; Abrahams et al., 1997; Bohbot et al., 1998). In contrast, the "response strategy" involves learning a series of stimulus-response associations such as a pattern of left and right turns from a given starting position. This strategy is inflexible in the sense that it does not allow deriving a direct path to a target location (O'Keefe and Nadel, 1978). The response strategy relies on the striatum, which includes the caudate nucleus in humans (Packard et al., 1989; Packard and Knowlton, 2002; White and McDonald, 2002).

In a previous study (Bohbot et al., 2007), we tested healthy young adult participants on a virtual navigation task that can be solved using either a spatial or response strategy. We found that spatial learning positively correlated with gray matter in the hippocampus, while response learning positively correlated with caudate nucleus gray matter. Furthermore, an inverse relationship was found between gray matter in the hippocampus and caudate nucleus. In other words, those who had more gray matter in the hippocampus had less gray matter in the caudate nucleus and vice versa. In addition, participants' peak hippocampal values correlated with gray matter in a network of regions anatomically connected to the hippocampus, such as the perirhinal, entorhinal and parahippocampal cortices, the orbitofrontal cortex, and the amygdala. There was also a significant correlation with gray matter in the contralateral hippocampus.

Several studies have examined the neural correlates of spatial memory in older adults. Using manual segmentation, Chen et al. (2010) and Head and Isom (2010) found that performance on a virtual spatial memory task correlated with total volume of the hippocampus. Head and Isom (2010) additionally found a positive correlation between caudate nucleus volume and performance on a virtual route learning task, a task known to utilize response strategies.

In the present study, we investigated whether performance on our navigation task that distinguishes between spontaneous spatial and response strategies correlated with gray matter in the hippocampus and caudate nucleus in healthy older adults, using the technique of voxel-based morphometry (VBM). We hypothesized that older adults who use spatial strategies would have more gray matter in the hippocampus while those who use response strategies would have more gray matter in the caudate nucleus. Furthermore, similar to results reported in Bohbot et al. (2007), we hypothesized that those with more gray matter in the hippocampus would have more gray matter in the associated network of neuroanatomically connected regions. Since gray matter in the hippocampus is associated with healthy cognition in aging, the variability in navigational strategies could potentially help distinguish a healthy older adult from an older adult at risk for cognitive deficits. Identifying such risk factors can have a profound impact on the well-being of older adults. This is especially relevant considering the current international demographics showing a growing aging population. By the year 2050, 16% of the world population will be over the age of 65. In the US, 20% of the population is expected to be over the age 65 by 2050 and in Japan, 38% of the population is expected to be over 65 by 2050. Consequently, the current paper may bring novel insights into healthy and unhealthy aging that can help define early detection methods in view of early intervention to promote healthy aging.

## MATERIALS AND METHODS

### PARTICIPANTS

Forty-five healthy older adults (mean age = 64.38 ± 4.0; 23 women and 22 men) participated in the study. All participants were right-handed and had normal or corrected vision. All participants were screened for any history of neurological or psychiatric disorders, alcohol, or drug abuse using a pre-screening questionnaire. All participants underwent a neuropsychological assessment to control for dementia, depression, and mild cognitive impairment (**Table 1**). Informed consent was obtained from all participants in accordance with the guidelines of the local ethics committee. The study was approved by the Research Ethics Board at the Douglas Mental Health University Institute and the Montreal Neurological Institute.

### BEHAVIORAL TASKS

#### *Concurrent spatial discrimination learning task*

The Concurrent Spatial Discrimination Learning Task (CSDLT) was created using the editor program of Unreal Tournament 2003 (Epic Games, Raleigh, NC). The task is situated in a radial maze surrounded by an enriched environment made up of a landscape and proximal and distal landmarks such as plants and hills (**Figure 1**). It consists of a center platform from which branch out 12 pathways. At the end of each pathway, there is a set of stairs that leads to a small pit where, in some of the arms, an object is located. The 12 arms of the maze are divided up into six adjacent pairs of arms. Within each pair of arms, one arm always contains an object while the other is always empty. During the experimental encoding phase (Stage 1), participants are repeatedly presented with the six pairs of arms in a pseudo-random order. They are asked to learn which arm contains an object within each pair of arms and to go down that arm to retrieve the object. Upon descending the stairs at the end of the pathway and entering the pit, participants are automatically brought back to the center platform and presented with the next pair of arms. The number of correct arms the participant visits within each trial is measured as choice accuracy. One trial consists of the presentation of all six pairs of arms. Participants are trained until a choice accuracy criterion of 11/12 is reached within two consecutive trials. A minimum of six trials is administered to all participants.

Upon reaching criterion, participants proceed to a test phase aimed as dissociating the strategies used during the encoding phase of the task. The test or probe phase (Stage 2), is also called the "recombined pairs" condition because, during this phase, the arms presented to the participants are rearranged into novel pairs; however, the reward contingency remains the same. In other words, during the recombined pairs condition, the objects are placed at the end of the same arms as during the encoding phase. Four pairs of recombined arms are presented twice in a pseudo-random order. Only four recombined pairs allowed for the presentation of adjacent arms with only one arm containing an object. The recombined pairs condition was designed in such a way that successful performance on this stage requires that individuals be flexible at using the information they learned during the encoding phase of the task, evidenced by the fact that they know the spatial relationship between the object and environmental landmarks (i.e., the spatial strategy). In other words, when the pairs of arms that are presented are recombined, participants who know the relationship between the target objects and landmarks are capable of discerning the target arm from the non-target arm. In contrast, people who did not show flexibility

**Table 1 | Older adult participant demographics and test means [SEM].**

| PARTICIPANT CHARACTERISTICS | |
|---|---|
| *N* | 45 |
| Women:Men | 23:22 |
| Age (years) | 64.38 ± 4.05 |
| IQ | 107.5 ± 13.12 |
| Education (years) | 15.48 ± 2.45 |
| Handedness | Right |
| **NEUROPSYCHOLOGICAL TEST SCORES** | |
| MMSE | 29.21 ± 0.91 |
| MoCA | 27.48 ± 1.65 |

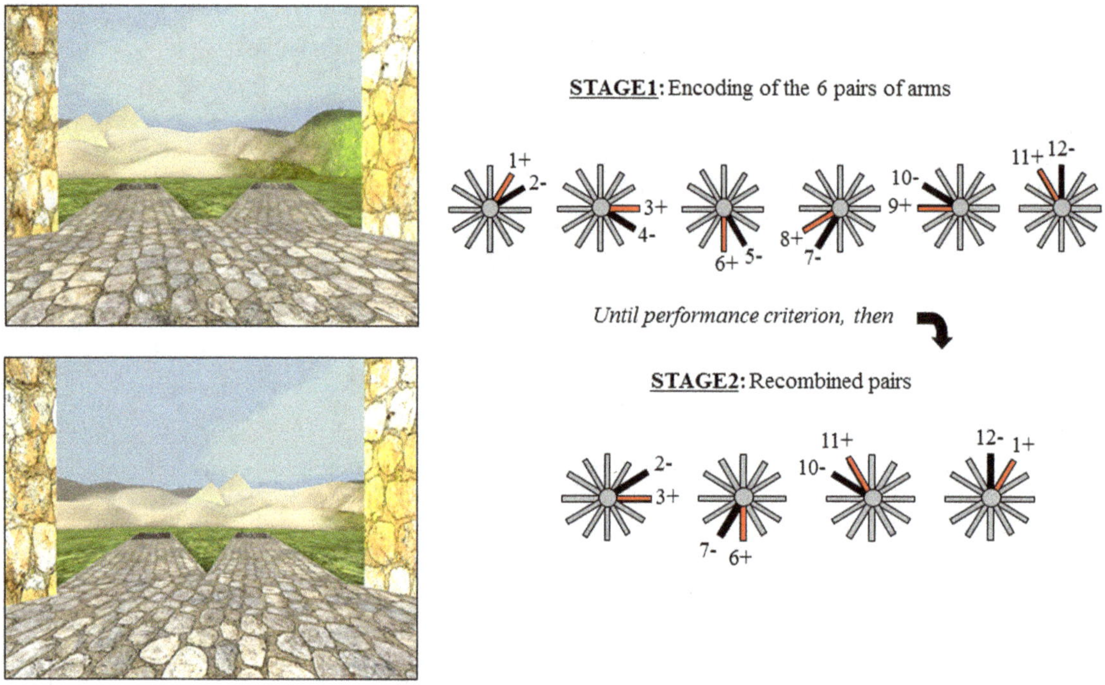


**FIGURE 1 | The two stages of the virtual radial maze with a schematic representation of the behavioral paradigm.** Example of a pair of arms presented during encoding (Stage 1) and a recombined pair during Stage 2.

during the recombined pairs have acquired the task by using a response strategy, i.e., "when I see the hills, take the arm to the left." In this case, since the pairs of presented arms were rearranged, "when I see the hills, take the arm to the left" in this recombined pairs stage is not the same arm as in the encoding stage. Thus, the recombined pairs stage allows us to distinguish between participants who are flexible and used a spatial strategy and those who are inflexible and used a response strategy in an objective fashion.

#### *Rey auditory verbal learning test*

The Rey Auditory Verbal Learning Test (RAVLT) is a standard neuropsychological memory test (Lezak, 1995). A list of 15 words (list A) is read for five trials and after each trial the participant is asked to verbally recall as many words as they can remember. Next, an interference trial is provided whereby a different list of 15 words (list B) is read to the participant and again the participant is asked to recall as many words as they can remember. Following this interference trial, the participant is asked to recall as many words as they can from list A. Finally, after a 30-min delay, the participant is again asked to remember as many words as they can from list A. Performance was assessed with the number of words recalled after interference (AI) and after the 30-min delay (delayed recall).

#### *Rey-osterrieth complex figure*

In the Rey-Osterrieth Complex Figure task (RO) (Osterrieth, 1944), participants are asked to copy a complex figure in as much detail as possible. After a 30-min delay, participants are asked to redraw the complex figure from memory in as much detail as they can.

### MAGNETIC RESONANCE IMAGING (MRI) SCANNING PROTOCOL

Structural MRI scans were obtained at the Montreal Neurological Institute with a 1.5T Siemens Sonata MRI scanner. Participants were comfortably placed in the scanner with their heads immobilized using an air cushion. An anatomical scan of ~15 min was taken for each participant. A 3D gradient echo acquisition is used to collect 160 contiguous 1 mm T1–weighted images in the sagittal plane (TR = 22, TE = 10, flip angle = 30°, 140 1 mm sagittal slices). The rectangular field of view (FOV) for the sagittal images is 256 mm (SI) by 224 mm (AP).

### MRI DATA ANALYSIS

VBM was used to investigate morphological differences between the different groups. MRI scans were spatially normalized by linear transformation into a standard stereotaxic Talairach space (Talairach and Tournoux, 1988). They were corrected for intensity non-uniformity (shading artifact) using the N3 software package (Sled et al., 1998). Each voxel was automatically labeled as white matter, gray matter, cerebrospinal fluid, or background using Intensity Normalized Stereotaxic Environment for the Classification of Tissues (INSECT) (Zijdenbos et al., 2002). The skull and dura were then masked from the brain. The gray matter was smoothed using a 8 mm full-width at half-maximum (FWHM) Gaussian kernel. Generalized linear model was used to correlate performance on the CSDLT with gray matter in our regions of interest, namely the hippocampus and caudate nucleus

(Worsley et al., 2002). After this initial analysis, results were used to regress gray matter values from our peak voxel in the hippocampus against the whole brain. This analysis allowed us to examine areas in the brain that co-vary with gray matter in the hippocampus.

Outputs of the statistical analyses were displayed as a statistical map overlaid on an MRI scan. For results within the hippocampus, statistical maps were overlaid on an MRI scan of a spatial learner, categorized by performance on the recombined pairs condition. The statistical maps show regions of gray matter that correlate with our variable of interest. Based on our a priori hypothesis, an uncorrected $p$-value of 0.001 ($N = 45$, $t = 3.29$) was used for voxels in the predicted regions of interest, namely, the hippocampus and caudate nucleus. For the whole brain, a Bonferroni correction for multiple comparisons was used to calculate the $t$-statistical threshold ($t = 5.47$ at $p < 0.05$).

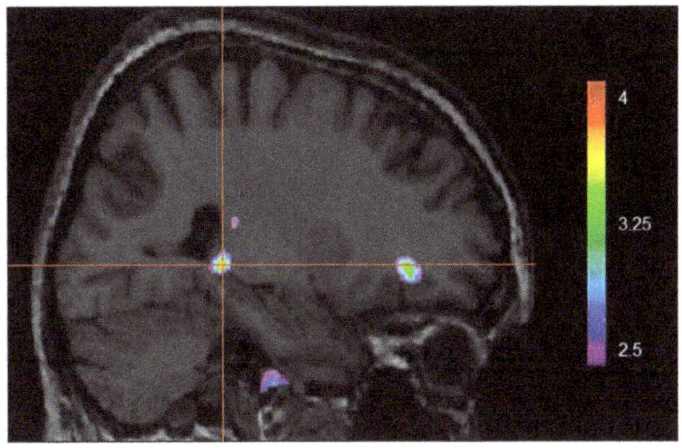


**FIGURE 2 | Whole brain regression analysis with scores on recombined pairs condition of CSDLT (Stage 2).** Results are superimposed onto an anatomical MRI and displayed in the sagittal plane. Results show that gray matter in the hippocampus significantly co-vary with spatial navigational strategies (MNI space coordinates $x = 26.0$, $y = -37.8$, $z = -3.2$; $t = 3.53$, $p < 0.0005$).

## RESULTS

### BEHAVIORAL

All participants were able to learn the reward contingency of the arms during the encoding phase of the CSLDT. On average participants required $10.02 \pm 4.15$ trials to reach criteria. Average performance on Stage 2 was $5.55 \pm 1.96$ out of 8. On the RAVLT, participants were able to recall an average of $10.83 \pm 2.76$ of the 15 words AI and $10.37 \pm 3.38$ after the 30-min delay. After the 30-min delay of the RO, participants had an average score of $18.14 \pm 6.83$ out of 32. Performance on Stage 2 of the CSDLT did not correlate with performance on the RAVLT (AI: $r = 0.012$, $p > 0.05$; Delayed recall: $r = 0.093$, $p > 0.05$) or RO ($r = -0.155$, $p > 0.05$). There was also no correlation between performance on Stage 2 of the CSDLT and age ($r = -0.061$, $p > 0.05$), years of education ($r = 0.019$, $p > 0.05$), or sex ($t = 1.19$, $p > 0.05$).

### VBM

Using VBM, performance on the CSDLT was regressed against gray matter in the brain. Performance during the recombined pairs condition (Stage 2) of the CSDLT positively correlated with gray matter in the right hippocampus (MNI space coordinates $x = 26.0$, $y = -37.8$, $z = -3.2$; $t = 3.53$, $p < 0.0005$), suggesting that healthy older adults who have higher scores on the recombined pairs condition and thus use spatial strategies, have more gray matter in the hippocampus (**Figure 2**). The correlation between the peak gray matter value in the hippocampus and performance on the recombined pairs condition of the CSDLT was $r = 0.478$, $p < 0.001$ (**Figure 3**). No areas of the brain, including the caudate nucleus, were found to negatively correlate with the performance on the recombined pairs condition of the CSDLT. In other words, we did not find a correlation between low score on the recombined pairs condition, indicative of a response strategy and gray matter in the caudate nucleus ($p > 0.001$, uncorrected). The number of trials to reach criteria did not correlate with gray matter in the hippocampus or caudate nucleus.

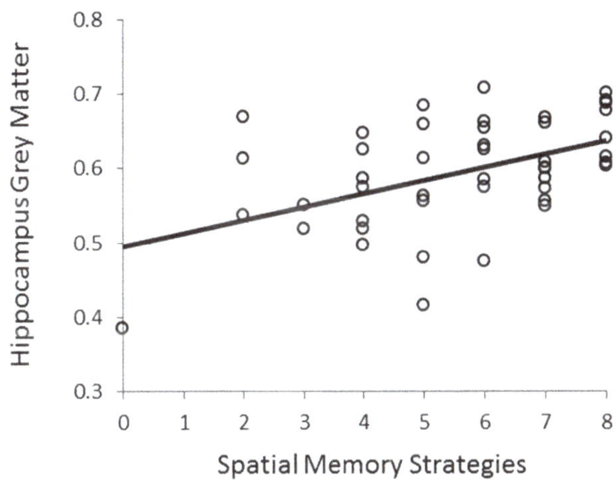


**FIGURE 3 | Correlation between scores on the recombined pairs condition (Stage 2) of the CSDLT and gray matter values extracted from the peak voxel (MNI space coordinates $x = 26.0$, $y = -37.8$, $z = -3.2$) in the right posterior hippocampus ($r = 0.478$, $p < 0.001$).** This graph shows that a better spatial memory score is associated with increased gray matter in the hippocampus.

Gray matter values extracted from our peak voxel in the hippocampus (from the first analysis) were used to regress against the entire MRI volume in all participants. Results showed a network of regions known to be anatomically linked to the hippocampus co-varying with the peak voxel in the right hippocampus (**Figure 4**). Consistent with our earlier findings (Bohbot et al., 2007), with increasing gray matter in the hippocampus, there was increased gray matter in the contralateral hippocampus, the right orbitofrontal cortex, bilateral amygdala, and bilateral parahippocampal cortex.

### NEUROANATOMICAL CORRELATES OF NEUROPSYCHOLOGICAL MEASURES

Performance AI and delayed recall on the RAVLT did not correlate with hippocampus gray matter. Similarly, delayed recall on the RO did not correlate with gray matter in the hippocampus

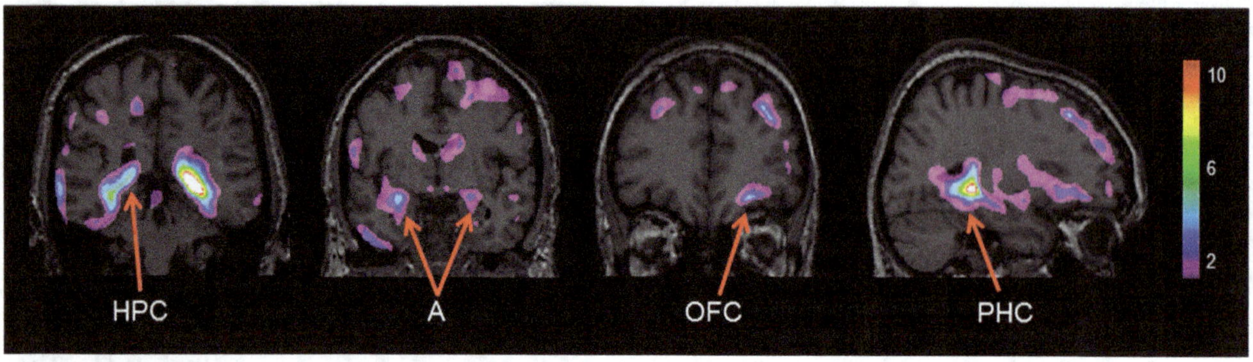


**FIGURE 4 | Regions of the brain that co-varied with our peak hippocampal gray matter value ($x = 26.0$, $y = -37.8$, $z = -3.2$).** A, Amygdala; HPC, hippocampus; PHC, parahippocampal cortex; OFC, orbitofrontal cortex. The color bar illustrates the range of $t$ statistical values.

suggesting that spatial memory is more sensitive to gray matter differences in the hippocampus than other types of memory measured with standard Neuropsychological tests.

## DISCUSSION

In the present study, we examined the relationship between performance on a virtual navigation task and gray matter in the hippocampus in healthy older adults. With VBM, we showed that the spontaneous use of spatial memory strategies positively correlates with gray matter in the hippocampus. In contrast, the use of response strategies negatively correlates with gray matter in the hippocampus. When the peak value in the hippocampus, the area in the hippocampus which most highly correlated with spatial memory, was used as a seed voxel to correlate with gray matter in the whole brain, positive correlations were observed in regions that are anatomically and functionally linked to the hippocampus, such as the contralateral hippocampus, the right orbitofrontal cortex, bilateral amygdala, and bilateral parahippocampal cortex.

While some studies in the literature reported a significant relationship between hippocampal volume and spatial memory (Chen et al., 2010; Head and Isom, 2010), others have failed to demonstrate this effect (Driscoll et al., 2003; Moffat et al., 2007). One factor that may help shed light on this issue concerns the fact that none of these studies involved tasks that assessed spontaneous navigational strategies (when both spatial and response strategies can be used in the same task). Indeed, ours is the first structural MRI study to utilize a task in older adults that distinguishes between navigational strategies. This is a notable distinction because both human and non-human animal studies showed that with aging, there is a decreased use of spatial strategies and increased use of response strategies (Barnes et al., 1980; Rapp et al., 1997; Rodgers et al., 2010; Etchamendy et al., 2011). Therefore, older adults tested on the virtual Water Maze (e.g., Moffat et al., 2007) may have performed well on that task despite the fact that they would have used a response strategy dependent on the caudate nucleus when tested on another task allowing for both strategies (Etchamendy and Bohbot, 2007). If this is the case, an association between task performance and hippocampal volume would not necessarily be found. On the other hand, as mentioned above, some spatial memory tasks that did not measure spontaneous navigational strategies were sensitive to gray matter in the hippocampus (Chen et al., 2010; Head and Isom, 2010). Further research would be needed in order to shed light on this issue. For instance, some of these spatial tasks may have been sufficiently complex to detect a learning deficit in participants favoring response strategies, thereby inadvertently dissociating between spatial and response strategies. In support of this hypothesis, we previously reported a correlation between spatial strategies and wayfinding performance in healthy older adults (Etchamendy et al., 2012). This would be consistent with our results that demonstrate that in fact only older adults using spatial strategies, and not those using response strategies, have more gray matter in the hippocampus.

The study by Head and Isom (2010) reported a correlation between caudate nucleus volume and route learning. Route learning is a form of response learning that involves learning a sequence of movements in response to specific stimuli. However, we did not observe a negative correlation between performance and caudate nucleus gray matter with the current task, suggesting that it may not be sensitive enough to detect variability in the gray matter of the caudate nucleus of our population. Interestingly, Kennedy et al. (2009) demonstrated a non-linear decline in hippocampus volume as a function of age, where the rate of hippocampus atrophy accelerates with age, while Raz et al. (2003) showed that in the caudate nucleus, there is a linear decline in volume with aging. Therefore, within an older adult population, there may be more variability in the volume of the hippocampus than in the volume of the caudate nucleus, making it easier to detect morphological differences within the hippocampus. Recruiting participants in a wider age range may help increase sensitivity to morphological differences in the caudate nucleus. Indeed, the age range of the participants in the Head and Isom (2010) study was 56–86 years, while in the current study it was 60–75 years. Therefore, a wider age range of participants may be needed to uncover the relationship between gray matter in the caudate nucleus and response strategies in our task.

We observed an association between the aging hippocampus and response strategies. However, the causal relationship cannot be determined in this study, i.e., the use of response strategies may be the consequence of decreased gray matter in the hippocampus or it may be the cause of a decrease gray matter in the hippocampus, i.e., "use it or loose it." In other words, biological factors such as genes (Banner et al., 2011) may have a negative impact on the hippocampus leading to an increase use in response strategies. Alternatively, environmental factors such as repetition (which leads to habit) (Iaria et al., 2003), stress (Schwabe et al., 2008), or reward (Del Balso et al., 2010) could promote response strategies at the expense of spatial strategies associated with the hippocampus. It is most likely a combination of both. Importantly, the fact that we found an association between response strategies and the aging hippocampus opens new possibilities for spatial memory-based cognitive interventions toward healthy aging (Bohbot et al., 2011). We have previously shown that strategy use can alter gray matter in the mouse hippocampus (Lerch et al., 2011). In that study, mice trained to use spatial strategies showed increased gray matter in the hippocampus relative to mice trained on the response strategy. Preliminary findings in older adults replicated these findings, demonstrating increased gray matter in the hippocampus after the administration of spatial memory training (Fouquet et al., 2011).

The relationship between navigational strategy and the hippocampus in young adults was previously investigated in Iaria et al. (2003) and Bohbot et al. (2007). Iaria et al. (2003) found that in a task where both strategies can be used, 50% of young adults spontaneously used a spatial strategy while 50% used a response strategy. Furthermore, individuals who used a spatial strategy showed significant fMRI activity in the hippocampus, while those who used a response strategy showed significant fMRI activity in the caudate nucleus, relative to baseline. Bohbot et al. (2007) found that the spontaneous use of spatial strategies was associated with increased gray matter in the hippocampus. The same technique of VBM was used to analyze the results in both Bohbot et al. (2007) and the current study. However, a different navigation task was used to assess navigational strategy. In Bohbot et al. (2007), the 4-on-8 virtual maze task was used while in the current study the CSDLT was used. Consistent results were obtained in the two studies.

Similar to Bohbot et al. (2007), a number of brain areas anatomically linked to the hippocampus correlated with gray matter values extracted from our peak voxel in the hippocampus in older adults, such as the orbitofrontal cortex, the parahippocampal cortex, and the amygdala. It is possible that the co-activity of this network of regions during navigation leads to increased gray matter. It has been suggested that the orbitofrontal cortex in rodents is involved in spatial memory (Vafaei and Rashidy-Pour, 2004) and learning reward expectancy in a spatial context (Young and Shapiro, 2011). Indeed, orbitofrontal cortex neurons respond when a rodent enters an arm that is expected to contain a reward. The parahippocampal cortex is known to be involved in navigation and its functions involve scene processing and spatial learning (Bohbot et al., 1998; Epstein, 2008). In rodents, the amygdala is associated with the hippocampus in place preference learning when it is associated with reward (Gaskin and White, 2006).

We also investigated the relationship between neuropsychological performance and gray matter in the hippocampus. Previous studies have found a correlation between the RAVLT and volume of the left hippocampus (Hackert et al., 2002; Chen et al., 2010), however we did not find this effect in our study. The inconsistency from the literature may arise from a cohort effect. The current sample population is composed of high functioning older adults with no detectable cognitive impairment. The RAVLT and RO may therefore not be sensitive enough to detect differences in gray matter in a more homogeneous population. These results suggest that spatial memory strategies are more sensitive to structural differences in the hippocampus than standard neuropsychological tests. In fact, a prospective study showed that patients with dementia had deficits in spatial cognition that preceded conversion to dementia by 3 years. In the same cohort, verbal memory, and working memory deficits were detected only 1 year before patients were diagnosed with dementia (Johnson et al., 2009), further demonstrating the sensitivity of spatial memory.

In conclusion, our present findings are consistent with the literature reporting that in healthy older adults there is a positive correlation between spatial memory and gray matter in the hippocampus. Furthermore, our results showed that those who have lower hippocampal gray matter are actually using another form of navigational strategy, the response strategy. With whole brain analysis, we observed that individuals with more gray matter in the hippocampus had more gray matter in anatomically and functionally connected cortical areas, namely the contralateral hippocampus, the right orbitofrontal cortex, bilateral amygdala, and bilateral parahippocampal cortex. Future studies will be needed to examine whether an intervention method focusing on spatial memory training can increase gray matter in the hippocampus and anatomically connected areas. Promoting the use of spatial strategies can be a potential avenue for intervention methods against hippocampal atrophy (Fotuhi et al., 2012). As lower hippocampal volume is a risk factor for cognitive decline as well as a number of disorders including Alzheimer's disease (Convit et al., 1997; Rusinek et al., 2003; Tapiola et al., 2008), promoting the use of spatial memory can potentially have protective effects against cognitive deficits in normal aging as well as risks of degenerative disorders of the hippocampus.

## REFERENCES

Abrahams, S., Pickering, A., Polkey, C. E., and Morris, R. G. (1997). Spatial memory deficits in patients with unilateral damage to the right hippocampal formation. *Neuropsychologia* 35, 11–24.

Antonova, E., Parslow, D., Brammer, M., Dawson, G. R., Jackson, S. H., and Morris, R. G. (2009).

Age-related neural activity during allocentric spatial memory. *Memory* 17, 125–143.

Banner, H., Bhat, V., Etchamendy, N., Joober, R., and Bohbot, V. D. (2011). The BDNF val66met polymorphism is associated with reduced fMRI activity in the hippocampus and increased use of caudate nucleus-dependent strategies in a human virtual navigation. *Eur. J. Neurosci.* 33,968–977.

Barnes, C. A., Nadel, L., and Honig, W. K. (1980). Spatial memory deficit in senescent rats. *Can. J. Psychol.* 34, 29–39.

Bohbot, V. D., Andersen, N., Trowbridge, A., Sham, R., Konishi, K., Dahmani, L., et al. (2011). *A Spatial Memory Intervention Program Aimed at Stimulating the Hippocampus While Controlling for Caudate Nucleus-Dependent Response Strategies led to Significant Improvements on Independent Virtual Navigation Tasks in Healthy Elderly Society for Neuroscience 2011 Abstracts* (Washington, DC, USA).

Bohbot, V. D., Kalina, M., Stepankova, K., Spackova, N., Petrides, M., and Nadel,

L. (1998). Spatial memory deficits in patients with lesions to the right hippocampus and to the right parahippocam- pal cortex. *Neuropsychologia* 36, 1217–1238.

Bohbot, V. D., Lerch, J., Thorndycraft, B., Iaria, G., and Zijdenbos, A. P. (2007). Gray matter differ- ences correlate with spontaneous strategies in a human virtual navigation task. *J. Neurosci.* 27, 10078–10083.

Burns, P. C. (1999). Navigation and the mobility of older drivers. *J. Gerontol. B Psychol. Sci. Soc. Sci.* 54, S49–S55.

Chen, K. H., Chuah, L. Y., Sim, S. K., and Chee, M. W. (2010). Hippocampal region-specific con- tributions to memory performance in normal elderly. *Brain Cogn.* 72, 400–407.

Convit, A., De Leon, M. J., Tarshish, C., De Santi, S., Tsui, W., Rusinek, H., et al. (1997). Specific hip- pocampal volume reductions in individuals at risk for Alzheimer's disease. *Neurobiol. Aging* 18, 131–138.

delpolyi, A. R., Rankin, K. P., Mucke, L., Miller, B. L., and Gorno-Tempini, M. L. (2007). Spatial cognition and the human navigation network in AD and MCI. *Neurology* 69, 986–997.

Del Balso, D., Casey, K., Conrad, K., Leyton, M., and Bohbot, V. D. (2010). *SubstanceAbuseisAssociated withResponseStrategiesinaHuman Virtual Navigation Task Society for Neuroscience 2010 Abstracts* (San Diego, CA, USA).

Driscoll, I., Hamilton, D. A., Petropoulos, H., Yeo, R. A., Brooks, W. M., Baumgartner, R. N., et al. (2003). The aging hippocampus: cognitive, biochemical and struc- tural findings. *Cereb. Cortex* 13, 1344–1351.

Epstein, R. A. (2008). Parahippocampal and retrosplenial contributions to human spatial naviga- tion. *Trends Cogn. Sci.* 12, 388–396.

Etchamendy, N., and Bohbot, V. D. (2007). Spontaneous navigational strategies and performance in the virtual town. *Hippocampus* 17, 595–599.

Etchamendy, N., Konishi, K., Pike, B. G., Marighetto, A., and Bohbot, V. D. (2011). Evidence for a virtual human analog of a rodent relational memory task: a study of aging and fMRI in young adults. *Hippocampus* 22, 869–880.

Etchamendy, N., Konishi, K., Pike, G. B., Marighetto, A., and Bohbot, V. D. (2012). Evidence for a virtual human analog of a rodent relational memory task: a study of aging and fMRI in young adults. *Hippocampus* 22, 869–880.

Fotuhi, M., Do, D., and Jack, C. (2012). Modifiable factors that alter the size of the hippocampus with ageing. *Nat. Rev. Neurol.* 8, 189–202.

Fouquet, C., Konishi, K., Dahmani, L., Kurdi, V., Sham, R., Anderson, N., et al. (2011). *A Spatial Memory Intervention Program Aimed at Stimulating the Hippocampus While Controlling for Caudate Nucleus-Dependent Response Strategies Increased fMRI Activity and Grey Matter in the Human Hippocampus and Neocortex. Society for Neuroscience 2011 Abstracts* (Washington, DC, USA).

Gaskin, S., and White, N. M. (2006). Cooperation and competition between the dorsal hippocampus and lateral amygdala in spatial dis- crimination learning. *Hippocampus* 16, 577–585.

Hackert, V. H., den Heijer, T., Oudkerk, M., Koudstaal, P. J., Hofman, A., and Breteler, M. M. (2002). Hippocampal head size associated with verbal memory performance in nondemented elderly. *Neuroimage* 17, 1365–1372.

Head, D., and Isom, M. (2010). Age effects on wayfinding and route learning skills. *Behav. Brain Res.* 209, 49–58.

Hort, J., Laczo, J., Vyhnalek, M., Bojar, M., Bures, J., and Vlcek, K. (2007). Spatial navigation deficit in amnestic mild cognitive impair- ment. *Proc. Natl. Acad. Sci. U.S.A.* 104, 4042–4047.

Iaria, G., Palermo, L., Committeri, G., and Barton, J. J. (2009). Age dif- ferences in the formation and use of cognitive maps. *Behav. Brain Res.* 196, 187–191.

Iaria, G., Petrides, M., Dagher, A., Pike, B., and Bohbot, V. D. (2003). Cognitive strategies dependent on the hippocampus and caudate nucleus in human navigation: vari- ability and change with practice. *J. Neurosci.* 23, 5945–5952.

Johnson, D. K., Storandt, M., Morris, J. C., and Galvin, J. E. (2009). Longitudinal study of the tran- sition from healthy aging to Alzheimer disease. *Arch. Neurol.* 66, 1254–1259.

Kennedy, K. M., Erickson, K. I., Rodrigue, K. M., Voss, M. W., Colcombe, S. J., Kramer, A. F., et al. (2009). Age-related differ- ences in regional brain volumes: a comparison of optimized voxel- based morphometry to manual volumetry. *Neurobiol. Aging* 30, 1657–1676.

Klein, D. A., Steinberg, M., Galik, E., Steele, C., Sheppard, J. M., Warren, A., et al. (1999). Wandering behaviour in community-residing persons with dementia. *Int. J. Geriatr. Psychiatry* 14, 272–279.

Lerch, J. P., Yiu, A. P., Martinez-Canabal, A., Pekar, T., Bohbot, V. D., Frankland, P. W., et al. (2011). Maze training in mice induces MRI-detectable brain shape changes specific to the type of learning. *Neuroimage* 54, 2086–2095.

Lezak, M. D. (1995). *Neuropsychological Assessment, 3rd Edn.* New York, NY: Oxford University Press.

Marighetto, A., Etchamendy, N., Touzani, K., Torrea, C. C., Yee, B. K., Rawlins, J. N., et al. (1999).

Knowing which and knowing what: a potential mouse model for age-related human declarative memory decline. *Eur. J. Neurosci.* 11, 3312–3322.

Moffat, S. D., Elkins, W., and Resnick, S. M. (2006). Age differences in the neural systems supporting human allocentric spatial navigation. *Neurobiol. Aging* 27, 965–972.

Moffat, S. D., Kennedy, K. M., Rodrigue, K. M., and Raz, N. (2007). Extrahippocampal contri- butions to age differences in human spatial navigation. *Cereb. Cortex* 17, 1274–1282.

Morris, R. G., Garrud, P., Rawlins, J. N., and O'Keefe, J. (1982). Place navigation impaired in rats with hippocampal lesions. *Nature* 297, 681–683.

O'Keefe, J., and Nadel, L. (1978). *The Hippocampus as a Cognitive Map.* Oxford: Clarendon Press.

Osterrieth, P. A. (1944). Le test de copie d'une figure complexe. *Arch. Psychol.* 30, 206–356.

Packard, M. G., Hirsh, R., and White, N. M. (1989). Differential effects of fornix and caudate nucleus lesions on two radial maze tasks: evi- dence for multiple memory systems. *J. Neurosci.* 9, 1465–1472.

Packard, M. G., and Knowlton, B. J. (2002). Learning and memory func- tions of the Basal Ganglia. *Annu. Rev. Neurosci.* 25, 563–593.

Packard, M. G., and McGaugh, J. L. (1996). Inactivation of hip- pocampus or caudate nucleus with lidocaine differentially affects expression of place and response learning. *Neurobiol. Learn. Mem.* 65, 65–72.

Rapp, P. R., Kansky, M. T., and Roberts, J. A. (1997). Impaired spatial infor- mation processing in aged monkeys with preserved recognition mem- ory. *Neuroreport* 8, 1923–1928.

Raz, N., Rodrigue, K. M., Kennedy, K. M., Head, D., Gunning-Dixon, F., and Acker, J. D. (2003). Differential aging of the human striatum: longitudinal evidence. *AJNR Am. J. Neuroradiol.* 24, 1849–1856.

Rodgers, M. K., Sindone, J. A. 3rd., and Moffat, S. D. (2010). Effects of age on navigation strategy. *Neurobiol. Aging* 33, 202.e15–202.e22.

Rusinek, H., De Santi, S., Frid, D., Tsui, W. H., Tarshish, C. Y., Convit, A., et al. (2003). Regional brain atrophy rate predicts future cog- nitive decline: 6-year longitudinal MR imaging study of normal aging. *Radiology* 229, 691–696.

Schwabe, L., Dalm, S., Schachinger, H., and Oitzl, M. S. (2008). Chronic stress modulates the use of spatial and stimulus-response learn- ing strategies in mice and man. *Neurobiol. Learn. Mem.* 90, 495–503.

Sled, J. G., Zijdenbos, A. P., and Evans, A. C. (1998). A nonparamet-ric method for automatic correction of intensity nonuniformity in MRI data. *IEEE Trans. Med. Imaging* 17, 87–97.

Talairach, J., and Tournoux, P. (1988). *Co-Planar Stereotaxic Atlas of the Human Brain.* New York, NY: Thieme.

Tapiola, T., Pennanen, C., Tapiola, M., Tervo, S., Kivipelto, M., Hanninen, T., et al. (2008). MRI of hippocam- pus and entorhinal cortex in mild cognitive impairment: a follow-up study. *Neurobiol. Aging* 29, 31–38.

Vafaei, A. A., and Rashidy-Pour, A. (2004). Reversible lesion of the rat's orbitofrontal cortex interferes with hippocampus-dependent spa- tial memory. *Behav. Brain Res.* 149, 61–68.

White, N. M., and McDonald, R. J. (2002). Multiple parallel mem- ory systems in the brain of the rat. *Neurobiol. Learn. Mem.* 77, 125–184.

Wood, E. R., and Dudchenko, P. A. (2003). Aging, spatial behavior and the cognitive map. *Nat. Neurosci.* 6, 546–548.

Worsley, K. J., Liao, C. H., Aston, J., Petre, V., Duncan, G. H., Morales, F., et al. (2002). A general statistical analysis for fMRI data. *Neuroimage* 15, 1-15.

# 13

# Friend or foe? Decoding the facilitative and disruptive effects of emotion on working memory in younger and older adults

**Linda Truong* and Lixia Yang***

*Department of Psychology, Ryerson University, Toronto, ON, Canada*

**Edited by:**
*Natalie Ebner, University of Florida, USA*

**Reviewed by:**
*Hakan Fischer, Stockholm University, Sweden*
*Jana Nikitin, University of Zurich, Switzerland*
*Paul Verhaeghen, Georgia Institute of Technology, USA*

***Correspondence:**
*Linda Truong and Lixia Yang, Department of Psychology, Ryerson University, 350 Victoria Street, Toronto, ON M5B 2K3, Canada*
*e-mail: ltruong@psych.ryerson.ca; lixiay@psych.ryerson.ca*

A growing body of work on emotion-cognition interactions has revealed both facilitative and disruptive effects of emotion on working memory in younger adults. These differing effects may vary by the goal relevancy of emotion within a task. Additionally, it is possible that these emotional effects would be larger for older adults, considering findings of preserved emotional processing with age. To test these hypotheses, the current study examined the effects of emotional content and aging on working memory for target information in the presence of distraction. Thirty-six younger (ages 18–29) and 36 older adults (ages 65–87) completed a delayed-response working memory task. Participants viewed two target words intermixed with two distracter words, and then judged whether a subsequently presented probe word was one of the target words. The emotional content (valence and arousal) of targets and distracters was systematically manipulated. Results indicated that emotional targets facilitated working memory in both age groups. In contrast, emotional distracters disrupted performance. Negative distracters were particularly disruptive for older adults, but younger adults did not show an emotional interference effect. These findings help clarify discrepancies in the literature and contribute to the sparse research on emotional working memory in older adults.

**Keywords: aging, emotions, working memory, goal relevance, distraction, interference resolution**

## INTRODUCTION

The ability to successfully complete a task—such as driving—requires focused attention on task-relevant information, like traffic lights, and limited attention to task-irrelevant distraction, such as roadside advertisements. Similarly, successful working memory performance consists of briefly maintaining relevant target information while ignoring interference from irrelevant distraction. Research suggests that working memory declines with normal aging, resulting in slower and less accurate responses in older adults (e.g., Rypma and D'Esposito, 2000; Gazzaley et al., 2005). According to the inhibitory deficit theory, age-related deficits in inhibition—the ability to avoid or remove distracting information from working memory—reduces the ability to focus attention on task-relevant information, thus lowering overall working memory performance (i.e., slower and/or less accurate responses) (Hasher and Zacks, 1988). In contrast to this decline, processing of emotional information is preserved in old age (see Scheibe and Carstensen, 2010 for a review). A body of research suggests a tendency for older adults to attend to, and remember, positive information relative to neutral and negative information, termed an age-related "positivity effect" (Mather and Carstensen, 2005; see Reed and Carstensen, 2012 for a review). Several theories have been proposed to account for this age-related preference toward positive information (Murphy and Isaacowitz, 2008 for a meta-analysis that did not find evidence of this preference). According to the socioemotional selectivity theory (Carstensen et al., 1999), the preserved emotional processing and functioning in old age is due to a motivational shift toward emotional regulation goals (i.e., achieving positive affect) as a result of increasingly limited time horizons with age. The dynamic integration theory (Labouvie-Vief, 2003) proposes that older adults increasingly prefer positive over negative information, due to greater cognitive demands required to process the latter. Taken together, these findings raise an important question: how is working memory influenced by emotional information in older adults? Specifically, would older adults' preserved emotional processing lead to working memory enhancements or would it further impair performance?

Some insights into these questions can be gained from a theory about working memory and emotion interactions: the dual-competition model (DCM; Pessoa, 2008, 2009). This model states that biases toward emotional information influence the allocation of processing resources. When emotional information is relevant to a task goal, performance is facilitated due to the additional resources that are recruited for emotional processing. However, this bias toward emotional information can be impairing if it conflicts with a task goal, thus depleting resources needed for executive control processes in working memory, as in the case of task-irrelevant emotional information (e.g., emotional distracter items). Thus, DCM predicts that working memory performance will be disrupted in the face of task-irrelevant emotional information. The DCM can be used to interpret the results of studies that have examined emotional working memory in both older and younger adults. For example, one study compared maintenance of affective (emotional intensity of emotional images) vs. visual information (brightness intensity of neutral images) over a delay period with both younger and older adults (Mikels et al., 2005). Results revealed an age-related working memory deficit for visual maintenance, but no such deficit was found for maintenance of emotional intensity. Interestingly, older adults actually outperformed younger adults on trials where positive affect was maintained. In contrast, younger adults performed better on negative relative to positive trials. These results suggest that older adults' preserved emotional processing—of positive information, in particular—can offset their working memory declines, resulting in maintained or even enhanced performance. Similarly, another study by Mammarella et al. (2013a) found that age-related deficits in working memory were reduced when the task contained emotional information. This study examined performance on an operation span task in which participants maintained a set of neutral or emotional target words in working memory while performing math operations. Results indicated larger age differences for neutral words, but reduced or eliminated age differences for positive and negative words, respectively. A similar study also found better working memory performance for positive and negative words, relative to neutral words, in older adults (Mammarella et al., 2013b). Such findings also extend to paradigms using emotional pictures. Borg et al. (2011) compared performance on two working memory tasks with emotional pictures in younger and older adults. In the first task, participants were shown two negative and two neutral pictures, presented sequentially. The task was to maintain these four target pictures during a delay, after which a probe picture appeared. Participants had to indicate whether this probe was an old (i.e., from the target set) or a new picture they had not seen before. For both age groups, accuracy on this task was better when target stimuli were negative vs. neutral. Taken together, these findings showed little age differences in emotional working memory, suggesting that performance on task-relevant emotional information is relatively preserved in older adults.

It should be noted that previous studies have primarily focused on analyzing the effect of emotional task-*relevant* information—little attention has been paid to the potential effects of task-*irrelevant* emotional information. The few existing studies have been primarily conducted with younger adults. In one such study, it was found that emotional distracters presented during a delay period can impair younger adults' working memory performance for target items (e.g., Dolcos and McCarthy, 2006). It is unknown whether detrimental effects of emotion would be found or perhaps magnified for older adults. The second working memory task in Borg et al. (2011) sheds a light on this. In this task, participants were asked to bind four target pictures (negative or neutral) with their respective presentation locations and then identify whether a subsequently presented probe picture was presented in its original location. Results revealed no emotional effects on younger adults' performance. However, older adults performed worse for negative vs. neutral pictures. It was interpreted that resources devoted to processing negative information may have limited the availability of resources needed for effortful processing in working memory (i.e., binding) in older adults. Thus, the emotional aspects of the negative pictures may have diverted resources away from the primary binding task. However, another study did not find any effects of emotional pictures on a 2-back task (which consists of both target and distracter items) in older adults (Döhnel et al., 2008). Thus, it remains unclear when emotional information hinders older adults' working memory.

The current study took a novel approach to directly examine whether the effects of emotional content vary depending on the goal-relevancy of the emotional content. Examining the effect of emotional distracters is particularly important considering findings that older adults' working memory deficits are due to a specific decline in the inhibition of distracters, rather than the ability to attend to and maintain goal-relevant content (Gazzaley et al., 2005). In the current study, we modified the delayed-response working memory paradigm used by Gazzaley et al. (2005) in which both targets and distracters were presented within a memorandum set. Younger and older participants viewed four sequentially presented words: two were cued as targets and two were cued as distracters, by different colored fonts. After a delay, a probe word (could be a target, a distracter, or a new control probe) appeared. Participants' task was to indicate whether this probe was a word that was cued as a target from the current memorandum set. For some trials, targets were emotional words presented with neutral distracter words; for others, targets were neutral and distracters were emotional. These trials were compared to trials where both targets and distracters were neutral words, to evaluate the emotional effect of task-relevant (i.e., targets) vs. task-irrelevant (i.e., distracter) information. The critical manipulation was the emotional content—as indexed by both the valence (positive, negative, neutral) and arousal (high vs. low)—of targets and distracters. Arousal was manipulated in this study given the evidence of distinct neural networks involved in processing arousing vs. valenced information (Kensinger and Corkin, 2004) and differential effects of low vs. high arousal valenced information (Leclerc and Kensinger, 2008). The arousal levels of stimuli were systematically manipulated so that half of the words were high arousal and half were low arousal within each of the three valence categories. This allowed us to evaluate valence effects by controlling for the level of arousal.

This study aimed to address three questions: (1) Does emotional target information facilitate working memory? (2) Does emotional distracter information hinder working memory? (3) Do these effects change with age? Based on predictions derived from the dual-competition model (Pessoa, 2008, 2009) and the literature reviewed earlier, several hypotheses were proposed. First, it was expected that emotional content would be facilitative to working memory (i.e., faster and/or more accurate responses) for goal-relevant target information and would reduce age differences in working memory, in line with previous studies (e.g., Mikels et al., 2005; Mammarella et al., 2013a). In contrast, performance would be disrupted (i.e., slower and/or less accurate responses) by emotional distracters (e.g., Dolcos and McCarthy, 2006); we hypothesized that a detrimental effect due to emotional content would be more evident in older adults. Older adults' limited ability to inhibit distracter information (e.g., Yang and Hasher, 2007) may result in increased demand for cognitive resources to successfully resolve interference arising from these distracters. However, based on the dual-competition model, resources for interference resolution may be further limited when they are prioritized to be diverted toward the processing of emotional information (Pessoa, 2008, 2009). As such, we hypothesized that disruptive effects of emotional distracters would be more evident in older vs. younger adults. Finally, we also hypothesized that older adults would show enhanced attention to positive information, in line with findings of an age-related positivity bias (Mather and Carstensen, 2005). Specifically, we expected that this enhanced attention would result in facilitative effects of positive target information but also disruptive effects from positive distracter information.

## MATERIALS AND METHODS

### PARTICIPANTS

Thirty-six healthy younger adults (ages 18–29, $M = 19.69$, $SD = 2.84$; 3 males) and 36 healthy older adults (ages 65–87, $M = 73.25$, $SD = 6.37$; 6 males) participated in this study. Younger adults were recruited from the undergraduate participant pool at Ryerson University. They received course credit as compensation. Older adults were recruited from the Ryerson Senior Participant Pool at Ryerson University and received $10 per hour for participation. Four older adults were replaced: three for low accuracy in the working memory task (< 80%; see Results) and one due to computer malfunctions. All participants were tested at the Cognitive Aging Laboratory of Ryerson University and provided informed consent prior to commencing the study. All procedures in the study were conducted according to regulatory standards and were approved by the Research Ethics Board at Ryerson University.

We excluded participants who: (a) learned English after the age of 6; (b) scored less than 20 on the Shipley Institute of Living Vocabulary (Shipley, 1940); (c) scored greater than 26 on the Beck Anxiety Inventory (BAI; Beck et al., 1988), suggesting severe anxiety symptoms; (d) scored greater than 29 on the Beck Depression Inventory (BDI; Beck et al., 1996), suggesting severe depressive symptoms; (e) had previous neurological disorders (e.g., stroke, dementia, prolonged periods of unconsciousness, and head injury); or (f) uncontrolled medical conditions (e.g., diabetes, cholesterol, and cardiovascular diseases). Older adults were screened with the Short Blessed Test (SBT; Katzman et al., 1983) for dementia-related cognitive impairments and all participants in the final sample scored above the cut-off score of 6 ($M = 0.78$, $SD = 1.35$). All demographic and health information were collected through a background information questionnaire. There were age differences in several demographic and cognitive measures (see **Table 1**). Older adults had more years of education and also learned English at a younger age than did younger adults. Older adults scored higher on the Shipley Institute of Vocabulary Test and on the positive affect scale of the Positive and Negative Affect Schedule (PANAS; Watson et al., 1988), but scored lower on the BAI, the BDI, and the Digit-Symbol Substitution Task (DSST; Wechsler, 1981) than did younger adults. These age differences are typically found in research examining cognitive aging and emotion (e.g., Isaacowitz et al., 2008).

**Table 1 | Participant characteristics.**

| Measure | Younger adults | Older adults |
|---|---|---|
| | *M (SD)* | *M (SD)* |
| Years of education** | 13.00 (1.74) | 17.53 (4.11) |
| Age learned english* | 1.13 (1.92) | 0.14 (0.83) |
| Digit-Symbol Substitution Task[a]** | 82.86 (15.37) | 68.78 (14.97) |
| PANAS-positive affect[b]** | 27.22 (7.91) | 33.83 (6.40) |
| PANAS-negative affect[b] | 15.19 (5.48) | 13.61 (4.14) |
| Shipley vocabulary ** | 27.50 (3.00) | 37.36 (1.93) |
| Beck Anxiety Inventory** | 12.67 (7.61) | 6.19 (5.67) |
| Beck Depression Inventory** | 10.83 (6.67) | 5.06 (4.65) |
| Health rating[c] | 7.79 (1.13) | 8.25 (1.27) |

*[a]Digit-Symbol scores were based on the number of correct solutions within a 2-min time limit;*
*[b]PANAS, the Positive and Negative Affect Schedule;*
*[c]Health ratings were self-reported based on a 1 ("poor") to 10 ("excellent") Likert-type scale;*
*$^{*}p < 0.01$, $^{**}p < 0.001$.*

### STIMULI

All stimuli for the delayed-response working memory task in this experiment were programmed with E-prime 1.0 and presented on a 17 inch computer screen. The stimuli consisted of a total of 329 words selected from the Affective Norms of English Words (ANEW) database (Bradley and Lang, 1999). The ANEW database contains normed ratings of arousal (1 for low arousal to 9 for high arousal) and valence (1 for negative valence to 9 for positive valence). Of the 329 words selected, 240 words were used for memoranda (targets or distracters), 20 for new control words, 48 for buffer/filler trials, and 21 for practice trials.

#### *Memoranda*

A total of 240 words were selected to be targets ($N = 120$) and distracters ($N = 120$) and consisted of 48 positive words (valence $M = 7.44$, range: 6.59–8.39), 48 negative words (valence $M = 2.86$, range: 1.57–3.50), and 144 neutral words (valence $M = 4.98$, range: 4.00–6.00). Half of the words for each valence category were high in arousal (HA; arousal range: 4.51–7.45) and the other half were low in arousal (LA; arousal range: 2.39–4.48), resulting in a total of 6 word lists (one HA and one LA list for each of the three valence categories). All valence categories in the LA list were matched for arousal ($ps > 0.10$); positive and negative HA lists were matched for arousal ($p = 0.90$) and both were higher in arousal than the neutral HA list ($ps < 0.001$). Each of these six lists was then divided into two sets: one set that served as targets and one set that served as distracters. These two sets were matched on word frequency ($M = 42.21$; range 1–294) and word length (i.e., the number of letters) ($M = 6.26$; range: 3–11) ($ps > 0.21$).

Each trial consisted of a set of four memoranda: two target and two distracter words. The combination of words used in each trial varied according to trial type: (1) positive targets paired with neutral distracters (posT/neuD); (2) negative targets paired with neutral distracters (negT/neuD); (3) neutral targets paired with neutral distracters (neuT/neuD); (4) neutral targets paired with positive distracters (neuT/posD); and (5) neutral targets paired with negative distracters (neuT/negD). In each trial, one target/distracter was HA and the other target/distracter was LA. Within each trial, targets and distracters were roughly matched on arousal, frequency, and word length. For example, a neuT/negD trial consisted of one neutral HA target, one neutral LA target, one negative HA distracter, and one negative LA distracter. There were 12 trials for each trial type, resulting in a total of 60 trials. The trials were presented in a pseudorandomized order such that no more than three trials of the same trial type occurred consecutively. The sequencing of memoranda within a trial was also pseudorandomized: half of the trials combined either two targets or two distracters in a row (e.g., distracter-distracter-target-target) and the other half with intermixed targets and distracters (e.g., distracter-target-distracter-target).

### *Probes*

After a brief delay following presentation of the memoranda, a probe word was presented. Probes belonged to one of six categories: (1) HA targets; (2) LA targets; (3) HA distracters; (4) LA distracters; (5) HA new control probes; and (6) LA new control probes. Target and distracter probes were from the current trial's memoranda set. New control probes were one of 20 additional words: 4 positive words (valence $M = 7.41$, range: 7.07–7.66), 4 negative words (valence $M = 2.80$, range: 2.73–2.90), and 12 neutral words (valence $M = 5.08$, range: 4.32–5.85), selected from ANEW (Bradley and Lang, 1999); half of the words in each valence category were HA (arousal $M = 5.70$, range: 4.66–6.41) and half were LA (arousal $M = 3.91$, range: 3.18–4.29). The new control probes matched those of the distracters on valence within a trial set (e.g., a neuT/negD trial had a new control probe that was also negative).

The six probe categories occurred equally often for each trial type. The selection of probes (i.e., which target word served as the target probe for a particular trial) was counterbalanced with a Latin Square design, resulting in six counterbalance conditions. In addition, the order within a memoranda set of targets and distracter probes was also counterbalanced such that each appeared equally often at each of the four possible positions (e.g., a HA target cue appeared in the first to fourth position equally).

### PROCEDURE

Upon arrival at the laboratory, participants read and signed an informed consent, and then completed the computerized delayed-response working memory task. Participants were seated centrally in front of the computer screen at a reading distance. They were instructed to keep their eyes on the screen at all times during the working memory task. The task instructions indicated which words they should remember (i.e., targets) and which they should ignore (i.e., distracters), as cued by either blue or red font color, counterbalanced across participants. Each trial began with a fixation cross presented for 500 ms, followed by a memoranda set. Each set contained two target and two distracter words, each presented sequentially for 800 ms with an inter-stimulus interval of 200 ms. After a 500 ms delay, a probe word (in black font) was presented for 2000 ms. Participants were instructed to press a key labeled "YES" (the "/" key) if the probe was a target word from the current set. If the probe was a distracter or a new control word, participants were instructed to press the "NO" key (the "Z" key). Participants were instructed to respond as quickly and accurately as possible. Following their responses, an accuracy feedback screen ("Correct," "Incorrect," or "No response detected") was presented for 800 ms (see **Figure 1**).

The working memory task consisted of a practice block (5 trials; approximately 35 s, with an option to be repeated if needed) and an experimental block (72 trials: 60 experimental, six buffer, and six filler trials; approximately 8.5 min). Buffer trials occurred at the beginning and end of the block to reduce primacy and recency effects and filler trials were randomly intermixed with experimental ones. All buffer and filler trials consisted of target probes, requiring "yes" responses, in order to minimize response bias by balancing the number of "yes" responses with those of "no" responses to make them approximately the same (i.e., 44% "yes" responses). In addition, no more than three "yes" or "no" responses occurred in a row throughout the task.

After the working memory task, participants completed the DSST, a measure of perceptual-motor speed for 2 min. They then completed the PANAS, a self-reported assessment of positive and negative affect. At the end, participants completed a variety of paper-and-pencil tests and questionnaires, including the Shipley Institute of Vocabulary Test, the BAI, the BDI, and a background information questionnaire, to determine their eligibility. Older adults then completed the SBT. Finally, participants were

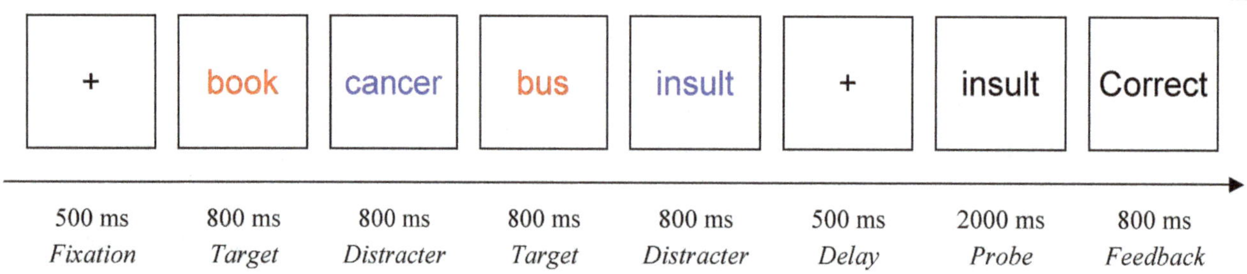


**FIGURE 1 | Working memory task procedure (a neuTnegD trial with a negative distracter probe).** In this example trial, the participant correctly responded "NO" to the distracter probe and received a feedback screen indicating that the response was correct.

debriefed and paid or granted course credit. The total duration of the experiment was approximately 1 h.

## RESULTS

To examine differential emotional effects of goal-relevant target vs. goal-irrelevant distracting information, response times (RTs) and accuracy in the working memory task were analyzed with mixed analyses of variance (ANOVAs). These analyses were conducted separately for target probe responses (reported as target identification, requiring "yes" responses) and responses to distracter and control probes (reported as interference scores, requiring "no" responses). Only RTs for correct responses were included in the RT analyses. RTs were also trimmed by excluding those that were beyond 2.5 *SD*s away from the mean for each participant in each condition, resulting in an exclusion of 6% of data points. To ensure sufficient correct trials for meaningful RT data in each condition, we replaced three individuals with overall accuracy scores lower than 80% ($M = 74.33$, $SD = 5.69$, range: 68–79).

### EFFECTS OF EMOTIONAL CONTENT ON TARGET IDENTIFICATION

To examine the effects of emotional content (i.e., arousal and valence) on the identification of target probes, a 2 × 2 × 3 mixed ANOVA with Age (younger, older) as a between-subjects variable, Arousal (high, low) and Valence (positive, negative, neutral) as within-subjects variables, was conducted on RTs and accuracy to target probes that require "yes" responses. The data for three younger and two older adults were excluded in the RT analysis because of missing data points due to RT trimming or lack of correct responses in a condition.

#### *RT analysis*

**Figure 2** displays the results of the RT analysis. The mixed ANOVA revealed a main effect of Age, $F_{(1, 65)} = 11.13, p = 0.001$, $\eta_p^2 = 0.15$. Overall, younger adults ($M = 739.59$, $SD = 154.08$) were faster than older adults ($M = 875.70$, $SD = 178.61$). The main effect of Arousal was significant, $F_{(1, 65)} = 5.01$, $p = 0.03$, $\eta_p^2 = 0.07$. This arousal effect was qualified by an Age by Arousal interaction, $F_{(1, 65)} = 4.32$, $p = 0.04$, $\eta_p^2 = 0.06$. The arousal effect was only significant for younger, $t_{(32)} = -2.85$, $p = 0.01$, but not for older adults ($p = 0.90$). The Arousal by Valence interaction was also significant, $F_{(2, 130)} = 6.64, p = 0.002, \eta_p^2 = 0.09$, with faster RTs to high arousal than to low arousal for positive, $t_{(66)} = -4.21, p < 0.001$, but not for negative ($p = 0.70$) or neutral target probes ($p = 0.90$). This benefit of arousal for positive targets was found for both younger, $t_{(32)} = -2.54, p = 0.02$, and older, $t_{(33)} = -3.59, p = 0.001$, adults. All other effects were not significant (*F*s < 1.30, *p*s > 0.28).

#### *Accuracy analysis*

The same mixed ANOVA on accuracy revealed a main effect of Valence, $F_{(2, 140)} = 5.79, p = 0.004, \eta_p^2 = 0.08$, with lower accuracy for neutral ($M = 0.92$, $SD = 0.16$) than for both positive ($M = 0.97$, $SD = 0.08$), $t_{(71)} = 2.82$, $p = 0.006$, and negative words ($M = 0.97$, $SD = 0.11$), $t_{(71)} = 2.88$, $p = 0.005$; the latter two did not differ from each other, $t_{(71)} = -0.21$, $p = 0.84$. This suggested a facilitative effect of emotional valence. In addition, the main effect of Arousal was marginally significant, $F_{(1, 70)} = 3.15$, $p = 0.08$, $\eta_p^2 = 0.04$, with higher accuracy for high arousal targets ($M = 0.97$, $SD = 0.09$) than for low arousal targets ($M = 0.94$, $SD = 0.01$), suggesting a trend toward a facilitative effect of emotional arousal (**Figure 3**). All other effects were not significant (*F*s < 0.31, *p*s > 0.73).

Overall, these findings indicated age-related slowing but preserved accuracy for target identification in working memory, possibly due to age-related shifts toward prioritization of accuracy over speed (Salthouse, 1979). The results also revealed that arousal facilitated the speed in identifying positive targets and valence facilitated target identification accuracy. In summary, emotional content (arousal or valence) facilitated target identification by making responses either faster or more accurate and the effects were largely similar across the two age groups.

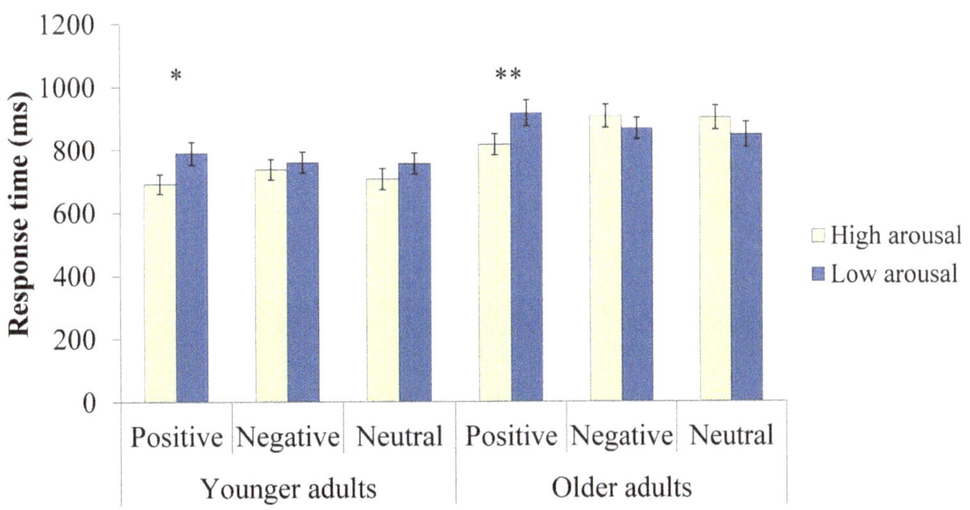


**FIGURE 2 | Response times for correct target identification responses.** Error bars represent standard errors. $^*p < 0.05$; $^{**}p < 0.01$.

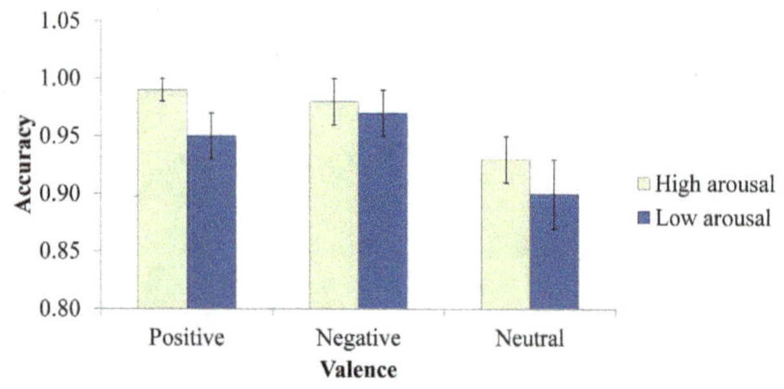


**FIGURE 3 | Accuracy for target identification responses.** Error bars represent standard errors.

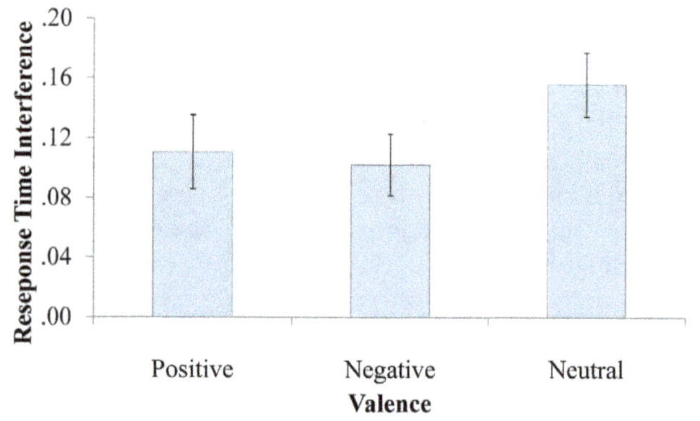


**FIGURE 4 | Response time interference scores.** Error bars represent standard errors.

## EFFECTS OF EMOTIONAL CONTENT ON INTERFERENCE OF DISTRACTERS

Following some previous work (Yang and Hasher, 2007), interference was operationally defined as performance differences in responding to distracter vs. matched control probes. This definition is based on the assumption that both distracter and control probes require the same "no" response (i.e., correct rejection of the probe as a target). The primary difference is that distracter probes were presented earlier during encoding. If participants successfully inhibited distracters, we would expect minimal interference at retrieval/probe responding; thus, performance would be very similar to that for control probes (newly presented words). However, if participants were not efficiently inhibiting or deleting the distracter from working memory, these distracter probes may result in false alarms (i.e., incorrectly identifying a distracter as a target probe) or slower rejection responses, thus increasing the performance difference between distracter and the matched control probes.

For the RT analysis, interference was indexed with proportional RT difference scores, calculated by subtracting the RTs to control probes from RTs to the matched distracters (distracters—controls), which was then divided by the RTs to control probes. A similar calculation was applied to the accuracy data, by subtracting the accuracy to distracter probes from that to matched controls, and then divided by the accuracy to controls. Thus, larger scores in both RT and accuracy indicated greater interference. These proportional interference scores controlled for potential age-related differences in response times and accuracy. These interference scores were analyzed with 2 × 2 × 3 mixed ANOVAs with Age (younger, older) as a between-subjects variable, and Arousal (high, low) and Valence (positive, negative, neutral) as within-subjects variables. For the RT analysis only, the data for one younger and four older adults were not included due to missing data points as a result of RT trimming or lack of correct responses in a condition.

### *RT analysis*

The mixed ANOVA revealed a marginal main effect of Valence, $F_{(2, 130)} = 2.62$, $p = 0.08$, $\eta_p^2 = 0.04$. Follow-up paired *t*-tests indicated slightly less interference for negative ($M = 0.10$, $SD = 0.17$) vs. neutral ($M = 0.16$, $SD = 0.17$) probes, $t_{(66)} = -1.79$, $p = 0.08$. All other effects were not significant ($Fs < 2.24$, $ps > 0.14$). The RT interference scores across valence are displayed in **Figure 4**.

### *Accuracy analysis*

**Figure 5** displays the results of the accuracy analysis. The ANOVA revealed an Age by Valence interaction, $F_{(2, 140)} = 3.89, p = 0.02$, $\eta_p^2 = 0.05$. There was a trend toward a main effect of Valence for older, $F_{(2, 70)} = 2.49$, $p = 0.09$, but not for younger adults, $F_{(1.63, 57.10)} = 0.83$, $p = 0.42$ (Greenhouse-Geisser correction). Guided by our hypotheses, we conducted planned comparisons. The results revealed that older adults experienced greater interference from negative ($M = 0.12$, $SD = 0.16$) than neutral ($M = 0.02$, $SD = 0.23$), $t_{(35)} = 2.25, p = 0.03$, and positive probes ($M = 0.03$, $SD = 0.23$), $t_{(35)} = -1.87$, $p = 0.07$; the latter two did not differ, $p = 0.89$. Follow-up independent samples *t*-tests for each valence also indicated age differences for negative probes only: older adults ($M = 0.12$, $SD = 0.16$) experienced greater interference from negative distracters than younger adults ($M = 0.02$, $SD = 0.12$), $t_{(64.49)} = -2.98$, $p = 0.004$. As a matter of fact, older adults experienced significant interference from negative probes, $t_{(35)} = 4.42$, $p < 0.001$, whereas younger adults did not, $t_{(35)} = 0.96$, $p = 0.35$. This age difference was not present for positive or neutral interference scores, $ts > 0.44$, $ps > 0.56$. All other effects were not significant ($Fs < 1.06$, $ps > 0.35$).

## DISCUSSION

To our knowledge, this is the first study to examine how the effects of emotional content on working memory vary according to goal relevancy and age. Consistent with our hypotheses, the overall results suggest that working memory is facilitated (i.e., faster and more accurate responses) by the emotional content of goal-relevant target information. In addition, working memory can be disrupted (i.e., larger interference) by the emotional content of goal-irrelevant distraction. However, this disruptive effect appears to be limited to negatively-valenced stimuli and occurs only for older adults. These results add novel contributions to our understanding of facilitative and disruptive emotional effects on working memory by manipulating and distinguishing between goal-relevant and goal-irrelevant information.

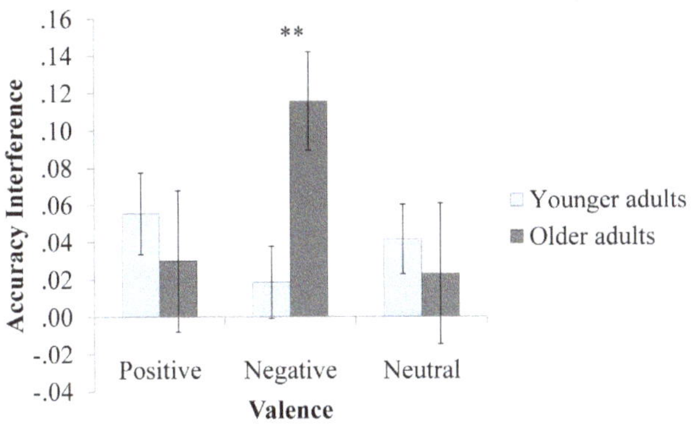


**FIGURE 5 | Accuracy interference scores.** Error bars represent standard errors. $^{**}p < 0.01$.

### EMOTIONAL TARGET INFORMATION FACILITATES WORKING MEMORY

The dual-competition model (DCM; Pessoa, 2008, 2009) posits that emotional information receives prioritized processing, which can be beneficial when the information is relevant to current goals. Our study found support for this prediction as responses were faster or more accurate to emotional/high arousing relative to neutral/low arousing goal-relevant target words. These results are consistent with studies that have found facilitative effects of emotion on working memory (Mammarella et al., 2013a). However, the facilitative effect of arousal only occurred for response speed, and was significant only for positive, but not for negative, target words. This appears to conflict with predictions from the DCM of enhanced processing for high arousal negative information (e.g., threat-relevant stimuli). We advise caution when interpreting this result, as performance was close to ceiling for negative targets, which may have limited our ability to find differences in performance between low and high arousal negative words. However, the findings of faster responses to positive high arousal targets are consistent with another study in which high arousal positive targets were detected faster amidst an array of neutral distracters (Leclerc and Kensinger, 2008). Taken together, it appears that high arousal positive goal-relevant stimuli can receive prioritized processing in competition against neutral distracters in the current paradigm.

In addition, the results indicated higher accuracy for emotional vs. neutral target word identification for both younger and older adults. There was also a pattern toward more accurate responses for high vs. low arousal words. These results are consistent with our hypotheses and other findings of attenuation of age differences when emotional materials are used (e.g., Mikels et al., 2005; Borg et al., 2011; Mammarella et al., 2013a). However, we found less evidence of a specific advantage for positive goal-relevant information in older adults, which we hypothesized based on literature pertaining to the positivity effect. Instead, our overall results indicated that emotional content in general, regardless of valence, appears to help younger and older adults to a similar extent. Together, these results may suggest that older adults are still capable of allocating resources to prioritize processing of emotional items, and thus show no impairment on working memory accuracy for target information.

### NEGATIVE DISTRACTER INFORMATION DISRUPTS WORKING MEMORY IN OLDER ADULTS

In contrast to the facilitative effects of emotion on working memory, there was some evidence supporting our hypothesis that emotional goal-irrelevant information can disrupt performance. Negative distracter stimuli caused greater interference in working memory, resulting in lower accuracy performance, but this was found for older adults only; no such effect occurred for younger adults. This finding converges, to some degree, with a large body of literature that suggests a shift toward a positivity bias in older adults vs. a negativity bias in younger adults (Reed and Carstensen, 2012). Although we hypothesized that older adults' enhanced attention to positive distracters would be detrimental to their working memory performance, our results suggested poorer performance due to negative distracters. Older adults were also less successful at resolving interference from negative distracters compared to younger adults. Poorer interference resolution involving negative distracters in older adults relative to younger adults is in line with research suggesting that younger and older adults differ in how negative information is processed, with greater attention toward negative information in younger adults and avoidance of negative information in older adults (Mather and Carstensen, 2003; Isaacowitz et al., 2006). A speculative interpretation of these findings may be derived based on the dual-competition model (DCM; Pessoa, 2008, 2009). DCM posits that task-irrelevant emotional stimuli can impair executive control by consuming resources needed for conflict resolution. If older adults have an "anti-negativity" bias, defined as avoidance of negative, relative to younger adults (e.g., Isaacowitz et al., 2006; Knight et al., 2007) or have particular difficulties processing cognitively-demanding negative information (Labouvie-Vief et al., 2010), it is possible that they did not devote sufficient resources to successfully encode negative words as distracters. This would result in a weaker representation of the negative word as a distracter item. When they encountered these words as probes during retrieval, resources may have been reallocated to prioritize the processing of these weak representations of negative information, at the expense of interference resolution. Thus, older adults' poorer performance with negative interference may be due to a "double-edged sword" of negative goal-irrelevant information, caused by both anti-negativity biases during encoding and competition between emotional information and executive control for limited resources at retrieval. In contrast, younger adults may have more resources to spare and appear to be more successful in processing negative content while simultaneously engaging in interference resolution. This is demonstrated in our study and others (Levens and Phelps, 2008) as an absence or reduction of interference arising from negative probes for younger adults.

Alternatively, disrupted performance from negative interference in older adults could also be explained as heightened attention to negative information in older adults. A negativity bias in older adults has been observed when cognitive resources are limited, often manipulated through divided or dual attention paradigms (Mather and Knight, 2005; Knight et al., 2007). Thus, it is possible that the working memory paradigm used in the current study sufficiently reduced or divided cognitive resources in older adults by requiring interference resolution, which resulted in greater attention toward negative information. This enhanced processing of negative information may have distracted older adults to a greater extent relative to positive and neutral information, resulting in increased false alarms to negative distracter probes.

### FUTURE OUTLOOK

Taken together, the results from this study provide evidence suggesting that the differential effects of emotion on working memory may vary by arousal, valence, age, and goal relevancy. However, there were several limitations of the current study. First, the irrelevant information in the working memory task (i.e., distracter words) was arbitrarily and externally assigned by experimenters. Thus, this paradigm does not inform us about the interference resolution of internally generated distractions, such as in proactive interference paradigms or when there is a mismatch between task goals and emotion regulation goals. Future research could address this question by modifying the paradigm to include internally generated distracter items to measure the impact of these items on working memory. Furthermore, it could also manipulate the match/mismatch of task vs. emotional goals by implementing task instructions that explicitly direct participants to engage in emotional processing, which contrasts with the more perceptually-based processing used in the current paradigm (i.e., cuing of target vs. distracter via different colored fonts).

The second limitation is our sample. The older sample has a larger age range (i.e., 22 years) than the younger sample (i.e., 11 years). This wider range in older adults may have introduced larger performance variability (e.g., Hultsch et al., 2002). We assume that any variability in the older adult group may also be reflective of aging more generally, as studies typically find that both inter- and intra-individual variability increases with age (e.g., Nelson and Dannefer, 1992; Shammi et al., 1998). As this study was a preliminary examination of emotion on working memory and aging, to better encompass any changes that may occur in later life, we followed a common approach in cognitive aging literature and did not set an upper age limit for the older group. Additionally, the low percentage of male participants (13% of the total sample) was another limitation of this sample. In consideration of research on gender differences in emotion regulation and processing (e.g., Gur and Gur, 2002; McRae et al., 2008), our findings may not be representative of emotion processing in males. As such, future studies should aim for more balanced numbers of female and male participants.

Finally, although we expected relatively high accuracy on this task based on results from other studies (e.g., Gazzaley et al., 2005), we also expected to find some evidence of age-related working memory declines. Aside from slower target identification, which could be attributed to age-related prioritization of accuracy over speed, there were no main effects of age. The lack of age differences suggests that this paradigm may not exert high demands on working memory. This may have limited our ability to find facilitative or disruptive effects of emotion. However, the lack of age differences may also suggest that the emotional nature of the task may have helped attenuate overall age-related working memory declines, as has been found in other studies (e.g., Mikels et al., 2005). To examine this, future studies could use a working memory paradigm that is more taxing and thus more sensitive at detecting age differences. Future research could also build on the results of this study by examining the neural mechanisms that contribute to the facilitative and disruptive effects of emotion in the aging brain. Such work could be informed by research on younger adults (Dolcos et al., 2011) that have identified multiple neural connections between areas implicated in emotion processing (e.g., ventral affective system) and cognitive control (e.g., dorsal executive system).

Overall, this study provided novel evidence in support of recent frameworks that specify the competitive advantage of emotional over non-emotional information (particularly for older adults; Carstensen et al., 1999) and the role of goal relevancy (Pessoa, 2008, 2009). It contributed to the sparse, but growing, literature on the important interactions between emotion and cognitive control in older adults (e.g., Pessoa, 2008; Dolcos et al., 2011). Such work helps identify situations in which older adults' preserved emotional processing could be a helpful "friend" vs. hindering "foe" to their declines in cognitive control.

## ACKNOWLEDGMENTS

We thank all research assistants involved in the completion of this project. This work was supported by a Natural Sciences and Engineering Research Council (NSERC) of Canada Discovery Grant (371762-2009) awarded to Lixia Yang.

## REFERENCES

Beck, A. T., Epstein, N., Brown, G., and Steer, R. A. (1988). An inventory for measuring clinical anxiety: psychometric properties. *J. Consult. Clin. Psychol.* 56, 893–897. doi: 10.1037/0022-006X.56.6.893

Beck, A. T., Steer, R. A., and Brown, G. K. (1996) *Manual for the Beck Depression Inventory-II*. San Antonio, TX: Psychological Corporation.

Borg, C., Leroy, N., Favre, E., Laurent, B., and Thomas-Antérion, C. (2011). How emotional pictures influence visuospatial binding in short-term memory in ageing and Alzheimer's disease? *Brain Cogn.* 76, 20–25. doi: 10.1016/j.bandc.2011.03.008

Bradley, M. M., and Lang, P. J. (1999). "Affective norms for English words (ANEW): stimuli, instruction manual and affective ratings," in *Technical Report C-1* (Gainesville, FL: The Center for Research in Psychophysiology, University of Florida).

Carstensen, L. L., Isaacowitz, D. M., and Charles, S. T. (1999). Taking time seriously: a theory of socioemotional selectivity. *Am. Psychol.* 54, 165–181. doi: 10.1037/0003-066X.54.3.165

Döhnel, K., Sommer, M., Ibach, B., Rothmayr, C., Meinhardt, J., and Hajak, G. (2008). Neural correlates of emotional working memory in patients with mild cognitive impairment. *Neuropsychologia* 46, 37–48. doi: 10.1016/j.neuropsychologia.2007.08.012

Dolcos, F., Iordan, A., and Dolcos, S. (2011). Neural correlates of emotion–cognition interactions: a review of evidence from brain imaging investigations. *J. Cogn. Psychol.* 23, 669–694. doi: 10.1080/20445911.2011.594433

Dolcos, F., and McCarthy, G. (2006). Brain systems mediating cognitive interference by emotional distraction. *J. Neurosci.* 26, 2072–2079. doi: 10.1523/JNEUROSCI.5042-05.2006

Gazzaley, A., Cooney, J. W., Rissman, J., and D'Esposito, M. (2005). Top-down suppression deficit underlies working memory impairment in normal aging. *Nat. Neurosci.* 8, 1298–1300. doi: 10.1038/nn1543

Gur, R. E., and Gur, R. C. (2002). Gender differences in aging: cognition, emotions, and neuroimaging studies. *Dialogues Clin. Neurosci.* 4, 197–210.

Hasher, L., and Zacks, R. T. (1988). "Working memory, comprehension, and aging: a review and a new view," in *The Psychology of Learning and Motivation: Advances in Research and Theory*, Vol. 22, ed G. H. Bower (New York, NY: Academic Press), 193–225.

Hultsch, D. F., MacDonald, S. W. S., and Dixon, R. A. (2002). Variability in reaction time performance of younger and older adults. *J. Gerontol. B Psychol. Sci. Soc. Sci.* 57, 101–115. doi: 10.1093/geronb/57.2.P101

Isaacowitz, D. M., Toner, K., Goren, D., and Wilson, H. R. (2008). Looking while unhappy: mood-congruent gaze in young adults, positive gaze in older adults. *Psychol. Sci.* 19, 848–853. doi: 10.1111/j.1467-9280.2008.02167.x

Isaacowitz, D. M., Wadlinger, H. A., Goren, D., and Wilson, H. R. (2006). Is there an age-related positivity effect in visual attention? A comparison of two methodologies. *Emotion* 6, 511–516. doi: 10.1037/1528-3542.6.3.511

Katzman, R., Brown, T., Fuld, P., Peck, A., Schechter, R., and Schimmel, H. (1983). Validation of a short orientation-memory-concentration test of cognitive impairment. *Am. J. Psychiatry* 140, 734–739.

Kensinger, E. A., and Corkin, S. (2004). Two routes to emotional memory: distinct neural processes for valence and arousal. *Proc. Natl. Acad. Sci. U.S.A.* 101, 3310–3315. doi: 10.1073/pnas.0306408101

Knight, M., Seymour, T. L., Gaunt, J. T., Baker, C., Nesmith, K., and Mather, M. (2007). Aging and goal-directed emotional attention: distraction reverses emotional biases. *Emotion* 7, 705–714. doi: 10.1037/1528-3542.7.4.705

Labouvie-Vief, G. (2003). Dynamic integration: affect, cognition, and the self in adulthood. *Curr. Dir. Psychol. Sci.* 12, 201–206. doi: 10.1046/j.0963-7214.2003.01262.x

Labouvie-Vief, G., Grühn, D., and Studer, J. (2010). "Dynamic integration of emotion and cognition: equilibrium regulation in development and aging," in *The Handbook of Lifespan Development*, eds R. M. Lerner, M. E. Lamb, and A. M. Freund (Hoboken: John Wiley and Sons, Inc.), 79–115.

Leclerc, C. M., and Kensinger, E. A. (2008). Effects of age on detection of emotional information. *Psychol. Aging* 23, 209–215. doi: 10.1037/0882-7974.23.1.209

Levens, S. M., and Phelps, E. A. (2008). Emotion processing effects on interference resolution in working memory. *Emotion* 8, 267–280. doi: 10.1037/1528-3542.8.2.267

Mammarella, N., Borella, E., Carretti, B., Leonardi, G., and Fairfield, B. (2013a). Examining an emotion enhancement effect in working memory: evidence from age-related differences. *Neuropsychol. Rehabil.* 23, 416–428. doi: 10.1080/09602011.2013.775065

Mammarella, N., Fairfield, B., Di Domenico, A., Borella, E., and Carretti, B. (2013b). Is working memory affective in dementia of alzheimer's type? *Neurosci. Discov.* 1, 1–4. doi: 10.7243/2052-6946-1-4

Mather, M., and Carstensen, L. L. (2003). Aging and attentional biases for emotional faces. *Psychol. Sci.* 14, 409–415. doi: 10.1111/1467-9280.01455

Mather, M., and Carstensen, L. L. (2005). Aging and motivated cognition: the positivity effect in attention and memory. *Trends Cogn. Sci.* 9, 496–502. doi: 10.1016/j.tics.2005.08.005

Mather, M., and Knight, M. (2005). Goal-directed memory: the role of cognitive control in older adults' emotional memory. *Psychol. Aging* 20, 554–570. doi: 10.1037/0882-7974.20.4.554

McRae, K., Ochsner, K. N., Mauss, I. B., Gabrieli, J. J. D., and Gross, J. J. (2008). Gender differences in emotion regulation: an fMRI Study of cognitive reappraisal. *Gr. Process. Intergr. Relat.* 11, 143–162. doi: 10.1177/1368430207088035

Mikels, J. A., Larkin, G. R., Reuter-Lorenz, P. A., and Cartensen, L. L. (2005). Divergent trajectories in the aging mind: changes in working memory for affective versus visual information with age. *Psychol. Aging* 20, 542–553. doi: 10.1037/0882-7974.20.4.542

Murphy, N. A., and Isaacowitz, D. M. (2008). Preferences for emotional information in older and younger adults: a meta-analysis of memory and attention tasks. *Psychol. Aging* 23, 263–286. doi: 10.1037/0882-7974.23.2.263

Nelson, E. A., and Dannefer, D. (1992). Aged heterogeneity: fact or fiction? the fate of diversity in gerontological research. *Gerontologist* 32, 17–23. doi: 10.1093/geront/32.1.17

Pessoa, L. (2008). On the relationship between emotion and cognition. *Nat. Rev. Neurosci.* 9, 148–158. doi: 10.1038/nrn2317

Pessoa, L. (2009). How do emotion and motivation direct executive control? *Trends Cogn. Sci.* 13, 160–166. doi: 10.1016/j.tics.2009.01.006

Reed, A. E., and Carstensen, L. L. (2012). The theory behind the age-related positivity effect. *Front. Psychol.* 3:339. doi: 10.3389/fpsyg.2012.00339

Rypma, B., and D'Esposito, M. (2000). Isolating the neural mechanisms of age-related changes in human working memory. *Nat. Neurosci.* 3, 509–515. doi: 10.1038/74889

Salthouse, T. A. (1979). Adult age and the speed-accuracy trade-off. *Ergonomics* 22, 811–821. doi: 10.1080/00140137908924659

Scheibe, S., and Carstensen, L. L. (2010). Emotional aging: recent findings and future trends. *J. Gerontol. Psychol. Sci.* 65B, 135–144. doi: 10.1093/geronb/gbp132

Shammi, P., Bosman, E., and Stuss, D. T. (1998). Aging and variability in performance. *Aging Neuropsychol. Cogn.* 5, 1–13. doi: 10.1076/anec.5.1.1.23

Shipley, W. C. (1940). A self-administering scale for measuring intellectual impairment and deterioration. *J. Psychol. Interdiscip. Appl.* 9, 371–337. doi: 10.1080/00223980.1940.9917704

Watson, D., Clark, L. A., and Tellegen, A. (1988). Development and validation of brief measures of positive and negative affect: the PANAS scales. *J. Pers. Soc. Psychol.* 54, 1063–1070. doi: 10.1037/0022-3514.54.6.1063

Wechsler, D. (1981). *Manual for the Wechsler Adult Intelligence Scale-Revised.* New York, NY: Psychological Corporation.

Yang, L., and Hasher, L. (2007). The enhanced effects of pictorial distraction in older adults. *J. Gerontol. B. Psychol. Sci. Soc. Sci.* 62, 230–233. doi: 10.1093/geronb/62.4.P230

14

# Virtual navigation strategies from childhood to senescence: evidence for changes across the life span

**Veronique D. Bohbot[1]*, Sam McKenzie[1], Kyoko Konishi[1], Celine Fouquet[1], Vanessa Kurdi[1], Russel Schachar[2], Michel Boivin[3] and Philippe Robaey[4]**

[1] Department of Psychiatry, Douglas Institute, McGill University, Verdun, QC, Canada
[2] Hospital for Sick Children, Toronto, ON, Canada
[3] Deptartment of Psychology, Université de Laval, Quebec, QC, Canada
[4] Department of Psychiatry, Ste-Justine Research Center, Montreal, QC, Canada

**Edited by:**
Thomas Wolbers, German Center for Neurodegenerative Diseases (DZNE), Germany

**Reviewed by:**
Jacques Micheau, University of Bordeaux 1, France
Jan M. Wiener, Bournemouth University, UK

***Correspondence:**
Veronique D. Bohbot, Faculty of Medicine, Department of Psychiatry, Douglas Mental Health University Institute, McGill University, FBC Building, 6875 boul. LaSalle, Verdun, QC H4H 1R3, Canada.
e-mail: veronique.bohbot@mcgill.ca

This study sought to investigate navigational strategies across the life span, by testing 8-years old children to 80-years old healthy older adults on the 4 on 8 virtual maze (4/8VM). The 4/8VM was previously developed to assess spontaneous navigational strategies, i.e., hippocampal-dependent spatial strategies (navigation by memorizing relationships between landmarks) versus caudate nucleus-dependent response strategies (memorizing a series of left and right turns from a given starting position). With the 4/8VM, we previously demonstrated greater fMRI activity and gray matter in the hippocampus of spatial learners relative to response learners. A sample of 599 healthy participants was tested in the current study. Results showed that 84.4% of children, 46.3% of young adults, and 39.3% of older adults spontaneously used spatial strategies ($p < 0.0001$). Our results suggest that while children predominantly use spatial strategies, the proportion of participants using spatial strategies decreases across the life span, in favor of response strategies. Factors promoting response strategies include repetition, reward and stress. Since response strategies can result from successful repetition of a behavioral pattern, we propose that the increase in response strategies is a biological adaptive mechanism that allows for the automatization of behavior such as walking in order to free up hippocampal-dependent resources. However, the down-side of this shift from spatial to response strategies occurs if people stop building novel relationships, which occurs with repetition and routine, and thereby stop stimulating their hippocampus. Reduced fMRI activity and gray matter in the hippocampus were shown to correlate with cognitive deficits in normal aging. Therefore, these results have important implications regarding factors involved in healthy and successful aging.

**Keywords: hippocampus, caudate nucleus, navigational strategy, spatial memory, twins, children, aging**

## INTRODUCTION

The human brain changes across the entire life span. Throughout childhood there are changes in the function and size of numerous brain structures which correlate with increased performance on tasks that are dependent upon these regions (Casey et al., 2002; Thomas et al., 2004; Menon et al., 2005). In contrast, decreases in memory and executive function have been observed with normal aging. These deficits have been associated with decreases in the volume of the hippocampus (Lupien et al., 1998; Small et al., 2002; Raz et al., 2004; Moffat et al., 2006) and frontal cortex (Raz et al., 1997; Grady and Craik, 2000; Cabeza, 2002). Despite known neural changes that happen during development and aging, very few human studies have examined the corresponding changes in behavior across the entire lifespan.

Navigation is often used as a model for learning because it is possible to dissociate different learning strategies which depend upon distinct memory systems. Many lines of research in rodents and humans have demonstrated that the hippocampus is required when one must learn the spatial relationships between multiple landmarks in the environment, i.e., when forming a cognitive map of the relationships between environmental landmarks (O'Keefe and Nadel, 1978; Packard et al., 1989; Bohbot et al., 2004). On the other hand, when stimulus-response associations must be made, i.e., by learning a series of specific movements from a given start position or stimulus, the striatum, formed of the caudate nucleus, putamen and nucleus accumbens, is necessary. Under certain experimental conditions, recruitment of the hippocampus has actually been shown to interfere with this form of learning (Packard et al., 1989; McDonald and White, 1993; Hartley et al., 2003). In young adult humans, the spontaneous use of a response strategy during virtual navigation has been associated with increased activity and gray matter of the caudate nucleus portion of the striatum, while the use of a spatial strategy has been related to increased activity and gray matter in the hippocampus (Iaria et al., 2003; Bohbot et al., 2007). Interestingly, a negative correlation between the gray matter of the caudate nucleus and hippocampus was observed (Bohbot et al., 2007), a finding that adds to the growing body of literature describing the fact that only one of the two structures is used at any given time, in a manner that appears competitive (Packard et al., 1989; McDonald and White, 1993; Gold, 2004).

Studies in rodents and humans have suggested that memory deficits in older adults are not uniform and may be specific to the decline of particular structures. In a study by Barnes et al. (1980), it was demonstrated that older rats employed a response strategy to a greater extent than younger rats in a T-maze. Similarly, after young and aged rats learn the location of a submerged platform in the Morris Water Maze, aged rats search more readily for a visible platform in a new location showing bias toward response strategies, as opposed to younger rats who ignore the visible platform and continue searching for the submerged platform in the old target location indicating a bias toward spatial strategies (Rapp et al., 1987). Another study (Nicolle et al., 2003) showed that aged mice were able to use a spatial strategy in the Morris Water Maze when forced to, but predominantly used a response strategy when given the choice. Structural and functional imaging studies have shown hippocampal decline in older adults (Jernigan et al., 2001; Raz et al., 2004; Jernigan and Gamst, 2005; Walhovd et al., 2005; Moffat et al., 2007; Head and Isom, 2010) as well as inferior performance when using processes which depend upon the hippocampus, such as spatial memory (Newman and Kaszniak, 2000; Moffat et al., 2006) and episodic memory (Maguire and Frith, 2003; Persson et al., 2006). Etchamendy et al. (2012) showed that human older adults tested on a virtual analog of a rodent radial task were impaired at using spatial relationships to solve the task, while response learning was intact.

A study (Leplow et al., 2003) has addressed the question of which memory system is spontaneously used in children. In this study, all the children over the age of 10 years old used a spatial strategy. However, it is unclear whether the paradigm used was equally sensitive to the two strategies. Other studies which have not tested for response strategies have found that the development of spatial competence emerges between seven and 8 years of age; about the same time that children can abstract spatial relationships to scaled models (Overman et al., 1996). It is unknown whether school-aged children would depend more on the information processing of the hippocampus or that of the caudate nucleus on a task which can be solved equally well using either learning strategy.

In order to assess the relative contribution of different memory systems across the lifespan, we administered a virtual navigation task that can be learned using either a spatial or response strategy to 299 children, 175 young adults, and 125 older adults. Based on previous studies in rodents and preliminary data with humans from our laboratory, we predicted that children would predominantly use spatial strategies and that response learning strategies would be increasingly used with age.

## METHODS

### PARTICIPANTS

Children participants were taken from a sample of 299 eight-years-old twins (monozygotic and dizygotic). Ninety-five young adults who took part in four ongoing studies were added to the sample of 80 young participants tested in two previously published studies (Iaria et al., 2003; Etchamendy et al., 2007) in which the same paradigm was used. Only data from the behavioral studies were used for the current study. In total, 175 young adults (84 men, 91 women, mean age: 25.6 ± 4.6 years, age range: 19–40) were tested. Participants were recruited through word of mouth. A sample of 125 older adults (50 men, 75 women, mean age: 66.5 ± 6.6 years, age range: 53–85) were recruited from newspaper and radio ads.

All participants were screened for neurological and psychiatric disorders, including depression. All older adult participants scored above the normative cutoff score for the Mini Mental State Examination (Iverson, 1998). All participants gave written consent to take part in the study. In the case of child participants, written consent was obtained from the parents. The study was approved by the Research Ethics Board at the Douglas Mental Health University Institute and the Sainte-Justine University Hospital Research Center. Participant recruitment and testing was in conformity with the local ethics committee requirements.

### 4 ON 8 VIRTUAL MAZE (4/8VM)

#### *Adult version*

A commercially available computer game (Unreal; Epic Games, Raleigh, NC) was used to create the virtual environments. The virtual tasks were presented on a 17′ computer screen. Before testing, the participants spent a few minutes moving in a virtual room that was different from the experimental environment to practice the motor aspects of the task. When the participants were comfortable using the keypad, the experimenter gave the instructions, and the experiment started.

The 4/8VM is composed of an eight-arm radial maze with a central starting location (**Figure 1**). The maze is surrounded by a landscape (mountains and sunset), two trees, and a short wall located between the landscape and the trees. At the end of each arm are stairs that lead to a pit where, in some of the arms, an object can be picked up. The location of the target objects cannot be seen from the center of the maze. Landmarks in the environment were not located directly in front of the target

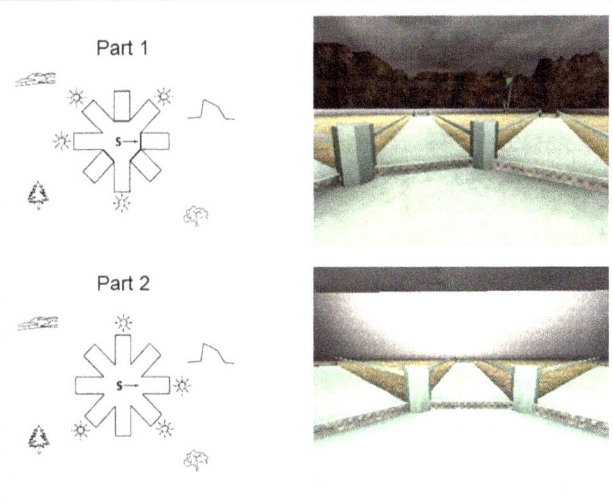


**FIGURE 1 | Schematic drawings (left) and first person views (right) of the adult 4/8VM environment.**

pathways, thereby avoiding the use of a beacon strategy. The participants used a keypad to move forward, left, and right within the environment and were instructed to not use the backwards key. Participants always started a trial at the center of the radial maze facing the same direction. The 4/8VM consisted of five trials, all of which are composed of two parts. In Part 1 of each trial, four arms were blocked with barriers and the remaining four arms were accessible and contain objects. In Part 2, all arms were accessible and the objects were located in the four arms that were previously blocked in Part 1. The participants were asked to retrieve all objects found in the accessible arms in Part 1 and to remember which arms they visited. In Part 2, they were asked to avoid the arms they previously visited in order to find the objects. Errors consisted of entering into an arm that did not contain an object or revisiting an arm. A trial was completed after all four objects were picked up. Among the five trials, there were three types of trials: type A, B, and C. In Part 1 of trial type A, arms 1, 3, 4, and 6 were accessible and contained objects; in Part 2, the four objects were located at the end of the four previously blocked arms (i.e., arms 2, 5, 7, and 8). In trial type B, a different sequence of accessible arms were used. In Part 1, arms 2, 3, 7, and 8 were accessible, and in Part 2 the objects were located at the end of arms 1, 4, 5, and 6. Trial type C was a probe trial. Part 1 of the probe was identical to part 1 of trial type A. In Part 2, however, the walls around the radial maze were raised to conceal the landscape, and the trees were removed so that no landmarks were visible. During part 2 of the probe trial, all of the arms contained an object. The probe trial was used to distinguish whether participants used a spatial or response strategy to learn the task. If participants were using a spatial strategy in which the landmarks present in the environment were relevant to perform the task, removing the landscape and landmarks should result in an increase in errors. In contrast, if participants were using a response strategy, no increase in errors should occur during the probe trial, since participants would remember a pattern or series of turns in relation to a starting position without relying on the landmarks. To reach criterion and to be allowed to take part in the probe trial, participants were required to make no errors on Part 2 in one of the trials before the probe. The learning criterion was set to ensure that participants were able to learn the task before performing the probe trial which evaluates how they learned the task. Participants were presented with sequences in the order of trial type ABACA. For the young and older adults, data from several studies were combined in order to obtain a larger sample size. Although there were design differences for each of the studies, the portion of the 4/8VM used in the current paper was identical in all studies. In one study, 74 participants received the ABACA sequence whereas in another 50, 13 trials were administered after the ABACA sequence for a total of 18 trials. In the current paper only the ABACA sequence was considered. Participants who were not able to complete a trial without error within the first three trials were given up to two extra trials in order to reach criterion. The extra trials were trial type A.

As previously described (Iaria et al., 2003; Bohbot et al., 2007, 2011; Banner et al., 2011; Andersen et al., 2012), the participants were debriefed at the end of the experiment. They were asked to report how they solved the task from the beginning to the end of the experiment. Participants were classified based on their spontaneous navigational strategy. Participants were categorized as using a response strategy if they initially learned the task by associating the arms with numbers or letters, or by counting the arms (clockwise or counterclockwise) from a single starting point. If they initially used two or more landmarks and did not mention a response strategy, they were categorized as using a spatial strategy. Errors on the probe trial were used to confirm navigational strategies in an objective fashion, where spatial learners were expected to make more errors than response learners. A recent eye tracking paper further validated verbal reports as a method of categorization (Andersen et al., 2012). The study showed that spatial learners spend significantly more time looking at landmarks than response learners.

#### *Children's version*

The 4/8VM described above was also used to test children, however the following modifications were necessary in order to obtain a valid test measuring navigational strategies. The environment contained the same eight-arm radial arm maze surrounded by a landscape (mountains and sunset) and two trees, however, additional landmarks were added: a planet, a pyramid, and a pile of boxes. In addition, instead of presenting Part 1 and Part 2 as we did in one trial of the adult version, one trial in the children's version only consisted of Part 2 where all eight arms are accessible and four objects had to be found. Furthermore, only two types of trials were used for the children: trial types A and C (**Figure 2**). This modification was made gradually throughout 1.5 years of pilot studies in order to make the test more easily comprehensible and feasible to 8-years old children. In the children 4/8VM, participants were asked to retrieve all objects from the target arms out of the eight open arms. A trial was completed after all four objects were picked up. The target arms were the same arms as those used in the adult version (2, 5, 7, and 8). Due to time constraints, participants were given at most either 10 (version 1, $N = 51$) or 13 trials (version 2, $N = 209$) to learn the target arms (2, 5, 7, and 8) to criteria. As in the adult version, at the beginning

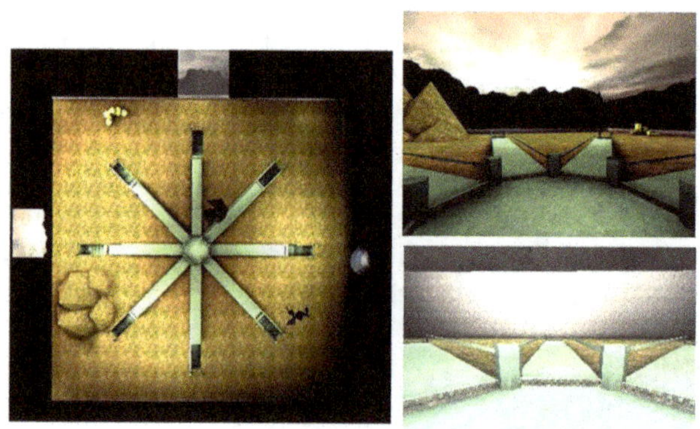

**FIGURE 2 | Top down (left) and first person (right) views of the children 4/8VM environment.**

of each trial, participants started in the center of the maze facing the same direction. To reach criteria, participants were required to have completed three out of four trials without error. Participants were therefore required to complete a minimum of three trials. For the participants who reached criteria, a second stage of the task, the probe trial (type C), was presented. In the probe trial, similar to the adult version, walls were raised to conceal the landscape and all landmarks were removed. An object was present in every arm. As in the adult version of this task, the purpose of the probe trial was to distinguish the participants who relied on landmarks (i.e., used a spatial strategy) from participants who learned the pattern of target arms irrespective of landmarks (i.e., used a response strategy).

After participants completed the virtual radial arm maze, they were asked how they found each of the objects, following a similar procedure as in adults. Participants were categorized as using a response strategy when they mentioned numbering or counting arms from a given start position, in order to find all the objects (i.e., "I went down the arm directly ahead, the one next to it, then skipped two arms to the right, then skipped one arm"). On the other hand, if participants mentioned at least two landmarks and did not mention using a pattern (i.e., "One was beside the pyramid, one on each side of the tree and one next to the Earth"), they were categorized as using a spatial strategy. The self-reports from the children were less detailed than those of the young and older adults. In order to prevent misclassifications, verbal reports that were ambiguous (e.g., when participants could only report a strategy to find one or two of the goal arms) or did not describe a strategy (e.g., "I just remembered where the arms were") were excluded. This method of categorization proved to be effective, as we were able to classify 86.48% of our participants.

Errors on the probe trial were used to confirm navigational strategies in an objective fashion. Again, participants using a spatial strategy were expected to make more errors that those using a response strategy, since they relied more on landmarks to find the objects.

In summary, as in the adult study, children were required to remember the position of four objects located in four of the eight arms during acquisition of the task and were required to reach criterion before the administration of the probe trial. The probe trial was used to assess navigational strategy and involved having to retrieve four objects in four of the eight arms in an environment devoid of landmarks and with a hidden landscape.

### ANALYSIS

All analyses were done using SPSS version 15.0 and Microsoft Office Excel 2003. For all participants, task performance was measured by analyzing the total number of errors made when participants had to remember which of the eight open arms contained objects (i.e., Part 2 of each trial). Part 1 errors were not taken into account because errors in a four-arm environment do not provide a sensitive measure of learning and memory for adults and because Part 1 was not administered to children.

During the probe trial, most of the participants in all age groups had the impulse to look around before making their selection and lost their initial heading. Consequently, the pattern of visited arms was used to score errors on the probe trial instead of using the actual arms in absolute space. This was assessed by rotating the pattern of visited arms until we obtained the best match. This method allowed us to distinguish individuals who had learned the pattern of arms (i.e., the response learners) from those who had used the spatial strategy. Specifically, we calculated a probe error term by considering what the number of errors would be if the goal arms were rotated to new positions around the radial arm maze. For example, the goal arms in absolute space were 2, 5, 7, and 8. If a participant initially turned 12.5° clockwise (one arm) and followed the learned relationships between the goal arms thereby making zero errors, they would enter arms 3, 6, 8, and 1, which, if errors were considered in absolute space, would result in three errors. The goal arms were rotated seven times for each possible initial shift in point of view. The best probe error term was then used for further data analysis for all participants. Based on all the possible combinations a participant can make, there is an 8.6% chance of getting two errors randomly, 11.4% chance of getting zero errors randomly, and 80% chance of making one error. Therefore, the mean rotational errors someone can make if they choose randomly is one. Verbal reports were scored by two independent raters showing a 99% agreement in the assessment of strategies for older adults, 93% for young adults and 93% for children.

## RESULTS

### PERFORMANCE

#### *Children*

Of these 299 children tested on the virtual radial arm maze, 281 had verbal report and we were able to assess spontaneous strategy in 243 children in total. Of the 299 original participants, 14 children were given the possibility to make 16 choices per trial instead of eight choices. Their verbal reports were analyzed but, to avoid any bias, their performance on the acquisition of the task was not included in the analysis. Among the remaining 285 children tested on the same version of the task (eight choices maximum per trial), 25 participants were excluded due to nausea ($N = 7$), failure to cooperate ($N = 10$), experimental error in administering the task ($N = 1$), and failure to complete the task within the allotted time ($N = 7$). The final sample used for analysis ($N = 260$) consisted of 134 boys and 126 girls and the average age for boys and girls combined was $8.43 \pm 0.11$ years old.

In total, of the 260 children who completed the study, 205 (78.8%) reached criteria, and 199 completed the probe; six participants who reached criteria did not complete the probe due to time constraints. Children made an average of 6.36 errors ($SD = 3.53$) on the first trial, 3.83 errors ($SD = 1.79$) on the second trial, and 3.05 errors ($SD = 2.08$) on the third trial. Of the 299 children tested, we were able to classify the spontaneous strategies of 243 participants. Of the 243 children, 205 used a spatial strategy (84.4%) and only 38 (15.6%) reported using a response strategy. Children's learning strategy had a profound effect on performance during the probe trial, confirming that our assessment of navigational strategy is consistent with errors on the probe trial. Those that reported using a response strategy made significantly fewer probe errors than those who reported using a spatial strategy, (response mean $= 0.69$, $SD = 0.59$; spatial mean $= 0.90$, $SD = 0.65$; one-tail independent samples $t$-test, $p < 0.05$), indicating that response learners relied less on environmental landmarks than spatial learners.

Note that among the 260 children included in the analysis, 51 children were given at most 10 trials (version 1) to reach criteria while 209 were given 13 trials (version 2) to reach criteria. The version of the task did not influence the proportion of children who reached criteria (80.4% in version 1 and 78.5% in version 2) or the average number of errors made during the first 3 trials ($4.6 \pm 1.7$ in version 1 and $4.4 \pm 1.7$ in version 2). The strategy spontaneously used by the children was also not affected by the version of the task. Spatial strategy was used by 93.2% of the children who were tested on version 1 and 82.01% of the children who were tested on version 2 (chi-square, $p > 0.05$). Taken together, these results indicate that the number of trials given to reach criteria did not influence neither the acquisition of the task nor the strategy used to solve it. Children data from both versions were therefore pooled together for the analyses.

#### Young adults

Of the 175 young adults, seven young adults did not meet criteria by the third trial. At the time of testing these participants were not given extra trials to learn the task before the probe, and therefore their probe performance were not considered in the analysis. Of the 175 young adults, error scores on the learning trials were not available for five participants, however, these participants reached criteria and therefore their strategy and probe scores were included in the analysis. In addition, eight participants did not perform the probe trial although criterion was met.

Young adults made an average of 1.54 errors ($SD = 2.27$) on the first trial (Trial type A), 0.45 errors ($SD = 1.15$) on the second trial (Trial type B), and 0.37 errors ($SD = 0.9$) on the third trial (Trial type A). Of the 175 young adults, 81 (46.3%) reported the use of a spatial strategy and 94 (53.7%) reported using a response strategy. These percentages are consistent with previous reports (Iaria et al., 2003; Etchamendy et al., 2007). Strategy predicted the number of errors made on the probe trial (one-tail independent samples $t$-test $t = -3.308$, $p < 0.001$), whereby response learners made fewer probe errors than spatial learners (response mean $= 0.18$, $SD = 0.45$, spatial mean $= 0.47$, $SD = 0.6$), confirming once again that our assessment of navigational strategy is consistent with errors on the probe trial.

#### Older adults

From the sample of 125 participants, 13 participants in total were excluded due to nausea ($N = 4$), failure to complete the task within the allotted time ($N = 5$) and failure to comprehend the task ($N = 4$). We were able to assess spontaneous strategy in 112 older adults (46 men, 66 women; mean age: $66.5 \pm 6.7$ years).

Of the 112 older adults, 32 subjects did not reach criteria within the first three trials and needed extra trials, of those 16 older adults never met criteria and did not do the probe trial. Older adults made an average of 2.92 errors ($SD = 2.88$) on the first trial (Trial type A), 2.37 errors ($SD = 2.58$) on the second trial (Trial type B), 1.82 errors ($SD = 2.6$) on the third trial (Trial type A). Of the 125 older adults tested, we were able to classify the spontaneous strategies of 112 participants. Of these 112 older adults, only 44 (39.3%) reported the use of a spatial strategy and 68 (60.7%) reported the use of a response strategy. Reported strategy predicted the number of probe errors (response mean $= 0.37$ errors, $SD = 0.55$; spatial mean $= 0.72$ errors; $SD = 0.70$; one-tail independent samples $t$-test $t = 2.76$, $p < 0.01$), confirming once again that our assessment of navigational strategy is consistent with errors on the probe trial. In the event that giving additional trials could influence navigational strategy, a separate analysis was performed with only the older adult participants who reached criteria in three trials. Results showed that the proportion of spatial and response learners did not differ from the whole group analysis: 62.4% used a response strategy and 37.6% used a spatial strategy. Therefore, giving older adult participants extra trials did not affect their navigational strategy. In support of these findings, giving extra trials to children did not increase their rate of using a response strategy. We further argue that a shift toward response strategies only occurs with over-training, after participants perform the task to criteria.

#### Children, young adults and older adults

When looking at all of the participants, 199 children, 160 young adults, and 96 older adults reached criteria and performed the probe trial. There was a significant difference in performance between children, young adults, and older adults on the first three learning trials [$F_{(2,\ 540)} = 298.76$; $p < 0.0001$]. During the learning trials, participants had to avoid the arms that they had previously visited in order to retrieve the objects. Young adults made significantly fewer errors than the older adults and both groups performed significantly better than the children (*post-hoc* tests: $p < 0.001$). All participants who met criteria obtained a perfect score in at least one learning trial before the probe. On the last trial, children that reached criteria and did the probe made no errors. Older adults made an average of 0.65 errors ($SD = 1.89$) and young adults made an average of 0.37 errors ($SD = 0.9$) on the last trial before the probe.

### STRATEGY

#### Children

Among the 199 children who reached criteria and did the probe, we were able to assess spontaneous strategy in 191 participants. Within these 191 children, we found that 83.3% were spatial learners and 16.7% were response learners. These proportions are similar to those found when looking at the 281 participants who had verbal report and no probe score. Strategy did not predict performance on the acquisition of the 4/8VM (before the probe trial). Strategy did not influence the number of errors made during the first three trials (independent samples $t$-test, $p > 0.05$). Similarly, strategy did not affect the number of trials needed to reach criteria (independent samples $t$-test, $p > 0.05$ in both versions of the task). There was no relationship between sex and strategy in the children population (chi-squared, $p > 0.05$).

#### Young adults

As in the children sample, strategy did not predict the number of errors made during the first three trials [$F_{(2,\ 167)} =$

0.065, $p > 0.05$]. There was no relationship between sex and strategy in the young adult population (chi-square, $p > 0.05$).

#### Older adults

Strategy had no effect on performance as measured by the number of errors made in the first three trials [$F_{(2, 107)} = 0.28$; $p > 0.05$]. Strategy also did not predict the decrease in errors between the first and second A trials ($t = 0.208$; $p > 0.05$). Strategy did not interact with older adults' ability to reach criteria by the third trial (chi-square; $p > 0.05$). There was no relationship between sex and strategy in the older adult population (chi-square, $p > 0.05$).

#### Comparison of the strategies of children, young adults, and older adults

A 3×2 chi-square (children, young adults, older adults × spatial, response) was used to compare the proportion of spatial and response learners across all age groups. The chi-squared analysis revealed a significant interaction [$\chi^2 = 94.69$, $p < 0.0001$] between age and strategy, with a decrease in the use of a spatial strategy throughout the lifespan: 84.4% of children, 46.3% of young adults, and only 39.3% of older adults reported the use of a spatial strategy (**Figure 3**). *Post-hoc* analysis revealed a significant difference in the proportion of spatial and response learners between children and young adults [$\chi^2 = 68.26$, $p < 0.0001$] and children and older adults [$\chi^2 = 74.38$, $p < 0.0001$]. There was no significant difference in the proportion of spatial and response learners between young and older adults [$\chi^2 = 1.361$, $p > 0.05$].

The probe trial was successful at discriminating between spatial and response strategies. A 3 × 2 ANOVA (age × strategy) revealed a significant main effect of strategy on probe performance [$F_{(2, 447)} = 9.96$, $p < 0.001$]. As anticipated, there was no interaction between age and strategy because response learners performed better than spatial learners on the probe trial across all ages [$F_{(1, 447)} = 0.221$, $p = 0.638$]. In order for the groups to be comparable, a normalized error term was calculated for each individual such that the average probe error equals one in each group. **Figure 4** shows the normalized probe errors according to strategy and age group.

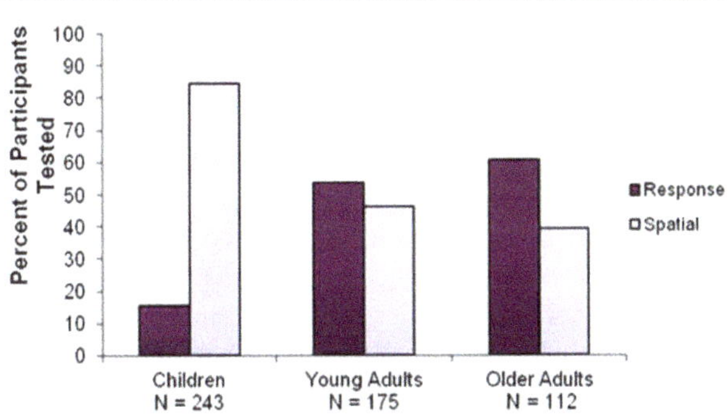


**FIGURE 3 | Percentage of participants using a spatial or response strategy according to age group.** This graph shows that the use of response strategies increases across the life span, at the expense of spatial strategies.

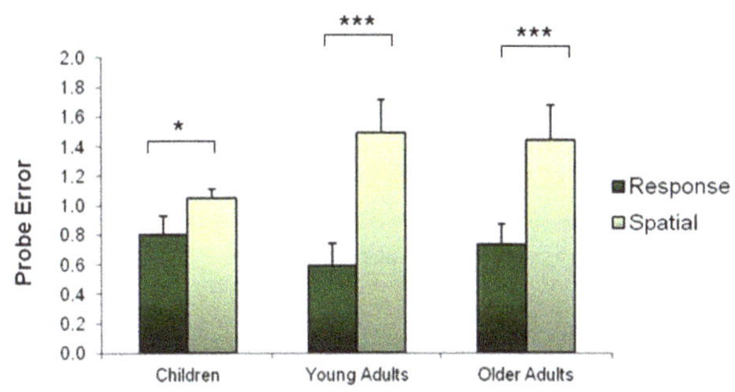


**FIGURE 4 | Normalized mean number of probe errors according to strategy and age group.** This graph shows that probe errors were effective at dissociating spatial and response strategies: spatial learners made more errors on the probe trial than response learners. Error bars represent standard error of the mean. *$p < 0.05$; ***$p < 0.001$.

## DISCUSSION

Our findings demonstrate a shift in navigational strategy across the lifespan (**Figure 3**). We found that 84% of children reported using a spatial strategy, indicating a clear bias compared to the 47% of young adults who reported using the same strategy. We also observed that 39% of older adults used a spatial strategy. Moreover, we found that response learners performed better on the probe than spatial learners in every age group, a finding which extends the results of previous studies carried out in young adults (Iaria et al., 2003; Bohbot et al., 2007) to children and older adults (**Figure 4**). These results suggest that, across all age groups, the probe trial was effective in discriminating spatial learners who relied on environmental landmarks from response learners who were not as affected by the removal of landmarks.

Young adults performed better than older adults on trials 1, 2, and 3, which is consistent with general navigational deficits that have been observed in normal aging (Marighetto et al., 1999; Driscoll et al., 2005). While some caudate nucleus-dependent deficits have been observed with aging (Barrash, 1994; Wilkniss et al., 1997; Meulenbroek et al., 2004; Raz and Rodrigue, 2006; Head and Isom, 2010), human and animal studies show that these deficits are milder or relatively spared in old age (Vasquez et al., 1983; Grady and Craik, 2000; Churchill et al., 2003). Bach et al. (1999) tested young and old mice on a Barnes circular maze and found that old mice had deficits in spatial memory compared to young mice. The same study also showed that on a cued version of the same task, a version that requires the formation of stimulus-response associations, aged mice performed similar to young mice, demonstrating the sparing of response learning with age. Interestingly, during learning, after the initial random exploration, aged mice adapted a serial search strategy that does not rely on the hippocampus while young mice adapted a spatial search strategy dependent on the hippocampus. Rapp et al. (1997) found similar results in monkeys where older monkeys used a serial search strategy compared to young monkeys. Authors also found that older monkeys were not affected by the removal of external maze cues, demonstrating their lack of reliance on spatial landmarks. Our study translates these results to humans and reveals a more complex picture for cognitive aging. The deficit seen in normal older adults in the current study is paralleled with a shift toward using response strategies, an effect first demonstrated in rats by Barnes et al. (1980). Response strategies are efficient when navigating in an environment where the start and target locations are constant, as in route learning paradigms (Hartley et al., 2003; Iaria et al., 2003; Head and Isom, 2010). In contrast, when the relationship between the start and target position changes and a novel path must be derived, response strategies are inefficient (Hartley et al., 2003; Driscoll et al., 2005). Deriving a novel path from different start and target locations requires knowledge of a cognitive map, making the use of spatial strategies more efficient. The drive toward efficiency may be an important underlying factor behind the shift in strategies with normal aging. With the repetition of a successful behavior, a response strategy emerges, leading to the automatization of behavior or habit formation (Iaria et al., 2003). However, this shift toward response strategies comes at a cost when a novel path must be derived using a cognitive map in order to navigate successfully.

Other lifestyle factors can produce a shift from using spatial strategies to response strategies with aging. For example, stress, as well as addiction related rewards such as nicotine, opiates, psychostimulants, and alcohol have been shown to affect the integrity of the hippocampus. Stress was reported to impair the hippocampus through the actions of glucocorticoids (Sapolsky et al., 1990; Sapolsky, 1994; McEwen and Sapolsky, 1995; Conrad et al., 1996; McKittrick et al., 2000; Kleen et al., 2006) and was shown to have an effect on navigational strategies. Schwabe et al. (2007, 2008, 2010, 2012) found that chronic stress, acute stress, and prenatal stress can increase the use of response strategies in people tested on a navigation task. Taking into consideration the inverse relationship between hippocampus and caudate nucleus gray matter (Bohbot et al., 2007) and the fact that rewards stimulate the caudate nucleus, we can expect the probability of using caudate nucleus-dependent response strategies to be higher in people exhibiting reward-seeking behaviors. Supportive evidence is found in a study showing that rewards lead to increased goal-oriented navigation and decreased free exploration, the latter of which is characteristic of spatial memory, in healthy adults performing a virtual water maze task (Adcock, 2010). These studies demonstrate that stress and reward can promote the use of response strategies.

Children, including both spatial and response learners had a higher number of probe errors than adult spatial and response learners. These data support the finding that children preferentially use their hippocampus to navigate, since high probe errors have been shown to be associated with greater hippocampal involvement (Iaria et al., 2003). Even the children that used caudate nucleus-dependent response strategies over hippocampus-dependent spatial strategies showed higher probe deficits as compared to young adults, suggesting that response learning may also be immature at 8 years of age. As an alternative to the view that the striatum is mature by childhood (Reber, 1992; Maybery and O'Brien-Malone, 1998), we propose that response learning, especially in difficult tasks, may also continue to develop through childhood and adolescence (Casey et al., 2002; Sowell et al., 2002; Thomas et al., 2004). Although children are capable of using patterns to learn, the pattern formation required in the current task that leads to the use of a response strategy, is much more sophisticated compared to a simple "egocentric" strategy, involving a single vector addition from a given position, reported in numerous children studies (Overman et al., 1996; Bremner and Bryant, 1977). As opposed to navigating toward a beacon, successful probe performance in our task requires participants to keep in memory a sequence of movements through virtual space. In other tasks that require more complex sequence learning, children have been shown to be impaired relative to adults and there is increased activation in the caudate nucleus when age is correlated with performance (Thomas et al., 2004). Though children may be capable of using an egocentric strategy from a very young age, even before the emergence of spatial strategies (Lehnung et al., 1998), the complex pattern of stimulus-response associations required in the current task seems to evolve later on.

Unlike previous reports that used tasks for which all adults used a spatial strategy (Bullens et al., 2010), we have shown that in learning situations where young adults are equally likely to adopt a spatial strategy or a response strategy, children are biased toward using spatial strategies. It is of interest that we found spatial strategies dominating in childhood, since these results show a bias toward hippocampal-based learning in the early stages of life, despite the immaturity of the hippocampus (Saitoh et al., 2001; Pine et al., 2002; Mulani et al., 2005; Lavenex et al., 2007). We recently replicated these findings in children using identical testing environments. We showed that 7–9 years old children use spatial strategies in greater proportions than older participants who in this case were older children 10–18 years of age (Lin et al., 2012). The caudate nucleus is a slow learning system that develops habits through repetition across a session (Iaria et al., 2003; Orban et al., 2006), days (Packard and McGaugh, 1996; Barnes et al., 2005), and potentially much longer periods of time depending on the complexity of the task. In childhood, most experiences are new and thus children have a smaller repertoire of habits because they have less experience in the world than adults. We hypothesize that this paucity of repetitive behavior is the reason we found a smaller proportion of children using caudate nucleus-dependant response learning and a greater percentage using hippocampal-based spatial learning. Interestingly, in young preweanling rats, the existence of place, head-direction, and grid cells have been shown even before rat pups begin exploring an environment. This finding demonstrates that the mechanisms necessary for building cognitive maps exist early on in development (Wills et al., 2010).

The traditional view that older adults tend to use response strategies because of an aging process, which negatively affects the hippocampus, suggests a compensatory mechanism for this shift in strategies (Etchamendy et al., 2012). We offer an alternate hypothesis whereby a shift in navigational strategy with time is a consequence of the increased use of the caudate nucleus-based response learning in older adults (Balram et al., 2010). We suggest that it is biologically adaptive for the caudate nucleus to automatize frequently repeated behavioral and cognitive processes such as learning how to walk, in order to free up cognitive resources (Albouy et al., 2008, 2012). This process, however, will result in a bias toward the memory encoding strategies dependent on the caudate nucleus and decrease the need to make novel relationships between multiple stimuli, a process which requires the hippocampus (Eichenbaum et al., 1992). With aging, people often gain expertise in a specific field through professional and personal life experiences. Gaining expertise, however, often involves carrying out processes faster and more efficiently. We argue that repetitive day-to-day behavior decreases the likelihood of experiencing difficult and long processes normally required for learning new things.

Normal aging is accompanied by a decrease in hippocampal volume and functional activity, which is associated with navigational deficits (Driscoll et al., 2005) in spatial memory tasks (Moffat et al., 2006; Antonova et al., 2009; Chen et al., 2010; Head and Isom, 2010). We suggest that decreases in hippocampal volume and activity could be a consequence of increased use of response strategies. In fact, recent studies by Rodgers et al. (2012) and Etchamendy et al. (2012) showed that a larger proportion of older adults use response strategies compared to young adults. When middle age healthy participants (mean age = $43.0 \pm 5.9$ years) were tested as a control group for patients with damage to the hippocampus in Bohbot et al. (2004), 85% used a response strategy on the 4/8VM. Although in the current study we did not find a direct difference in the proportion of spatial and response learners between young and older adults this may in part be due to stringent screening for various disorders, more common in older adults than in young adults. In Bohbot et al. (2004) healthy participants were recruited by word of mouth and were often spouses of the brain-damaged patients because they were balanced for age, education and socio-economic status. On the other hand, participants recruited for studies comparing young and older adults have to be screened for numerous factors. This screening process results in a greater exclusion rate in older adults than in young adults making the older adult population a very healthy sample, free of neurological, psychiatric, metabolic (e.g., heart attack, cholesterol, diabetes), and chronic diseases (e.g., cancer). As previously mentioned, the automatization of behavior may be a biologically adaptive mechanism that permits us to free up resources, such as hippocampal function. However, less hippocampal engagement may lead to decreased hippocampal gray matter and volume, which is associated with cognitive deficits in normal aging and is a risk factor for developing dementia (Lupien et al., 1998; Tisserand et al., 2004). This suggestion fits with the finding that years of education lowers the risk of developing dementia (Ravaglia et al., 2002; Karp et al., 2004; Caamano-Isorna et al., 2006), presumably because the hippocampus was involved in making novel relationships for a longer period of time while people were learning new information. Thus, having more years of education may play a role in delaying the shift toward response strategies. Similarly, James et al. (2011) found that people with a larger life space, measured by more movement through the Chicago area during their daily activities, have a decreased risk of developing dementia. Longitudinal studies of successful aging have also highlighted the importance of participating in everyday activities which require the learning of novel information (Hultsch et al., 1999), a finding which gives credence to the "use it or lose it" hypothesis presented here. In support of these studies, our mouse imaging study showed an inverse relationship between gray matter in the hippocampus and striatum when mice trained on a spatial memory version of the water maze were contrasted to mice trained on the response memory version in absence of the possibility of using spatial strategies because landmarks were hidden with a curtain (Lerch et al., 2011). In sum, the use of spatial strategies may have protective effects on the hippocampus.

In conclusion, with age, people who use response strategies to a great extent in their everyday life may be more at risk of developing cognitive deficits in normal aging and dementia (Dossa et al., 2010), through increased caudate-dependent learning and decreased hippocampal-dependent processing. An emphasis on cognitive mapping may increase the functioning and gray matter of the hippocampus, both of which increase the probability of healthy and successful aging. Thus, reversing the shift toward response strategies that comes with age with spatial memory training may be an effective method of prevention against cognitive decline and dementia.

## ACKNOWLEDGMENTS

This project was funded CIHR Grant, #64381, #82638, #86727, and CIHR New Emerging Team KIDNET. We wish to thank Louisa Dahmani for her help with the manuscript.

## REFERENCES

Adcock, A. (2010). "Memory in service of goals: affective neuromodulation and mnemonic salince maps," in *Cognitive Neuroscience Society 2010 Meeting Abstracts*, (Montreal, QC).

Albouy, G., Sterpenich, V., Balteau, E., Vandewalle, G., Desseilles, M., Dang-Vu, T., et al. (2008). Both the hippocampus and striatum are involved in consolidation of motor sequence memory. *Neuron* 58,261–272.

Albouy, G., Sterpenich, V., Vandewalle, G., Darsaud, A., Gais, S., Rauchs, G., et al. (2012). Neural corre- lates of performance variability dur- ing motor sequence acquisition. *Neuroimage* 60, 324–331.

Andersen, N. E., Dahmani, L., Konishi, K., and Bohbot, V. D. (2012). Eye tracking, strategies, and sex differences in virtual naviga- tion. *Neurobiol. Learn. Mem.* 97, 81–89.

Antonova, E., Parslow, D., Brammer, M., Dawson, G. R., Jackson, S. H., and Morris, R. G. (2009). Age- related neural activity during allo- centric spatial memory. *Memory* 17, 125–143.

Bach, M. E., Barad, M., Son, H., Zhuo, M., Lu, Y. F., Shih, R., et al. (1999). Age-related defects in spatial memory are correlated with defects in the late phase of hippocam- pal long-term potentiation *in vitro* and are attenuated by drugs that enhance the cAMP signaling path- way. *Proc. Natl. Acad. Sci. U.S.A.* 96, 5280–5285.

Balram, B., Etchamendy, N., and Bohbot, V. D. (2010). "Cultural differences in spontaneous virtual navigation strategies in aging: a higher proportion of Japanese people use spatial strategies com- pared to North Americans," in *Society for Neuroscience 2010 Abstracts*, (San Diego, CA).

Banner, H., Bhat, V., Etchamendy, N., Joober, R., and Bohbot, V. D. (2011). The brain-derived neurotrophic factor Val66Met polymorphism is associated with reduced functional magnetic res- onance imaging activity in the hippocampus and increased use of caudate nucleus-dependent strate- gies in a human virtual navigation task. *Eur. J. Neurosci.* 33,968–977.

Barnes, C. A., Nadel, L., and Honig, W. K. (1980). Spatial memory deficit in senescent rats. *Can. J. Psychol.* 34, 29–39.

Barnes, T. D., Kubota, Y., Hu, D., Jin, D. Z., and Graybiel, A. M. (2005). Activity of striatal neurons reflects dynamic encoding and recoding of procedural memories. *Nature* 437, 1158–1161.

Barrash, J. (1994). Age-related decline in route learning ability. *Dev. Neuropsychol.* 10, 189–201.

Bohbot, V. D., Gupta, M., Banner, H., and Dahmani, L. (2011). nucleus-dependent response strate- gies in a virtual navigation task are associated with lower basal corti- sol and impaired episodic mem- ory. *Neurobiol. Learn. Mem.* 96, 173–180.

Bohbot, V. D., Iaria, G., and Petrides, M. (2004). Hippocampal function and spatial memory: evidence from functional neuroimaging in healthy participants and performance of patients with medial temporal lobe resections. *Neuropsychology* 18, 418–425.

Bohbot, V. D., Lerch, J., Thorndycraft, B., Iaria, G., and Zijdenbos, A. P. (2007). Gray matter differ- ences correlate with spontaneous strategies in a human virtual navigation task. *J. Neurosci.* 27, 10078–10083.

Bremner, J. G., and Bryant, P. E. (1977). Place versus response as the basis of spatial errors made by young infants. *J. Exp. Child Psychol.* 23, 162–171.

Bullens, J., Igloi, K., Berthoz, A., Postma, A., and Rondi-Reig, L. (2010). Developmental time course of the acquisition of sequential ego- centric and allocentric navigation strategies. *J. Exp. Child Psychol.* 107, 337–350.

Caamano-Isorna, F., Corral, M., Montes-Martinez, A., and Takkouche, B. (2006). Education and dementia: a meta-analytic study. *Neuroepidemiology* 26, 226–232.

Cabeza, R. (2002). Hemispheric asym- metry reduction in older adults: the HAROLD model. *Psychol. Aging* 17, 85–100.

Casey, B. J., Thomas, K. M., Davidson, M. C., Kunz, K., and Franzen, P. L. (2002). Dissociating striatal and hippocampal function develop- mentally with a stimulus-response compatibility task. *J. Neurosci.* 22, 8647–8652.

Chen, K. H., Chuah, L. Y., Sim, K., and Chee, M. W. (2010). Hippocampal region-specific con- tributions to memory performance in normal elderly. *Brain Cogn.* 72, 400–407.

Churchill, J. D., Stanis, J. J., Press, C., Kushelev, M., and Greenough, W. (2003). Is procedural memory relatively spared from age effects? *Neurobiol. Aging* 24, 883–892.

Conrad, C., Galea, L., Kuroda, Y., and McEwen, B. (1996). Chronic stress impairs rat spatial memory on the Y maze, and this effect is blocked by tianeptine pretreatment. *Behav. Neurosci.* 110, 1321–1334.

Dossa, F., Tau, M., Etchamendy, N., and Bohbot, V. D. (2010). "The use of a hippocampal-dependent spatial memory strategy in aging is associated with reduced risks of dementia assessed with the MoCA in healthy older adults," in *Society for Neuroscience 2010 Abstracts*, (San Diego, CA).

Driscoll, I., Hamilton, D. A., Yeo, R. A., Brooks, W. M., and Sutherland, R. J. (2005). Virtual navigation in humans: the impact of age, sex, and hormones on place learning. *Horm. Behav.* 47, 326–335.

Eichenbaum, H., Otto, T., and Cohen, N. J. (1992). The hippocampus- what does it do? *Behav. Neural Biol.* 57, 2–36.

Etchamendy, N., Konishi, K., Pike, G. B., Marighetto, A., and Bohbot, V. D. (2012). Evidence for a virtual human analog of a rodent relational memory task: a study of aging and fMRI in young adults. *Hippocampus* 22, 869–880.

Etchamendy, N., Pike, B., Marighetto, A., Zijdenbos, A., and Bohbot, V. D. (2007). "Hippocampal contri- bution to memory accross mice and humans in an fMRI study," in *Society for Neuroscience 2007 Abstracts*, (San Diego, CA).

Gold, P. E. (2004). Coordination of multiple memory systems. *Neurobiol. Learn. Mem.* 82, 230–242.

Grady, C. L., and Craik, F. I. (2000). Changes in memory processing with age. *Curr. Opin. Neurobiol.* 10, 224–231.

Hartley, T., Maguire, E. A., Spiers, H. J., and Burgess, N. (2003). The well-worn route and the path less traveled: distinct neu- ral bases of route following and wayfinding in humans. *Neuron* 37, 877–888.

Head, D., and Isom, M. (2010). Age effects on wayfinding and route learning skills. *Behav. Brain Res.* 209, 49–58.

Hultsch, D. F., Hertzog, C., Small, B. J., and Dixon, R. A. (1999). Use it or lose it: engaged lifestyle as a buffer of cognitive decline in aging? *Psychol. Aging* 14, 245–263.

Iaria, G., Petrides, M., Dagher, A., Pike, B., and Bohbot, V. D. (2003). Cognitive strategies depen- dent on the hippocampus and caudate nucleus in human nav- igation: variability and change with practice. *J. Neurosci.* 23, 5945–5952.

Iverson, G. L. (1998). Interpretation of Mini-Mental State Examination scores in community-dwelling elderly and geriatric neuropsy- chiatry patients. *Int. J. Geriatr. Psychiatry* 13, 661–666.

James, B. D., Boyle, P. A., Buchman, A. S., Barnes, L. L., and Bennett, D. A. (2011). Life space and risk of Alzheimer disease, mild cognitive impairment, and cognitive decline in old age. *Am. J. Geriatr. Psychiatry* 19, 961–969.

Jernigan, T. L., Archibald, S. L., Fennema-Notestine, C., Gamst, A. C., Stout, J. C., Bonner, J., et al. (2001). Effects of age on tissues and regions of the cerebrum and cerebellum. *Neurobiol. Aging* 22, 581–594.

Jernigan, T. L., and Gamst, A. C. (2005). Changes in volume with age– consistency and interpretation of observed effects. *Neurobiol. Aging* 26, 1271–1274. discussion: 1275–1278.

Karp, A., Kareholt, I., Qiu, C., Bellander, T., Winblad, B., and Fratiglioni, L. (2004). Relation of education and occupation-based socioeconomic status to inci- dent Alzheimer's disease. *Am. J. Epidemiol.* 159, 175–183.

Kleen, J., Sitomer, M., Killeen, P., and Conrad, C. (2006). Chronic stress impairs spatial memory and moti- vation for reward without disrupt- ing motor ability and motivation to explore. *Behav. Neurosci.* 120, 842–851.

Lavenex, P., Banta Lavenex, P., and Amaral, D. G. (2007). Postnatal development of the primate hip- pocampal formation. *Dev. Neurosci.* 29, 179–192.

Lehnung, M., Leplow, B., Friege, L., Herzog, A., Ferstl, R., and Mehdorn, M. (1998). Development of spatial memory and spatial orientation in preschoolers and primary school children. *Br. J. Psychol.* 89(Pt 3), 463–480.

Leplow, B., Lehnung, M., Pohl, J., Herzog, A., Ferstl, R., and Mehdorn, M. (2003). Navigational place learning in children and young adults as assessed with a standardized loco- motor search task. *Br. J. Psychol.* 94(Pt3), 299–317.

Lerch, J. P., Yiu, A. P., Martinez- Canabal, A., Pekar, T., Bohbot, V. D., Frankland, P. W., et al. (2011). Maze training in mice induces MRI-detectable brain shape changes specific to the type of learning. *Neuroimage* 54, 2086–2095.

Lin, S. Y., Calcott, A., Germann, J., Konishi, K., Bohbot, V. D., and Lerch, J. P. (2012). "Decreased use of hippocampus–dependent spatial strategy in favor of cau- date nucleus-dependent response strategy from childhood to adoles- cence," in *Society for Neuroscience 2012 Abstracts*, (New Orleans, LA).

Lupien, S. J., de Leon, M., de Santi, S., Convit, A., Tarshish, C., Nair, N. P., et al. (1998). Cortisol levels during human aging predict hippocampal atrophy and memory deficits. *Nat. Neurosci.* 1, 69–73.

Maguire, E. A., and Frith, C. D. (2003). Aging affects the engage- ment of the hippocampus during autobiographical mem- ory retrieval. *Brain* 126(Pt 7), 1511–1523.

Marighetto, A., Etchamendy, N., Touzani, K., Torrea, C. C., Yee, B. K., Rawlins, J. N., et al. (1999). Knowing which and knowing what: a potential mouse model for age-related human declarative memory decline. *Eur. J. Neurosci.* 11, 3312–3322.

Maybery, M., and O'Brien-Malone, A. (1998). "Implicit and automatic processes in cognitive develop- ment," in *Implicit and Explicit Mental Processes*, eds K. Kirsner, C. Speelman, M. Mayberry, A. O'Brien-Malone, M. Anderson, and C. McLeod (Mahwah, NJ: Erlbaum), 149–170.

McDonald, R. J., and White, N. M. (1993). A triple dissociation of memory systems: hippocampus, amygdala, and dorsal striatum. *Behav. Neurosci.* 107, 3–22.

McEwen, B., and Sapolsky, R. (1995). Stress and cognitive function. *Curr. Opin. Neurobiol.* 5, 205–216.

McKittrick, C., Magariños, A., Blanchard, D., Blanchard, R., McEwen, B., and Sakai, R. (2000). Chronic social stress reduces dendritic arbors in CA3 of hip- pocampus and decreases binding to serotonin transporter sites. *Synapse* 36, 85–94.

Menon, V., Boyett-Anderson, J. M., and Reiss, A. L. (2005). Maturation of medial temporal lobe response and connectivity during memory encoding. *Brain Res. Cogn. Brain Res.* 25, 379–385.

Meulenbroek, O., Petersson, K. M., Voermans, N., Weber, B., and Fernandez, G. (2004). Age differences in neural correlates of route encoding and route recognition. *Neuroimage* 22, 1503–1514.

Moffat, S. D., Elkins, W., and Resnick, S. M. (2006). Age differences in the neural systems supporting human allocentric spatial navigation. *Neurobiol. Aging* 27, 965–972.

Moffat, S. D., Kennedy, K. M., Rodrigue, K. M., and Raz, N. (2007). Extrahippocampal contri- butions to age differences in human spatial navigation. *Cereb. Cortex* 17, 1274–1282.

Mulani, S. J., Kothare, S. V., and Patkar, D. P. (2005). Magnetic res- onance volumetric analysis of hip- pocampi in children in the age group of 6-to-12 years: a pilot study. *Neuroradiology* 47, 552–557.

Newman, M., and Kaszniak, A. (2000). Spatial memory and aging: per- formance on a human analog of the Morris water maze. *Aging Neuropsychol. Cogn.* 7, 86–93.

Nicolle, M. M., Prescott, S., and Bizon, J. L. (2003). Emergence of a cue strategy preference on the water maze task in aged C57B6 x SJL F1 hybrid mice. *Learn. Mem.* 10, 520–524.

O'Keefe, J., and Nadel, L. (1978). *The Hippocampus as a Cognitive Map.* Oxford: Clarendon Press.

Orban, P., Rauchs, G., Balteau, E., Degueldre, C., Luxen, A., Maquet, P., et al. (2006). Sleep after spatial learning promotes covert reorgani- zation of brain activity. *Proc. Natl. Acad. Sci. U.S.A.* 103, 7124–7129.

Overman, W. H., Pate, B. J., Moore, K., and Peuster, A. (1996). Ontogeny of place learning in children as measured in the radial arm maze, Morris search task, and open field task. *Behav. Neurosci.* 110, 1205–1228.

Packard, M. G., Hirsh, R., and White, N. M. (1989). Differential effects of fornix and caudate nucleus lesions on two radial maze tasks: evi- dence for multiple memory systems. *J. Neurosci.* 9, 1465–1472.

Packard, M. G., and McGaugh, J. L. (1996). Inactivation of hippocam- pus or caudate nucleus with lido- caine differentially affects expres- sion of place and response learning. *Neurobiol. Learn. Mem.* 65, 65–72.

Persson, J., Nyberg, L., Lind, J., Larsson, A., Nilsson, L. G., Ingvar, M., et al. (2006). Structure- function correlates of cognitive decline in aging. *Cereb. Cortex* 16, 907–915.

Pine, D. S., Grun, J., Maguire, E. A., Burgess, N., Zarahn, E., Koda, V., et al. (2002). Neurodevelopmental aspects of spatial navigation: a vir- tual reality fMRI study. *Neuroimage* 15, 396–406.

Rapp, P. R., Kansky, M. T., and Roberts, J. A. (1997). Impaired spatial information processing in aged monkeys with preserved recog- nition memory. *Neuroreport* 8, 1923–1928.

Rapp, P. R., Rosenberg, R. A., and Gallagher, M. (1987). An evalua- tion of spatial information process- ing in aged rats. *Behav. Neurosci.* 101, 3–12.

Ravaglia, G., Forti, P., Maioli, F., Sacchetti, L., Mariani, E., Nativio, V., et al. (2002). Education, occu- pation, and prevalence of dementia: findings from the Conselice study. *Dement. Geriatr. Cogn. Disord.* 14, 90–100.

Raz, N., Gunning, F. M., Head, D., Dupuis, J. H., McQuain, J., Briggs, S. D., et al. (1997). Selective aging of the human cerebral cor- tex observed *in vivo*: differential vulnerability of the prefrontal gray matter. *Cereb. Cortex* 7, 268–282.

Raz, N., and Rodrigue, K. M. (2006). Differential aging of the brain: pat- terns, cognitive correlates and mod- ifiers. *Neurosci. Biobehav. Rev.* 30, 730–748.

Raz, N., Rodrigue, K. M., Head, D., Kennedy, K. M., and Acker, J. D. (2004). Differential aging of the medial temporal lobe: a study of a five-year change. *Neurology* 62, 433–438.

Reber, A. (1992). The cognitive unconscious: an evolutionary perspective. *Conscious. Cogn.* 1, 93–133.

Rodgers, M. K., Sindone, J. A. 3rd., and Moffat, S. D. (2012). Effects of age on navigation strategy. *Neurobiol. Aging* 33, 202.e215–202.e222.

Saitoh, O., Karns, C. M., and Courchesne, E. (2001). Development of the hippocam- pal formation from 2 to 42 years: MRI evidence of smaller area dentata in autism. *Brain* 124(Pt 7), 1317–1324.

Sapolsky, R. (1994). The physiolog- ical relevance of glucocorticoid endangerment of the hippocampus. *Ann. N.Y. Acad. Sci.* 746, 294–304. discussion: 304–307.

Sapolsky, R., Uno, H., Rebert, C., and Finch, C. (1990). Hippocampal damage associated with pro- longed glucocorticoid exposure in primates. *J. Neurosci.* 10, 2897–2902.

Schwabe, L., Bohbot, V. D., and Wolf, O. T. (2012). Prenatal stress changes learning strategies in adulthood. *Hippocampus*. doi: 10.1002/hipo.22034. [Epub ahead of print].

Schwabe, L., Dalm, S., Schachinger, H., and Oitzl, M. S. (2008). Chronic stress modulates the use of spatial and stimulus-response learning strategies in mice and man. *Neurobiol. Learn. Mem.* 90, 495–503.

Schwabe, L., Oitzl, M. S., Philippsen, C., Richter, S., Bohringer, A., Wippich, W., et al. (2007). Stress mod- ulates the use of spatial versus stimulus-response learning strate- gies in humans. *Learn. Mem.* 14, 109–116.

Schwabe, L., Schachinger, H., de Kloet, E. R., and Oitzl, M. S. (2010). Stress impairs spatial but not early stimulus-response learning. *Behav. Brain Res.* 213, 50–55.

Small, S. A., Tsai, W. Y., DeLaPaz, R., Mayeux, R., and Stern, Y. (2002). Imaging hippocampal function across the human life span: is memory decline normal or not? *Ann. Neurol.* 51, 290–295.

Sowell, E. R., Trauner, D. A., Gamst, A., and Jernigan, T. L. (2002). Development of cortical and sub- cortical brain structures in child- hood and adolescence: a structural MRI study. *Dev. Med. Child Neurol.* 44, 4–16.

Thomas, K. M., Hunt, R. H., Vizueta, N., Sommer, T., Durston, S., Yang, Y., et al. (2004). Evidence of devel- opmental differences in implicit sequence learning: an fMRI study of children and adults. *J. Cogn. Neurosci.* 16, 1339–1351.

Tisserand, D. J., van Boxtel, M. P., Pruessner, J. C., Hofman, P., Evans, A. C., and Jolles, J. (2004). A voxel-based morphometric study to determine individual differences in gray matter density associated with age and cognitive change over time. *Cereb. Cortex* 14, 966–973.

Vasquez, B. J., Martinez, J. L. Jr., Jensen, R. A., Messing, R. B., Rigter, H., and McGaugh, J. L. (1983). Learning and memory in young and aged Fischer 344 rats. *Arch. Gerontol. Geriatr.* 2, 279–291.

Walhovd, K. B., Fjell, A. M., Reinvang, I., Lundervold, A., Dale, A. M., Eilertsen, D. E., et al. (2005). Effects of age on volumes of cortex, white matter and subcortical structures. *Neurobiol. Aging* 26, 1261–1270. discussion: 1275–1268.

Wilkniss, S. M., Jones, M. G., Korol, D. L., Gold, P. E., and Manning, C. A. (1997). Age-related differences in an ecologically based study of route learning. *Psychol. Aging* 12, 372–375.

Wills, T. J., Cacucci, F., Burgess, N., and O'Keefe, J. (2010). Development of the hippocampal cognitive map in preweanling rats. *Science* 328, 1573–1576.

15

# Age differences in medial prefrontal activity for subsequent memory of truth value

**Brittany S. Cassidy[1]*, Trey Hedden[2], Carolyn Yoon[3] and Angela H. Gutchess[1]**

[1] Department of Psychology, Brandeis University, Waltham, MA, USA
[2] Athinoula A. Martinos Center for Biomedical Imaging, Massachusetts General Hospital, Boston, MA, USA
[3] University of Michigan, Ann Arbor, MI, USA

***Edited by:***
*Natalie Ebner, University of Florida, USA*

***Reviewed by:***
*Hakan Fischer, Stockholm University, Sweden*
*Eric S. Allard, Boston College, USA*
*Kyungmi Kim, Yale University, USA*

****Correspondence:***
*Brittany S. Cassidy, Department of Psychology, Brandeis University, 415 South St., MS 062, Waltham, MA 02454, USA*
*e-mail: bcassidy@brandeis.edu*

Much research has demonstrated that aging is marked by decreased source memory relative to young adults, yet a smaller body of work has demonstrated that increasing the socioemotional content of source information may be one way to reduce age-related performance differences. Although dorsomedial prefrontal cortex (dmPFC) activity may support source memory among young and older adults, the extent to which one activates dorsal vs. ventral mPFC may reflect one's personal connection with incoming information. Because truth value may be one salient marker that impacts one's connection with information and allocation of attention toward incoming material, we investigated whether the perceived truth value of information differently impacts differences in mPFC activity associated with encoding source information, particularly with age. Twelve young (18–23 years) and 12 older adults (63–80 years) encoded true and false statements. Behavioral results showed similar memory performance between the age groups. With respect to neural activity associated with subsequent memory, young adults, relative to older adults, exhibited greater activity in dmPFC while older adults displayed enhanced ventromedial prefrontal cortex (vmPFC) and insula engagement relative to young. These results may potentially indicate that young adults focus on a general knowledge acquisition goal, while older adults focus on emotionally relevant aspects of the material. The findings demonstrate that age-related differences in recruitment of mPFC associated with encoding source information may in some circumstances underlie age-equivalent behavioral performance.

**Keywords: medial prefrontal cortex, truth value, aging, encoding, insula**

## INTRODUCTION

In addition to remembering the information itself, some of the most important choices in life require consideration of the context related to incoming information, often referred to as source memory (Johnson and Raye, 1981; Johnson et al., 1993). For example, the reliability of a source may be crucial when evaluating health claims (e.g., should you believe an endorsement that a dietary supplement can increase longevity if the endorser helped develop the supplement?). A small body of behavioral evidence shows that increasing task salience, or the degree of importance of a task to an individual, may reduce age differences in source memory (e.g., Rahhal et al., 2002; but see Siedlecki et al., 2005), in contrast with the age-related source memory impairments shown for tasks across several domains of stimuli that utilize less salient (e.g., focusing on perceptual information, as in Rahhal et al., 2002) and non-social material (e.g., Spencer and Raz, 1995). This suggests that for salient information (e.g., using affective or value-based information, as in Rahhal et al., 2002), older adults may not show the same pattern of age-related impairment that is typically found in tasks involving less salient information.

Purported truth might be one salient factor driving prioritization of information at encoding, and may reduce age differences in source memory, given the inherent value of knowing whether information is true. For instance, while both the *National Enquirer* and *The New York Times* are sources of information, people may perceive non-tabloid journalism as more truthful, and more deeply encode this information. These decisions occur in the interpersonal realm as well. You might, for example, learn the same piece of information from a gossiping co-worker known to spread rumors, or from a trusted friend; you may allocate more attention to your friend due to the perceived reliability of that source. This prioritization in encoding strategies suggests that source memory, or remembering the context in which information was presented, may directly relate to how we process information obtained from our daily interactions.

It is possible that the neural activity supporting age-equivalent source memory for socially salient material involves the interaction of cortical systems with the medial temporal lobe (MTL) that are distinct from the cortical-MTL interactions underlying non-social sources, which undergo age-related decline. Processing socially meaningful vs. non-social information recruits a reliable network of brain regions (Mitchell et al., 2002, 2005), and the engagement of medial prefrontal cortex (mPFC) in particular has been documented in a range of tasks involving socioemotional processing (Van Overwalle, 2009), including memory for information encoded during a social vs. a non-social orienting task (e.g., Mitchell et al., 2004).

Work exploring potential age differences in mPFC function during social tasks shows evidence for equivalent engagement for young and older adults (Gutchess et al., 2007; Beadle et al., 2012; Cassidy et al., 2012) as well as evidence for decreased activity with age (Moran et al., 2012). The diverging patterns of age effects on dorsomedial prefrontal cortex (dmPFC), however, may reflect when information is personally salient (Beadle et al., 2012; Cassidy et al., 2012) vs. when it is not (Moran et al., 2012). For instance, for the socially salient task involving self-referencing, young and older adults similarly recruit dmPFC for the processing of self- vs. other-related information (Gutchess et al., 2007) and for successful encoding of source materials presented in a self- vs. other-referential way (Leshikar and Duarte, 2013). However, older adults may not activate dmPFC to the level of young (e.g., Moran et al., 2012) unless a task explicitly involves socially and personally salient information.

Age-equivalent mPFC activity in personally salient social tasks may be concordant with behavioral data showing that socioemotional or value-rich materials reduce age-related performance differences (Fung and Carstensen, 2003; Carstensen and Mikels, 2005; Mather and Carstensen, 2005; May et al., 2005; Cassidy and Gutchess, 2012). Because older adults place higher priorities than young adults on value-rich, affective information (Fredrickson and Carstensen, 1990), they may perform as well as young adults on source memory tasks with value-rich material. For instance, although young adults recall perceptual and conceptual source information better than older adults, this age difference disappears when using sources relevant to emotional information (May et al., 2005) or truth value (Rahhal et al., 2002).

Recruitment of dmPFC for social tasks may also depend on one's orientation to the task, regardless of age. For instance, young adults show a dissociation in mPFC activity when thinking about similar or dissimilar others, such that dmPFC is engaged when abstractly thinking about a dissimilar other, while ventromedial prefrontal cortex (vmPFC) is recruited for thinking about self-similar others and emotional states (Mitchell et al., 2006a). This raises the possibility that age differences in mPFC activity may in part be due to differences in how young and older adults naturally orient to social tasks (e.g., they approach the learning of social information in an abstract way largely devoid of personal involvement, or with more of an emotional orientation). Supporting the idea of task orientation influencing mPFC activity, recent work has demonstrated that age differences in mPFC engagement toward processing valenced social material are driven by dmPFC in young adults, and by vmPFC in older adults (Cassidy et al., 2013). It is unknown, however, whether young and older adults display overall differences in neural activity, and specifically dissociations in dorsal and ventral mPFC activity, for salient tasks that are not overtly positive or negative.

A tendency to focus on value-rich and emotional information with age is reflective of Socioemotional Selectivity Theory, which posits that older adults tend to focus on processing information with enhanced value and socioemotional meaning due to the feeling that time in one's life is limited (Carstensen et al., 1999). In contrast, young adults are proposed to have a more general focus on acquiring knowledge. Illustrating this concept, older adults have been shown to remember more advertisements featuring emotionally meaningful messages, whereas young adults do not display a bias based on the type of presented material (Fung and Carstensen, 2003). If older adults approach tasks involving value-rich stimuli with an emotional orientation, then more vmPFC activity rather than dmPFC activity might be expected in older vs. young for such tasks. This is because ventral subregions of mPFC have been implicated in affective processing (Davidson and Irwin, 1999), including subsequent memory for emotional material (Dolcos et al., 2004), and for affective components, as opposed to cognitive components, in theory of mind tasks (Shamay-Tsoory and Aharon-Peretz, 2007). In contrast, dmPFC has been implicated in more complex cognitive operations (e.g., see Saxe, 2006).

Another distinction in dorsal and ventral mPFC activity involves the extent of their engagement during controlled and automatic processing tasks (Satpute and Lieberman, 2006; Lieberman, 2007). For instance, automatic processing has been likened to reflexive processing and with vmPFC activity during the formation of intuitions (Bechara et al., 1997). In contrast, controlled processing has been likened to reflective processing, and has been linked with increased dmPFC activity when using reappraisal to reduce emotional response to negative scenes (Ochsner et al., 2002). Older adults have larger memory deficits on tasks involving controlled processing, relative to automatic processing (Hasher and Zacks, 1979), perhaps because many tasks do not motivate older adults to access controlled processing resources (Germain and Hess, 2007). When motivated by socioemotional goals, however, older adults may be more likely to allocate the cognitive resources necessary for controlled processing toward their goal, as in the case of emotion regulation (Carstensen et al., 2003). Thus, in the case of a context where information is value-rich, but the task itself is not necessarily emotionally meaningful, we might expect young, but not older, adults to use controlled processing to encode information even if they are not instructed to do so, in the service of knowledge acquisition goals. In contrast, older adults may employ automatic processing during similar tasks. For a task involving value-rich stimuli, this might be reflected in enhanced vmPFC activity among older adults relative to young adults.

The present study explored whether young and older adults differentially engage dmPFC and vmPFC for the value-rich task of encoding truth value, be it inferred from a social source or explicitly stated. Our task involved learning the purported truth value of health-related statements, which provides a unique opportunity to appeal to the processing strategies of both young and older adults. Because health-related statements may hold particular importance for older adults, age differences in behavioral source memory for truth value may be reduced compared to the typical finding of deficits with age. Given previous findings of age differences in dmPFC and vmPFC activity as a function of the content of incoming salient information (Leclerc and Kensinger, 2008, 2010; Cassidy et al., 2013), we expected that young adults would show enhanced dmPFC activity relative to older adults for subsequent memory based on the idea that learning true and false statements might signal an inherent knowledge acquisition focus in the young. In contrast, we expected that older adults would exhibit increased vmPFC activity relative to young adults for subsequent memory, given that the more value-based aspects of health-related statements to older adults may make them more likely to approach the task with a socioemotional orientation. Given a potential socioemotional orientation among older adults, the insula, due to its broad role in emotional processing, was another neural region where increased activity might be expected in older vs. young adults for the encoding of truth value (Adolphs et al., 2000; Phan et al., 2002; Sanfey et al., 2003; Barrett et al., 2004; Craig, 2009; Wiech et al., 2010; Zaki et al., 2012). Insofar as the insula is engaged when making decisions in an emotional context (Sanfey et al., 2003), greater insula recruitment might be expected among individuals who orient to material in an emotional way (e.g., older adults) relative to those less likely to do so (e.g., young adults).

## METHODS

### PARTICIPANTS

Twelve right-handed University of Michigan students (18–23 years old, $M = 20.5$, $SD = 1.2$, 58% female) and twelve right-handed community dwelling older adults (63–80 years old, $M = 71.1$, $SD = 5.5$, 66% female) were recruited for the study. Older adults were screened for abnormal orientation scores (<27) using the Mini-Mental State Examination ($M = 28.7$, $SD = 1.1$), and had marginally more years of education ($M = 15.4$ years, $SD = 2.7$) than young adults ($M = 13.6$ years, $SD = 1.7$), $t_{(22)} = 1.95$, $p = 0.06$. To ensure the samples' comparability with those in the prior literature, participants completed a vocabulary measure (Shipley, 1986), digit and pattern comparison tasks (Salthouse and Babcock, 1991), forward and backward digit span measures (Wechsler, 1981), and a letter-number sequencing measure (Wechsler, 1997). Results are summarized in **Table 1**. Participants reported no history of psychiatric or neurological disorders and no history of drug or alcohol abuse at the time of testing. The University of Michigan Institutional Review Board approved the study, and written informed consent was obtained from all participants.

### STIMULI

The stimuli consisted of 240 true statements regarding health-related information for which participants were unlikely to have prior knowledge (e.g., "Women's hearts beat faster than men's"). Altering words in each true statement created factually untrue statements (e.g., "Men blink nearly twice as much as women"). After creating a factually untrue version of each statement, each statement was randomly assigned to one of two sets (Set A and Set B). For half of the participants, Set A consisted of true versions and Set B of false. For the other half of participants, Set A consisted of false versions and Set B of true. Thus, whether each participant saw a true or false version of any given statement was fully counterbalanced across participants. The order of statements from each set was randomly drawn for each participant. These statements have been used in prior aging research (Skurnik et al., 2005) and are available upon request. All stimuli were programmed and presented using E-Prime software (Psychological Software Tools, Pittsburgh, PA) and IFIS 9.0 (MRI Devices, Waukesha, WI).

**Table 1 | Means (*SD*) for cognitive measures.**

| Measure | Young adults | Older adults | *t* | *p*-value |
|---|---|---|---|---|
| Shipley vocabulary | 31.1 (3.6) | 37.3 (2.9) | −4.37 | <0.001 |
| Digit comparison | 28.6 (2.8) | 22.2 (4.0) | 4.10 | 0.001 |
| Pattern comparison | 24.2 (2.3) | 16.2 (4.7) | 4.70 | <0.001 |
| Forward digit span | 8.2 (1.3) | 7.9 (1.2) | 0.55 | 0.60 |
| Backward digit span | 6.4 (1.1) | 5.8 (1.7) | 0.78 | 0.45 |
| Letter-number sequencing | 5.4 (1.0) | 5.1 (0.9) | 0.86 | 0.40 |

### TRUTH JUDGMENT TASK

Participants were told they would see statements coupled with an indication of truth value, and would later be asked to remember if each statement was true or false. The task comprised a 2 (Truth Value: True/False) × 2 (Source Type: Inferred/Stated) design, in which source memory for different types of information was compared across age groups. Some statements were stated to be true or false (stated: "TRUE" or "FALSE"), without referencing a social source. Other statements were inferred to be true or false, based on the source (inferred: "PAT says:" or "CHRIS says:"). Prior to encoding, participants were introduced to two hypothetical individuals, Pat and Chris. One individual was described as being honest and trustworthy, and participants were told to assume that every statement obtained from this person was true. The other individual was described as very dishonest and untrustworthy, and participants were told to assume this person only made false statements. Half of the statements were true and the other half false, and each of these were randomly assigned to each participant for the corresponding inferred or stated source. Participants practiced the task and received feedback on their responses before completing the full encoding task in the scanner.

Statements and truth value indications were presented on the screen concurrently for 6 s (see **Figure 1**). Participants selected whether presented information was true or false via button press. Responses were monitored during scanning to ensure that participants were accurately reporting the truth status of statements. No participant exhibited difficulty with this aspect of the task. Each run contained 60 statements, pseudorandomly distributed among baseline periods of fixation ranging from 2 to 12 s. Condition order and baseline periods were determined using Optseq2 (http://surfer.nmr.mgh.harvard.edu/optseq).

Participants completed the source memory task outside the scanner approximately 15–20 min after structural scans and four encoding runs. Participants were reminded of the truth values associated with each person (e.g., "If you remember that Pat said it, it must be true; if Chris said it, it must be false."), were informed that they had seen all statements previously in the scanner, and were told that half the statements were true and half false. During the source memory task, participants saw each of the 240 statements displayed during encoding, with no indication of truth value. Participants indicated whether they were confident a statement was true, guessing that it was true, guessing

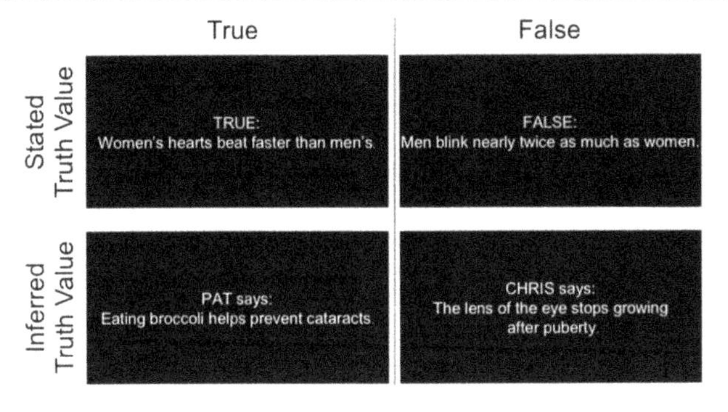


**FIGURE 1 | Examples of encoding stimuli used in each condition.**

it was false, or confident it was false, via a four-choice button press.

## IMAGE ACQUISITION

Data were acquired using a 3T GE LX MR scanner (GE Signa 9.0 VH3 software, General Electric, Milwaukee, WI) paired with a whole-head coil. Two hundred and seventy volumes were obtained in each of four functional runs, using a gradient-echo spiral acquisition sequence to measure blood oxygen level-dependent (BOLD) effects ($TR = 2000$ ms, $TE = 25$ ms, flip angle $= 80$, $64 \times 64$ matrix, FOV $= 200$ mm). Dummy scans were also acquired, but discarded for analyses. Thirty-two contiguous oblique slices were acquired parallel to the AC/PC line. T1 Structural images were acquired using a Spoiled GRASS sequence (FOV $= 24$ mm, $256 \times 192$ matrix), of 120 sagittal slices (0.9373 mm in-plane resolution) of 1.5 mm thickness.

## DATA ANALYSIS

### *Behavioral data*

Behavioral data were analyzed using an alpha level of 0.05. Responses to a statement involving a confident correct truth value attribution were classified as correct source memory for that statement. Guessing responses and incorrect attributions were classified as incorrect source memory for that statement, in keeping with prior research (Otten et al., 2001).

### *fMRI data*

Functional volumes were slice time corrected with an 8-point Hanning windowed sinc interpolation implemented in C++. Subject motion correction was performed using AIR 3.08 (Woods et al., 1992). Remaining analyses were performed using SPM2 (Wellcome Department of Cognitive Neurology, London, UK) and programs from the Gablab Toolbox (Massachusetts Institute of Technology, Cambridge, MA). The anatomical image was coregistered to the fifth functional volume and normalized to MNI space using a standard T1 template image with 2 $mm^3$ voxels. Normalization parameters determined from the anatomy were applied to functional volumes, which were then smoothed with a 6 mm isotropic Gaussian kernel. Effects for the eight stimulus conditions [i.e., 2 (Truth Value: True/False) × 2 (Source Type: Inferred/Stated) × 2 (Subsequent Memory: Correct/Incorrect)] were estimated using event-related regressors convolved with a canonical hemodynamic response function.

Results reported are from group-level, random effects analyses using an uncorrected threshold of $p = 0.005$ with a cluster size of $k > 11$, chosen to ensure that activations spanned at least two acquired contiguous voxels. Although we used a fairly liberal threshold, we took a whole-brain rather than a region of interest approach because relatively little prior work on this topic made it desirable to test a wider array of regions showing age-related changes in subsequent source memory in order to inform future work. Functional images from encoding were back-sorted for further analyses according to whether truth value was subsequently remembered (correct: high confidence correct responses only) or forgotten (incorrect: summing across guess responses and confident incorrect attributions). Subsequent memory contrasts (young > old, correct > incorrect source memory; old > young, correct > incorrect source memory) were used to initially analyze functional data and to identify regions demonstrating age differences where correct source memory produced increased engagement over incorrect source memory. The correct > incorrect source memory contrast was defined at the subject-level individually, and then entered in a group-level analysis for simple one-way group-wise differences. Locations of peak activation on the cortical surface were identified using SPM2, and Brodmann areas were obtained with MRIcron (Rorden and Brett, 2000). To characterize age differences in subsequent source memory from our whole-brain analysis, parameter estimates for each condition from each participant were extracted from the peak voxels of our a priori regions of interest (dmPFC, vmPFC, and insula) where significant activations emerged in the correct > incorrect source memory contrast.

# RESULTS

## BEHAVIORAL RESULTS

Proportions of recognition responses in each category (confident true, guessing true, guessing false, confident false) are shown in **Table 2**. From these responses, two behavioral measures were computed to assess memory performance. First, the proportion of correct source memory judgments (confident correct attributions; e.g., confident true when the statement was true) was calculated. Second, the false alarm rate was calculated as the proportion of statements incorrectly assigned a confident attribution (e.g., confident true when the statement was false). We analyzed these measures separately as dependent variables using a 2 (Age Group: young, old) × 2 (Source Type: inferred, stated) × 2 (Truth Value: true, false) mixed ANOVA.

For correct source memory judgments, there was a main effect of Truth Value, $F_{(1, 22)} = 45.84$, $p < 0.001$, $\eta_p^2 = 0.68$, such that participants correctly identified more true ($M = 0.71$, $SD = 0.18$) than false ($M = 0.53$, $SD = 0.20$) statements. There were no main effects of Age Group or Source Type. There was also a significant interaction between Source Type and Truth Value, $F_{(1, 22)} = 9.42$, $p < 0.01$, $\eta_p^2 = 0.30$. Contrasts showed that true statements coming from a stated source ($M = 0.73$, $SD = 0.19$) were better remembered than true statements coming from a inferred source ($M = 0.68$, $SD = 0.17$), $F_{(1, 22)} = 7.69$, $p < 0.01$, $\eta_p^2 = 0.26$. In contrast, accuracy in identifying false statements from inferred ($M = 0.54$, $SD = 0.20$) and stated

**Table 2 | Behavioral source memory performance [*M*, (*SD*)] for young (YA) and older (OA) adults.**

| | Confident true | | Guessing true | | Guessing false | | Confident false | |
|---|---|---|---|---|---|---|---|---|
| | **True** | **False** | **True** | **False** | **True** | **False** | **True** | **False** |
| **SOCIAL SOURCE** | | | | | | | | |
| YA | 0.70 (0.19) | 0.13 (0.06) | 0.15 (0.14) | 0.12 (0.11) | 0.10 (0.06) | 0.19 (0.09) | 0.06 (0.03) | 0.56 (0.16) |
| OA | 0.67 (0.16) | 0.13 (0.10) | 0.15 (0.12) | 0.12 (0.11) | 0.09 (0.06) | 0.21 (0.14) | 0.09 (0.07) | 0.53 (0.25) |
| **NON-SOCIAL SOURCE** | | | | | | | | |
| YA | 0.73 (0.22) | 0.13 (0.08) | 0.14 (0.12) | 0.14 (0.11) | 0.07 (0.09) | 0.20 (0.13) | 0.06 (0.07) | 0.54 (0.18) |
| OA | 0.73 (0.16) | 0.15 (0.12) | 0.13 (0.11) | 0.13 (0.11) | 0.08 (0.05) | 0.23 (0.12) | 0.06 (0.06) | 0.50 (0.22) |

*Correct source memory is the same as confident responses for the correct truth value (e.g., confident true for true statements). Incorrect source memory is the sum of guessing (true and false) and confident incorrect source attributions. No age group differences were significant in any condition.*

($M = 0.52$, $SD = 0.20$) sources did not differ, $F_{(1, 22)} = 1.33, p = 0.26$, $\eta_p^2 = 0.06$. No other interactions approached significance.

For false alarm rates, there was a main effect of Truth Value, $F_{(1, 22)} = 15.46$, $p < 0.001$, $\eta_p^2 = 0.41$. Participants were more likely to confidently remember an originally false statement as true than an originally true statement as false. No other effects approached significance.

The absence of behavioral interactions involving Source Type and Age Group suggests that source memory in aging does not depend on whether information was inferred via a person's reliability or explicitly stated. However, prior fMRI results have suggested that social information processing is neurally distinct from processing other types of information (Mitchell et al., 2002, 2004; Van Overwalle, 2009). We accordingly characterized our imaging data to determine if the processing mechanisms involved in encoding inferred vs. stated truth value were similarly distinct, and how aging might modulate the engagement of these regions.

## fMRI RESULTS

We identified brain regions showing age differences in response to overall subsequent memory, given the relatively low number of participants in this study ($Ns = 12$ for each age group) (correct > incorrect memory; see **Table 3**). This contrast captures regions that differ across age groups, but is conservative with respect to the source and truth of each statement. Parameter estimates from the peak voxel of these functionally defined regions were probed to characterize whether age differences in activity was driven by Source Type or Truth Value (**Figure 1**). However, specific contrasts involving these factors were not conducted due to low power and the lack of behavioral evidence for source memory differences with age depending on Source Type or Truth Value.

In a whole-brain analysis, this subsequent memory contrast yielded brain regions contributing to age differences in correct subsequent memory for source (**Table 2**). To probe the expected age differences related to socioemotional processing in the dmPFC, vmPFC, and insula, we focused on these regions. Parameter estimates of activation attributable to each condition were then extracted and compared in 2 (Age Group: young, old) × 2 (Source Type: inferred, stated) × 2 (Truth Value: true, false) mixed ANOVAs.

As defined by the contrast, young adults had increased activation compared to older adults in two regions of left dmPFC [**Figure 2A**; BA 6: $F_{(1, 22)} = 9.43$, $p < 0.01$, $\eta_p^2 = 0.30$; BA 8: $F_{(1, 22)} = 16.48, p < 0.001, \eta_p^2 = 0.43$]. Characterizing this effect further (and probing effects unrelated to the region-defining contrast), there were marginal Age Group by Truth Value interactions in both regions of dmPFC [BA 6: $F_{(1, 22)} = 3.01, p = 0.097, \eta_p^2 = 0.12$; BA 8: $F_{(1, 22)} = 3.43$, $p = 0.08$, $\eta_p^2 = 0.14$]. Pairwise comparisons showed that in both dmPFC regions, this interaction appeared to be driven by enhanced activity in young relative to older adults when successfully encoding true (BA6: $p = 0.002$, BA 8: $p = 0.004$) vs. false (BA 6: $p = 0.40$, BA 8: $p = 0.70$) statements.

As defined by the contrast, older adults had increased vmPFC engagement compared to young adults in a region of left vmPFC [**Figure 2B**; $F_{(1, 22)} = 3.43$, $p = 0.002$, $\eta_p^2 = 0.35$]. Examination of parameter estimates for effects unrelated to the region-defining contrast showed that unlike the marginal Age Group by Truth Value interactions in dmPFC activity, vmPFC showed a marginal Age Group by Source Type interaction, $F_{(1, 22)} = 3.46, p = 0.08$, $\eta_p^2 = 0.14$. Young adults engaged vmPFC more for the successful encoding of truth value from stated vs. socially-inferred sources, $F_{(1, 11)} = 4.35$, $p = 0.06$, $\eta_p^2 = 0.28$, while older adults, showed no such difference, $F < 1$, $p = 0.93$. There was also a marginal main effect of Source Type, such that all participants tended to recruit vmPFC for the successful encoding of stated vs. inferred truth value, $F_{(1, 22)} = 3.11$, $p = 0.09$, $\eta_p^2 = 0.12$. Finally, older adults had increased neural activity relative to young adults (as defined by the contrast) in the right insula (**Figure 2C**), $F_{(1, 22)} = 9.55$, $p < 0.01$, $\eta_p^2 = 0.30$, for the successful encoding of truth value. Unlike the marginal Truth Value by Age Group interactions in dmPFC and Source Type by Age Group interaction exhibited in vmPFC during the task, no interactions were present in insula recruitment.

## DISCUSSION

Previous research on source memory and aging has detailed decreases in older adults' behavioral performance (Chalfonte and Johnson, 1996), and neural activity (Mitchell et al., 2006b; Dennis et al., 2008) when compared to a young cohort, indicating overall age-related decline in encoding source information. However, a smaller body of behavioral work suggests that

**Table 3 | Age differences in brain activity for correct > incorrect source memory.**

| Region | BA | k | Activation Peak (x, y, z) | | | t |
|---|---|---|---|---|---|---|
| **(A) YOUNG > OLD, CORRECT > INCORRECT SOURCE MEMORY** | | | | | | |
| L dorsomedial prefrontal cortex | 6/8 | 68 | −14 | 32 | 54 | 5.70 |
| L dorsomedial prefrontal cortex | 6 | 33 | −14 | 12 | 66 | 3.60 |
| R amygdala | | 28 | 20 | −2 | −24 | 3.87 |
| R superior frontal gyrus | 6 | 14 | 14 | −16 | 78 | 3.52 |
| L precuneus | 19 | 15 | −30 | −72 | 32 | 3.25 |
| L inferior frontal gyrus | 9 | 14 | −52 | 20 | 24 | 3.08 |
| **(B) OLD > YOUNG, CORRECT > INCORRECT SOURCE MEMORY** | | | | | | |
| L ventromedial prefrontal cortex | 10/11 | 66 | −16 | 56 | −2 | 4.01 |
| L medial prefrontal cortex | 10 | | −8 | 52 | −4 | 3.16 |
| L anterior cingulate gyrus | 32 | | −14 | 46 | −4 | 3.08 |
| R insula | | 37 | 44 | −6 | −2 | 3.26 |
| R precuneus | 7 | 224 | 16 | −66 | 52 | 5.81 |
| L dorsolateral prefrontal cortex | 9/46 | 75 | −40 | 36 | 36 | 5.36 |
| L middle frontal gyrus | 46 | | −46 | 36 | 24 | 4.10 |
| L precentral gyrus | 4 | 50 | −52 | −16 | 28 | 4.69 |
| R middle frontal gyrus | 8 | 180 | 26 | 36 | 40 | 4.69 |
| R cingulate gyrus | 32 | | 18 | 22 | 36 | 3.43 |
| L cingulate gyrus | 31 | 25 | −20 | −28 | 40 | 4.48 |
| L insula | | 12 | −28 | −22 | 24 | 4.08 |
| R inferior parietal lobule | 40 | 64 | 68 | −26 | 26 | 3.77 |
| R superior parietal lobe | 5 | 40 | 20 | −52 | 58 | 3.66 |
| R thalamus | | 19 | 10 | −38 | 10 | 3.59 |
| R middle frontal gyrus | 6 | 13 | 26 | 4 | 42 | 3.58 |
| L inferior parietal lobule | 40 | 20 | −34 | −42 | 48 | 3.57 |
| R inferior frontal gyrus | 47 | 27 | 36 | 36 | 2 | 3.56 |
| L superior parietal lobule | 5 | 12 | −22 | −46 | 68 | 3.53 |
| R posterior cingulate gyrus | 29 | 18 | 6 | −50 | 4 | 3.53 |
| R superior frontal gyrus | 6 | 20 | 8 | −10 | 70 | 3.52 |
| R insula | | 15 | 38 | 22 | 6 | 3.45 |
| R inferior temporal gyrus | 20 | 24 | 50 | −34 | −14 | 3.41 |
| R fusiform gyrus | 37 | 12 | −12 | 58 | 20 | 3.26 |
| L postcentral gyrus | 40 | 15 | −54 | −22 | 14 | 3.26 |
| R middle frontal gyrus | 10 | 28 | 32 | 56 | 22 | 3.24 |
| R superior frontal gyrus | 10 | | 22 | 62 | 24 | 3.05 |
| R superior frontal gyrus | 9 | 11 | 10 | 56 | 30 | 3.06 |

*The data show regions emerging in the contrast with an overall threshold of $p < 0.005$ and an extent threshold of 11 voxels. Regions listed without a cluster size are subsumed by the larger cluster listed directly above. A priori regions of interest are listed first. Other regions are listed from highest to lowest t-value. L, Left; R, right; k, cluster size.*

increasing the salience of stimuli can reduce age-related source memory impairments (Rahhal et al., 2002; May et al., 2005), and that older adults' memory may be enhanced when information is initially encoded in a salient way (Cassidy and Gutchess, 2012). The current study extended this idea by asking if the value-rich task of encoding truth value would be represented by differential activation of mPFC with age, despite potential age-equivalent memory performance. If young adults rely more on knowledge acquisition goals when learning salient information, greater activity in *dorsal* mPFC would be expected, whereas greater activity in *ventral* mPFC and in the insula would be expected for older adults, representing an approach to the task that reflects more socioemotional processing. Our findings are consistent with these expectations, suggesting that in these circumstances, age-equivalent performance may be supported by differential neural recruitment.

The demonstrated dorsal-ventral shift in encoding-related activity with age could also be reflective of overall changes in processing focus, as posited by Socioemotional Selectivity Theory (Carstensen et al., 1999). This theory puts forth the idea that with increasing age, people shift from a focus on acquiring knowledge to a focus on enhancing the emotional meaning in one's life. Thus, a changing focus in older adults toward material with enhanced emotional meaning might be reflected in enhanced activity in regions supporting affective processing (i.e., vmPFC) relative to young. In contrast, regions implicated in the encoding

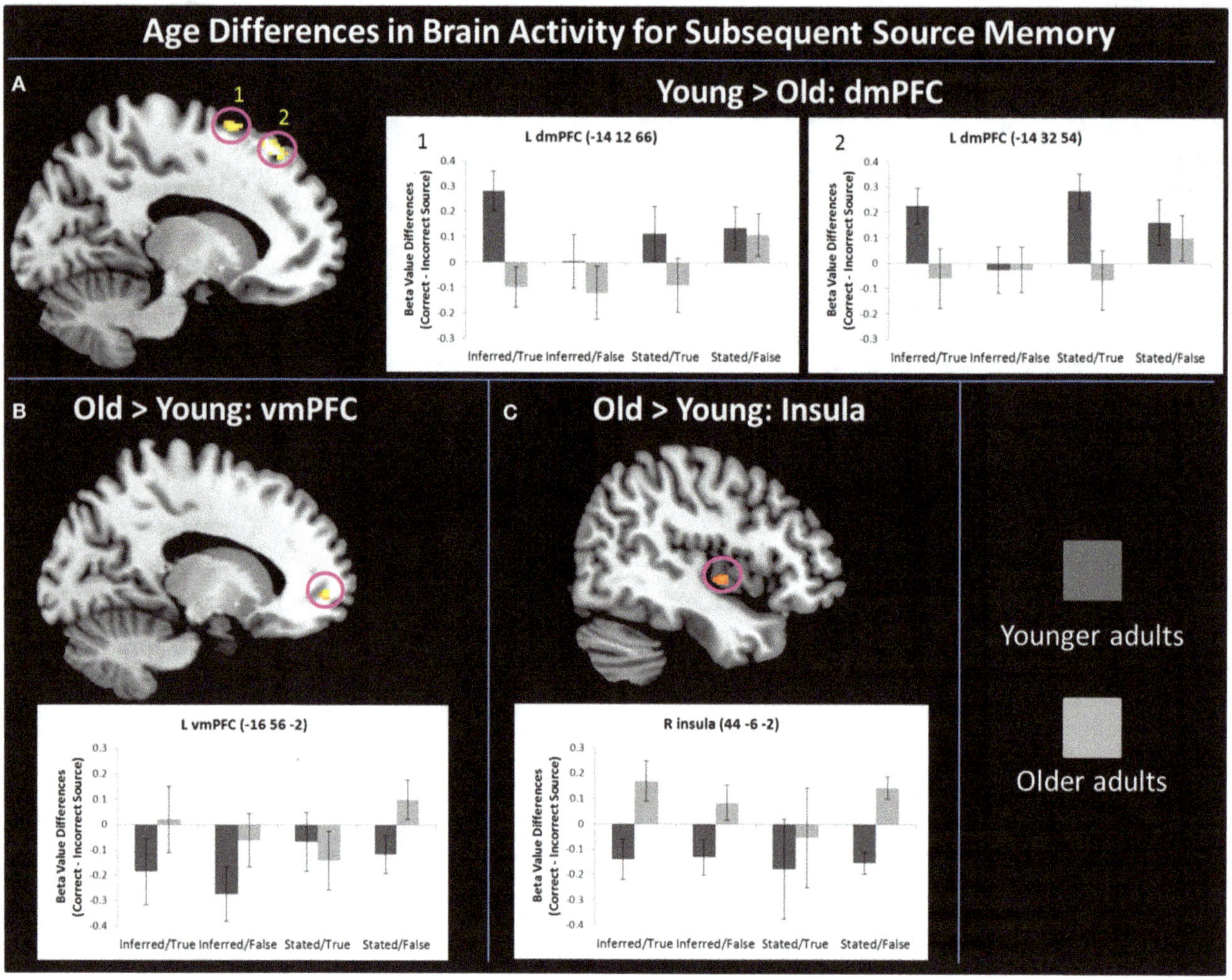


**FIGURE 2 | Age differences for correct—incorrect source memory for truth value existed in mPFC, such that young adults had enhanced activity over older adults in two regions of left dmPFC (A), while older adults had increased recruitment over young in left vmPFC (B).** Older adults also had enhanced activity relative to young adults for subsequent memory of truth value in the right insula **(C)**. Error bars represent standard error of the mean.

of value-rich information (i.e., dmPFC) may be more active in young than older adults, as young adults may try to optimize their likelihood of acquiring knowledge.

The current findings revealed enhanced overall dmPFC activity in young relative to older adults. While older adults have shown dmPFC activity similar to young adults during socially self-relevant processing (Gutchess et al., 2007; Beadle et al., 2012; Cassidy et al., 2012), age-related decreases have been observed in tasks involving social, but not-explicitly self-related, material (Moran et al., 2012). Given that the current task did not place older adults within such a social task, we might not expect them to activate dmPFC to the same extent as young. Increased dmPFC processing among young compared to older adults may also indicate the use of relatively more controlled processing to encode information. Additional research is needed to clarify this possibility.

Exploratory analyses provided further insight into whether stated or inferred truth value, or the truth value of information itself, drove age differences in dmPFC activity. An exploratory characterization of the greater activity in dmPFC among young adults revealed a trend toward increased activity among young over older adults during encoding of veridical, but not false, information regardless of the source. Albeit speculative, such an interaction might be expected for this task because being told that information is true might trigger allocation of attention for prioritized encoding. Enhanced dmPFC activity in young over older adults, especially for encoding true statements, may therefore reflect the overall knowledge acquisition focus among young adults posited by Socioemotional Selectivity Theory (Carstensen et al., 1999).

Older adults, in contrast, tend toward an enhanced focus on salient and emotionally meaningful material (Fredrickson and Carstensen, 1990; Carstensen and Turk-Charles, 1994; Fung et al., 1999; Carstensen et al., 2000; Carstensen and Mikels, 2005), which we suggest may be reflected in their recruitment of vmPFC and insula for subsequent memory relative to young adults. If older adults approach a task involving salient material with a focus, conscious or not, on the personally relevant or emotional aspects of the presented information, then we might expect increased engagement of vmPFC (e.g., Mitchell et al., 2006a). Previous work with young adults has shown that vmPFC is more active for tasks involving more self-similar, and thereby potentially more personally salient, information, vs. self-dissimilar social material, and work in aging has also shown that age-related biases toward positively valenced social information might be primarily reflected in vmPFC (Cassidy et al., 2013), rather than dmPFC activity. Thus, a tendency to focus on salient socioemotional material with age may result in more activation of neural regions sensitive to emotional processing during tasks that involve the encoding of value-rich material, such as truth value. Age-related increases in vmPFC engagement may also reflect the idea that, with age, enhanced focus on value-rich material may result in the recruitment of brain regions supporting more affective vs. cognitive processing.

Our findings are consistent with a growing body of work showing that for young adults (Mitchell et al., 2004; Gilron and Gutchess, 2012), and healthy older adults (Leshikar and Duarte, 2013), mPFC engagement may underlie subsequent memory for value-rich information. This is in contrast to prior literature on the encoding of non-social source material, which shows that age-related impairments in encoding source information stem from MTL dysfunction, particularly in the hippocampus (Mitchell et al., 2000; Dennis et al., 2008). Notably, we did not find age differences in hippocampal function for the task in the present study. However, our results are *consistent* with a recent study on source memory in aging that also utilized socially relevant stimuli (Leshikar and Duarte, 2013), and with work suggesting that face-trait associations are preserved in individuals with substantial hippocampal damage (Todorov and Olson, 2008). A critical follow-up to the present experiment would be to compare directly, memory for socially salient with non-social source information collected within the same task. Such a task could provide evidence that different cortical networks may interact with MTL memory systems for social vs. non-social information across age.

Importantly, the demonstrated age differences in how young and older adults recruit mPFC for encoding truth value may reflect how such information was presented to them. Although Pat and Chris were presented as sources of information, participants never learned additional behavioral information about Pat and Chris aside from learning that one was more trustworthy than the other. Speculatively, in aging, explicit person representations and comparisons may drive dmPFC activity in socially salient tasks. It could be that a lack of explicit person representation involved in assessing abstract factual statements may explain why young adults had enhanced dmPFC activity compared to older adults for the encoding of truth value. Thus, we might expect to see interactions with age in dmPFC activity for source memory related to people, but not for more abstract material. At the same time, a focus on the emotional value of health information, something that might have increased salience with age, may have led to the demonstrated age difference in vmPFC activity seen in the current task. These ideas could be further tested in future work that directly compares neural responses to both abstract and concrete social and non-social sources.

Also consistent with age differences in socioemotional orientation to the task, older adults had increased insula activity relative to young adults. However, our exploratory analysis of parameter estimates showed that enhanced activation of the right insula was not characterized specifically by the truth value of information or by the social source. Speculatively, enhanced insula activity in older relative to young adults for subsequent memory for truth value may be indicative of more emotional initial responses to incoming information (Critchley et al., 2004; Tsakiris et al., 2007; Craig, 2009; Zaki et al., 2012) rather than treating incoming material as facts that must be acquired for the pursuit of knowledge.

Limitations of the present work include the sample sizes of the young and older adult cohorts as well as the threshold for fMRI analyses. Although exploring memory for truth value from the lens of aging is an important topic with both social and public health implications, the limited statistical power due to small sample sizes restricted the present analyses from utilizing direct contrasts of potential interactions (e.g., a direct contrast exploring brain regions that might be differentially engaged with age based on whether truth value was inferred or stated), and thus the reported marginal interactions between conditions as well as null results must be interpreted with caution. Although we investigated this in an exploratory way by characterizing our regions of interest for potential differences in activity by truth value and source type, we recognize that future work should test this in a direct manner. Nonetheless, the marginal interactions we report could be fruitful for the generation of future hypotheses, and the reported effect sizes for these interactions suggest a potentially significant effect if larger sample sizes were to be employed. Moreover, the small sample sizes used here could have masked potential age differences in our behavioral data, which in turn could have guided analyses of the imaging data. Because other studies found similar behavioral performance among young and older adults for socioemotionally salient material (e.g., May et al., 2005), it is unclear whether increasing our sample size would yield age differences in memory, particularly as our means were quite similar across the age groups.

Another potential limitation of the current work involved the different age ranges of our young (5 year span) compared to older (17 year span) adult samples. This could be problematic insofar as it could have led to more age-related variance in the older vs. young adults. This notable limitation is indicative of recruitment difficulties in aging research, as fewer older adults volunteer for fMRI studies than young. Moreover, the older adults who volunteer for fMRI studies tend to be active and highly educated, allowing for the possibility that more sedentary older adults may show different patterns of brain activation. Incorporating a wider range of ages in a lifespan sample could be helpful to address these issues in future work.

Studying how young and older adults subsequently remember truth value and its underlying neural mechanism may help to clarify a public health issue of critical importance. Older adults have increased vulnerability to fraud compared to young adults (Lormel, 2001; Telemarketing fraud against older Americans,

2007; Ruffman et al., 2012). Deficits in source memory processes may in part contribute to this enhanced vulnerability because in order to successfully navigate through one's environment, one must not only consider and remember snippets of information, but also *where* the information came from. That is, failing to remember that a "fact" came from an unreliable source may lead to suboptimal decision making. For instance, one may make a bad financial investment after being given information from an untrustworthy source, or may adopt a political opinion while forgetting to consider that a biased source was reporting the information in the first place. The observed age differences in mPFC activity in response to encoding truth value may indicate that approaching the learning of social source information with a goal of acquiring knowledge could be a strategy more typical of young adults that combats against fraud vulnerability, as opposed to encoding incoming information in a more emotional way, a strategy more typical of older adults.

In summary, the current work demonstrated that for the salient task of encoding truth value of health statements, young and older adults show differential recruitment of dmPFC and vmPFC, despite showing similar behavioral performance. It would be worthwhile for future work to test explicitly how age differences in information processing styles may be associated with age-related increases in vulnerability to fraud and deception.

## ACKNOWLEDGMENTS

We thank Cory Crane for assistance in data collection. Research funding was provided by the Stephen M. Ross School of Business at the University of Michigan, and NIH grant K01 AG040197 (supporting Trey Hedden).

## REFERENCES


Adolphs, R., Damasio, H., Tranel, D., Cooper, G., and Damasio, A. (2000). A role for somatosensory cortices in the visual recognition of emotion as revealed by three-dimensional lesion mapping. *J. Neurosci.* 20, 2683–2690.

Barrett, L., Quigley, K., Bliss-Moreau, E., and Aronson, K. (2004). Interoceptive sensitivity and self-reports of emotional experience. *J. Pers. Soc. Psychol.* 87, 684–697. doi: 10.1037/0022-3514.87.5.684

Beadle, J., Yoon, C., and Gutchess, A. (2012). Age-related neural differences in affiliation and isolation. *Cogn. Affect. Behav. Neurosci.* 12, 269–279. doi: 10.3758/s13415-012-0085-y

Bechara, A., Damasio, H., Tranel, D., and Damasio, A. (1997). Deciding advantageously before knowing the advantageous strategy. *Science* 275, 1293–1294. doi: 10.1126/science.275.5304.1293

Carstensen, L., Fung, H., and Charles, S. (2003). Socioemotional selectivity theory and the regulation of emotion in the second half of life. *Motiv. Emot.* 27, 103–123. doi: 10.1023/A:1024569803230

Carstensen, L., Isaacowitz, D., and Charles, S. (1999). Taking time seriously: a theory of socioemotional selectivity. *Am. Psychol.* 54, 165–181. doi: 10.1037/0003-066X.54.3.165

Carstensen, L., and Mikels, J. (2005). At the intersection of emotion and cognition. *Curr. Dir. Psychol. Sci.* 14, 117–121. doi: 10.1111/j.0963-7214.2005.00348.x

Carstensen, L., Pasupathi, M., Mayr, U., and Nesselroade, J. (2000). Emotional experience in everyday life across the adult lifespan. *J. Pers. Soc. Psychol.* 79, 644–655. doi: 10.1037/0022-3514.79.4.644

Carstensen, L., and Turk-Charles, S. (1994). The salience of emotion across the adult life span. *Psychol. Aging* 9, 259–264. doi: 10.1037/0882-7974.9.2.259

Cassidy, B., and Gutchess, A. (2012). Social relevance enhances memory for impressions in older adults. *Memory* 20, 332–345. doi: 10.1080/09658211.2012.660956

Cassidy, B., Leshikar, E., Shih, J., Aizenman, A., and Gutchess, A. (2013). Valence-based age differences in medial prefrontal activity during impression formation. *Soc. Neurosci.* 8, 462–473. doi: 10.1080/17470919.2013.832373

Cassidy, B., Shih, J., and Gutchess, A. (2012). Age-related changes to the neural correlates of social evaluation. *Soc. Neurosci.* 7, 552–564. doi: 10.1080/17470919.2012.674057

Chalfonte, B., and Johnson, M. (1996). Feature memory and binding in young and older adults. *Mem. Cogn.* 24, 403–416. doi: 10.3758/BF03200930

Craig, A. (2009). How do you feel–now? The anterior insula and human awareness. *Nat. Rev. Neurosci.* 10, 59–70. doi: 10.1038/nrn2555

Critchley, H., Wiens, S., Rotshtein, P., Ohman, A., and Dolan, R. (2004). Neural systems supporting interoceptive awareness. *Nat. Neurosci.* 7, 189–195. doi: 10.1038/nn1176

Davidson, R., and Irwin, W. (1999). The functional neuroanatomy of emotion and affective style. *Trends Cogn. Sci.* 3, 11–21. doi: 10.1016/S1364-6613(98)01265-0

Dennis, N., Hayes, S., Prince, S., Madden, D., Huettel, S., and Cabeza, R. (2008). Effects of aging on the neural correlates of successful item and source memory encoding. *J. Exp. Psychol. Learn. Mem. Cogn.* 34, 791–808. doi: 10.1037/0278-7393.34.4.791

Dolcos, F., LaBar, K., and Cabeza, R. (2004). Dissociable effects of arousal and valence on prefrontal activity indexing emotional evaluation and subsequent memory: an event-related fMRI study. *Neuroimage* 23, 64–74. doi: 10.1016/j.neuroimage.2004.05.015

Fredrickson, B., and Carstensen, L. (1990). Choosing social partners: how old age and anticipated endings make people more selective. *Psychol. Aging* 5, 335–347. doi: 10.1037/0882-7974.5.3.335

Fung, H., and Carstensen, L. (2003). Sending memorable messages to the old: age differences in preferences and memory for advertisements. *J. Pers. Soc. Psychol.* 85, 163–178. doi: 10.1037/0022-3514.85.1.163

Fung, H., Carstensen, L., and Lutz, A. (1999). Influence of time on social preferences: implications for lifespan development. *Psychol. Aging* 14, 595–604. doi: 10.1037/0882-7974.14.4.595

Germain, C. M., and Hess, T. M. (2007). Motivational influences on controlled processing: moderating distractibility in older adults. *Neuropsychol. Dev. Cogn. B Aging Neuropsychol. Cogn.* 14, 462–486. doi: 10.1080/13825580600611302

Gilron, R., and Gutchess, A. (2012). Remembering first impressions: effects of intentionality and diagnosticity of subsequent memory. *Cogn. Affect. Behav. Neurosci.* 12, 85–98. doi: 10.3758/s13415-011-0074-6

Gutchess, A., Kensinger, E., and Schacter, D. (2007). Aging, self-referencing, and medial prefrontal cortex. *Soc. Neurosci.* 2, 117–133. doi: 10.1080/17470910701399029

Hasher, L., and Zacks, R. (1979). Automatic and effortful processes in memory. *J. Exp. Psychol. Gen.* 108, 356–388. doi: 10.1037/0096-3445.108.3.356

Johnson, M., Hashtroudi, S., and Lindsay, D. (1993). Source monitoring. *Psychol. Bull.* 114, 3–28. doi: 10.1037/0033-2909.114.1.3

Johnson, M., and Raye, C. (1981). Reality monitoring. *Psychol. Rev.* 88, 67–85. doi: 10.1037/0033-295X.88.1.67

Leclerc, C., and Kensinger, E. (2008). Age-related differences in medial prefrontal activation in response to emotional images. *Cogn. Affect. Behav. Neurosci.* 8, 153–164. doi: 10.3758/CABN.8.2.153

Leclerc, C., and Kensinger, E. (2010). Age-related valence-based reversal in recruitment of medial prefrontal cortex on a visual search task. *Soc. Neurosci.* 5, 560–576. doi: 10.1080/17470910903512296

Leshikar, E., and Duarte, A. (2013). Medial prefrontal cortex supports subsequent memory for self-referenced materials in young and older adults. *Cogn. Affect. Behav. Neurosci.* 1–17. doi: 10.3758/s13415-013-0198-y. [Epub ahead of print].

Lieberman, M. (2007). Social cognitive neuroscience: a review of core processes. *Annu. Rev. Psychol.* 58, 259–289. doi: 10.1146/annurev.psych.58.110405.085654

Lormel, D. (2001). *Fraud Against the Elderly. Federal Bureau of Investigation.* Available online at: http://www.fbi.gov/news/testimony/fraud-against-the-elderly

Mather, M., and Carstensen, L. (2005). Aging and motivated cognition: the positivity effect in attention and memory. *Trends Cogn. Sci.* 9, 496–502. doi: 10.1016/j.tics.2005.08.005

May, C., Rahhal, T., Berry, E., and Leighton, E. (2005). Aging, source memory, and emotion. *Psychol. Aging* 20, 571–578. doi: 10.1037/0882-7974.20.4.571

Mitchell, J., Heatherton, T., and Macrae, C. (2002). Distinct neural systems subserve person and object knowledge. *Proc. Natl. Acad. Sci. U.S.A.* 99, 15238–15243. doi: 10.1073/pnas.232395699

Mitchell, J., Macrae, C., and Banaji, M. (2004). Encoding-specific effects of social cognition on the neural correlates of subsequent memory. *J. Neurosci.* 24, 4912–4917. doi: 10.1523/JNEUROSCI.0481-04.2004

Mitchell, J., Macrae, C., and Banaji, M. (2005). Forming impressions of people versus inanimate objects: social-cognitive processing in the medial prefrontal cortex. *Neuroimage* 26, 251–257. doi: 10.1016/j.neuroimage.2005.01.031

Mitchell, J., Macrae, C. N., and Banaji, M. R. (2006a). Dissociable medial prefrontal contributions to judgments of similar and dissimilar others. *Neuron* 50, 655–663. doi: 10.1016/j.neuron.2006.03.040

Mitchell, K., Raye, C., Johnson, M., and Greene, E. (2006b). An fMRI investigation of short-term source memory in young and older adults. *Neuroimage* 30, 627–633. doi: 10.1016/j.neuroimage.2005.09.039

Mitchell, K., Johnson, M., Raye, C., and D'Esposito, M. (2000). fMRI evidence of age-related hippocampal dysfunction in feature binding in working memory. *Brain Res. Cogn. Brain Res.* 10, 197–206. doi: 10.1016/S0926-6410(00)00029-X

Moran, J., Jolly, E., and Mitchell, J. (2012). Social-cognitive deficits in normal aging. *J. Neurosci.* 32, 5553–5561. doi: 10.1523/JNEUROSCI.5511-11.2012

Ochsner, K., Bunge, S., Gross, J., and Gabrieli, J. (2002). Rethinking feelings: an fMRI study of the cognitive regulation of emotion. *J. Cogn. Neurosci.* 14, 1215–1229. doi: 10.1162/089892902760807212

Otten, L., Henson, R., and Rugg, M. (2001). Depth of processing effects on neural correlates of memory encoding: relationship between findings from across- and within-task comparisons. *Brain* 124, 399–412. doi: 10.1093/brain/124.2.399

Phan, K., Wager, T., Taylor, S., and Liberzon, I. (2002). Functional neuroanatomy of emotion: a meta-analysis of emotion activation studies in PET and fMRI. *Neuroimage* 16, 331–348. doi: 10.1006/nimg.2002.1087

Rahhal, T., May, C., and Hasher, L. (2002). Truth and character: sources that older adults can remember. *Psychol. Sci.* 13, 101–105. doi: 10.1111/1467-9280.00419

Rorden, C., and Brett, M. (2000). Stereotaxic display of brain lesions. *Behav. Neurol.* 12, 191–200. doi: 10.1155/2000/421719

Ruffman, T., Murray, J., Halberstadt, J., and Vater, T. (2012). Age-related differences in deception. *Psychol. Aging* 27, 543–549. doi: 10.1037/a0023380

Salthouse, T., and Babcock, R. (1991). Decomposing adult age differences in working memory. *Dev. Psychol.* 27, 763–776. doi: 10.1037/0012-1649.27.5.763

Sanfey, A., Rilling, J., Aronson, J., Nystrom, L., and Cohen, J. (2003). The neural basis of economic decision-making in the ultimatum game. *Science* 300, 1755–1758. doi: 10.1126/science.1082976

Satpute, A., and Lieberman, M. (2006). Integrating automatic and controlled processes into neurocognitive models of social cognition. *Brain Res.* 1079, 86–97. doi: 10.1016/j.brainres.2006.01.005

Saxe, R. (2006). Uniquely human social cognition. *Curr. Opin. Neurobiol.* 16, 235–239. doi: 10.1016/j.conb.2006.03.001

Shamay-Tsoory, S., and Aharon-Peretz, J. (2007). Dissociable prefrontal networks for cognitive and affective theory of mind: a lesion study. *Neuropsychologia* 45, 3054–3067. doi: 10.1016/j.neuropsychologia.2007.05.021

Shipley, W. (1986). *Shipley Institute of Living Scale*. Los Angeles, CA: Western Psychological Services.

Siedlecki, K., Salthouse, T., and Berish, D. (2005). Is there anything special about the aging of source memory? *Psychol. Aging* 20, 19–32. doi: 10.1037/0882-7974.20.1.19

Skurnik, I., Yoon, C., Park, D., and Schwarz, N. (2005). How warnings about false claims become recommendations. *J. Consum. Res.* 31, 713–724. doi: 10.1086/426605

Spencer, W., and Raz, N. (1995). Differential effects of aging on memory for content and context: a meta-analysis. *Psychol. Aging* 10, 527–539. doi: 10.1037/0882-7974.10.4.527

Telemarketing fraud against older Americans. (2007). *Federal Trade Commission*. Available online at: http://www.ftc.gov/reports/Fraud/fraudcon.shtm

Todorov, A., and Olson, I. (2008). Robust learning of affective trait associations with faces when the hippocampus is damaged, but not when the amygdala and temporal pole are damaged. *Soc. Cogn. Affect. Neurosci.* 3, 195–203. doi: 10.1093/scan/nsn013

Tsakiris, M., Hesse, M., Boy, C., Haggard, P., and Fink, G. (2007). Neural signatures of body ownership: a sensory network for bodily self-consciousness. *Cereb. Cortex* 17, 2235–2244. doi: 10.1093/cercor/bhl131

Van Overwalle, F. (2009). Social cognition and the brain: a meta-analysis. *Hum. Brain Mapp.* 30, 829–858. doi: 10.1002/hbm.20547

Wechsler, D. (1981). *Wechsler Adult Intelligence Scale–Revised Manual*. New York, NY: Psychological Corporation.

Wechsler, D. (1997). *Wechsler Memory Scale, 3rd Edn*. San Antonio, TX: The Psychological Corporation.

Wiech, K., Lin, C., Brodersen, K., Bingel, U., Ploner, M., and Tracey, I. (2010). Anterior insula integrates information about salience into perceptual decisions about pain. *J. Neurosci.* 30, 16324–16331. doi: 10.1523/JNEUROSCI.2087-10.2010

Woods, R., Cherry, S., and Mazziotta, J. (1992). Rapid automated algorithm for aligning and reslicing PET images. *J. Comput. Assist. Tomogr.* 16, 620–633. doi: 10.1097/00004728-199207000-00024

Zaki, J., Davis, J., and Ochsner, K. (2012). Overlapping activity in anterior insula during interoception and emotional experience. *Neuroimage* 62, 493–499. doi: 10.1016/j.neuroimage.2012.05.012

# 16

# Facial age affects emotional expression decoding

**_Mara Fölster[1]*, Ursula Hess[2] and Katja Werheid[1]_**

[1] *Clinical Gerontopsychology, Department of Psychology, Humboldt-Universität zu Berlin, Berlin, Germany*
[2] *Social and Organizational Psychology, Department of Psychology, Humboldt-Universität zu Berlin, Berlin, Germany*

**Edited by:**
*Natalie Ebner, University of Florida, USA*

**Reviewed by:**
*Natalie Ebner, University of Florida, USA*
*Derek Isaacowitz, Northeastern University, USA*
*Jessica Komes, Friedrich Schiller University, Germany*

***Correspondence:**
*Mara Fölster, Clinical Gerontopsychology, Department of Psychology, Humboldt-Universität zu Berlin, Rudower Chaussee 18, 12489 Berlin, Germany*
*e-mail: mara.foelster@hu-berlin.de*

Facial expressions convey important information on emotional states of our interaction partners. However, in interactions between younger and older adults, there is evidence for a reduced ability to accurately decode emotional facial expressions. Previous studies have often followed up this phenomenon by examining the effect of the observers' age. However, decoding emotional faces is also likely to be influenced by stimulus features, and age-related changes in the face such as wrinkles and folds may render facial expressions of older adults harder to decode. In this paper, we review theoretical frameworks and empirical findings on age effects on decoding emotional expressions, with an emphasis on age-of-face effects. We conclude that the age of the face plays an important role for facial expression decoding. Lower expressivity, age-related changes in the face, less elaborated emotion schemas for older faces, negative attitudes toward older adults, and different visual scan patterns and neural processing of older than younger faces may lower decoding accuracy for older faces. Furthermore, age-related stereotypes and age-related changes in the face may bias the attribution of specific emotions such as sadness to older faces.

**Keywords: emotional facial expressions, facial expression decoding, older face, aging, own-age advantage, response bias, expressivity**

## INTRODUCTION

Facial expressions convey important information on emotional states of our interaction partners (Ekman et al., 1982). Thus, the correct interpretation of facial expressions may facilitate emotional understanding and enhance the quality of interpersonal communication.

Recent evidence suggests that the correct interpretation of emotional expressions may be negatively affected in older age due to processes related to both the sender and the observer. The majority of the extant research has focused on the influence of the observers' age and concludes that older observers have deficits in the decoding of specific emotions (see Ruffman et al., 2008; Isaacowitz and Stanley, 2011, for reviews).

The age of those showing the facial expressions was initially less often considered. As a possible reason, the influential model of face processing by Bruce and Young (1986) postulated that the decoding of facial expressions is robust to the idiosyncratic features of a given face, which might be influenced by age, sex or other factors. However, this proposition has been subject to controversial debate (e.g., Schweinberger and Soukup, 1998; Schyns and Oliva, 1999; Kaufmann and Schweinberger, 2004; Calder and Young, 2005; Aviezer et al., 2011; Barret et al., 2011). Instead, it is likely that wrinkles, folds and the sag of facial musculature in the older face affect the interpretation of facial expressions. This assumption has been confirmed by recent results of decoding accuracy varying with the age of the face (Malatesta et al., 1987b; Borod et al., 2004; Ebner and Johnson, 2009, 2010; Murphy et al., 2010; Richter et al., 2011; Riediger et al., 2011; Hess et al., 2012; Ebner et al., 2012, 2013; Hühnel et al., 2014). Previous reviews have mainly focused on the age of the observer (Ruffman et al., 2008; Isaacowitz and Stanley, 2011) or on age-of-face effects on face identity recognition (e.g., Rhodes and Anastasi, 2012). Adding to this work, the present review is the first to focus on the influence of facial age on expression decoding and its possible underlying mechanisms, taking into account most recent work on this subject published after these previous reviews. Our aim was to compile and evaluate findings, thereby focusing on the question to which extent methodological differences between studies may account for inconsistent results. Further, we wish to identify unresolved research questions and suggest topics for future research. We will first give a very brief overview of the influence of the observers' age on decoding accuracy and the mechanisms underlying these effects. However, as this research has already been reviewed elsewhere (Ruffman et al., 2008; Isaacowitz and Stanley, 2011), we will mainly focus on the influence of the faces' age.

## INFLUENCE OF THE OBSERVERS' AGE

An age-related decline in decoding facial expressions has been repeatedly reported (e.g., Calder et al., 2003; Ruffman et al., 2008; Isaacowitz and Stanley, 2011). However, recent evidence suggests that this decline is confined to specific emotions. An overview of mechanisms underlying emotion-specific effects of the observers' age on facial expression decoding is given in **Figure 1** (right part). Some studies found an age-related deficit in decoding negative, but not positive emotional expressions (Phillips et al., 2002; Williams et al., 2006; Keightley et al., 2007; Ebner and Johnson, 2009). In addition, older observers had a greater bias toward thinking that individuals were feeling happy when they were displaying either enjoyment or non-enjoyment smiles (Slessor et al., 2010; but see Riediger et al., under review). These results have been accounted for by an information processing bias by older observers, leading to increased attention

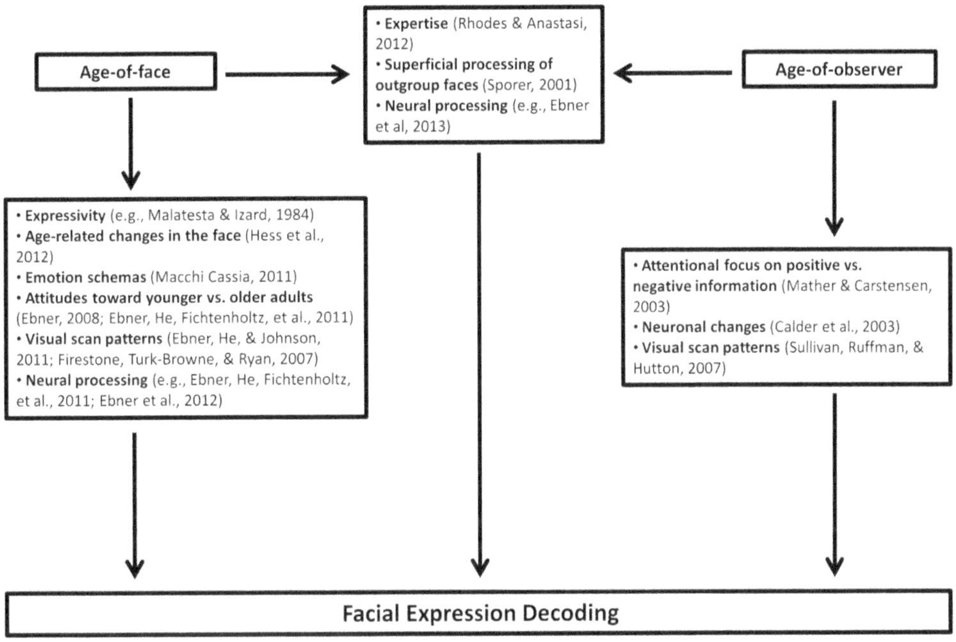


**FIGURE 1 | Overview of mechanisms underlying effects of the age of the face (left part) and the age of the observer (right part) as well as own-age effects (central part) on facial expression decoding.**

toward positive compared to negative information (Mather and Carstensen, 2003). This explanation is based on the socioemotional selectivity theory (SST, Carstensen and Charles, 1998), stating that older persons are, due to their limited future time perspective, inclined to engage in tasks related to emotional balance and well-being. Younger persons, in contrast, favor information seeking over emotionally rewarding goals and, thus, may be more inclined to attend to other persons' negative emotional states (Carstensen and Mikels, 2005). However, Isaacowitz and Stanley (2011) argued that the preserved ability to decode happiness may as well be due to the relative ease of the task, when happiness is the only positive response option. Supporting this assumption, age effects for positive emotions emerged when the task was more difficult (Isaacowitz et al., 2007). Further evidence against the SST-based account is that the majority of research on emotional prosody and body language suggests that older observers have difficulties to decode positive as well as negative emotions (emotional prosody: Taler et al., 2006; Ruffman et al., 2009a,b; Lambrecht et al., 2012, body language: Ruffman et al., 2009a,b, but see Montepare et al., 1999, for an exception).

Further conflicting the SST-based account, some studies found an age-related improvement in decoding disgust, together with no age differences for happiness and an age-related deficit in decoding sadness (Suzuki et al., 2007), or anger, fear and sadness (Calder et al., 2003). There are two alternative explanations for these findings.

The first explanation is based on observed age differences in visual scan patterns: older observers focus primarily on the lower part of the face and neglect the upper part (Wong et al., 2005; Sullivan et al., 2007). As the upper part plays a more important role for expressions of anger, fear and sadness, but not for disgust and happiness (Calder et al., 2000), this may explain why older observers are especially impaired in decoding these emotions. In line with this explanation, older observers' poor performance for decoding anger, fear and sadness correlated with fewer fixations to the top half of faces (Wong et al., 2005). However, Ebner et al. (2011c) found that visual scan patterns were independent of the observers' age, but rather varied with the expression. Thus, evidence for age differences in visual scan patterns is mixed. Furthermore, as already mentioned above, older observers' difficulties are not restricted to decoding facial expressions, but also emerge when decoding emotional prosody and bodily expression, at least rendering visual scan patterns as sole underlying mechanism unlikely.

The second explanation states that the brain regions that are responsible for decoding emotions, differ between the various emotions and that these regions are also differently affected by age-related changes (Ruffman et al., 2008; Ebner and Johnson, 2009; Ebner et al., 2012). As the frontal region, which is especially important for anger and sadness (Murphy et al., 2003), and the amygdala, which is important for fear (Murphy et al., 2003; Adolphs et al., 2005), are particularly affected by age-related changes (Jack et al., 1997; Bartzokis et al., 2003), a stronger age-related decline in decoding these emotions is predicted. In contrast, the basal ganglia, playing an important role for disgust (Phan et al., 2002), are less strongly affected by age-related changes (Raz, 2000; Williams et al., 2006), possibly resulting in a relatively preserved ability to decode disgust. Wong et al. (2005) further suggested that age-related declines in the frontal eye field, an area in the frontal lobe, may lead to deficits in visual attention, possibly leading to dysfunctional visual scan patterns. In addition, recent fMRI studies investigating brain activity in younger and older observers while viewing emotional faces suggest functional brain changes with age (Williams et al., 2006; Keightley et al., 2007). Although the pattern of results is somewhat mixed, older observers showed less amygdala activation (Gunning-Dixon et al., 2003; Fischer et al., 2005, 2010), but more prefrontal cortex activation (Gunning-Dixon et al., 2003; Fischer et al., 2010) compared to younger observers when viewing emotional faces. Fischer et al. (2005) suggested that this may represent an attempt to compensate for diminished functions in other brain regions than the frontal brain. Williams et al. (2006) further argued that this may reflect a shift from automatic processing to a more controlled processing of emotional information, possibly enabling older observers to better selectively control reactions to negative stimuli and finally leading to better emotional well-being. However, it may also be important to consider the valence of the facial expressions, and to differentiate between dorsomedial (dmPFC) and ventromedial prefrontal cortex (vmPFC). A recent study (Ebner et al., 2012) suggests that the vmPFC is more involved in affective and evaluative processing, whereas the dmPFC is involved in cognitively more complex processing. This functional dissociation seems to be largely comparable between younger and older observers. However, older observers showed increased dmPFC activity to negative faces, but decreased dmPFC to positive faces, possibly representing more controlled processing of negative compared to positive faces in older observers (Ebner et al., 2012).

## INFLUENCE OF THE FACES' AGE

Concerning the age of the face, the majority of previous research found that posed emotional facial expressions were decoded less accurately in older compared to younger faces, irrespective of the target emotion (Borod et al., 2004; Riediger et al., 2011; Ebner et al., 2012, 2013) or with the exception of happiness (Ebner and Johnson, 2009; Ebner et al., 2011c), which may be due to ceiling effects. Hess et al. (2012) confirmed this finding with artificially created face stimuli displaying identical expressions for younger and older faces. As an exception, Ebner et al. (2010) found no age difference for posed fear expressions, but for happiness, anger, sadness, disgust, and neutrality expressions. Taken together, these results suggest that decoding emotional expressions is more difficult in older compared with younger faces. However, results obtained with spontaneous, dynamic expressions yielded a more heterogeneous pattern of results. Whereas Richter et al. (2011) confirmed the generally lower decoding accuracy for older faces, and Murphy et al. (2010) found a more accurate differentiation between posed and spontaneous dynamic smiles in younger than older faces, Riediger et al. (under review) found no main effect of facial age on the differentiation between spontaneous and posed dynamic smiles, Malatesta et al. (1987b) found no significant age difference on decoding emotional facial expressions and Hühnel et al. (2014) found even higher decoding accuracy for older faces displaying sadness. In the following, we will discuss possible mechanisms underlying these results. An overview of these studies is given in **Table 1** and an overview of the underlying mechanisms is given in **Figure 1** (left part).

### EXPRESSIVITY

One possible explanation for reduced decoding accuracy for older faces may be that there actually is a difference in the way older and younger adults express emotions in their faces. Supporting this assumption, older adults performed worse than younger adults when following muscle-by-muscle instructions for constructing facial prototypes of emotional expressions (Levenson et al., 1991). Thus, due to age-related changes in flexibility and controllability of muscle tissue, the intentional display of facial emotions may become less successful with age and displays of unintended blended emotions may become more likely (Ebner et al., 2011c). In line with this assumption, observers more accurately judged whether videotaped speakers were telling the truth or lying when the speakers were older than when they were younger (Ruffman et al., 2012). Borod et al. (2004) further argued that an age-related decline in the frontal lobe may change emotional facial expressions, as frontal structures are especially important for the production of facial expressions and are highly vulnerable to aging.

Notably, these explanations may only account for age effects in posed expressions. For spontaneous expressions, results rather point to the assumption that younger and older adults do not differ in expressivity. In several studies, younger and older adults were filmed while reliving an emotional event or watching emotional film clips. Afterwards, their facial reactions were analyzed with objective coding systems such as FACS (Ekman et al., 1978), or MAX (Izard, 1979). An overview of these studies is given in **Table 2**. Although an early study suggested that older adults display more masked, that is, dissimulated, mixed and fragmented facial expressions than younger adults (Malatesta and Izard, 1984), later studies did not confirm these age differences in expressivity (Levenson et al., 1991; Tsai et al., 2000; Kunz et al., 2008), or even found higher expressivity for older faces (Malatesta-Magai et al., 1992). Thus, intentional displays of emotions may become less successful with age, but spontaneous emotional facial reactions seem to remain equally expressive throughout the life span. Besides, lower decoding accuracy for older faces cannot be fully explained by age differences in expressivity, because this effect has also been found when artificially created face stimuli controlled for expressivity were used (Hess et al., 2012).

Nevertheless, analyses of spontaneous facial expressions suggest that there may be age-related "dialects," that is, slight differences in the way older and younger adults express certain emotions. For example, older adults expressed sadness mainly through a lowered head, whereas younger adults also showed lowered brows (Malatesta and Izard, 1984). While reliving anger and sadness eliciting episodes, younger adults showed longer durations of shame, contempt and joy expressions, which may be interpreted as a cynical, self-conscious, perhaps mocking facial presentation that is common in younger adults (Magai et al., 2006). Older adults, on the other hand, showed more knitted brows, possibly indexing a generalized distress configuration in a regulated form, serving to indicate that negative emotion is present, but protecting social partners from emotional contagion (Magai et al., 2006). Notably, these age differences were not related to a corresponding age difference in experienced emotions

**Table 1 | Summary of research on age-of-face effects on decoding accuracy.**

| Authors | Age-of-face | Stimuli description/database | Target emotions | Observers | Dependent variables | Main age-of-face results |
|---|---|---|---|---|---|---|
| Borod et al., 2004 | 30 YA,<br>30 MA,<br>30 OA, only females | Still posed expressions, developed for this study | Happiness, pleasant surprise, sadness, disgust, neutrality | 12 YA,<br>12 MA,<br>12 OA, only females | Multiple choice emotion identification<br>Confidence of rating | OA faces were rated less accurately and with less confidence than YA faces<br>No own-age effect |
| Ebner et al., 2011c | 8 YA and 8 OA per emotion | Still posed expressions [FACES developed by Ebner et al., 2010] | Happiness, anger, fear, sadness, disgust, neutrality | 30 YA,<br>30 OA | Multiple choice emotion identification<br>Visual scan patterns | Higher accuracy for YA than OA faces for anger, fear, disgust, sadness and neutrality<br>No age-of-face effect for happiness<br>No own-age effect<br>Both YA and OA looked longer at own-age than other-age faces<br>Longer looking at own-age faces predicted better own-age expression identification |
| Ebner and Johnson, 2009 | 8 YA and 8 OA per emotion | Still posed expressions [FACES developed by Ebner et al., 2010] | Happiness, anger, neutrality | 32 YA,<br>24 OA | Multiple choice emotion identification<br>Self-reported contact to YA and OA | Higher decoding accuracy for YA than OA faces for anger and neutrality<br>No age-of-face effect for happiness<br>No own-age effect<br>The more contact observers reported with the own age group, the less they were able to identify expressions of the other age group<br>No relationship between own-age contact and own-age decoding accuracy |

*(Continued)*

**Table 1 | Continued**

| Authors | Age-of-face | Stimuli description/database | Target emotions | Observers | Dependent variables | Main age-of-face results |
|---|---|---|---|---|---|---|
| Ebner et al., 2012[1] | 16 YA and 16 OA per emotion | Still posed expressions [FACES developed by Ebner et al., 2010] | Happiness, anger, neutrality | 30 YA, 32 OA | Multiple choice emotion identification<br>fMRI data | Higher accuracy for YA than OA faces<br>No age-of-face by emotion interaction<br>No own-age effect<br>Functional dissociation between vmPFC (affective processing) and dmPFC (cognitive control)<br>Greater dmPFC activity for OA compared to YA faces |
| Ebner et al., 2010 | 58 YA, 56 MA, 57 OA | Still posed expressions (development and validation of FACES in this study) | Happiness, anger, fear, sadness, disgust, neutrality | 52 YA, 51 MA, 51 OA | Multiple choice emotion identification<br>Age estimation | Higher accuracy for YA than OA faces for happiness, anger, sadness, disgust, and neutrality<br>No age-of-face effect for fear<br>No own-age effect<br>Happy faces were perceived as younger and fearful faces as older than faces with other expressions |
| Hess et al., 2012 | 6 YA, 6 OA | Morphed identical facial expressions to neutral faces from Minear and Park (2004) | Happiness, anger, sadness | 65 YA | Continuous emotion rating | OA faces were rated as more intense on inaccurate emotions, but as less intense on accurate emotions than YA faces |
| Hühnel et al., 2014 | 4 YA, 4 OA | Videos of adults talking about biographic episodes (without sound) | Happiness, anger, sadness, disgust | 39 YA, 39 OA, only females | Continuous emotion rating<br>Mimicry measured via facial EMG | Higher accuracy for YA than OA faces for happiness and disgust<br>Higher accuracy for OA than YA faces for sadness<br>No age-of-face effect for anger<br>No own-age effect<br>No age-of-face effects on mimicry |
| Malatesta et al., 1987a | 14 OA | Photos of posed expressions | Happiness, anger, sadness, fear, neutrality | 30 YA | Multiple choice emotion identification<br>Personality test results of posers | Emotions rated in the neutral face were congruent with the posers' dominant trait emotions |

*(Continued)*

**Table 1 | Continued**

| Authors | Age-of-face | Stimuli description/database | Target emotions | Observers | Dependent variables | Main age-of-face results |
|---|---|---|---|---|---|---|
| Malatesta and Izard, 1984 | 10 YA, 10 MA, 10 OA, only females | Videos of women talking about biographic episodes (without sound) | Happiness, anger, sadness, fear, affection | 30 adults (no specification of age) | MAX-Coding of facial expressions<br>Multiple choice emotion identification | MAX-Coding: see **Table 2**<br>OA faces received less anger, but more sadness attributions than YA faces |
| Malatesta et al., 1987b | 10 YA, 10 MA, 10 OA, only females | Videos of women talking about biographic episodes (without sound) | Sadness, fear, anger | 10 YA, 10 MA, 10 OA, only females | Multiple choice emotion identification<br>Rating of intensity of dominant emotion | No significant age-of-face effect on decoding accuracy<br>Own-age bias in decoding accuracy<br>Trend for more frequent attribution of sadness to OA than YA faces |
| Matheson, 1997 | 10 YA<br>10 OA, chronic pain patients | Videos of patients undergoing motion tests | Posed, masked and true pain, neutrality | 39 YA, 24 OA | Rating of intensity of experienced pain | More pain attribution to OA, for all experimental conditions |
| Murphy et al., 2010 | 13 YA, 11 OA, only females | Videos of women talking about an imagined pleasant scenario (posed smile), pleasant biographical experience/response to winning a prize (spontaneous smile) | Posed smile, spontaneous smile | 23 YA, 26 OA | Multiple choice rating of posed vs. spontaneous smile | Higher accuracy for YA than OA faces<br>No own-age effect |
| Richter et al., 2011 | 4 YA, 4 OA, only females | Videos of women talking about biographic episodes (played with vs. without sound) | Happiness, anger, sadness | 48 YA, 35 OA, only females | Continuous emotion rating, correlation of observers' and actors' ratings of felt emotions | Higher accuracy for YA than OA faces, no interaction with emotion<br>Younger observers showed an own-age advantage when videos were played with, but not without sound |
| Riediger et al., 2011 | 58 YA, 56 MA, 57 OA | Still posed expressions [FACES developed by Ebner et al., 2010] | Happiness, anger, sadness, fear, disgust, neutrality | 52 YA, 51 MA, 51 OA | Continuous emotion rating | OA faces were rated as more intense on inaccurate emotions, but as less intense on accurate emotions<br>Own-age effect for happiness and anger<br>Attribution of more inaccurate neutrality, anger, and sadness to OA than YA faces |

*(Continued)*

**Table 1 | Continued**

| Authors | Age-of-face | Stimuli description/database | Target emotions | Observers | Dependent variables | Main age-of-face results |
|---|---|---|---|---|---|---|
| Riediger et al., under review, Study 2 | 16 YA and 16 OA per smile type | Videos of adults watching amusing film clips (spontaneous smile), or posing smiles | Posed smile, spontaneous smile | 48 YA, 49 OA | Multiple choice rating of posed vs. spontaneous positive-affect smile | More frequent attribution of positive-affect smile to OA than YA faces, effect was more pronounced for YA than OA observers<br>Own-age advantage in decoding posed smiles for both YA and OA, and in decoding spontaneous smiles for OA<br>No main effect of facial age on decoding accuracy |

*YA, younger adults; MA, middle-aged adults; OA, older adults; [1] As Ebner et al. (2013) report identical emotion decoding data to Ebner et al. (2012), the former study is not mentioned in the table.*

(Malatesta and Izard, 1984; Magai et al., 2006). However, it is unclear whether these differences are actually due to the participants' age, or whether these are cohort-specific differences. Thus, long-term studies examining several cohorts in different ages would be necessary to follow up this question.

### AGE-RELATED CHANGES IN THE FACE

Decoding accuracy for older faces may also be reduced due to age-related changes in the face such as wrinkles and folds (see Albert et al., 2007; Porcheron et al., 2013; for overviews of age-related changes in the face). The wrinkles and folds in the older face may resemble emotional facial expressions and lead to the impression of a permanent affective state (Hess et al., 2008). These background affects may make older adults' facial expressions more ambiguous and reduce the signal clarity (Ebner and Johnson, 2009; Hess et al., 2012). Thus, when emotional expressions were rated on multiple intensity scales for target as well as non-target emotions instead of forced-choice scales, raters attributed less of the target emotions, but more non-target emotions to older faces (Riediger et al., 2011; Hess et al., 2012). Further supporting this account, no age-of-target effects emerged for decoding emotional prosody (Dupuis and Pichora-Fuller, 2011), suggesting that lowered decoding accuracy for older targets may be specific to faces.

These age-related changes in the face may also systematically bias emotional attributions. Hess et al. (2008) suggested that facial expressions and morphological features can have similar effects on emotional attributions ("functional equivalence hypothesis"). Thus, age-related changes in the face may both reduce the signal clarity and bias emotional attributions. Physiognomic features that are frequently found in older faces, such as for example down-turned corners of the mouth may be misinterpreted as emotional expressions. Supporting this assumption, older faces received more sadness attributions than younger faces (Malatesta and Izard, 1984).

However, so far it is unclear whether these effects are due to general aging effects *per se* (e.g., loss of muscle tone) or due to trace emotions (Malatesta et al., 1987a). Interestingly, emotions participants attributed to older senders' neutral expressions were congruent with senders' dominant trait emotions (Malatesta et al., 1987a). Thus, frequently experienced emotions may leave a trace on the face ("habitual emotional expressions"), so that in older age, the neutral expression resembles these emotions. However, to our knowledge, this result has not yet been replicated. Clearly, more research on the relationship between emotionality and age-related changes in the face is needed. Here, long-term studies may constitute a valuable extension of previous research.

### EMOTION SCHEMAS

As an alternative explanation for reduced decoding accuracy for older faces, Ebner et al. (2011a) suggested that facial expression prototypes are more likely young faces. The authors argue that emotion schemas may be developed in childhood from the young faces of parents and TV and movie depictions of facial expressions, where older individuals are underrepresented (Signorielli, 2004). Thus, emotion schemas may be better calibrated to decode

**Table 2 | Summary of research on age differences in facial expressivity.**

| Authors | Age-of-face | Emotion induction | Target emotions | Coding system | Other dependent variables | Main results |
|---|---|---|---|---|---|---|
| Kunz et al., 2008 | 46 YA, 61 OA | Pressure stimulation, electrical stimulation | Pain | FACS (Ekman et al., 1978) | Self-reported pain | No age differences in facial expressions or self-reported pain |
| Levenson et al., 1991 | 20 OA, 62 YA | Muscle-by-muscle instruction for posing expressions<br>Reliving biographical episodes | Happiness, anger, sadness, fear, disgust, surprise | FACS (Ekman et al., 1978) | Self-reported experienced emotions<br>ANS activity | OA performed worse than YA when posing facial expressions and experienced the emotions to a lower degree than YA<br>Spontaneous expressions and experiences of target emotions were comparable between YA and OA |
| Magai et al., 2006 | 32 YA, 32 MA, 32 OA | Reliving biographical episodes | Anger, sadness | MAX (Izard, 1979) | Self-reported experienced emotions | YA showed more shame, contempt and joy than OA<br>OA showed more knitted brows than YA<br>OA experienced more interest than YA and MA, no age differences for the remaining emotions<br>Greater heterogeneity in experienced emotions in OA than YA, but this was due to age differences in chosen topics |
| Malatesta and Izard, 1984 | 10 YA, 10 MA, 10 OA, only females | Reliving biographical episodes | Happiness, anger, sadness, fear, affection | MAX (Izard, 1979) | Self-reported experienced emotions | OA showed more masked, mixed and fragmented partial expressions than YA<br>OA showed more anger and contempt, less sadness than YA<br>No age differences in experienced emotions |
| Malatesta-Magai et al., 1992 | 80 YA, 80 OA | Reliving biographical episodes | Anger, sadness, fear, interest, affection | MAX (Izard, 1979) | Self-reported experienced emotions | OA showed more anger, sadness, fear and interest than YA<br>OA experienced more interest, no age differences for the remaining emotions |
| Tsai et al., 2000 | 48 YA, 48 OA | Watching emotional film clips | Sadness, amusement | Coding system by Gross and Levenson (1993) | Self-reported experienced emotions<br>Cardiovascular response | No age difference in facial expressions<br>No age difference in experienced emotions<br>Smaller cardiovascular reactions in OA than YA |

*YA, younger adults; MA, middle-aged adults; OA, older adults.*

emotions in younger than older faces. A strong effect of the frequency of contact with faces of specific age groups has been confirmed for face identity recognition (Harrison and Hole, 2009). Furthermore, studies investigating the ability to discriminate among individual faces suggest that early in childhood, perceptual processes become tuned to adult faces as the faces children have been most frequently exposed to since birth (see Macchi Cassia, 2011, for a review). Thus, 3-year old children who had frequent contact with elderly people showed no processing advantage for younger over older adult faces, whereas non-experienced children did (Proietti et al., 2013). However, these processes may still be modulated by experience with faces of different age groups during adulthood (Macchi Cassia, 2011). As not only younger, but also older adults substantially differ in the amount of contact with older people (Wiese et al., 2012), emotion schemas for older faces may still vary in older observers.

Pertaining to decoding accuracy, this explanation still needs empirical investigation. Future studies could examine a sample with frequent contact with older adults during childhood, for example children that grew up in multi-generational homes. If this sample showed less difference in decoding accuracy between younger and older faces than a control group, this would support the hypothesis of less elaborated emotion schemas as an underlying mechanism. Furthermore, the influence of experience with older faces during early and late adulthood may be investigated by examining individuals of varying age and with varying amount of contact with older adults.

### ATTITUDES TOWARD OLDER ADULTS

An alternative explanation may be that younger adults are preferred over older adults (Ebner and Johnson, 2009). Although there are both positive and negative elements in age stereotypes (e.g., Hummert et al., 2004; Kornadt and Rothermund, 2011), both younger and older adults showed more positive implicit attitudes (Ebner et al., 2011b) and explicit evaluations (Ebner, 2008) of younger than older faces. In addition, young adults implicitly associated themselves more closely with the concept of being young than old (Wiese et al., 2013b).

Furthermore, as individuals resort on stereotype knowledge about social groups when decoding ambiguous facial expressions of strangers (Hess and Kirouac, 2000), stereotypes may also, just like age-related changes in the face, bias the attribution of emotions. For example, if individuals hold the stereotype of older persons being less satisfied, they may be more prone to attribute sadness and less prone to attribute happiness to an older compared to a younger face. Higher decoding accuracy for emotions corresponding to stereotypes and lower decoding accuracy for emotions contradicting stereotypes may result. This may not that much apply to the posed expressions typically used in emotion decoding studies, which are rather unambiguous, but more to spontaneous expressions that we encounter in everyday life, which can be mixtures of several emotions, or be masked behind socially more desirable emotions. In line with this assumption, for spontaneous expressions, Hühnel et al. (2014) did not replicate the pattern of generally lower decoding accuracy for older faces. Instead, happiness and disgust were more accurately decoded in younger faces, whereas sadness was more accurately decoded in older faces. Also, the previously mentioned result that older faces received more sadness attributions (Malatesta and Izard, 1984) may not only be due to age-related changes in the face, but also to age-related stereotypes. In this vein, observers attributed more pain (Matheson, 1997), but less anger (Malatesta and Izard, 1984) to older faces. In addition, individuals displaying a happy facial expression were perceived as younger than individuals displaying a fearful, angry, disgusted or sad expression (Voelkle et al., 2012). In the same vein, Bzdok et al. (2012) found a negative association between the perceived age and happiness of faces. Although this pattern of results is somewhat mixed, it seems that youth is more likely associated with happiness, whereas older age is more likely associated with sadness.

However, aging stereotypes in emotional domains were not found in explicit measures, possibly because they are socially undesirable. When participants were directly asked to describe "typical" younger and older individuals, relatively neutral stereotypes in social and emotional domains were found (Boduroglu et al., 2006). Also, not all studies using spontaneous expressions found emotion-specific effects of the faces' age on decoding accuracy (Malatesta et al., 1987b; Richter et al., 2011). Furthermore, contradicting the assumed association between youth and happiness, Riediger et al. (under review) found a more frequent attribution of positive emotions to smiles shown by older compared to younger individuals. Clearly, more research is needed, using more subtle or implicit measures for age-related stereotypes, such as IAT (implicit association test), and relating them to attributed emotions.

### VISUAL SCAN PATTERNS

There is some evidence that visual scan patterns may differ, depending on the age of the face that is being observed. Specifically, both younger and older observers looked longer at the eye region of older than younger neutral faces, and longer at the mouth region of younger than older neutral faces (Firestone et al., 2007). Considering the above mentioned higher importance of the eye region for expressions of anger, fear, and sadness, and the mouth region for sadness and disgust, one could expect higher decoding accuracy for younger than older faces for disgust and happiness, but not for anger, fear and sadness. However, among the studies examining age-of-face effects on decoding accuracy, only one was in line with this pattern (Hühnel et al., 2014). The majority of previous research found lower decoding accuracy for older faces, independent of the type of expression. Furthermore, other studies found that visual scan patterns were independent of the faces' age (He et al., 2011) or depended on the type of expression (Ebner et al., 2011c). Thus, Ebner et al. (2011c) only confirmed the result of longer looking at the eye region of older than younger faces for expressions of anger. For disgust, the opposite pattern with longer looking at the lower half of older than younger faces was found. There were no age differences for happy, fearful, sad or neutral faces. Thus, the result of different visual scan patterns for younger than older faces may not be generalizable across all facial expressions. In addition, whereas young observers' expression identification of young faces was better the longer they looked at the upper half of faces, older observers' expression identification of young faces was better the longer they looked at the lower half of faces (Ebner et al., 2011c). Thus, the assumption of one visual scan pattern leading to higher accuracy for both younger and older observers and younger and older faces might not always be appropriate.

Considering these mixed results, more research on this topic, relating visual scan patterns for faces with varying age and facial expressions to decoding accuracy is needed to decide whether visual scan patterns may account for age-of-face effects on decoding accuracy. So far, evidence rather contradicts the assumption of visual scan patterns as an underlying mechanism.

### NEURAL PROCESSING

To our knowledge, previous EEG studies only examined the neural processing of neutral, but not emotional younger and older faces (e.g., Wiese et al., 2008, 2012; Ebner et al., 2011b; Wolff et al., 2012). These studies revealed that the age of the face influenced both early and late ERP components (Ebner et al., 2011b), suggesting that age already influences early processing stages. For older faces, enlarged amplitudes of the N170, a negative deflection over occipito-temporal sites, have been found (Wiese et al., 2008, 2012), suggesting that structural encoding may be more difficult for older faces. Further, enlarged Late Positive Potentials (LPP, a positive deflection over parietal sites) for older faces suggest more controlled processing of older than younger faces (Ebner et al., 2011b). This latter assumption is further supported by recent fMRI results of greater dmPFC activation for older than younger emotional faces (Ebner et al., 2012). However, so far only very little research on neural processing of younger and older emotional faces has been conducted, allowing no definite conclusion on neural processing as an underlying mechanism. Thus, further research examining the relation of neural processing of emotional younger and older faces to decoding accuracy is needed.

## OWN-AGE ADVANTAGE

Apart from the above mentioned main effects of the ages of the observer and the face, age congruence between the observer and the face might influence decoding accuracy as well. As emotions are less accurately decoded in out-group than in-group faces (Thibault et al., 2006) and age is an important social category, one could expect an own-age advantage in face processing.

In line with this assumption, participants tended to look longer at own-age faces and longer looking at own-age faces predicted better own-age expression identification (Ebner et al., 2011c); they were more distracted by own-age faces (Ebner and Johnson, 2010) and fMRI-Studies report different activities for own-age than other-age faces (Wright et al., 2008; Ebner et al., 2011a, 2013), possibly indexing a preference for and more interest in own-age faces. Some EEG-studies report partly comparable own-age and own-race effects on ERPs for neutral faces (Wiese et al., 2008; Ebner et al., 2011b; but see Wiese, 2012; Wiese et al., 2013a, for partly different ERP correlates). Furthermore, several studies found that participants remembered own-age faces better than other-age faces (see Rhodes and Anastasi, 2012, for a meta-analysis). There are two main explanations for this latter finding. Firstly, social cognitive theories suggest that faces of out-group members are cognitively disregarded and more superficially processed than faces of in-group members (Sporer, 2001). Secondly, more experience or contact with members of the own age group may lead to higher perceptual expertise with own-age faces (Rhodes and Anastasi, 2012) and to higher familiarity with the expressive style of the own age group (Malatesta et al., 1987b). So far, evidence is more in line with the latter explanation, as the amount of contact appears to be related to face identity recognition (Harrison and Hole, 2009; Wiese et al., 2012, 2013b; Wolff et al., 2012) and facial expression decoding accuracy (Ebner and Johnson, 2009) of other-age faces. Hugenberg and colleagues (Hugenberg et al., 2010, 2013) suggested an integration of both theories in the Categorization- Individuation Model, which may also be useful to explain the own-age advantage. According to this model, own-group biases may be due to the combined influence of social categorization, the motivation to individuate and perceptual experience (Hugenberg et al., 2010). An overview of possible mechanisms underlying own-age effects on decoding accuracy is given in **Figure 1** (central part).

It is likely to assume that these in-group effects in face processing also influence facial expression decoding. Usually, facial expressions of in-group members are more accurately decoded than expressions of out-group members, even if group membership is manipulated (Thibault et al., 2006; Young and Hugenberg, 2010). In addition, automatic affective responses to other persons' emotional expressions are congruent for ingroup members, but incongruent for outgroup members (Weisbuch and Ambady, 2008). In an early study, Malatesta et al. (1987b) confirmed an own-age advantage in facial expression decoding accuracy. In addition, Riediger et al. (under review) reported an own-age effect on the ability to differentiate between spontaneous and posed smiles. Surprisingly though, the majority of the extant research found no own-age advantage (Borod et al., 2004; Ebner

**Box 1 | Questions for future research.**

Are age-related dialects for facial expressions due to aging effects *per se* (such as changes in flexibility and controllability of muscle tissue), or due to cohort-specific differences (such as differences in display rules)?
Does the frequency of contact to older adults during childhood and adulthood modulate age-of-face effects on decoding accuracy?
Are age-related changes in facial physiognomic features that resemble certain emotions due to aging effects *per se* (such as loss of muscle tone) or due to frequently experienced emotions, leaving a trace on the face?
Are age-related response biases in emotion decoding tasks related to implicit and explicit stereotypes of aging?
Is the lower decoding accuracy for older faces related to more negative attitudes toward older than younger adults?
Do visual scan patterns differ for younger and older emotional faces? If yes, might this effect explain age-of-face effects on decoding accuracy?
Are age-of-face effects on expression decoding related to differences in neural processing of younger and older emotional faces?
What is the time course of neural processing of age and emotional expression of a face?
Does the age of the target affect emotion decoding in other emotion channels than facial expressions, such as emotional prosody or body language?
Does the lower decoding accuracy for older faces affect the quality of interpersonal interactions and relationships for older adults?

and Johnson, 2009; Murphy et al., 2010; Ebner et al., 2011c, 2012, 2013; Hühnel et al., 2014) or an own-age advantage that was confined to specific emotions (Riediger et al., 2011). Thus, age congruence between the observer and sender of facial expressions seems to play a minor role for facial expression decoding, and the features that are important for identity recognition of faces may not be identical to those that are important for decoding facial expressions (Ebner and Johnson, 2009).

## CONCLUSIONS AND FUTURE DIRECTIONS

To sum up, the age of the face seems to play an important role for the interpretation of facial expressions. Posed expressions are less accurately decoded in older compared with younger faces. However, for spontaneous expressions, results are rather mixed. As a possible explanation, older adults are less expressive when posing emotional expressions, but equally expressive when spontaneously showing emotions. Yet at the same time, age stereotypes and age-related changes in physiognomic features of the face may bias the attribution of certain emotions. Contrariwise, age congruence between observer and sender of facial expressions may only play a minor role for expression decoding.

Concerning the underlying mechanisms, more research is needed to decide which of the suggested mechanisms are likely to underlie age-of-face effects on decoding accuracy. Age differences in expressivity are unlikely to be the sole underlying mechanism, as age-of-face effects have also been found when expressivity was controlled for (Hess et al., 2012). Further, previous research rather argues against visual scan patterns as an underlying mechanism. For the remaining mechanisms, i.e., age-related changes in the face, emotion schemas, attitudes toward older adults, and neural processing, more research is needed to judge the applicability of these accounts. It is unlikely to assume only one single mechanism driving age-of-face effects. Rather, multiple mechanisms seem to affect decoding accuracy.

One of the aims of the present review was to outline promising areas of future research. Although several mechanisms have been proposed to underlie age-of-face effects on decoding accuracy, only very little research directly tested the influence of these mechanisms. Thus, in our view, the most important objective for future research in this area will be to directly examine the influence of each of these variables on decoding accuracy for younger and older faces. An overview of some interesting questions for future research is given in **Box 1**. For example, further EEG and fMRI studies would be suited to relate neural processing of younger and older emotional faces to decoding accuracy. In addition, long-term studies on age-related changes in the face and their relation to frequently experienced emotions, and on changes in emotion schemas, which may be related to contact frequency with different age groups, may shed further light on gradual evolvement of these mechanisms. Further research is also needed on the relationship between age-related stereotypes and decoding biases. Furthermore, so far the question whether age-of-target effects are specific for facial expressions, or whether they also emerge in other emotion channels, is not yet fully resolved, as there is only one previous study analyzing age-of-target effects on decoding emotional prosody (Dupuis and Pichora-Fuller, 2011). Finally, future studies may examine whether the lower decoding accuracy for older faces affects the quality of interpersonal interactions and relationships. Thus, we think that exploring age-of-face effects on facial expression decoding and the underlying mechanisms is a promising and interesting area for future research.

## ACKNOWLEDGMENTS

This research was supported by grant WE 4836/1-1 from the German Research Foundation.

## REFERENCES


Adolphs, R., Gosselin, F., Buchanan, T. W., Tranel, D., Schyns, P., and Damasio, A. R. (2005). A mechanism for impaired fear recognition after amygdala damage. *Nature* 433, 68–72. doi: 10.1038/nature03086

Albert, A. M., Ricanek, K., and Patterson, E. (2007). A review of the literature on the aging adult skull and face: implications for forensic science research and applications. *Forensic Sci. Int.* 172, 1–9. doi: 10.1016/j.forsciint.2007.03.015

Aviezer, H., Bentin, S., Dudarev, V., and Hassin, R. R. (2011). The automaticity of emotional face-context integration. *Emotion* 11, 1406–1414. doi: 10.1037/a0023578

Barret, L. F., Mesquita, B., and Gendron, M. (2011). Context in emotion perception. *Curr. Dir. Psychol. Sci.* 20, 286–290. doi: 10.1177/0963721411422522

Bartzokis, G., Cummings, J. L., Sultzer, D., Henderson, V. W., Nuechterlein, K. H., and Mintz, J. (2003). White matter structural integrity in healthy aging adults and patients with Alzheimer disease: a magnetic resonance imaging study. *Arch. Neurol.* 60, 393–398. doi: 10.1001/archneur.60.3.393

Boduroglu, A., Yoon, C., Luo, T., and Park, D. C. (2006). Age-related stereotypes: a comparison of American and Chinese cultures. *Gerontology* 52, 324–333. doi: 10.1159/000094614

Borod, J., Yecker, S., Brickman, A., Moreno, C., Sliwinski, M., Foldi, N., et al. (2004). Changes in posed facial expression of emotion across the adult life span. *Exp. Aging Res.* 30, 305–331. doi: 10.1080/03610730490484399

Bruce, V., and Young, A. (1986). Understanding face recognition. *Br. J. Psychol.* 77, 305–327. doi: 10.1111/j.2044-8295.1986.tb02199.x

Bzdok, D., Langner, R., Hoffstaedter, F., Turetsky, B. I., Zilles, K., and Eickhoff, S. B. (2012). The modular neuroarchitecture of social judgments on faces. *Cereb. Cortex* 22, 951–961. doi: 10.1093/cercor/bhr166

Calder, A. J., Keane, J., Manly, T., Sprengelmeyer, R., Scott, S., Nimmo-Smith, I., et al. (2003). Facial expression recognition across the adult life span. *Neuropsychologia* 41, 195–202. doi: 10.1016/S0028-3932(02)00149-5

Calder, A. J., and Young, A. W. (2005). Understanding the recognition of facial identity and facial expression. *Nat. Rev. Neurosci.*6, 641–651. doi: 10.1038/nrn1724

Calder, A. J., Young, A. W., Keane, J., and Dean, M. (2000). Configural information in facial expression perception. *J. Exp. Psychol. Hum. Percept. Perform.* 26, 527–551. doi: 10.1037/0096-1523.26.2.527

Carstensen, L. L., and Charles, S. T. (1998). Emotion in the second half of life. *Curr. Dir. Psychol. Sci.* 7, 144–149. doi: 10.1111/1467-8721.ep10836825

Carstensen, L. L., and Mikels, J. A. (2005). At the intersection of emotion and cognition—aging and the positivity effect. *Curr. Dir. Psychol. Sci.* 14, 117–121. doi: 10.1111/j.0963-7214.2005.00348.x

Dupuis, K., and Pichora-Fuller, M. K. (2011). Recognition of emotional speech for younger and older talkers: behavioural findings from the toronto emotional speech set. *Canadian Acoustics* 39, 182–183. Available online at: http://jcaa.caa-aca.ca/index.php/jcaa/article/view/2471

Ebner, N. C. (2008). Age of face matters: age-group differences in ratings of young and old faces. *Behav. Res. Methods* 40, 130–136. doi: 10.3758/BRM.40.1.130

Ebner, N. C., Gluth, S., Johnson, M. R., Raye, C. L., Mitchell, K. J., and Johnson, M. K. (2011a). Medial prefrontal cortex activity when thinking about others depends on their age. *Neurocase* 17, 260–269. doi: 10.1080/13554794.2010.536953

Ebner, N. C., He, Y., Fichtenholtz, H. M., McCarthy, G., and Johnson, M. K. (2011b). Electrophysiological correlates of processing faces of younger and older individuals. *Soc. Cogn. Affect. Neurosci.* 6, 526–535. doi: 10.1093/scan/nsq074

Ebner, N. C., He, Y., and Johnson, M. K. (2011c). Age and emotion affect how we look at a face: visual scan patterns differ for own-age versus other-age emotional faces. *Cogn. Emot.* 25, 983–997. doi: 10.1080/02699931.2010.540817

Ebner, N. C., and Johnson, M. K. (2009). Young and older emotional faces: are there age group differences in expression identification and memory? *Emotion* 9, 329–339. doi: 10.1037/a0015179

Ebner, N. C., and Johnson, M. K. (2010). Age-group differences in interference from young and older emotional faces. *Cogn. Emot.* 24, 1095–1116. doi: 10.1080/02699930903128395

Ebner, N. C., Johnson, M. K., and Fischer, H. (2012). Neural mechanisms of reading facial emotions in young and older adults. *Front. Psychol.* 3:223. doi: 10.3389/fpsyg.2012.00223

Ebner, N. C., Johnson, M. R., Rieckmann, A., Durbin, K. A., Johnson, M. K., and Fischer, H. (2013). Processing own-age vs. other-age faces: neuro-behavioral correlates and effects of emotion. *Neuroimage* 78, 363–371. doi: 10.1016/j.neuroimage.2013.04.029

Ebner, N. C., Riediger, M., and Lindenberger, U. (2010). FACES- a database of facial expressions in young, middle-aged, and older women and men: development and validation. *Behav. Res. Methods* 42, 351–362. doi: 10.3758/BRM.42.1.351

Ekman, P., Friesen, W. V., and Ellsworth, P. (1982). "Does the human face provide accurate information?" in *Emotion in the Human Face*, ed P. Ekman (New York, NY: Cambridge University Press), 56–97.

Ekman, P., Friesen, W. V., and Hager, J. C. (1978). *Facial Action Coding System (FACS)*. Palo Alto, California: Consulting.

Firestone, A., Turk-Browne, N. B., and Ryan, J. D. (2007). Age-related deficits in face recognition are related to underlying changes in scanning behavior. *Aging Neuropsychol. Cogn.* 14, 594–607. doi: 10.1080/13825580600899717

Fischer, H., Nyberg, L., and Bäckman, L. (2010). Age-related differences in brain regions supporting successful encoding of emotional faces. *Cortex* 46, 490–497. doi: 10.1016/j.cortex.2009.05.011

Fischer, H., Sandblom, J., Gavazzeni, J., Fransson, P., Wright, C. I., and Bäckman, L. (2005). Age-differential patterns of brain activation during perception of angry faces. *Neurosci. Lett.* 386, 99–104. doi: 10.1016/j.neulet.2005.06.002

Gross, J. J., and Levenson, R. W. (1993). Emotional suppression—physiology, self-report, and expressive behavior. *J. Pers. Soc. Psychol.* 64, 970–986. doi: 10.1037/0022-3514.64.6.970

Gunning-Dixon, F. M., Gur, R. C., Perkins, A. C., Schroeder, L., Turner, T., Turetsky, B. I., et al. (2003). Age-related differences in brain activation during emotional face processing. *Neurobiol. Aging* 24, 285–295. doi: 10.1016/S0197-4580(02)00099-4

Harrison, V., and Hole, G. J. (2009). Evidence for a contact-based explanation of the own-age bias in face recognition. *Psychon. Bull. Rev.* 16, 264–269. doi: 10.3758/PBR.16.2.264

He, Y., Ebner, N. C., and Johnson, M. K. (2011). What predicts the own-age bias in face recognition memory? *Soc. Cogn.* 29, 97–109. doi: 10.1521/soco.2011.29.1.97

Hess, U., Adams, R. B., and Kleck, R. E. (2008). "The devil is in the details: the meanings of faces and how they influence the meanings of facial expressions," in *Affective Computing: Focus on Emotion Expression, Synthesis, and Recognition*, ed J. Or (I-techonline/I-Tech), 45–56. Available online at: http://www.intechopen.com/books/affective_computing/the_devil_is_in_the_details_-_the_meanings_of_faces_and_how_they_influence_the_meanings_of_facial_. doi: 10.5772/6187

Hess, U., Adams, R. B. J., Simard, A., Stevenson, M. T., and Kleck, R. E. (2012). Smiling and sad wrinkles: age-related changes in the face and the perception of emotions and intentions. *J. Exp. Soc. Psychol.* 48, 1377–1380. doi: 10.1016/j.jesp.2012.05.018

Hess, U., and Kirouac, G. (2000). "Emotion expression in groups," in *Handbook of Emotions*, ed M. Lewis (New York, NY: Guilford Press), 368–381.

Hugenberg, K., Wilson, J. P., See, P. E., and Young, S. G. (2013). Towards a synthetic model of own group biases in face memory. *Vis. Cogn.* 21, 1392–1417. doi: 10.1080/13506285.2013.821429

Hugenberg, K., Young, S. G., Bernstein, M. J., and Sacco, D. F. (2010). The categorization-individuation model: an integrative account of the other-race recognition deficit. *Psychol. Rev.* 117, 1168–1187. doi: 10.1037/a0020463

Hühnel, I., Fölster, M., Werheid, K., and Hess, U. (2014). Empathic reactions of younger and older adults: no age related decline in affective responding. *J. Exp. Soc. Psychol.* 50, 136–143. doi: 10.1016/j.jesp.2013.09.011

Hummert, M. L., Garstka, T. A., Ryan, E. B., and Bonnesen, J. L. (2004). "The role of age stereotypes in interpersonal communication," in *Handbook of Communication and Aging Research, 2nd Edn*, eds J. F. Nussbaum and J. Coupland (Mahwah, NJ: Lawrence Erlbaum), 91–114.

Isaacowitz, D. M., Löckenhoff, C. E., Lane, R. D., Wright, R., Sechrest, L., Riedel, R., et al. (2007). Age differences in recognition of emotion in lexical stimuli and facial expressions. *Psychol. Aging* 22, 147–159. doi: 10.1037/0882-7974.22.1.147

Isaacowitz, D. M., and Stanley, J. T. (2011). Bringing an ecological perspective to the study of aging and recognition of emotional facial expressions: past, current, and future methods. *J. Nonverbal Behav.* 35, 261–278. doi: 10.1007/s10919-011-0113-6

Izard, C. E. (1979). *The Maximally Discriminitive Facial Movements Coding System, MAX*. Newark, DE: University of Delaware.

Jack, C. R., Petersen, R. C., Xu, Y. C., Waring, S. C., O'Brien, P. C., Tangalos, E. G., et al. (1997). Medial temporal atrophy on MRI in normal aging and very mild Alzheimer's disease. *Neurology* 49, 786–794. doi: 10.1212/WNL.49.3.786

Kaufmann, J. M., and Schweinberger, S. R. (2004). Expression influences the recognition of familiar faces. *Perception* 33, 399–408. doi: 10.1068/p5083

Keightley, M. L., Chiew, K. S., Winocur, G., and Grady, C. L. (2007). Age-related differences in brain activity underlying identification of emotional expressions in faces. *Soc. Cogn. Affect. Neurosci.* 2, 292–302. doi: 10.1093/scan/nsm024

Kornadt, A. E., and Rothermund, K. (2011). Contexts of aging: assessing evaluative age stereotypes in different life domains. *J. Gerontol. B Psychol. Sci. Soc. Sci.* 66, 547–556. doi: 10.1093/geronb/gbr036

Kunz, M., Mylius, V., Schepelmann, K., and Lautenbacher, S. (2008). Impact of age on the facial expression of pain. *J. Psychosom. Res.* 64, 311–318. doi: 10.1016/j.jpsychores.2007.09.010

Lambrecht, L., Kreifelts, B., and Wildgruber, D. (2012). Age-related decrease in recognition of emotional facial and prosodic expressions. *Emotion* 12, 529–539. doi: 10.1037/a0026827

Levenson, R. W., Carstensen, L. L., Friesen, W. V., and Ekman, P. (1991). Emotion, physiology, and expression in old age. *Psychol. Aging* 6, 28–35. doi: 10.1037/0882-7974.6.1.28

Macchi Cassia, V. (2011). Age biases in face processing: the effects of experience across development. *Br. J. Psychol.* 102, 816–829. doi: 10.1111/j.2044-8295.2011.02046.x

Magai, C., Consedine, N. S., Krivoshekova, Y. S., Kudadjie-Gyamfi, E., and McPherson, R. (2006). Emotion experience and expression across the adult life span: insights from a multimodal assessment study. *Psychol. Aging* 21, 303–317. doi: 10.1037/0882-7974.21.2.303

Malatesta, C. Z., Fiore, M. J., and Messina, J. J. (1987a). Affect, personality, and facial expressive characteristics of older people. *Psychol. Aging* 2, 64–69. doi: 10.1037/0882-7974.2.1.64

Malatesta, C. Z., Izard, C. E., Culver, C., and Nicolich, M. (1987b). Emotion communication skills in young, middle-aged, an older women. *Psychol. Aging* 2, 193–203. doi: 10.1037/0882-7974.2.2.193

Malatesta, C. Z., and Izard, C. E. (1984). "The facial expression of emotion: young, middle-aged, and older adult expressions," in *Emotion in Adult Development*, eds C. Z. Malatesta and C. E. Izard (London: Sage Publications), 253–273.

Malatesta-Magai, C., Jonas, R., Shepard, B., and Culver, L. C. (1992). Type A behavior pattern and emotion expression in younger and older adults. *Psychol. Aging* 7, 551–561. doi: 10.1037/0882-7974.7.4.551

Mather, M., and Carstensen, L. L. (2003). Aging and attentional biases for emotional faces. *Psychol. Sci.* 14, 409–415. doi: 10.1111/1467-9280.01455

Matheson, D. H. (1997). The painful truth: interpretation of facial expressions of pain in older adults. *J. Nonverbal Behav.* 21, 223–238. doi: 10.1023/A:1024973615079

Minear, M., and Park, D. C. (2004). A lifespan database of adult facial stimuli. *Behav. Res. Methods Instrum. Comput.* 36, 630–633. doi: 10.3758/BF03206543

Montepare, J., Koff, E., Zaitchik, D., and Albert, M. (1999). The use of body movements and gestures as cues to emotions in younger and older adults. *J. Nonverbal Behav.* 23, 133–152. doi: 10.1023/A:1021435526134

Murphy, F. C., Nimmo-Smith, I., and Lawrence, A. D. (2003). Functional neuroanatomy of emotions: a meta-analysis. *Cogn. Affect. Behav. Neurosci.* 3, 207–233. doi: 10.3758/CABN.3.3.207

Murphy, N. A., Lehrfeld, J. M., and Isaacowitz, D. M. (2010). Recognition of posed and spontaneous dynamic smiles in young and older adults. *Psychol. Aging* 25, 811–821. doi: 10.1037/a0019888

Phan, K. L., Wager, T., Taylor, S. F., and Liberzon, I. (2002). Functional neuroanatomy of emotion: a meta-analysis of emotion activation studies in PET and fMRI. *Neuroimage* 16, 331–348. doi: 10.1006/nimg.2002.1087

Phillips, L. H., MacLean, R. D. J., and Allen, R. (2002). Age and the understanding of emotions: neuropsychological and sociocognitive perspectives. *J. Gerontol. B. Psychol. Sci. Soc. Sci.* 57, P526–P530. doi: 10.1093/geronb/57.6.P526

Porcheron, A., Mauger, E., and Russell, R. (2013). Aspects of facial contrast decrease with age and are cues for age perception. *PLoS ONE* 8:e57985. doi: 10.1371/journal.pone.0057985

Proietti, V., Pisacane, A., and Macchi Cassia, V. (2013). Natural experience modulates the processing of older adult faces in young adults and 3-year-old children. *PLoS ONE* 8:e57499. doi: 10.1371/journal.pone.0057499

Raz, N. (2000). "Aging of the brain and its impact on cognitive performance: integration of structural and functional findings," in *The Handbook of Aging and Cognition, 2nd Edn*, eds F. I. M. Craik and T. A. Salthouse (Mahwah, NJ: Lawrence Erlbaum), 1–90.

Rhodes, M. G., and Anastasi, J. S. (2012). The own-age bias in face recognition: a meta-analytic and theoretical review. *Psychol. Bull.* 138, 146–174. doi: 10.1037/a0025750

Richter, D., Dietzel, C., and Kunzmann, U. (2011). Age differences in emotion recognition: the task matters. *J. Gerontol. B Psychol. Sci. Soc. Sci.* 66, 48–55. doi: 10.1093/geronb/gbq068

Riediger, M., Voelkle, M. C., Ebner, N. C., and Lindenberger, U. (2011). Beyond "happy, angry, or sad?" Age-of-poser and age-of-rater effects on multi-dimensional emotion perception. *Cogn. Emot.* 25, 968–982. doi: 10.1080/02699931.2010.540812

Ruffman, T., Halberstadt, J., and Murray, J. (2009a). Recognition of facial, auditory, and bodily emotions in older adults. *J. Gerontol. B Psychol. Sci. Soc. Sci.* 64, 696–703. doi: 10.1093/geronb/gbp072

Ruffman, T., Sullivan, S., and Dittrich, W. (2009b). Older adults' recognition of bodily and auditory expressions of emotion. *Psychol. Aging* 24, 614. doi: 10.1037/a0016356

Ruffman, T., Henry, J. D., Livingstone, V., and Phillips, L. H. (2008). A meta-analytic review of emotion recognition and aging: implications for neuropsychological models of aging. *Neurosci. Biobehav. Rev.* 32, 863–881. doi: 10.1016/j.neubiorev.2008.01.001

Ruffman, T., Murray, J., Halberstadt, J., and Vater, T. (2012). Age-related differeces in deception. *Psychol. Aging* 27, 543–549. doi: 10.1037/a0023380

Schweinberger, S. R., and Soukup, G. R. (1998). Asymmetric relationships among perceptions of facial identity, emotion, and facial speech. *J. Exp. Psychol. Hum. Percept. Perform.* 24, 1748–1765. doi: 10.1037/0096-1523.24.6.1748

Schyns, P. G., and Oliva, A. (1999). Dr. Angry and Mr. Smile: when categorizazion flexibly modifies the perception of faces in rapid visual presentations. *Cognition* 69, 243–265. doi: 10.1016/S0010-0277(98)00069-9

Signorielli, N. (2004). Aging on television: messages relating to gender, race, and occupation in prime time. *J. Broadcast. Electron. Media* 48, 279–301. doi: 10.1207/s15506878jobem4802_7

Slessor, G., Miles, L. K., Bull, R., and Phillips, L. H. (2010). Age-related changes in detecting happiness: discriminating between enjoyment and nonenjoyment smiles. *Psychol. Aging* 25, 246–250. doi: 10.1037/a0018248

Sporer, S. L. (2001). Recognizing faces of other ethnic groups: an integration of theories. *Psychol. Pub. Policy Law* 7:36. doi: 10.1037/1076-8971.7.1.36

Sullivan, S., Ruffman, T., and Hutton, S. B. (2007). Age differences in emotion recognition skills and the visual scanning of emotion faces. *J. Gerontol. B Psychol. Sci. Soc. Sci.* 62, P53–P60. doi: 10.1093/geronb/62.1.P53

Suzuki, A., Hoshino, T., Shigemasu, K., and Kawamura, M. (2007). Decline or improvement? Age-related differences in facial expression recognition. *Biol. Psychol.* 74, 75–84. doi: 10.1016/j.biopsycho.2006.07.003

Taler, V., Baum, S., and Saumier, D. (2006). "Perception of linguistic and affective prosody in younger and older adults," in *Paper presented at the Twenty-eighth Annual Conference of the Cognitive Science Society*, (Vancouver), 2216–2221.

Thibault, P., Bourgeois, P., and Hess, U. (2006). The effect of group-identification on emotion recognition: the case of cats and basketball players. *J. Exp. Soc. Psychol.* 42, 676–683. doi: 10.1016/j.jesp.2005.10.006

Tsai, J. L., Levenson, R. W., and Carstensen, L. L. (2000). Autonomic, subjective, and expressive responses to emotional films in older and younger Chinese Americans and European Americans. *Psychol. Aging* 15, 684–693. doi: 10.1037/0882-7974.15.4.684

Voelkle, M. C., Ebner, N. C., Lindenberger, U., and Riediger, M. (2012). Let me guess how old you are: effects of age, gender, and facial expression on perceptions of age. *Psychol. Aging* 27, 265–277. doi: 10.1037/a0025065

Weisbuch, M., and Ambady, N. (2008). Affective divergence: automatic responses to others' emotions depend on group membership. *J. Pers. Soc. Psychol.* 95, 1063–1079. doi: 10.1037/a0011993

Wiese, H. (2012). The role of age and ethnic group in face recognition memory: ERP evidence from a combined own-age and own-race bias study. *Biol. Psychol.* 89, 137–147. doi: 10.1016/j.biopsycho.2011.10.002

Wiese, H., Komes, J., and Schweinberger, S. R. (2012). Daily-life contact affects the own-age bias and neural correlates of face memory in elderly participants. *Neuropsychologia* 50, 3496–3508. doi: 10.1016/j.neuropsychologia.2012.09.022

Wiese, H., Komes, J., and Schweinberger, S. R. (2013a). Ageing faces in ageing minds: a review on the own-age bias in face recognition. *Vis. Cogn.* 21, 1337–1363. doi: 10.1080/13506285.2013.823139

Wiese, H., Wolff, N., Steffens, M. C., and Schweinberger, S. R. (2013b). How experience shapes memory for faces: an event-related potential study on the own-age bias. *Biol. Psychol.* 94, 369–379. doi: 10.1016/j.biopsycho.2013.07.001

Wiese, H., Schweinberger, S. R., and Hansen, K. (2008). The age of the beholder: ERP evidence of an own-age bias in face memory. *Neuropsychologia* 46, 2973–2985. doi: 10.1016/j.neuropsychologia.2008.06.007

Williams, L. M., Brown, K. J., Palmer, D., Liddell, B. J., Kemp, A. H., Olivieri, G., et al. (2006). The mellow years? Neural basis of improving emotional stability over age. *J. Neurosci.* 26, 6422–6430. doi: 10.1523/JNEUROSCI.0022-06.2006

Wolff, N., Wiese, H., and Schweinberger, S. R. (2012). Face recognition memory across the adult life span: event-related potential evidence from the own-age bias. *Psychol. Aging* 27, 1066–1081. doi: 10.1037/a0029112

Wong, B., Cronin-Golomb, A., and Neargarder, S. (2005). Patterns of visual scanning as predictors of emotion identification in normal aging. *Neuropsychology* 19, 739–749. doi: 10.1037/0894-4105.19.6.739

Wright, C. I., Negreira, A., Gold, A. L., Britton, J. C., Williams, D., and Barrett, L. F. (2008). Neural correlates of novelty and face-age effects in young and elderly adults. *Neuroimage* 42, 956–968. doi: 10.1016/j.neuroimage.2008.05.015

Young, S. G., and Hugenberg, K. (2010). Mere social categorization modulates identification of facial expressions of emotion. *J. Pers. Soc. Psychol.* 99, 964–977. doi: 10.1037/a0020400

# 17

# Remote spatial memory in aging: all is not lost

**R. Shayna Rosenbaum[1,2]*, Gordon Winocur[2,3,4,5], Malcolm A. Binns[2,6] and Morris Moscovitch[2,3,7]**

[1] Neuroscience Graduate Diploma Program, Department of Psychology, York University, Toronto, ON, Canada
[2] Rotman Research Institute, Baycrest, Toronto, ON, Canada
[3] Department of Psychology, University of Toronto, Toronto, ON, Canada
[4] Department of Psychiatry, University of Toronto, Toronto, ON, Canada
[5] Department of Psychology, Trent University, Peterborough, ON, Canada
[6] Dalla Lana School of Public Health, University of Toronto, Toronto, ON, Canada
[7] Department of Psychology, Baycrest, Toronto, ON, Canada

**Edited by:**
*Thomas Wolbers, University of Edinburgh, UK*

**Reviewed by:**
*Eric Blalock, University of Kentucky, USA*
*Sue Becker, McMaster University, Canada*

***Correspondence:**
*R. Shayna Rosenbaum, Department of Psychology, Neuroscience Graduate Diploma Program, York University, 4700 Keele St., Toronto, ON M3J 1P3, Canada.*
*e-mail: shaynar@yorku.ca*

The ability to acquire and retain spatial memories in order to navigate in new environments is known to decline with age, but little is known about the effect of aging on representations of environments learned long ago, in the remote past. To investigate the status of remote spatial memory in old age, we tested healthy young and older adults on a variety of mental navigation tests based on a large-scale city environment that was very familiar to participants but rarely visited by the older adults in recent years. We show that whereas performance on a route learning test of new spatial learning was significantly worse in older than younger adults, performance was comparable or better in the older adults on mental navigation tests based on a well-known environment learned long ago. An exception was in the older adults' ability to vividly re-experience the well-known environment, and recognize and represent the visual details contained within it. The results are seen as analogous to the pattern of better semantic than episodic memory that has been found to accompany healthy aging.

**Keywords: aging, hippocampus, landmark recognition, mental navigation, recollection, remote memory, route learning, spatial memory**

## INTRODUCTION

Healthy aging is characterized by a variety of neural changes, with the hippocampus among the most prominent brain structures to be affected (e.g., Jernigan et al., 2001; Raz et al., 2005; Park and Reuter-Lorenz, 2009). These changes are accompanied by difficulties in forming and retaining new spatial memories of allocentric relations among locations (e.g., Barnes, 1979; Winocur and Gagnon, 1998; Head and Isom, 2010; Harris and Wolbers, 2012). Whereas the hippocampus is needed to support such spatial representations (e.g., O'Keefe and Dostrovsky, 1971; Morris et al., 1982; Wolbers and Büchel, 2005; Nedelska et al., 2012; but see Corkin, 2002), it does not appear to be needed for all aspects of remote spatial memory for environments encountered long ago[1] (Rosenbaum et al., 2000, 2004, 2007; Maguire et al., 2006). However, there is little information about the effects of aging on remote spatial memory. The current study examines the integrity of remote spatial memory in healthy young and older adults.

The ability to flexibly represent the external world in order to navigate efficiently between spatial locations in both new and familiar environments is essential for independent living. Despite its importance, there is a long-standing debate about the neural substrate of allocentric spatial memory for large-scale environments, particularly those that were experienced long ago. Central to this debate is the role of the hippocampus. A long-standing theory is that the hippocampus is always necessary for supporting allocentric spatial memory ("cognitive maps") to navigate an environment, no matter how long ago that memory was acquired, as opposed to egocentric representations of the environment within body-centered coordinates (O'Keefe and Nadel, 1978; Bird and Burgess, 2008). A derivative of this theory views scene construction as the central role of the hippocampus. Scene construction involves the retrieval and integration of relevant details into a coherent spatial framework within which details of personal memories can be re-experienced and manipulated into imagined new experiences (Byrne et al., 2007; Hassabis et al., 2007; Hassabis and Maguire, 2009). Based on these theories, one might predict that both recent and remote spatial memory and navigation that rely on allocentric cues would be affected by hippocampal damage. An alternative prediction is that deficits in scene construction may only impair the detailed perceptual representations of an environment, such as is required to recall or imagine scenes, but not for navigation.

Another view that may be considered complementary is that the hippocampus has a time-limited role in representing coarse, schematic, or semantic-like aspects of spatial memory, but is needed always for representing rich, detailed episodic-like aspects (Rosenbaum et al., 2001; Moscovitch et al., 2005; Winocur et al., 2010a). By schematic representations, we mean map-like representations that contain information about landmarks, their location, and relation to one another, which are needed for

[1] The term "remote" is used to describe memories that are temporally distant and is not used in the current paper in reference to spatial distance.

navigation[2]. From our view, this schematic representation is impoverished with respect to perceptual details that are incidental to navigation, such as the appearance of houses (Rosenbaum et al., 2000) and even of the landmarks themselves. We consider these more detailed aspects as part of the representation that allows for a rich re-experiencing of an environment. The distinction between schematic and detailed spatial representations, which may or may not be orthogonal to allocentric vs. egocentric frameworks, is based on findings from lesion and neuroimaging studies. Amnesic people with hippocampal lesions show evidence of relatively preserved navigation but impaired memory for perceptual details of environments learned long ago (Teng and Squire, 1999; Rosenbaum et al., 2000, 2005; Maguire et al., 2006). These findings are consistent with evidence from neuroimaging studies showing a relative lack of hippocampal activation for mental navigation in the same environments (Rosenbaum et al., 2004, 2007; Hirshhorn et al., 2012). The hippocampus is known to suffer structural and functional decline with age. Similar to hippocampal amnesic patients, older adults show a decline in autobiographical episodic memory for both recent and remote events and associated recollection processes, but relative preservation of semantic memory and associated familiarity (e.g., Davidson and Glisky, 2002; Levine et al., 2002; Piolino et al., 2006).

The changes in declarative/relational memory that do occur appear to relate to significant atrophic changes in hippocampal volume associated with aging (Yonelinas et al., 2007). Aging has also been associated with spatial disorientation in recently encountered environments in both animals and humans in relation to hippocampal volume loss (e.g., Driscoll et al., 2006; Moffat, 2009). A study of older adults suggests that this impairment extends to the re-experiencing of familiar routes from an environment that was traveled extensively in the past, which is correlated with neuropsychological tests of hippocampal function and autobiographical episodic memory (Hirshhorn et al., 2011). Nevertheless, the ability to represent the spatial distance between landmarks located in the same environment does not appear to be affected, though comparison of the older adults' remote spatial memory performance was not made with a younger group. In a more direct investigation, aged rats with prior exposure to a complex "village" environment showed significantly better memory for allocentric spatial relations among locations contained within that environment than age-matched rats who were naïve to the environment (Winocur et al., 2010a). The experienced aged rats performed slightly worse than they had as young rats during initial training, but better than a separate group of young rats not previously exposed to the environment, indicating both preserved remote spatial memory and impaired new spatial learning in old age.

Overall, the findings suggest that spatial representations of well-learned environments formed long ago are relatively impervious to the effects of aging and, together with earlier findings of similar preservation in young rats with hippocampal lesions (Winocur et al., 2005, 2010a), do not depend on the hippocampus. To our knowledge, however, systematic examination of remote spatial memory in young vs. older adults has not been attempted in humans. If the hippocampus, which functionally declines with age, is not needed for various aspects of remote spatial memory, particularly those which support navigation, then aging should not affect performance on spatial memory tasks based on an environment that was extensively navigated in the past, even if it affects spatial learning in newly encountered environments. Retention and retrieval of perceptual details of an environment, whether experienced recently or long ago, however, should be impaired in older adults as these always are dependent on the hippocampus. The data presented in the current study support these predictions.

## MATERIALS AND METHODS

### PARTICIPANTS

A group of 14 healthy older adults aged 65–85 years (half male; 13 right-handed) were recruited from the Baycrest participant pool for monetary compensation. Comparisons were made with a group of 14 young adults aged 18–30 years (half male; 13 right-handed) recruited from the Baycrest participant pool for monetary compensation and the York University Undergraduate Research Participant Pool for course credit. Demographic information and other descriptive data are summarized in **Table 1**. Participants were matched for years of education, fluent in English, free from a history of neurological and psychiatric illness, and lived in Toronto for a minimum of 10 years. None of the older participants met criteria for dementia based on the MMSE or MoCA. The study received approval from the York University and Baycrest research ethics boards.

### MATERIALS AND PROCEDURE

Participants' remote spatial memory was tested for mental navigation amid landmarks and for the visual identity of those

**Table 1 | Demographic characteristics of the younger and older participants.**

| | | Younger | | Older | |
|---|---|---|---|---|---|
| | | Mean | SD | Mean | SD |
| Age (years) | | 22.21 | 4.00 | 72.21 | 6.31 |
| Education (years) | | 14.36 | 1.15 | 15.29 | 1.98 |
| Living in Toronto (years) | | 18.21 | 4.66 | 50.5 | 16.16 |
| Visit frequency[a] | | 3.82 | 1.38 | 2.71 | 1.12 |
| Navigation ability[b] | New environments | 3.54 | 1.15 | 4.04 | 0.89 |
| | Familiar environments | 4.43 | 0.85 | 4.5 | 0.65 |

*Note: SD, standard deviation.*

[a] *Based on scale ranging from 1 to 5, where 1 = no more than once a year, 2 = 1 to 2 times per year, 3 = once a month, 4 = once a week, and 5 = more than once a week.*

[b] *Based on subjective ratings on a Likert scale, ranging from 1 (difficulty navigating/always disoriented) to 5 (navigates with ease/never disoriented).*

[2] At the moment, we do not know how integrated the information on the map is and what kind of fine-grained information this kind of map can support. It is possible that this representation contains a series of local map-like representations or route knowledge that is strung together.

landmarks located in a city environment (downtown Toronto, approximately 5 square km). The environment was experienced approximately 2–3 times per week for at least 10 years by all participants and up to 45 years ago by the older participants. Most of the older participants rarely experienced the environment in the last 5 years. The tasks were designed to simulate the demands of negotiating through large-scale space, with mental navigation tasks varying in terms of their demands on allocentric (tasks 1–4) vs. egocentric processing (tasks 5 and 6; see Ciaramelli et al., 2010, for a detailed rationale for task classification). Comparisons in remote spatial memory performance were made with spatial memory acquisition on a route learning test. Tasks were presented in a fixed order, as follows.

### Mental navigation tests (Toronto Public Places Test; TPPT)

***Proximity judgments.*** In a test of relative distance judgments, participants indicated which of two Toronto landmarks was closest to a third reference landmark. The actual distance among the 10 sets of landmarks for each environment varied from trial to trial, and half of the trials were more demanding (i.e., the difference in distance between the reference landmark and either of the choice landmarks was less than 1 km).

***Distance judgments.*** Participants were asked to provide numerical judgments of absolute distance between each of 10 pairs of landmarks located in downtown Toronto in their preferred unit of measure (i.e., km or miles). A sample trial was administered prior to testing in order to give the participants an indication of scale. The actual distances between landmarks were varied and randomly intermixed across trials. The mean deviation of the judged distances from the actual distances in km was calculated for each trial and averaged to derive absolute error scores.

***Vector mapping.*** In a test of allocentric distance and head-direction between landmarks, participants were asked to draw arrows indicating the correct distance and direction from a location specified by a mark to an unmarked landmark on 10 maps of downtown Toronto that included lines indicating northern and southern downtown city limits. Deviation of estimates from actual directions in degrees and distances in km was calculated for each trial and averaged to derive absolute error scores.

***Landmark sequencing.*** Ten randomly ordered names of landmarks located along a north-south route were presented, and participants were to order the landmarks in the sequence that would be passed during a mental walk of the route.

***Blocked routes.*** Participants were asked to simulate taking shortcuts in a task requiring a change of route from the most direct route between a pair of landmarks. There was a total of 5 such trials, each consisting of 2 to 4 choice points at which to turn right or left, for a maximum score ranging from 11 to 16 per participant. Partial points were given for impoverished descriptions of routes that otherwise led to the specified destination. At the end of the task, participants were additionally asked whether they felt that they were remembering the simulated navigation episodes from a first-person perspective (i.e., as being actually involved in the episode; e.g., driving or walking on the streets) or from a third-person perspective (i.e., as being an observer of the episode, or adopting a survey perspective), and whether they had experienced the routes as vivid and rich in detail while mentally navigating them.

### Landmark appearance

Participants were asked to distinguish between photographs of downtown Toronto landmarks and of buildings that are structurally similar to those located in downtown Toronto but that have never been encountered by the participants. The stimulus set included a total of 25 landmarks and 25 distractors. All photographs were taken from an unobstructed view and were digitally scanned and adjusted for luminance and contrast. For each photograph, participants were to decide if the landmark is familiar, and if so, to identify it by name and location or by some other means if necessary (e.g., type of building, decade in which it was established, function).

### Baycrest route learning test

A route learning test previously found to be sensitive to hippocampal function in Alzheimer's disease (Rosenbaum et al., 2005) was adapted for the present study to assess spatial acquisition. Participants were taken on a novel route through two floors of Baycrest, where the Rotman Research Institute is located. Four of the older participants had visited Baycrest prior to the current study, and none had traversed the particular test route. There were 16 choice points along the route where participants had to decide whether to turn right or left or to continue straight. The route covered three floors of the hospital, and participants relied on an elevator to travel between floors. Four legs of the route included large windows with views to distal outdoor cues; the remainder of the route did not include views to the outside.

***Procedure.*** The learning phase involved a 15-min experimenter-led tour of the route. Participants were instructed to pay attention to the route and its visual features as reminders of where to turn because they would later be asked to lead the experimenter on the same route. While on the tour, the experimenter did not point out landmarks or turns, other than the destination floor when the elevator was taken. During the test phase, the participant led the experimenter through the route, with errors recorded and corrected to maintain the flow of the route. After a 30 min filled break, during which the landmark appearance test was administered, participants were asked to lead the experimenter through the route a final time.

## STATISTICAL ANALYSES

Most of the tasks (Proximity Judgments, Landmark Sequencing, Blocked Routes, Landmark Identification, and Baycrest Route Learning) generated error count data as the outcome variable of interest. For these measures we entered number of errors as the dependent variable in a Poisson regression to examine differences between the younger and older participants. We adjusted the null hypothesis tests using the deviance scaling option to compensate for under- or over-dispersion. An offset variable was included for the Blocked Routes test to accommodate differences in the total number of streets used for each trial per participant. The remaining tasks (Distance Judgments, Vector Mapping, and Landmark Recognition) generated outcome variables with reasonably bell-shaped distributions, and these were entered into an analysis of variance (ANOVA) with Group (young vs. old) as a between-subject factor. In order to examine the effects of differences in exposure to downtown Toronto on the main effect of age, the number of years living in Toronto and frequency of recent visits to the downtown core (i.e., within the past 5 years) were included individually as covariates in all models. Finally, correlations in performance on the experimental measures, stratified by age, were calculated. All hypothesis tests are performed at an alpha level of 5%.

## RESULTS

As indicated by the descriptive data in **Table 1**, the young adults visited downtown Toronto more frequently within the past 5 years compared to the older adults, whereas the older adults lived in Toronto for a significantly longer time than the young adults. Although each of the variables were included separately as covariates in the analyses, the lack of overlap in groups on the latter variable may present a challenge to interpreting conditional age effects in test performance. Surprisingly, subjective ratings of navigation ability were lower for the young adults compared to the older adults for new environments and indistinguishable for familiar environments. Participants' performance on all spatial memory tests is presented in **Table 2**.

### MENTAL NAVIGATION TESTS (TPPT)

#### *Proximity judgments*

Poisson regression on error count (collapsed across easy and difficult trials) revealed no significant effect of group, $p = 0.88$, even when taking into account frequency of visits, $p = 0.86$. It remains possible that older participants perform worse when number of years living in Toronto was taken into account, though this sample produced equivocal results, $X^2(1, N = 28) = 1.98, p = 0.16$.

#### *Distance judgments*

ANOVA on mean deviation of estimates from actual distance (in km) revealed no significant effect of group, $p = 0.2$. Likewise, analysis of covariance (ANCOVA) revealed no significant effect of frequency of visits or number of years living in Toronto, $p > 0.26$ in both cases, even when an outlier was withheld from the analyses.

#### *Vector mapping*

ANOVA on deviation of estimates from actual distance (in km) revealed no significant effect of group, $p = 0.15$. ANCOVA revealed no significant effect of group when number of years living in Toronto was taken into account, $p = 0.32$, even when an outlier was withheld from the analyses. There was a marginally significant effect when frequency of visits was taken into account, $F_{(1,\,26)} = 3.92$, $p = 0.06$, suggesting that the older adults performed better than the younger adults in estimating vector distance.

ANOVA on mean deviation of estimates from actual direction (in degrees) revealed a significant effect of group, $F_{(1,\,26)} = 4.59$, $p = 0.04$, such that older adults performed better than younger adults. ANCOVA revealed the effect of group to be larger when frequency of visits was taken into account, $F_{(1,\,26)} = 8.66$, $p = 0.007$[3]. This result is presented in **Figure 1A**.

[3]Withholding data from an influential participant reduced the effect of group to marginal. This was true both without and with the frequency of visits covariate, $p > 0.06$ in both cases, with the effect continuing to be in the predicted direction.

**Table 2 | Performance of young and older participants on experimental tasks.**

| Experimental task | | Young | | Old | | *p*-value | *d* | pd | $e^{\beta}$ |
|---|---|---|---|---|---|---|---|---|---|
| | | Mean | SD | Mean | SD | | | | |
| **MENTAL NAVIGATION** | | | | | | | | | |
| Proximity | error | 1.21 | 1.42 | 1.14 | 0.95 | 0.88 | 0.06 | −0.06 | 1.06 |
| Distance | deviation (km) | 1.99 | 2.66 | 1.04 | 0.7 | 0.2 | 0.49 | – | – |
| Vector | deviation (km) | 0.36 | 0.19 | 0.28 | 0.11 | 0.06† | 0.51‡ | – | – |
| | deviation (°) | 17.47 | 7.29 | 12.38 | 5.12 | 0.007† | 0.81 | – | – |
| Sequencing | error | 1.43 | 1.45 | 0.93 | 1 | 0.33 | 0.4 | −0.35 | 1.54 |
| Blocked Route | error | 3.64 | 2.6 | 2.61 | 1.06 | 0.0005† | 0.52‡ | −0.28 | 1.99 |
| **LANDMARK APPEARANCE** | | | | | | | | | |
| Recognition | hits – fa | 17.64 | 2.62 | 13.21 | 4.56 | 0.004 | 1.19 | – | – |
| | hits + fa | 26.93 | 4.5 | 24.07 | 5.94 | 0.04* | 0.54 | – | – |
| Identification | error | 16.25 | 3.79 | 13.69 | 2.68 | 0.07 | 0.78 | −0.16 | 0.77 |
| **ROUTE LEARNING** | | | | | | | | | |
| Immediate | error | 1.29 | 1.14 | 5.21 | 2.08 | <0.0001 | −2.34 | 3.04 | 0.25 |
| Delayed | error | 0.07 | 0.27 | 0.64 | 0.74 | 0.01 | −1.02 | 8.14 | 0.11 |

*Note: fa, false alarm; SD, standard deviation; pd, proportional difference,* $\frac{mean^{old} - mean^{young}}{mean^{young}}$; $e^{\beta}$, *multiplicative effect of age on error rate.*
**Influential observation withheld; †effect of group, conditional on a covariate (see text); ‡better performance in older adults.*

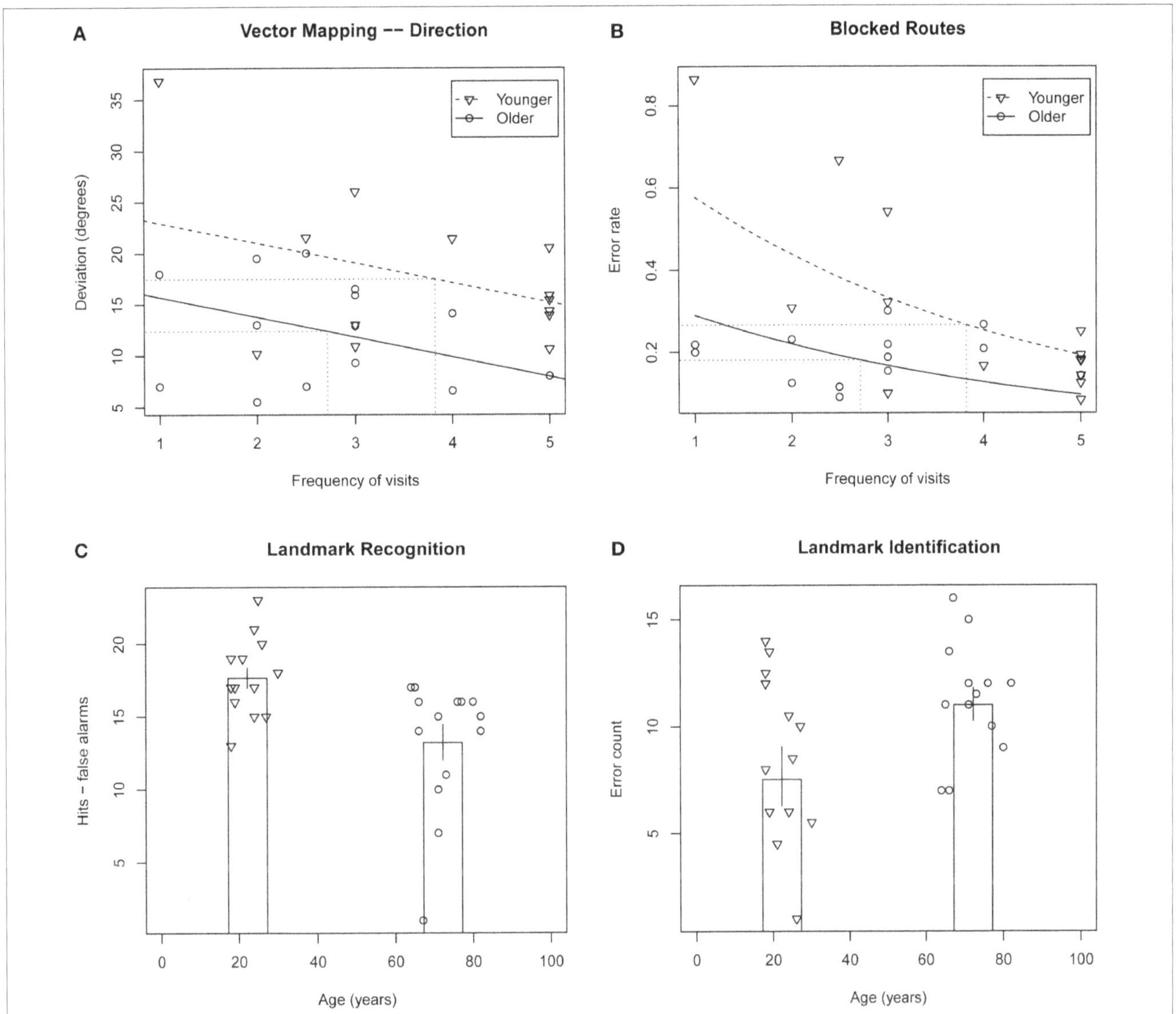


**FIGURE 1 | Top row: scatterplots of mental navigation performance versus frequency of visits to Toronto for vector mapping—direction deviation (A) and blocked routes error rate (B), tasks on which older adults performed significantly better than younger adults.** Fitted models for younger and older adults are indicated by dashed and solid lines, respectively, and averages for the two groups are indicated by dotted lines. Bottom row: scatterplots of performance on landmark recognition **(C)** and landmark identification **(D)** versus age. Column height indicates average performance for each of the two groups. Error bars indicate ± one standard error.

#### *Landmark sequencing*

Poisson regression on error count revealed no significant effect of group, $p = 0.33$, even when frequency of visits and number of years living in Toronto were taken into account.

#### *Blocked routes*

Poisson regression on error count when adjusting for the difference in total number of streets between participants revealed that the effect of group was marginal, $X^2(1, N = 28) = 3.18, p = 0.07$, with older participants performing better than younger participants. This observed effect was enhanced when frequency of visits was taken into account, $X^2(1, N = 28) = 12.3$, $p < 0.0005$ (see **Figure 1B**).

### SUBJECTIVE RE-EXPERIENCING

With respect to the participants' subjective report, significantly fewer older (7/14) than younger adults (14/14) reported adopting a first-person perspective during navigation in the blocked route task, Fisher's Exact Test, $p = 0.006$. More striking was the finding that 12/14 older adults but only 2/14 younger adults reported that their re-experiencing of the routes in memory lacked vividness and perceptual detail, Fisher's Exact Test, $p = 0.0004$.

### LANDMARK APPEARANCE

#### *Landmark recognition*

ANOVA on error count for hits minus false alarms revealed a significant effect of group, $F_{(1, 26)} = 9.93$, $p < 0.004$, with the older participants less able to discriminate between target and distractor landmarks than the younger participants (presented in **Figure 1C**). ANCOVA revealed the effect of group to remain even when frequency of visits and number of years living in Toronto were taken into account, $p > 0.58$ in both cases[4]. ANOVA performed for the sum of hits and false alarms was equivocal with respect to an effect of age group, $F_{(1, 26)} = 2.06$, $p = 0.16$, that was found to be significant when a participant with an unusually high number of false alarms was withheld, $F_{(1, 26)} = 4.61$, $p < 0.04$. The effect indicated a conservative response bias in the older adults and a non-conservative response bias in the younger adults.

#### *Landmark identification*

Poisson regression on error count revealed a marginally significant effect of group, $F_{(1, 25)} = 3.32$, $p = 0.07$, with the older participants identifying fewer Toronto landmarks than the younger participants[5] (**Figure 1D**). There was no effect of frequency of visits or number of years living in Toronto.

### BAYCREST ROUTE LEARNING TEST

Poisson regression on error count for immediate learning of the new route (sum of runs 1 and 2) revealed an effect of group, $X^2$ $(1, N = 28) = 25.46$, $p < 0.0001$, such that the older adults performed significantly worse than the young adults. The same was true for delayed learning of the route, $X^2$ $(1, N = 28) = 6.02$, $p < 0.01$, with the older adults performing significantly worse than the young adults.

### CORRELATIONS

Correlational analyses indicated a positive correlation in new route learning between the two trials of the immediate condition, $r_{(26)} = 0.56$, $p = 0.003$, and a negative correlation between the rates of learning from the first to second trial of the immediate condition and from the immediate condition to the delay condition, $r_{(26)} = -0.54$, $p = 0.004$. New route learning in the delay condition was negatively correlated with landmark recognition for hits minus false alarms, $r_{(26)} = -0.48$, $p = 0.01$, and positively correlated for hits plus false alarms, $r_{(26)} = 0.4$, $p = 0.04$. Participants' subjective reports of navigation ability in new environments was positively correlated with their subjective reports of navigation ability in old environments, $r_{(26)} = 0.55$, $p = 0.004$, and negatively correlated with landmark recognition for hits minus false alarms, $r_{(26)} = -0.42$, $p = 0.03$. Correlations among the mental navigation tests of remote spatial memory were mostly positive, ranging from $r_{(26)} = 0.43$ to $0.57$, $p = 0.03$ to $0.003$. Finally, landmark recognition was positively correlated with landmark identification, $r_{(26)} = 0.55$, $p = 0.004$, whereas landmark identification was negatively correlated with vector mapping–distance, $r_{(26)} = -0.55$, $p = 0.004$, and landmark sequencing, $r_{(26)} = -0.42$, $p = 0.03$.

[4]The age effect remained, even when withholding a potentially influential participant.

[5]Data were not available for one of the older adults.

## DISCUSSION

The current study investigated whether the changes in memory that accompany aging affect spatial representations formed long ago (i.e., 10 years ago or more). Older adults performed at least as well as younger adults on a wide range of mental navigation tests of remote spatial memory, even when amount of exposure to downtown Toronto was taken into account. No effect of age was found on proximity judgments, distance judgments, and landmark sequencing, and older adults outperformed younger adults on vector mapping and blocked routes. However, only half of the older adults, as compared to most of the younger adults, reported imagining the routes from a first-person perspective, and nearly all of the older adults, and hardly any of the young adults, reported that their imagined routes lacked perceptual richness and a feeling of re-experiencing. This age difference in self report was accompanied by significantly worse performance in the older adults in visually recognizing and identifying the landmarks for which intact spatial judgments had been made. Preserved performance in older adults was also in stark contrast to significantly worse navigation along a new route, both immediately after learning and following a 30-min delay. These results lend support to the view that the hippocampus is necessary for the establishment of spatial memories and for retaining and retrieving visual and experiential details even of representations formed long ago. However, it does not appear to be needed for representing the schematic attributes that are likely to have been extracted over many years navigating a large-scale environment.

Healthy aging is most often associated with a decline in memory and other cognitive processes, but some types of memory remain unchanged or even improve with age (e.g., Grady and Craik, 2000; Park and Reuter-Lorenz, 2009). In remote memory, episodic memory appears to be most vulnerable to the effects of aging, whereas semantic memory appears to resist such effects. Our work with humans and rats suggests similar distinctions in remote spatial memory. Here we showed that extensive navigation in a city environment over a long period of time leads to long-standing representations of spatial locations that resist disruption from aging. Comparable or better performance was found in old vs. young adults on a range of remote spatial memory tasks previously identified as more likely to be solved in an allocentric reference frame (proximity judgments, distance judgments, vector mapping) as well as those more likely to be solved in an egocentric reference frame (landmark sequencing, blocked routes; see Rosenbaum et al., 2004; Ciaramelli et al., 2010).

The current study does not provide direct evidence of a neuroanatomical substrate for remote spatial memory, but the results in the older adults closely resemble findings in patients with hippocampal damage or degeneration (Teng and Squire, 1999; Rosenbaum et al., 2000, 2005; Maguire et al., 2006). Patients with large bilateral medial temporal lobe (MTL) lesions that affect the hippocampus are able to negotiate their way in most places within premorbidly familiar environments and make a variety of judgments about the spatial relations contained within them. These findings suggest that, with sufficient time and experience, spatial memories can exist independently of the hippocampus and MTL. In the current study, correlations among the mental navigation tests did not appear to distinguish between tasks pre-classified as allocentric or egocentric, pointing to a blend of reference frames or a separate common strategy to sustain spatial memory performance in the face of other areas of cognitive decline associated with aging. These strategies, and resulting gist-like or schematic representations, may be supported by extra-hippocampal regions specialized for the initial coding of different information about environments within allocentric or egocentric frameworks, or in the integration or translation of the two frameworks. These regions include parahippocampal cortex within the MTL and regions of retrosplenial cortex and posterior parietal cortex to which the MTL regions are strongly interconnected (for a review, see Epstein, 2008). This possibility has been supported by evidence of co-activation of these regions during tests of spatial memory and navigation in neuroimaging experiments (Rosenbaum et al., 2004, 2007; Spiers and Maguire, 2006) and in studies with rats (Maviel et al., 2004; Frankland and Bontempi, 2005; Teixeira et al., 2006).

An alternative account of our findings is that both schematic and detailed, episodic-like aspects of remote spatial memories (discussed below) continue to depend on the hippocampus and that a gist is what survives following partial hippocampal damage. As mentioned, however, studies of patients with extensive damage to the hippocampus bilaterally indicate that even they can navigate in premorbidly learned environments and perform normally on tests of remote spatial memory similar to the ones included in the current study (Teng and Squire, 1999; Rosenbaum et al., 2000). Indeed, a functional neuroimaging study indicated that the little hippocampal tissue that remains in one such case (K.C.) was not differentially activated as he performed remote spatial memory tasks (Rosenbaum et al., 2007). Another possibility is that gist-like spatial memories rely on the hippocampus in older adults, as this structure is not severely damaged as is the case in the amnesic patients that have been studied. But, here again, neuroimaging studies indicate that even young adults do not differentially activate the hippocampus on these tasks (Rosenbaum et al., 2004).

Our results resemble findings in rats which showed that extensive experience in a complex maze as young rats enabled them to retain memory for efficient navigation to specific locations when they got old (Winocur et al., 2010a). Probe trials indicated that the rats' successful performance was, indeed, based on the application of allocentric spatial strategies and not on the use of non-spatial local cues or procedural learning. There are limits to how far we can extend this interpretation to older adults because there were some key differences. Unlike the older adults in the present study who performed normally on these spatial tasks, the aged rats performed slightly worse compared to when they were young. A possible account is that the older adults continued to visit downtown Toronto in recent years, whereas the aged rats were completely restricted from entering the environment for 15 months, about half a rat's lifespan. By contrast, older adults in the present study visited Toronto infrequently and significantly less often than did the young adults in the 5 years preceding the study. In fact, taking frequency of visits into account revealed better performance in the older than in the younger adults, suggesting that the older adults may have used a variety of non-hippocampal strategies to supplement their performance.

Findings of intact performance do not appear to be explained by the number of years that participants lived in Toronto, which was significantly greater for older than younger participants. There may be a minimum amount of experience and/or time (visiting once a week for no more than 10 years) needed for the formation and maintenance of a robust and presumably flexible representation of a real-world environment, but it appears that not much is gained beyond that minimum. Nevertheless, there are other potential confounds that we were unable to control or verify that relate to the nature of exposure to downtown Toronto. For example, the purpose of navigating in downtown Toronto (e.g., location of one's work, home, leisure activities), means of travel (walking, driving, taking public transit), and size or part of downtown Toronto in which one frequents may covary with age. These and other variables may influence the initial encoding and re-encoding of the environment as well as the quality of the representation itself.

Although age differences in representing spatial relations among landmarks and the routes between them were not apparent or favoured older adults, differences did emerge in subjective reports of the experiential quality of mentally navigating the routes. Whereas all of the young adults reported imagining the routes from a first-person perspective, half of the older adults reported a third-person perspective. Even more striking was the finding that the majority of the older participants reported that their re-experiencing of mentally navigating the route lacked vividness and richness of perceptual detail. Hirshhorn et al. (2011) reported a similar paucity of re-experiencing well-known Toronto routes in older adults who otherwise appeared to make accurate proximity judgments based on the same Toronto environment. Importantly, only re-experiencing of routes was correlated with autobiographical episodic memory and other neuropsychological tests of hippocampal function. Although we did not directly investigate the experiential and perceptual qualities of spatial judgments on vector mapping, a task that was also performed better by the older participants, it is possible that perceptual richness and re-experiencing interfered with efficient mental navigation in the younger participants.

The finding that aspects of mental navigation amid spatial locations were intact in the older adults contrasts with impaired recognition of landmarks that occupy those locations, reflecting both a difficulty discriminating between Toronto landmarks and similar-looking foil landmarks, and an overall conservative response rate. The data also suggested worse performance in older than younger adults in providing identifying information (name or other distinctive details) for landmarks that were accurately recognized as being located in Toronto. This additional finding suggests some modality-specific loss of distinctive visual information that enables naming. Object recognition impairment has also been reported in aged rats (Burke et al., 2010; see also McTighe et al., 2010), although these results may also reflect an age-related aversiveness to novelty. The recognition deficit appears to be independent of impaired spatial learning in the rats and resembles impaired pattern separation between stimuli that share visual features in rats and humans with perirhinal cortex lesions (Burke et al., 2011; for a review, see Graham et al., 2010). Similarly, the landmark recognition deficit described here resembles findings of impaired perceptual discrimination of complex scenes in relation to hippocampal and parahippocampal cortex lesions (Graham et al.). Indeed, we found a similar impairment of Toronto landmark recognition in a former taxi driver who had developed Alzheimer's disease (patient S.B.) in the context of reduced hippocampal and ventral visual cortex volumes (Rosenbaum et al., 2005). This contrasts with intact landmark recognition reported in the former taxi driver T.T. who was post-encephalitic and had bilateral hippocampal damage but intact perirhinal and parahippocampal cortices (Maguire et al., 2006). Park et al. (2004) and Schiavetto et al. (2002) have demonstrated that even when behavioural discrimination of faces, places, and other objects is not required, such object categories are not differentiated in ventral visual cortex to the same extent in old compared to young adults. It remains for future research to determine if the decline in landmark recognition is a consequence of such a lack of neural specificity.

It is possible that detailed knowledge of well-known city landmarks is not essential for navigation, especially when aerial views are presented to capture the landmarks in their entirety, and may, instead be treated as episodic-like details. It is unknown if visual recognition of landmarks is related to re-experiencing those landmarks and other visual features along an imagined route. In a recent study of remote spatial memory in patients with parietal lesions, we found a similar effect of age on the likelihood of reporting detailed, personal episodes associated with Toronto landmarks during a recognition task (Ciaramelli et al., 2010). Impaired autobiographical episodic memory for details of personal events was also found to co-occur with impaired landmark recognition in S.B. (Rosenbaum et al., 2005) and impaired recognition of neighbourhood houses in K.C. (Rosenbaum et al., 2000). In both patients, the impairment was in the context of intact remote memory for spatial locations but impaired learning of new routes. Findings that the perception of spatial elements and vivid recollections of those elements in remote memory are compromised in healthy and pathological aging and in amnesia suggest that the hippocampus is needed for linking different types of spatial details with each other and these to a rich episode.

Finally, we successfully replicated a consistent finding in the literature of impaired spatial learning in aging, which has been demonstrated in rats (Barnes, 1979; Gallagher and Pelleymounter, 1988; Winocur and Gagnon, 1998; Winocur et al., 2010a) and in humans, primarily based on virtual environments (Antonova et al., 2009; Head and Isom, 2010; Etchamendy et al., 2012; Rodgers et al., 2012; see Evans et al., 1984 and Cushman et al., 2008 for findings in real-world environments). The older adults in the current study committed significantly more errors than the young adults in the form of incorrect turns on two trials of an immediate learning condition as well as after a 30-min delay, though both groups showed improvement across trials. Interestingly, older participants seemed not to be cognizant of their deficient learning as they gave similar ratings of good navigational ability in both new and old environments. Both new route learning in the delay condition and ratings of navigational ability in new environments were negatively correlated with the ability to recognize well-known Toronto landmarks. Difficulties perceiving or encoding the appearance of newly encountered landmarks may have hindered route learning in the older adults, though work with rats described above would predict otherwise (see Burke et al., 2011).

Amnesia resulting from hippocampal damage is characterized by a profound inability to form and retain new spatial memories (e.g., Smith and Milner, 1981; Maguire et al., 1996, 2006; Holdstock et al., 2000; Rosenbaum et al., 2000; but see Corkin, 2002). This is supported by data from cellular recordings in animals (O'Keefe and Dostrovsky, 1971; Best et al., 2001; Moser et al., 2008) and humans (Ekstrom et al., 2003), animal lesion studies (Morris et al., 1982; Hampton et al., 2004; Lavenex et al., 2006), and human neuroimaging studies (Spiers and Maguire, 2006; Igloi et al., 2010). Findings like these contributed to the development of Cognitive Map Theory, which specifies that allocentric spatial memory for configural relations among objects located in the environment is uniquely dependent on the hippocampus (O'Keefe and Nadel, 1978; Bird and Burgess, 2008). This theory, and the related scene construction view of hippocampal function, accommodate findings in healthy aging, Alzheimer's disease, and hippocampal amnesia of impaired autobiographical episodic memory (Bright et al., 2006; Gilboa et al., 2006; Kirwan et al., 2008; Rosenbaum et al., 2008) and the construction of scenes and future events (Hassabis et al., 2007; Addis et al., 2011), which inherently involve a spatial framework (Byrne et al., 2007). The hippocampus is believed to sustain and guide this organizing principle, either by virtue of its purported role in processing spatial information or by some general binding process (Rosenbaum et al., 2009; Race et al., 2011). However, these theories do not take into consideration that detailed spatial memories change with time and experience and therefore cannot account for the preserved spatial memories that support navigation in older adults and other people whose hippocampal function is compromised.

Only the Transformation Hypothesis of spatial memory (Winocur et al., 2010b; Winocur and Moscovitch, 2011; see also Rosenbaum et al., 2001 and Moscovitch et al., 2005) can account for both the preserved and impaired spatial memories that we reported. The Transformation Hypothesis is based on the distinction between detailed or episodic-like spatial representations, which are impaired in aging and in hippocampal amnesia no matter how long ago the memories were acquired, and schematic/generic spatial representations of environments, which are resistant to the effects of aging and amnesia after they have been assimilated and stored over time. Spatial memories, like other types of declarative or relational memories, may change over time into a schematic or gist-like form. This process may resemble the "semanticization" of episodic memories in humans, whereby memory traces of repeated events become integrated with pre-existing knowledge in neocortex, stripped of contextual details that would allow for rich re-experiencing of the event. The hippocampus may be needed for the maintenance and retrieval of spatial details that are embedded within an episodic representation but not for a spatial layout that has been experienced in many different ways across a multitude of episodes. However, when fine discrimination is needed to distinguish routes or landmarks from one another, perirhinal cortex may also play a role even for remote memories of those routes or landmarks (Burke et al., 2011). Our findings provide evidence that older adults benefit from spatial-relational cues that are extracted over many different encounters with an environment as they do from the semantic gist that is extracted over repeated and varied experiences.

## ACKNOWLEDGMENTS

This work was supported by grants from the Natural Sciences and Engineering Research Council of Canada and a Sloan Research Fellowship to R. Shayna Rosenbaum and Canadian Institutes of Health Research (Grant #: MGP 6694) to R. Shayna Rosenbaum, Gordon Winocur, and Morris Moscovitch. The authors gratefully acknowledge the technical assistance of Nicholas Hill, Janet Roberts, and Audrey Wong. We also thank Thomas Wolbers, Eric Blalock, and Sue Becker for their valuable comments.

## REFERENCES

Addis, D. R., Roberts, R. P., and Schacter, D. L. (2011). Age-related neural changes in autobio- graphical remembering and imagining. *Neuropsychologia* 49, 3656–3669.

Antonova, E., Parslow, D., Brammer, M., Dawson, G. R., Jackson, S. H., and Morris, R. G. (2009). Age- related neural activity during allo- centric spatial memory. *Memory* 17, 125–143.

Barnes, C. A. (1979). Memory deficits associated with senescence: a neuro-physiological and behavioral study in the rat. *J. Comp. Physiol. Psychol.* 93, 74–104.

Best, P. J., White, A. M., and Minai, A. (2001). Spatial processing in the brain: the activity of hippocampal place cells. *Annu. Rev. Neurosci.* 24, 459–486.

Bird, C. M., and Burgess, N. (2008). The hippocampus and memory: insights from spatial processing. *Nat. Rev. Neurosci.* 9, 182–194.

Bright, P., Buckman, J., Fradera, A., Yoshimasu, H., Colchester, A. C., and Kopelman, M. D. (2006). Retrograde amnesia in patients with hippocampal, medial temporal, temporal lobe, or frontal pathology. *Learn. Mem.* 13, 545–557.

Burke, S. N., Wallace, J. L., Hartzell, A. L., Nematollahi, S., Plange, K., and Barnes, C. A. (2011). Age- associated deficits in pattern sepa- ration functions of the perirhinal cortex: a cross-species consensus. *Behav. Neurosci.* 125, 836–847.

Burke, S. N., Wallace, J. L., Nematollahi, S., Uprety, A. R., and Barnes, C. A. (2010). Pattern separation deficits may contribute to age-associated recognition impairments. *Behav. Neurosci.* 124, 559–573.

Byrne, P., Becker, S., and Burgess, N. (2007). Remembering the past and imagining the future: a neural model of spatial memory and imagery. *Psychol. Rev.* 114, 340–375.

Ciaramelli, E., Rosenbaum, R. S., Solcz, S., Levine, B., and Moscovitch, M. (2010). Mental time travel in space: damage to posterior parietal cortex prevents egocentric navigation and re-experiencing of remote spatial memories. *J. Exper. Psychol. Learn. Mem. Cogn.* 36, 619–634.

Corkin, S. (2002). What's new with the amnesic patient H.M.? *Nat. Rev. Neurosci.* 3, 153–160.

Cushman, L. A., Stein, K., and Duffy, C. J. (2008). Detecting naviga- tional deficits in cognitive aging and Alzheimer disease using virtual real- ity. *Neurology* 71, 888–895.

Davidson, P. S., and Glisky, E. L. (2002). Neuropsychological corre- lates of recollection and familiarity in normal aging. *Cogn. Affect. Behav. Neurosci.* 2, 174–186.

Driscoll, I., Howard, S. R., Stone, J. C., Monfils, M. H., Tomanek, B., Brooks, W. M., and Sutherland, R. J. (2006). The aging hippocampus: a multi-level analysis in the rat. *Neuroscience* 139, 1173–1185.

Ekstrom, A. D., Kahana, M. J., Caplan, J. B., Fields, T. A., Isham, E. A., Newman, E. L., and Fried, I. (2003). Cellular networks under- lying human spatial navigation. *Nature* 425, 184–188.

Epstein, R. A. (2008). Parahippocampal and retrosplenial contributions to human spatial navigation. *Trends Cogn. Sci.* 12, 388–396.

Etchamendy, N., Konishi, K., Pike, G. B., Marighetto, A., and Bohbot, V. D. (2012). Evidence for a virtual human analog of a rodent relational memory task: a study of aging and fMRI in young adults. *Hippocampus* 22, 869–880.

Evans, G. W., Brennan, P. L., Skorpanich, M. A., and Held, D. (1984). Cognitive mapping and elderly adults: verbal and location memory for urban landmarks. *J. Gerontol.* 39, 452–457.

Frankland, P. W., and Bontempi, B. (2005). The organization of recent and remote memories. *Nat. Rev. Neurosci.* 6, 119–130.

Gallagher, M., and Pelleymounter, M. A. (1988). Spatial learning deficits in old rats: a model for memory declineintheaged. *Neurobiol. Aging* 9, 549–556.

Gilboa, A., Winocur, G., Rosenbaum, R. S., Poreh, A., Gao, F., Black, S. E., Westmacott, R., and Moscovitch, M. (2006). Hippocampal contributions to recollection in retrograde and anterograde memory. *Hippocampus* 16, 966–980.

Grady, C. L., and Craik, F. I. (2000). Changes in memory processing with age. *Curr. Opin. Neurobiol.* 10, 224–231.

Graham, K. S., Barense, M. D., and Lee, A. C. (2010). Going beyond LTM in the MTL: a synthesis of neuropsychological and neuroimag- ing findings on the role of the medial temporal lobe in memory and perception. *Neuropsychologia* 48, 831–853.

Hampton, R. R., Hampstead, B. M., and Murray, E. A. (2004). Selective hip- pocampal damage in rhesus mon- keys impairs spatial memory in an open-field test. *Hippocampus* 14, 808–818.

Harris, M. A., and Wolbers, T. (2012). Ageing effects on path integra- tion and landmark navigation. *Hippocampus* 22, 1770–1780.

Hassabis, D., Kumaran, D., Vann, S. D., and Maguire, E. A. (2007). Patients with hippocampal amne- sia cannot imagine new experiences. *Proc. Natl. Acad. Sci. U.S.A.* 104, 1726–1731.

Hassabis, D., and Maguire, E. A. (2009). The construction system of the brain. *Philos. Trans. R. Soc. Lond. B Biol. Sci.* 364, 1263–1271.

Head, D., and Isom, M. (2010). Age effects on wayfinding and route learning skills. *Behav. Brain Res.* 209, 49–58.

Hirshhorn, M., Grady, C. L., Rosenbaum, R. S., Winocur, G., and Moscovitch, M. (2012). An fMRI study of the hippocampus and other structures involved in memory for a recently learned environment. *Hippocampus* 22, 842–852.

Hirshhorn, M., Newman, L., and Moscovitch, M. (2011). Detailed descriptions of routes traveled, but not map-like knowledge, correlates with tests of hippocampal function in older adults. *Hippocampus* 21, 1147–1151.

Holdstock, J. S., Mayes, A. R., Cezayirli, E., Isaac, C. L., Aggleton, J. P., and Roberts, N. (2000). A comparison of egocentric and allocentric spatial memory in a patient with selective hippocam- pal damage. *Neuropsychologia* 38, 410–425.

Igloi, K., Doeller, C. F., Berthoz, A., Rondi-Reig, L., and Burgess, N. (2010). Lateralized human hippocampal activity predicts navigation based on sequence or place memory. *Proc. Natl. Acad. Sci. U.S.A.* 107, 14466–14471.

Jernigan, T. L., Archibald, S. L., Fennema-Notestine, C., Gamst, A. C., Stout, J. C., Bonner, J., and Hesselink, J. R. (2001). Effects of age on tissues and regions of the cerebrum and cerebellum. *Neurobiol. Aging* 22, 581–594.

Kirwan, C. B., Bayley, P. J., Galvan, V. V., and Squire, L. R. (2008). Detailed recollection of remote autobiographical memory after damage to the medial temporal lobe. *Proc. Natl. Acad. Sci. U.S.A.* 105, 2676–2680.

Lavenex, P. B., Amaral, D. G., and Lavenex, P. (2006). Hippocampal lesion prevents spatial relational learning in adult macaque monkeys. *J. Neurosci.* 26, 4546–4558.

Levine, B., Svoboda, E., Hay, J. F., Winocur, G., and Moscovitch, M. (2002). Aging and autobiographical memory: dissociating episodic from semantic retrieval. *Psychol. Aging* 17, 677–689.

Maguire, E. A., Burke, T., Phillips, J., and Staunton, H. (1996). Topographicaldisorientation following unilateral temporal lobe lesions in humans. *Neuropsychologia* 34, 993–1001.

Maguire, E. A., Nannery, R., and Spiers, H. J. (2006). Navigation around London by a taxi driver with bilat- eral hippocampal lesions. *Brain* 129, 2894–2907.

Maviel, T., Durkin, T. P., Menzaghi, F., and Bontempi, B. (2004). Sites ofneocortical reorganization critical for remote spatial memory. *Science* 305, 96–99.

McTighe, S. M., Cowell, R. A., Winters, B. D., Bussey, T. J., and Saksida, L. M. (2010). Paradoxical false mem- ory for objects after brain damage. *Science* 330, 1408–1410.

Moffat, S. D. (2009). Aging and spatial navigation: what do we know and where do we go? *Neuropsychol. Rev.* 19, 478–489.

Morris, R. G. M., Garrud, P., Rawlins, J. N. P., and O'Keefe, J. (1982). Place navigation impaired in rats with hippocampal lesions. *Nature* 297,681–683.

Moscovitch, M., Rosenbaum, R. S., Gilboa, A., Addis, D. R., Westmacott, R., Grady, C., McAndrews, M. P., Levine, B., Black, S., Winocur, G., and Nadel, L. (2005). Functional neuroanatomy of remote episodic, semantic and spatial memory: a unified account based on multiple trace theory. *J. Anat.* 207, 35–66.

Moser, E. I., Kropff, E., and Moser, M. B. (2008). Place cells, grid cells, and the brain's spatial representa- tion system. *Annu. Rev. Neurosci.* 31, 69–89.

Nedelska, Z., Andel, R., Laczó, J., Vlcek, K., Horinek, D., Lisy, J., Sheardova, K., Bures, J., and Hort, J. (2012). Spatial navigation impairment is proportional to right hippocampal volume. *Proc. Natl. Acad. Sci. U.S.A.* 109, 2590–2594.

O'Keefe, J., and Dostrovsky, J. (1971). The hippocampus as a spatial map. Preliminary evidence from unit activity in the freely-moving rat. *Brain Res.* 34, 171–175.

O'Keefe, J., and Nadel, L. (1978). *The Hippocampus as a Cognitive Map.* Oxford: Clarendon.

Park, D. C., Polk, T. A., Park, R., Minear, M., Savage, A., and Smith, M. R. (2004). Aging reduces neural spe- cialization in ventral visual cortex. *Proc. Natl. Acad. Sci. U.S.A.* 101, 13091–13095.

Park, D. C., and Reuter-Lorenz, P. (2009). The adaptive brain: aging and neurocognitive scaffolding. *Annu. Rev. Psychol.* 60, 173–196.

Piolino, P., Desgranges, B., Clarys, D., Guillery-Girard, B., Taconnat, L., Isingrini, M., and Eustache, F. (2006). Autobiographical memory, autonoetic consciousness, and self- perspective in aging. *Psychol. Aging* 21, 510–525.

Race, E., Keane, M. M., and Verfaellie, M. (2011). Medial temporal lobe damage causes deficits in episodic memory and episodic future think- ing not attributable to deficits in narrative construction. *J. Neurosci.* 31, 10262–10269.

Raz, N., Lindenberger, U., Rodrigue, K. M., Kennedy, K. M., Head, D., Williamson, A., Dahle, C., Gerstorf, D., and Acker, J. D. (2005). Regional brain changes in aging healthy adults: general trends, individual differences and modifiers. *Cereb. Cortex* 15, 1676–1689.

Rodgers, M. K., Sindone, J. A. 3rd., and Moffat, S. D. (2012). Effects of age on navigation strategy. *Neurobiol. Aging* 202, e15–e22.

Rosenbaum, R. S., Gao, F., Richards, B., Black, S. E., and Moscovitch, M. (2005). "Where to?" Remote memory for spatial relations and landmark identity in former taxi drivers with Alzheimer's disease and encephalitis. *J. Cogn. Neurosci.* 17, 446–462.

Rosenbaum, R. S., Gilboa, A., Levine, B., Winocur, G., and Moscovitch, M. (2009). Amnesia as impair- ment of detail generation and binding: evidence from personal, fictional, and semantic narra- tives in K.C. *Neuropsychologia* 47, 2181–2187.

Rosenbaum, R. S., Moscovitch, M., Foster, J. K., Schnyer, D. M., Gao, F. Q., Kovacevic, N., Verfaellie, M., Black, S. E., and Levine, B. (2008). Patterns of autobiographical mem- ory loss in medial temporal lobe amnesic patients. *J. Cogn. Neurosci.* 20, 1490–1506.

Rosenbaum, R. S., Priselac, S., Köhler, S., Black, S. E., Gao, F., Nadel, L., and Moscovitch, M. (2000). Remote spatial memory in an amnesic per- son with extensive bilateral hip- pocampal lesions. *Nat. Neurosci.* 3, 1044–1048.

Rosenbaum, R. S., Winocur, G., Grady, C. L., Ziegler, M., and Moscovitch, M. (2007). Memory for familiar environments learned in the remote past: fMRI studies of healthy people and an amnesic person with extensive bilateral hip- pocampal lesions. *Hippocampus* 17, 1241–1251.

Rosenbaum, R. S., Winocur, G., and Moscovitch, M. (2001). New views on old memories: re-evaluating the role of the hippocampal complex. *Behav. Brain Res.* 127, 183–197.

Rosenbaum, R. S., Ziegler, M., Winocur, G., Grady, C. L., and Moscovitch, M. (2004). "I have often walked down this street before": fMRI studies on the hip- pocampus and other structures during mental navigation of an old environment. *Hippocampus* 14, 826–835.

Schiavetto, A., Köhler, S., Grady, C. L., Winocur, G., and Moscovitch, M. (2002). Neural correlates of memory for object identity and object location: effects of aging. *Neuropsychologia* 40, 1428–1442.

Smith, M. L., and Milner, B. (1981). The role of the right hippocam- pus in the recall of spatial location. *Neuropsychologia* 19, 781–793.

Spiers, H. J., and Maguire, E. A. (2006). Thoughts, behaviour, and brain dynamics during navigation in the real world. *NeuroImage* 31, 1826–1840.

Teng, E., and Squire, L. R. (1999). Memory for places learned long ago is intact after hippocampal damage. *Nature* 400, 675–677.

Teixeira, C. M., Pomedi, S. R., Maei, H. R., Kee, N., and Frankland, P. W. (2006). Involvement of the anterior cingulate cortex in the expression of remote spatial memory. *J. Neurosci.* 26, 7555–7564.

Winocur, G., and Gagnon, S. (1998). Glucose treatment attenuates spa- tial learning and memory deficits of aged rats on tests of hippocam- pal function. *Neurobiol. Aging* 19, 233–241.

Winocur, G., and Moscovitch, M. (2011). Memory transformation and systems consolidation. *J. Int. Neuropsychol. Soc.* 17, 766–780.

Winocur, G., Moscovitch, M., and Bontempi, B. (2010a). Memory formation and long-term retention in humans and animals: convergence towards a transformation account of hippocampal-neocortical inter- actions. *Neuropsychologia* 48, 2339–2356.

Winocur, G., Moscovitch, M., Rosenbaum, R. S., and Sekeres, M. (2010b). A study of remote spa- tial memory in aged rats. *Neurobiol. Aging* 31, 143–150.

Winocur, G., Moscovitch, M., Fogel, S., Rosenbaum, R. S., and Sekeres, M. (2005). Preserved spatial memory after hippocampal lesions: effects of extensive experience in a com- plex environment. *Nat. Neurosci.* 8, 273–275.

Wolbers, T., and Büchel, C. (2005). Dissociable retrosplenial and hippocampal contributions to successful formation of survey representations. *J. Neurosci.* 25, 3333–3340.

Yonelinas, A. P., Widaman, K., Mungas, D., Reed, B., Weiner, M. W., and Chui, H. C. (2007). Memory in the aging brain: doubly dis- sociating the contribution of the hippocampus and entorhi- nal cortex. *Hippocampus* 17, 1134–1140.

18

# Age-associated changes in the hippocampal-ventral striatum-ventral tegmental loop that impact learning, prediction, and context discrimination


***Marsha R. Penner** and **Sheri J. Y. Mizumori****

*Laboratory of Neural Systems, Decision Science, Learning and Memory, Department of Psychology, University of Washington, Seattle, WA, USA*



**Edited by:**
*Paul A. Dudchenko, University of Stirling, UK*

**Reviewed by:**
*Daniel Ortuño-Sahagun, Centro Universitario de Ciencias Biológicas y Agropecuarias, Mexico*
*David Bett, University of Edinburgh, UK*



***Correspondence:**
*Sheri J. Y. Mizumori, Department of Psychology, University of Washington, Box 351525 Guthrie Hall, Seattle, WA 98195, USA.*
*e-mail: mizumori@uw.edu*



Studies of the neural mechanisms of navigation and context discrimination have generated a powerful heuristic for understanding how neural codes, circuits, and computations contribute to accurate behavior as animals traverse and learn about spatially extended environments. It is assumed that memories are updated as a result of spatial experience. The mechanism, however, for such a process is not clear. Here we suggest that one revealing approach to study this issue is to integrate our knowledge about limbic system mediated navigation and context discrimination with knowledge about how midbrain neural circuitry mediates decision-making. This perspective should lead to new and specific neural theories about how choices that we make during navigation determine what information is ultimately learned and remembered. This same circuitry may be involved when past experiences come to bias future spatial perceptions and response selection. With old age come not only important changes in limbic system operations, but also significant decline in the function of midbrain regions that underlie accurate and efficient decisions. Thus, suboptimal accuracy of spatial context-based decision-making may be, at least in part, responsible for the common observation of spatial memory decline in old age.



**Keywords: adaptive navigation, context discrimination, decision-making, error prediction, hippocampus, ventral striatum, ventral tegmental area**


## INTRODUCTION

Cognitive map theory (O'Keefe and Nadel, 1978), which was based on the discovery of place cells in the hippocampus (O'Keefe and Dostrovsky, 1971), suggested that the hippocampus is important for the representation of experiences that occur within a spatial context (Nadel, 2008). These ideas have since been elaborated on, and one current assertion, discussed herein, is that the hippocampus does not just represent context, but also works to discriminate *between* contexts and to determine when a salient feature of a context have changed (Mizumori et al., 1999, 2007a). There is a growing body of experimental evidence providing support for this idea. Moreover, convergent evidence suggests a key role for the hippocampus in age-related impairments of context-based learning and memory. For example, work with rodent, primate, and human subjects shows that a compromised hippocampus results in spatial memory deficits that could be accounted for by poorer analysis of contextual details. These deficits are proposed to have a significant impact on context-dependent decision-making processes.

## WHAT IS CONTEXT?

Although there may be some disagreement regarding what features make up or define a context, everyone would probably agree that a context is a multifaceted entity, and that everything we experience takes place within a context. According to Nadel (2008) the features that define a context must be relatively stable, meaning that their relationship to each other remains, even when there is no one there to experience them. Context, as we will use the term in the following discussion, refers to stable background stimuli, such as the geometrical features of a testing room, as well as more abstract features, such as the task demands and internal state that come to help make some aspects of a context more salient than others (see Smith and Mizumori, 2006a).

The detection of changes in context is necessary for both optimal learning and the selection of appropriate behaviors within a given context. In order to determine if a salient feature of a particular context has changed, match–mismatch comparisons are made (**Figure 1**). This allows an organism to determine how similar the current context is to the context the animal was expecting based on past experience (see Mizumori et al., 2007a).

## THE HIPPOCAMPUS AND CONTEXT

There is growing evidence that the hippocampus has a special role in learning and memory because it functions to distinguish meaningful contexts, and in that way determine the saliency of different contexts (e.g., Mizumori et al., 1999; Smith and Mizumori, 2006a; Mizumori et al., 2007a; Penner and Mizumori, 2012). This function is critical for the formation of new episodic memories because it separates in time and space one meaningful event from the next. Such "chunking" of memories could facilitate long-term information storage according to memory schemas (Tse et al., 2007; Bethus et al., 2010).

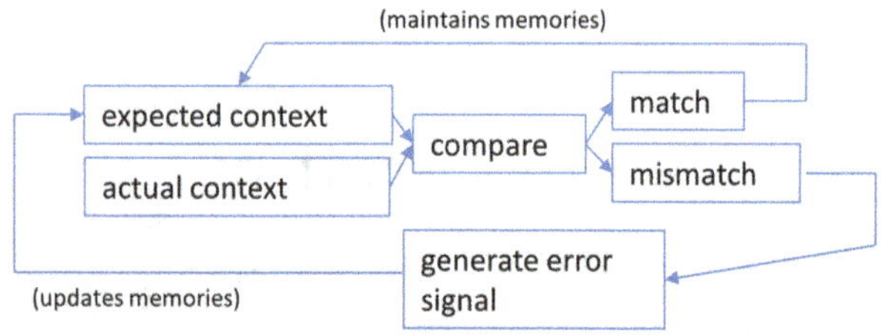


**FIGURE 1 | A schematic illustration of the steps involved in a context prediction error analysis.** Information about expected features of a given context are compared against actual contextual features experienced by the animal. If they are perceived to be the same, a "match" signal is generated that maintains (or possibly strengthens) the neural network that underlies the current active memory. Pattern completion computations may predominate in such a determination of a match (see text for discussion). If a "mismatch" is detected, the result is hippocampal output that reflects the error in prediction. In this case, pattern separation computations may prevail over pattern completion computations. The impact of a context prediction error signal is to ultimately update long-term memories that will define the expected contextual features the next time an animal enters the same situation.

Studies of the predominant type of neural representation by hippocampal pyramidal neurons, location-selective firing (O'Keefe and Dostrovsky, 1971; O'Keefe and Nadel, 1978), have provided insight into the mechanisms by which the hippocampus analyzes context information to result in context prediction error signals. As decades of research have shown (summarized in Mizumori et al., 2007a), "place fields" of recorded "place cells" are dynamic and integrated representations of multiple types of information, from sensory, motivational, and behavioral, to mnemonic. For example, changing any modality of cues, the motivational state, or the behaviors needed to perform the task result in alterations of place field properties, a process commonly referred to as re-mapping. Thus, it is the combination of these different types of information that have come to define the meaning of "context" when referring to hippocampal processing. The relative contributions of these different input types vary with task demands, and this is evidenced by findings across many laboratories that place fields change when rats use identical environmental information to solve tasks according to different strategies (e.g., Ferbinteanu and Shapiro, 2003; Kennedy and Shapiro, 2004; Mizumori et al., 2004; Eschenko and Mizumori, 2007). To the extent that different cognitive strategies are mediated by different underlying memories, a particular pattern of activated place cells is thought to reflect one memory, and a different pattern of activated place cells corresponds to a different memory (e.g., Samsonovich and McNaughton, 1997). Thus, when one refers to place field re-mapping, implicit is the notion that each map is driven by a different memory.

Many cleverly designed studies have sought to determine the features and sensory inputs that affect re-mapping of hippocampal place fields. Early studies, for example, showed that place cells are sensitive to changes in the visual environment (e.g., Ranck, 1973; O'Keefe, 1976; Olton et al., 1978; Muller and Kubie, 1987) such as the geometric features of the environment (e.g., Gothard et al., 1996; O'Keefe and Burgess, 1996; Wiener, 1996). Other sensory inputs can also affect place activity, including olfactory cues (Save et al., 2000), auditory cues (O'Keefe and Conway, 1978; McEchron and Disterhoft, 1999), and somatosensory cues (Young et al., 1994). Based on this body of work, it is clear that hippocampal pyramidal neurons process multimodal sensory cue information. Hippocampal place fields are also sensitive to changes in a task's reward structure (Smith and Mizumori, 2006b; Wikenheiser and Redish, 2011). Smith and Mizumori (2006b) tested this idea by training rats to distinguish Context A from Context B according to where reward was expected to be found. Importantly, the motivational, sensory and behavioral requirements of task performance were explicitly held constant across the two contexts so that changes in place fields could be attributed to the recall of a different memory. Place fields were found to reorganize at the beginning of trials in Context B, a time when a match–mismatch comparison may be implemented, and a time when there may be uncertainty about the context. In a similar experiment, Wikenheiser and Redish (2011) demonstrated that changes in reward contingency can modulate the trial-to-trial variability of hippocampal place cell activity.

## FROM PREDICTION ERRORS TO CONTEXT DISCRIMINATION: A ROLE FOR THE HIPPOCAMPUS

What kind of computations take place in order for an organism to determine if a salient feature of the context has changed? When an organism's expectations about its experiences are violated, it is adaptive to update expectations so that adequate predictions can be made in the future. Once mismatches between expectations and outcomes no longer occur, learning is considered "complete." According to classic learning theories, learning is driven by errors in the ability to accurately predict the occurrence of rewards, referred to as "prediction errors" (Rescorla and Wagner, 1972; Pearce and Hall, 1980; Sutton, 1988). The most common examples are the Rescorla–Wagner (Rescorla and Wagner, 1972) and temporal difference learning models (Sutton, 1988; Sutton and Barto, 1998) which use errors to drive associative changes. When a large prediction error is generated, a correspondingly large change in associative strength occurs. In contrast, no change in associative strength will occur if the computed prediction error is zero (i.e., the outcome is accurately predicted). Importantly, the relative sign of the error determines whether associative strength is promoted or weakened. When an outcome is better than predicted, the error generated will be positive, resulting in a strengthening of the association between the cues and the outcome. Alternatively, when the outcome is worse than predicted, a negative error signal is generated, and the association will weaken.

The neural instantiation of a reward prediction error was first observed in the midbrain dopamine system (Schultz et al., 1997). Using Pavlovian reward predicting paradigms in monkeys and rodents, it has been shown that dopamine cells increase phasic discharge when new rewards are encountered (Schultz et al., 1997). As the animal learns to expect reward, however, dopamine cell responses to rewards decline (Fiorillo et al., 2003). When this is the case, dopamine cells come to respond not to the reward itself but rather to the cues that predict the reward, such as a tone or light. The finding that reward responses of dopamine cells change from the reward to the cues that predict rewards is mirrored by corresponding changes in the timing of dopamine release in the nucleus accumbens (Day et al., 2007).

#### ASSESSING VALUE

The dopaminergic system is also part of a neural network that assesses the value of behavioral outcomes—reward-induced excitation of dopamine neurons scales to the magnitude of rewards (Schultz et al., 1997). Thus, encounters with large rewards are accompanied by larger amplitude phasic dopamine responses than encounters with small amounts of reward. In addition, dopamine cells respond to unexpected reward absences (Schultz et al., 1997) by decreasing their firing rates. The reduction in firing to the absence of expected reward is greater if the expectation was for a large, and not small, reward. A schematic illustration of these different dopamine cell responses to reward can be found in **Figure 2** (left side of figure).

#### OTHER FUNCTIONS OF DOPAMINE

In addition to generating a reward prediction signal, midbrain dopamine neurons also transmit signals related to salient but non-rewarding experiences such as aversive and alerting events (e.g., Pezze et al., 2001; Pezze and Feldon, 2004; Redgrave and Gurney, 2006). Thus, it has been suggested that dopamine neurons represent a heterogeneous population of cells that are connected to anatomically and functionally distinct brain networks (Bromberg-Martin et al., 2010). This would imply that dopamine neurons can have distinct roles in motivational control; some dopamine neurons may encode motivational value, supporting brain networks for seeking, evaluation, and value learning while others encode motivational salience, supporting brain networks for orienting, cognition, and general motivation (e.g., Berridge, 2007; Smith et al., 2011). For both types of dopamine neurons, an alerting signal could prime these cells for rapid detection of potentially important cues, a computation that would be necessary for detecting salient aspects and/or changes in context (see Bromberg-Martin et al., 2010).

#### PREDICTION ERRORS IN OTHER BRAIN REGIONS

Neural correlates of reward prediction errors have also been observed outside of the midbrain, in the prefrontal cortex, orbitofrontal cortex, striatum, amygdala, reticular formation, and habenula (Nobre et al., 1999; Schultz and Dickinson, 2000; McClure et al., 2003; Satoh et al., 2003; Bayer and Glimcher, 2005; Fiorillo et al., 2005; Tobler et al., 2006; Yacubian et al., 2006; Belova et al., 2007; Matsumoto and Hikosaka, 2007; Roesch et al., 2007; Puryear and Mizumori, 2008). This suggests that a critical and common function of many brain areas is to provide an outcome expectancy signal or prediction. Evidence is accumulating that the hippocampus is another brain region that may generate error prediction signals.

#### HIPPOCAMPAL CONTEXT PREDICTION ERROR

It has been suggested that hippocampal neurons represent the contextual features of an environment for the purpose of computing the extent to which familiar contexts change (Nadel and Wilner, 1980; Nadel and Payne, 2002), or more specifically the extent to which expected and actual context features match (e.g., Mizumori et al., 1999; Anderson and Jeffery, 2003; Jeffery et al., 2004; Hasselmo, 2005; Smith and Mizumori, 2006a,b; Nadel, 2008). If the hippocampus determines that there was no change (e.g., a familiar context appears as expected), then the currently active neural network that defines the current memory will be strengthened so that it can continue to drive behavior. If, on the other hand, a mismatch signal is generated, it will alert other neural systems of the brain so that they become prepared for rapid and new learning (**Figure 1**). The mismatch could be considered an example of an error in predicting the contextual details of the current situation and is thus referred to here as a "context prediction error." Transmission of a context prediction error signal can inform distal brain areas that a change in the context has occurred. For example, upon receipt of the hippocampal message, midbrain structures may respond with changes in excitation or inhibition to determine the subjective value of the context prediction error signal. Similarly, the same hippocampal signal may enable plasticity mechanisms (perhaps in neocortex) that allow new information to be incorporated into existing memory schemas (e.g., Mizumori et al., 2007a,b; Tse et al., 2007; Bethus et al., 2010). In this way, hippocampal context analyses becomes critical for the formation of new episodic memories via a prediction signal that can provide a mechanism that separates in time and space one meaningful event from the next. **Figure 2** shows schematized hippocampal place field responses, based on the vast literature on place field responses to context changes (Mizumori et al., 2007b), that illustrate the relationship between hippocampus and dopamine neurons: when the hippocampus signals a change in context, dopamine cells encode reward value.

### HIPPOCAMPAL CHANGES IN THE AGED BRAIN

The natural environment in which we behave continually changes. Optimal learning and performance depends on our ability to detect changes in context with sufficient temporal and informational specificity so that decisions about future adaptive responses can be made. Alterations in the ability of the hippocampus to perform these operations will contribute to significant learning and memory deficits that are manifested by an inability to recognize that something important or salient has changed, as is often observed in aged subjects. There is abundant and consistent evidence from aged rodents, monkeys, and humans that behavioral deficits are often observed on tasks whose optimal solution requires the use of spatial information (Gallagher and Rapp, 1997; Rosenzweig and Barnes, 2003; Wilson et al., 2006). Although neurobiological differences certainly exist across species, the organizational and functional principles governing spatial information processing are strikingly similar from rat to human.

The hippocampal place cells of aged rats show changes that are likely to significantly impact memory and context analysis functions. The initial pioneering work of Barnes (1979) demonstrated significant age-related deficits in spatial memory function that correlated with changes in synaptic plasticity; modification of synaptic efficacy at the perforant path synapses in the dentate gyrus was found to be significantly impaired (Barnes, 1979). Subsequent to this work, Barnes et al. (1983) recorded CA1 place cell activity in adult and aged rats as they performed a forced-choice eight-arm maze task. Rats were not required to

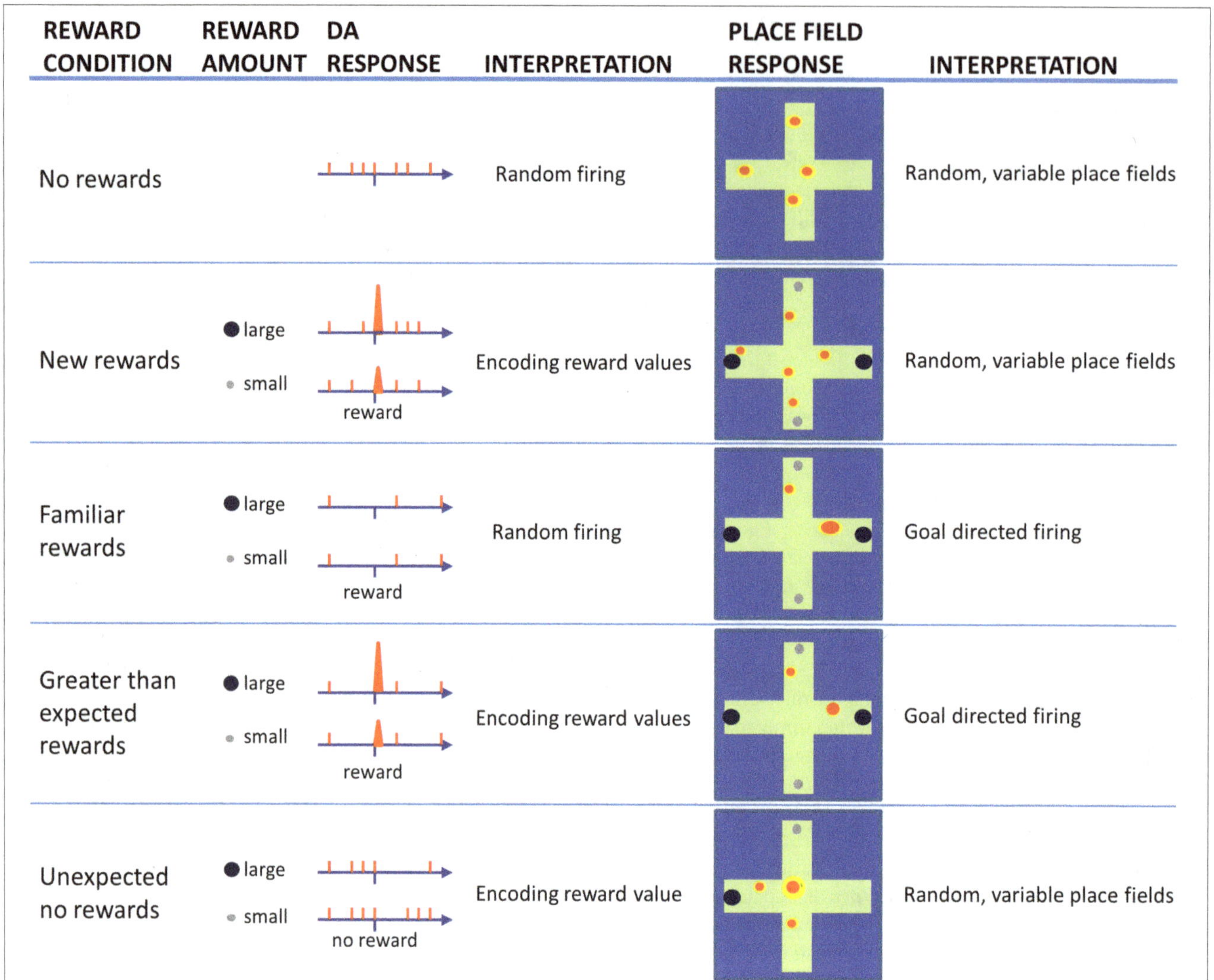


**FIGURE 2 | Schematic illustration of dopamine (DA) cell responses to encounters of large or small rewards as a rat solves a maze task under different reward conditions (left).** Consistent with the literature, DA cells appear to fire randomly at low rates as animals traverse a maze when no rewards are present (No reward). When a rat encounters reward for the first time (New rewards), DA cells exhibit phasic burst firing to a larger extent following encounters with large rewards than small rewards. In this case, DA cells are considered to be encoding reward values. When the reward-finding task is learned (Familiar rewards), DA cells should no longer fire upon reward encounters. If the rat then unexpectedly encounters reward, one will again observe burst firing by DA cells in proportion to the magnitude of reward (Greater than expected rewards). If a trained rats goes to a location that was previously associated with rewards, but the reward is unexpectedly absent (Unexpected no rewards), then DA cells are observed to show brief periods of inhibited firing that is proportional to the amount of reward expected. The right panels illustrate expected (based on the current literature) place field responses when recorded under the same varying reward conditions. During random activity on a maze, place fields exist but they tend to occur in somewhat random locations. On a trial when new rewards are first encountered, place fields may continue to occur in random locations since the new reward information has yet to update long-term memories. As a task is learned, and locations are associated with specific rewards, one may observe increased place field specificity, and the location of the field may skew toward the rewarded location. If animals encounter larger than expected rewards, the place fields may not change or they may become even more specific to reflect the increased significance of rewarded locations. If on the other hand, a reward is not found at a previously rewarded location, then one may observe place fields to move, or re-map, due to the elevated degree of uncertainty.

remember any spatial information but could access reward arms sequentially. Place fields in aged rats were found to be less place-specific and less reliable, in that they did not fire every time an animal ran through the field. These changes were suggested to contribute to the memory deficits observed in aged rats (Barnes et al., 1983).

Subsequent to this work, Barnes et al. (1997) demonstrated that when aged rats are brought into a familiar environment, they occasionally re-map. That is, there was an occasional global change in the place fields of most or all of the cells being recorded—some fields changed their preferred location within the environment, some cells stop firing in a previously preferred location (i.e., lose a place field), and some previously silent cells began firing (i.e., gained a place field). When this kind of re-mapping occurred during a recording session, the overall place fields appeared "noisy," as was initially demonstrated by Barnes

(Barnes et al., 1983). Importantly, when this re-mapping occurred it did so only when animals re-entered an environment it had previous experience with, never when an animal remained in the environment (Barnes et al., 1997).

Subsequent work, however, reported conflicting results in that the place fields of aged rats were shown to be just as place-specific and stable as those of adult rats, and under some conditions, more so (Markus et al., 1994; Mizumori et al., 1996; Shen et al., 1997; Tanila et al., 1997; Oler and Markus, 2000; Wilson et al., 2003). For example, Tanila et al. (1997) manipulated visual cues within the recording environment, and found that aged, memory-impaired rats were less likely than were adult rats or aged, memory intact rats to re-map in response to major changes in the environment. Thus, instead of being multi-stable, as reported by Barnes et al. (1997), the place cells of aged memory-impaired rats were often impervious to changes in the visual environment.

These results were subsequently reconciled by Wilson et al. (2004) who recorded place cells from aged and young rats as they repeatedly explored either a highly familiar environment or a novel environment. Initially, place cells in aged rats maintained their activity between the familiar and novel environments, suggesting that they were more rigid than those of the younger rats, as had been previously reported by others. However, Wilson et al. (2004) also observed that the rigidity of aged place cells was temporary. With additional experience, new representations of the novel environment could eventually be formed by aged rats, indicating a delay rather than an inability to detect a change in the environment. Finally, once these new spatial representations did develop, they were shown to be multi-stable across repeated exposures to the formerly novel environment. Thus, it appears that significant deficits in the ability of visual cues to control spatial representations of aged rats can manifests in at least three ways: rigidity, delayed control by external cues, and multi-stability (Wilson et al., 2004).

Environments or contexts are composed of more than just visual cues, and these other features can also exert control over place cell firing. Oler and Markus (2000) tested the idea that task demands, rather than spatial cue-based manipulations, would differentially impact changes in place field characteristics in young and aged rats. To test this idea, rats moved through a figure eight maze to retrieve chocolate rewards. The maze configuration was then changed to a plus maze configuration. Importantly, the maze remained in the same testing environment, so visual cues within the testing room remained unchanged. Rats were then required to run the plus maze, and after several laps, the maze was again restored to a figure eight configuration. Recordings from hippocampal place fields changed their spatial firing preference between the two maze configurations in younger rats, but this change did not occur in aged rats. Instead, place cells in the aged hippocampus retained their spatial firing pattern even though the task demands had changed. These results demonstrate that hippocampal place cells in young rats encode task-related information within a relatively stable spatial context while aged rats show deficits in encoding this information. The possibility remains that old rats were simply delayed in encoding changes in task demands, as described by Wilson et al. (2004). This idea has not yet been explicitly tested.

The work discussed thus far pooled data obtained from different subregions of the hippocampus (CA1 and CA3) in order to increase statistical power. It is now appreciated, however, that subareas of the hippocampus perform different information processing tasks and have different place field characteristics. These differences are a direct result of differences in their efferent and afferent projections, and this makes them differentially sensitive to context manipulations that produce re-mapping. For example, the CA3 subregion receives excitatory inputs from the mossy fibers of dentate granule cells, layer II of the entorhinal cortex, as well as a recurrent network of densely interconnected CA3 pyramidal cells, making it particularly suited for rapid learning of environment-specific features (Nakazawa et al., 2003). Work by several groups have shown that CA3 pyramidal cells exhibit an all-or-nothing change in their firing patterns when familiar environments are changed, or new environments are encountered (Lee et al., 2004; Leutgeb et al., 2004; Vazdarjanova and Guzowski, 2004; Miyashita et al., 2009). Conversely, area CA1 receives excitatory input from CA3 via Schaffer collaterals and the entorhinal cortex but has extremely limited intrinsic excitatory connections. When changes to familiar environments are encountered, area CA1 has been shown to display a gradual change in firing patterns. This has led some to suggest that area CA1 acts as a "comparator," in that it determines if a change in context has occurred by comparing the outputs of CA3 with direct inputs from the entorhinal cortex (Mizumori et al., 1999; Leutgeb et al., 2004; Vazdarjanova and Guzowski, 2004).

To test the idea that specific subregions of the hippocampus may be selectively vulnerable to effects of the normal aging processes, Wilson et al. (2004) compared the spatial firing patterns of CA1 and CA3 neurons in aged memory-impaired rats with those of young rats as they explored familiar and novel environments. Within area CA1, place cells in aged and young rats had similar firing characteristics in both familiar and novel environments. In contrast, within area CA3, aged rats showed place cells with higher firing rates when compared to young rats. In addition, CA3 place cells of aged rats failed to change their firing rates and place fields to the same degree that CA3 cells of young rats did when the rats were introduced to a novel environment. Thus, aged CA3 cells failed to rapidly encode new spatial information compared with young CA3 cells, suggesting a unique contribution of CA3 dysfunction to age-related memory impairment and context discrimination. In fact, these results are supported by the finding that a complete ensemble of CA3 pyramidal neurons are activated by a single exposure to a context, whereas CA1 cells require multiple exposures in order for a complete ensemble to be activated (Miyashita et al., 2009).

The dentate gyrus is another subregion of the hippocampus that is likely to contribute to a context discrimination function. Because sparse firing patterns are characteristic of dentate granule cells make it technically challenging to record from these cells, a relative dearth of *in vivo* electrophysiology data has been collected from this brain region. Other methods, including immediate-early gene imaging and fMRI studies have provided extensive evidence that this subarea of the hippocampus is particularly vulnerable to normative aging processes (Small et al., 2004; Penner et al., 2011).

## COMPUTATIONAL MECHANISMS THAT SUPPORT CONTEXT DISCRIMINIATION

Detecting a change in context is a necessary computation if one needs to discriminate contexts. Originating in the work of Marr (1971), pattern separation and completion computations are two functions that are widely attributed to specific subregions of the hippocampus (Marr, 1971; McNaughton and Morris, 1987; O'Reilly and McClelland, 1994; Samsonovich and McNaughton, 1997). Pattern completion is the process through which incomplete, noisy or degraded input are filled in based on representations that have previously been stored. In this way, complete episodes/memories can be recalled without a complete set of inputs. Pattern separation, on the other hand, is a computation that orthogonalizes similar inputs/representations. This functions to make similar inputs as dissimilar as possible, so that similar episodes/memories can be distinguished (Guzowski et al., 2004; Yassa and Stark, 2011). The interplay between these processes determines the extent to which hippocampal output signals a context prediction error: if pattern completion is greater than pattern separation, the hippocampal output signals a "match," whereas conditions in which pattern separation is greater than pattern completion should generate a mismatch (or prediction error) signal (Mizumori, 2008). Specific subareas of the hippocampus may compute the degrees of pattern separation and completion. Both theoretical models and experimental work suggest that the granule cells of the dentate gyrus perform pattern separation functions on the input received from the entorhinal cortex. Area CA3 is envisaged as an auto associative network and is therefore ideal for pattern completion functions on inputs received from the dentate gyrus and its own recurrent collaterals. Because of the unique pattern of excitatory inputs to area CA3, this subarea can also perform a pattern separation function. This function may be supported by a subset of neurons within the entorhinal cortex that bypass the dentate gyrus, and thus provide direct input to area CA3. This weaker input can compete with the input from mossy fibers of the dentate gyrus, and thus area CA3 may be well equipped to perform both pattern completion and pattern separation functions (Guzowski et al., 2004; Yassa and Stark, 2011).

In sum, the result of pattern separation and pattern completion computations determines the extent to which hippocampus generates a context prediction signal that can be broadcast to other brain regions for the purposes of modifying behavior that is appropriate for the current context. The work discussed here suggests that aged rats show impairments in both pattern separation and pattern completion computations, resulting in hippocampal representations of contexts that can be either too rigid, or too plastic. Impaired pattern completion in aged rats might cause the occasional retrieval of an incorrect map (especially for CA3 place fields) upon entry to a familiar environment, while impaired pattern separation in aged rats might prevent the formation of a new map in response to environmental changes (Yassa and Stark, 2011).

As discussed above, studies of place cell firing characteristics between adult and aged rats initially produced conflicting results. In some cases, it appeared that hippocampal cells engaged in too much pattern separation, resulting in multi-stable or unstable place fields, while in other instances, it appeared that the reverse was true (e.g., Barnes et al., 1997; Tanila et al., 1997). These results were subsequently reconciled (Wilson et al., 2004, 2005), especially in the case when recordings from CA3 and CA1 were analyzed separately (Wilson et al., 2005). These processes have since been investigated in human subjects (e.g., Bakker et al., 2008; Lacy et al., 2011), and recent work has shown age-related changes in these processes (Stark et al., 2010; Yassa et al., 2011a,b; Holden et al., 2012). For example, Yassa et al. (2011a) tested the ability of young and aged adults to discriminate between novel, familiar or similar objects and with measuring BOLD activity in the hippocampus during performance of the task. They observed a behavioral impairment in pattern separation for the aged adults compared to the young controls. These findings were related to an increase in CA3/dentate gyrus activity, a finding reminiscent of animal work showing hyperactivity in area CA3 (Wilson et al., 2004). In addition, Yassa et al. (2011a) found that larger changes in the input (greater dissimilarity) were necessary in order for aged adults to successfully encode new information as distinct from previously learned information.

## TARGETS OF THE CONTEXT PREDICTION SIGNAL

The hippocampus is hypothesized to provide a context prediction error signal to other areas of the brain in order to determine if expectations about the current context have been met, or if they need to be updated. The hippocampus is directly connected to both the ventral striatum (also known as the nucleus accumbens) and the prefrontal cortex, and these structures are therefore direct recipients of the hippocampal context prediction error. In addition, the hippocampus regulates activity within the ventral tegmental area (VTA) via its effects on the ventral striatum (Yang and Mogenson, 1987; Floresco et al., 2001) and via the lateral septum (Luo et al., 2011). The following discussion will focus on contextual information processing within the hippocampal-ventral striatal-VTA loop (Voorn et al., 2004; Pennartz et al., 2009, 2011; Humphries and Prescott, 2010).

### HIPPOCAMPUS-VENTRAL STRIATUM INTERACTIONS

The ventral striatum is often referred to a limbic-motor interface (Mogenson et al., 1980). It receives convergent glutamatergic input from multiple sensory and association areas of the neocortex, and the limbic system, including the hippocampus and related structures (for review see Humphries and Prescott, 2010). The nucleus accumbens, the main structure of the ventral striatum, can be divided into core and shell subregions, which differ significantly in terms of their cellular morphology, neurochemistry, and patterns of projections. The shell receives hippocampal input predominantly from ventral CA1 and subiculum, whereas the core receives it from dorsal CA1 and subiculum and from parahippocampal regions (Voorn et al., 2004).

The ventral striatum is not only important for processing spatial and contextual cues (Annett et al., 1989; Seamans and Phillips, 1994; Floresco et al., 1997; Ferretti et al., 2010), but also processes information relevant to effort and cost-based decision-making (e.g., Aberman et al., 1998; Aberman and Salamone, 1999; Hauber and Sommer, 2009; Day et al., 2011). The ability to make these kinds of decisions is essential if animals are to make adaptive behavioral choices within a given context. The ventral striatum appears strategically positioned to play a key role in context-dependent value-based decisions given the convergent evidence from a variety of maze studies, including the spatial version of the Morris swim task (Setlow and McGaugh, 1998; Sargolini et al., 2003), the radial maze (Gal et al., 1997; Smith-Roe et al., 1999), a spatial version of the hole board task (Maldonado-Irizarry and Kelley, 1995), as well as a task in which the animals are required to discriminate a spatial displacement of objects (Annett et al., 1989; Seamans and Phillips, 1994; Ferretti et al., 2010).

To investigate the idea that the ventral striatum associates spatial context with reward information, Lavoie and Mizumori (1994) recorded neural activity in the ventral striatum while rats navigated an eight-arm radial maze for food reward. This study demonstrated, for the first time, spatial firing correlates within the ventral striatum. The mean place specificity for all ventral striatal neurons was significantly lower than that typically observed in the hippocampus (Barnes et al., 1990), indicating that while ventral striatal neurons discharge with spatial selectivity, they are not as selective as those observed from hippocampal neurons. The moderate spatial selectivity likely reflects the integration of spatial with other non-spatial information within the ventral striatum, including reward and movement. The fact that single ventral striatal neurons encode multiple types of information supports the view that spatial, reward, and movement information may be integrated at the level of individual ventral striatal neurons (Lavoie and Mizumori, 1994; Pennartz et al., 2011). Recent evidence suggests that spatial information within the ventral striatum is derived from the hippocampus. Ito et al. (2008) showed that an interruption of information sharing between the hippocampus and shell of the nucleus accumbens disrupted the acquisition of context-dependent retrieval of cue information, suggesting that the shell, in particular, may provide a site at which spatial and salient cue information may be integrated.

## FROM THE VENTRAL STRIATUM TO MIDBRAIN

Signals originating in the nucleus accumbens impact VTA dopamine neurons via two main routes (**Figure 3**): a direct inhibitory GABAergic synaptic input from the accumbens itself (e.g., Heimer et al., 1991; Kalivas et al., 1993) or an indirect route that includes the ventral pallidum and the pedunculopontine nucleus (PPTg; e.g., Floresco et al., 2003; Zweifel et al., 2009). The direct route may relay information about the expected features of a context while the indirect route may relay information about the actual context features (Humphries and Prescott, 2010; Penner and Mizumori, 2012). Since the direct projection is inhibitory onto dopamine cells, and the indirect route is excitatory, hippocampal signals indicating that a familiar context has not changed (i.e., there is no mismatch of expected and actual context information) would result in equal input from direct (−) and indirect (+) pathways. The result is that dopamine cells should show no change in baseline responding when rewards are encountered. Indeed, under such circumstances dopamine cells do not respond to rewards (e.g., Schultz et al., 1997). In the event that hippocampus signals a change in context (i.e., a mismatch between expected and actual contextual features) the indirect input would be stronger than the direct input. The resultant increased excitability after input from the indirect pathway could make more likely a dopamine cell response to a subsequent reward encountered. Indeed dopamine cells are known to increase responding to rewards after a context change (e.g., Schultz et al., 1997; Puryear et al., 2010). Thus dopamine neurons may be placed on high alert after a change in context is detected, and in that way be better prepared to determine the subjective value of the hippocampal prediction error signal.

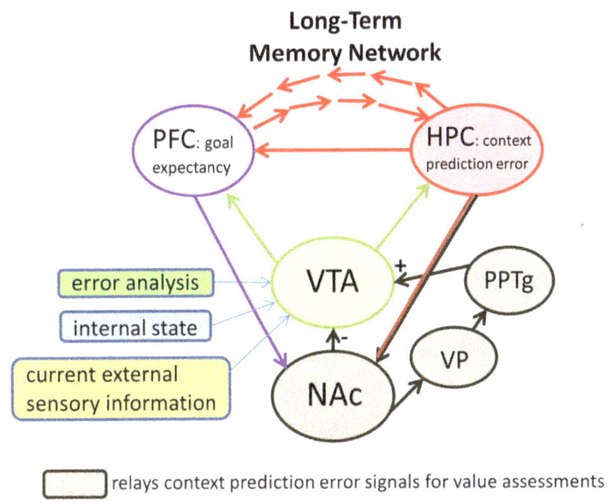


**FIGURE 3 | A proposed neural circuit illustrating that midbrain (dopamine) systems and the prefrontal cortex (PFC) are key brain areas that evaluate the significance of hippocampal (HPC) context prediction error signals for the purpose of directing future behaviors and updating long-term memories.** Direct HPC output arrives in the midbrain system via projections to the ventral striatum (i.e., the nucleus accumbens, or NAc). The NAc determines whether the outcomes of behavior are as predicted based on an animal's expectations for a given context. If the outcome is as expected, NAc continues exerting inhibitory control (−) over ventral tegmental area (VTA) neurons. In this case, encounters with rewards do not result in dopamine cell firing. In constrast, context prediction error signals from the HPC to the NAc may preferentially excite (+) VTA neurons via an indirect pathway that includes the ventral pallidum (VP) and the pedunculopontine nucleus (PPTg). The result of this elevated excitation may be a depolarization of VTA neurons such that they are more likely to fire when subsequent reward information arrives in VTA. Also influencing the likelihood that dopamine cells will fire in response to future rewards are specific computations that reflect negative reward prediction errors (reward prediction error analysis), information about the animal's current motivational and behavioral state (internal state), and additional information about the current salient cues (current external sensory information). The latter appears to involve at least the PPTg. The impact of the prefrontal cortex on VTA function is not clear. One possibility is that it provides the midbrain circuitry with information about what to expect in terms of goals based on past experience. The summed input to the VTA results in an output that reflects the subjective value of context prediction error signals.

## AGING OF THE VENTRAL STRIATUM

There is a limited literature investigating the effects that the normal aging process has on function of the ventral striatum. Much of what is known has come from human work. For example, Schott et al. (2007) used fMRI to investigate the neural mechanisms underlying reward prediction and reward outcome processing in young and elderly healthy subjects. Young adults showed a pattern of midbrain and ventral striatal activation for cues that predicted monetary reward when compared with cues that predicted neutral feedback. In contrast, healthy aged subjects showed the opposite pattern: an absent reward prediction response in the face of mesolimbic activation to reward feedback itself. This may reflect a reduced ability of older subjects to accurately estimate expected rewards. These results support other behavioral results indicating that older adults have deficits in learning from positive feedback (e.g., Mell et al., 2005).

### HIPPOCAMPAL-VTA INTERACTIONS

The VTA and hippocampus reciprocally interact such that novel, context information detected by the hippocampus enhances VTA dopamine release. This in turn enables encoding of new information into long-term memory (Lisman and Grace, 2005; Bethus et al., 2010). Input from the VTA to the hippocampus is direct (Gasbarri et al., 1994), whereas hippocampal output to VTA is indirect, arriving via the lateral septum (Luo et al., 2011) and the ventral striatum (Yang and Mogenson, 1987; Floresco et al., 2001). As evidence of the functional significance of VTA-hippocampus interactions, the VTA has been shown to regulate hippocampal activity and spatial learning (Martig et al., 2009; Martig and Mizumori, 2011a,b) and encoding of hippocampus-dependent memories (Rossato et al., 2009). In addition, the hippocampus has been shown to regulate dopamine responses to novelty (Legault and Wise, 2001) and analogous to hippocampal place fields, phasic reward responses of putative dopamine neurons in VTA are sensitive to changes in the visuo-spatial context (Puryear et al., 2010).

Recent work by Luo et al. (2011) has identified a circuit from area CA3 of the dorsal hippocampus to the VTA that uses the lateral septum as a relay. When area CA3 is stimulated, dopaminergic neurons within the VTA are excited, while non-DA neurons are inhibited. The observed excitation of dopamine neurons is likely mediated by disinhibition because local antagonism of GABA receptors can block the response to CA3 stimulation. Conversely, inactivating components of this circuit blocked evoked responses in VTA and also had a significant impact on reinstatement of drug-seeking by contextual stimuli. Thus, the link between the hippocampus and the VTA may be an important substrate by which information about the environmental context regulates goal-directed behavior. Efficient reward-seeking requires that environmental stimuli be interpreted, allowing accurate predictions about when and where reward can be expected. It is possible that dorsal CA3 conveys information to VTA about the current context as a whole, which allows rapid activation of dopamine neurons to promote salience attribution to conditioned contexts. Such processing is important for cognitive function by providing adjustments in behavior in response to changing real-world environments.

### AGING OF THE DOPAMINE SYSTEM

A number of age-related changes in the dopamine system have been demonstrated (for review, see Backman et al., 2006, 2010). Most of this work has been done in non-human primate and human subjects and have for the most part focused on changes that occur in the striatal and frontal cortical areas of the brain. For example, dopamine concentration (Goldman-Rakic and Brown, 1981), transporter availability and binding potential (e.g., Volkow et al., 1998a,b; Mozley et al., 2001), and dopamine D1 and D2 receptor density (e.g., Volkow et al., 1996; Wang et al., 1998; Backman et al., 2000) all decline with age. In addition, work by Kaasinen et al. (2000) found significant age-related declines of D2/3 receptors in all brain regions studied, including the frontal cortical areas, and the hippocampus (Kaasinen et al., 2000). Importantly, for all of the studies mentioned here, these changes occur in the absence of pathological aging, such as Parkinson's and Alzheimer's disease. Treatment of aged monkeys with a D2 receptor agonist reduces the decline in performance on a delayed memory task (Arnsten and Goldman-Rakic, 1985). In addition, imaging of D2 receptors in humans has found a correlation between receptor availability and performance on attention and response inhibition tasks and on the Wisconsin Card Sorting Task, and have also shown that striatal D2 receptor binding accounts for a greater amount of variation in performance on processing speed and episodic memory tasks than does chronological age (Volkow et al., 1998a; Backman et al., 2000). Based on these findings, it has been proposed that age-related deficits in learning are the result of a decline in dopaminergic function in older age (Nieuwenhuis et al., 2002; Backman et al., 2006, 2010). To date, data on the effects that the normal aging process may have on the midbrain, especially the VTA itself are sparse. However, there is some evidence indicating that significant age-associated changes in dopamine transporter activity within the VTA (e.g., Cruz-Muros et al., 2009).

## THE IMPACT OF AGING ON CONTEXT-DEPENDENT DECISION-MAKING BEHAVIORS

Decision-making is the process of choosing an option or course of action from among a set of alternatives. This process depends on the decision-maker's estimate of the outcome of the different options (Rangel et al., 2008). Because memory has a significant impact on the ability of an organism to make the "best" decision in a given context, it may not be surprising that aging affects decision-making behaviors. Determining the subjective value of behavioral outcomes requires an assessment of the extent to which expected rewards are actually received. While it is true that a number of factors are likely to contribute to the definition of one's expectations for behavioral outcomes, the most obvious factor is whether there is an expectation based on past experience. Presumably if there is no history of obtaining rewards in a particular context, then there should be no expectation for a reward. If, however, there is some kind of expectation of reward because of past experiences, then the degree of expectation (i.e., subjective goal values) can be enhanced or reduced (Schultz et al., 2008). The ability to learn from feedback and adaptively change behavior according to positive and negative outcomes is significantly impaired in aged subjects (Samanez-Larkin et al., 2007; Zamarian et al., 2008; Eppinger et al., 2010, 2011; Herbert et al., 2011). In addition, older adults are impaired at learning if reward delivery is probabilistic, a time when predicted outcomes are unreliable. When, however, reward contingencies are deterministic (certain) older adults are able to learn as well as young adults.

Older adults' learning impairments under reward uncertainty may reflect deficits in the ability to form and update value (outcome) representations using prediction error signals. Since learning and the formation of new memories is driven by the ability to respond to prediction error signals, it would be expected that individuals (e.g., aged adults) who suffer from responding appropriately to error signals would also show impaired learning and memory.

Assessments of subjective goal values, then, may change when hippocampus generates context error signals. The ultimate dopamine cell response to such hippocampal input reflects a subjective value that can be ascribed to the context change. How subjective value is computed is not understood. One factor that is sure to come into play is efficient learning strategies within a given context. For example, if an aged organism is unable to learn about the reward contingencies within a given environment, perhaps because of insufficient or erroneous prediction codes, then adaptive choices within a given context will be impaired. It appears that regulation of the dopamine cell phasic firing by hippocampus may control the "teaching" signal that is often attributed to dopamine neurons (e.g., Luo et al., 2011), a signal that informs neural circuitry that makes decisions about the selection of future responses.

## SUMMARY AND SUGGESTIONS FOR FUTURE WORK

The work presented here highlights a fundamental role for the hippocampus in context discrimination. While the hippocampus may be especially important for detecting and responding to the spatial features of context, it is becoming increasingly clear that the hippocampus is also sensitive to non-spatial aspects of a context, including other sensory cues, task demands, and internal factors such as hunger or thirst. When salient aspects of a context change, the hippocampus is in a unique position to broadcast a teaching signal in the form of a context prediction error signal to other brain areas to which it is closely connected, including the ventral striatum and VTA. These brain regions then assist the hippocampus in determining if salient features of a context have, in fact, changed. Functional changes in the hippocampus that occur during the normal aging process result in significant deficits in the ability to accurately determine if a change in context has occurred. For example, an age-related deficit in the ability to discriminate contexts by the hippocampus will result in inefficient signals that would normally prepare other connected brains regions (e.g., the midbrain, ventral striatum, and prefrontal cortex) for the plasticity required to adaptively respond. Although not discussed here, additional brain regions are likely to contribute to the learning and memory deficits observed in aged subjects. For example, the prefrontal cortex, dorsal striatum, and amygdala are likely to contribute to context discrimination processes under certain conditions.

Dopamine signaling within the VTA has a significant impact on the ability of both the ventral striatum and the hippocampus to integrate reward and spatial information. Changes in dopaminergic signaling, then, are also important for determining if salient changes in context have occurred. Although not discussed, there is experimental evidence that other neuromodulatory systems, including acetylcholine and serotonin are affected by normative aging processes (see Wilson et al., 2006; Eppinger et al., 2011) and may contribute to a failure to accurately detect contextual changes. In addition, although it is clear that many changes in dopamine signaling occur, evidence remains relatively sparse in terms of how age affects information processing within the VTA itself. Thus, this is a particular area of research ripe for further investigation.

## ACKNOWLEDGMENTS

We thank Dr. Van Redila, Valerie Tryon and Jack Clearman for helpful comments on a previous version. This work is funded by NIMH grant MH58755.

## REFERENCES

Aberman, J. E., and Salamone, J. D. (1999). Nucleus accumbens dopamine depletions make rats more sensitive to high ratio require- ments but do not impair primary food reinforcement. *Neuroscience* 92,545–552.

Aberman, J. E., Ward, S. J., and Salamone, J. D. (1998). Effects of dopamine antagonists and accumbens dopamine depletions on time-constrained progressive-ratio performance. *Pharmacol. Biochem. Behav.* 61, 341–348.

Anderson, M. I., and Jeffery, K. J. (2003). Heterogeneous mod- ulation of place cell firing by changes in context. *J. Neurosci.* 23, 8827–8835.

Annett, L. E., McGregor, A., and Robbins, T. W. (1989). The effects of ibotenic acid lesions of the nucleus accumbens on spatial learning and extinction in the rat. *Behav. Brain Res.* 31, 231–242.

Arnsten, A. F., and Goldman-Rakic, P. S. (1985). Catecholamines and cog- nitive decline in aged nonhuman primates. *Ann. N.Y. Acad. Sci.* 444, 218–234.

Backman, L., Ginovart, N., Dixon, A., Wahlin, T. B., Wahlin, A., Halldin, C., and Farde, L. (2000). Age-related cognitive deficits medi- ated by changes in the striatal dopamine system. *Am. J. Psychiatry* 157, 635–637.

Backman, L., Lindenberger, U., Li, S. C., and Nyberg, L. (2010). Linking cognitive aging to alterations in dopamine neurotransmitter func- tioning: recent data and future avenues. *Neurosci. Biobehav. Rev.* 34, 670–677.

Backman, L., Nyberg, L., Lindenberger, U., Li, S. C., and Farde, L. (2006). The correlative triad among aging, dopamine, and cogni- tion: current status and future prospects. *Neurosci. Biobehav. Rev.* 30,791–807.

Bakker, A., Kirwan, C. B., Miller, M., and Stark, C. E. (2008). Pattern sep- aration in the human hippocampal CA3 and dentate gyrus. *Science* 319, 1640–1642.

Barnes, C. A. (1979). Memory deficits associated with senescence: a neurophysiological and behavioral study in the rat. *J. Comp. Physiol. Psychol.* 93, 74–104.

Barnes, C. A., McNaughton, B. L., Mizumori, S. J., Leonard, B. W., and Lin, L. H. (1990). Comparison of spatial and temporal charac- teristics of neuronal activity in sequential stages of hippocampal processing. *Prog. Brain Res.* 83, 287–300.

Barnes, C. A., McNaughton, B. L., and O'Keefe, J. (1983). Loss of place specificity in hippocampal com- plex spike cells of senescent rat. *Neurobiol. Aging* 4, 113–119.

Barnes, C. A., Suster, M. S., Shen, J., and McNaughton, B. L. (1997). Multistability of cognitive maps in the hippocampus of old rats. *Nature* 388, 272–275.

Bayer, H. M., and Glimcher, P. W. (2005). Midbrain dopamine neu- rons encode a quantitative reward prediction error signal. *Neuron* 47, 129–141.

Belova, M. A., Paton, J. J., Morrison, E., and Salzman, C. D. (2007). Expectation modulates neural responses to pleasant and aver- sive stimuli in primate amygdala. *Neuron* 55, 970–984.

Berridge, K. C. (2007). The debate over dopamine's role in reward: the case for incentive salience. *Psychopharmacology (Berl.)* 191, 391–431.

Bethus, I., Tse, D., and Morris, R. G. (2010). Dopamine and memory: modulation of the persistence of memory for novel hippocam- pal NMDA receptor-dependent paired associates. *J. Neurosci.* 30, 1610–1618.

Bromberg-Martin, E. S., Matsumoto, M., and Hikosaka, O. (2010). Dopamine in motivational control: rewarding, aversive, and alerting. *Neuron* 68, 815–834.

Cruz-Muros, I., Afonso-Oramas, D., Abreu, P., Perez-Delgado, M. M., Rodriguez,

M., and Gonzalez- Hernandez, T. (2009). Aging effects on the dopamine transporter expression and compensatory mechanisms. *Neurobiol. Aging* 30, 973–986.

Day, J. J., Jones, J. L., and Carelli, R. M. (2011). Nucleus accumbens neu- rons encode predicted and ongoing rewardcostsinrats.*Eur. J. Neurosci.* 33,308–321.

Day, J. J., Roitman, M. F., Wightman, M., and Carelli, R. M. (2007). Associative learning mediates dynamic shifts in dopamine signal- ing in the nucleus accumbens. *Nat. Neurosci.* 10, 1020–1028.

Eppinger, B., Hammerer, D., and Li, C. (2011). Neuromodulation of reward-based learning and decision making in human aging. *Ann. N.Y. Acad. Sci.* 1235, 1–17.

Eppinger, B., Herbert, M., and Kray, J. (2010). We remember the good things: age differences in learn- ing and memory. *Neurobiol. Learn. Mem.* 93, 515–521.

Eschenko, O., and Mizumori, S. J. (2007). Memory influences on hip- pocampal and striatal neural codes: effects of a shift between task rules. *Neurobiol. Learn. Mem.* 87, 495–509.

Ferbinteanu, J., and Shapiro, M. L. (2003). Prospective and retrospec- tive memory coding in the hip- pocampus. *Neuron* 40, 1227–1239.

Ferretti, V., Roullet, P., Sargolini, F., Rinaldi, A., Perri, V., Del Fabbro, M., Costantini, V. J., Annese, V., Scesa, G., De Stefano, M. E., Oliverio, A., and Mele, A. (2010). Ventral striatal plasticity and spatial memory. *Proc. Natl. Acad. Sci. U.S.A.* 107, 7945–7950.

Fiorillo, C. D., Tobler, P. N., and Schultz, W. (2003). Discrete coding of reward probability and uncer- taintybydopamineneurons. *Science* 299, 1898–1902.

Fiorillo, C. D., Tobler, P. N., and Schultz, W. (2005). Evidence that the delay-period activity of dopamine neurons corresponds to reward uncertainty rather than backpropagating TD errors. *Behav. Brain Funct.* 1, 7.

Floresco, S. B., Seamans, J. K., and Phillips, A. G. (1997). Selective roles for hippocampal, prefrontal cor- tical, and ventral striatal circuits in radial-arm maze tasks with or without a delay. *J. Neurosci.* 17, 1880–1890.

Floresco, S. B., Todd, C. L., and Grace, A. A. (2001). Glutamatergic afferents from the hippocampus to the nucleus accumbens regulate activity of ventral tegmental area dopamine neurons. *J. Neurosci.* 21, 4915–4922.

Floresco, S. B., West, A. R., Ash, B., Moore, H., and Grace, A. A. (2003) Afferent modulation of dopamine neuron firing differentially regulates tonic and phasic dopamine trans- mission.*Nat. Neurosci.* 6, 968–973.

Gal, G., Joel, D., Gusak, O., Feldon, J., and Weiner, I. (1997). The effects of electrolytic lesion to the shell subterritory of the nucleus accumbens on delayed non- matching-to-sample and four-arm baited eight-arm radial-maze tasks. *Behav. Neurosci.* 111, 92–103.

Gallagher, M., and Rapp, P. R. (1997). The use of animal models to study the effects of aging on cognition. *Annu. Rev. Psychol.* 48, 339–370.

Gasbarri, A., Packard, M. G., Campana, E., and Pacitti, C. (1994). Anterograde and retro- grade tracing of projections from the ventral tegmental area to the hippocampal formation in the rat. *Brain Res. Bull.* 33, 445–452.

Goldman-Rakic, P. S., and Brown, R. M. (1981). Regional changes of monoamines in cerebral cor- tex and subcortical structures of agingrhesus monkeys.*Neuroscience* 6, 177–187.

Gothard, K. M., Skaggs, W. E., Moore, K. M., and McNaughton, B. L. (1996). Binding of hippocampal CA1 neural activity to multiple ref- erence frames in a landmark-based navigation task. *J. Neurosci.* 16, 823–835.

Guzowski, J. F., Knierim, J. J., and Moser, E. I. (2004). Ensemble dynamics of hippocampal regions CA3andCA1. *Neuron* 44, 581–584.

Hasselmo, M. E. (2005). The role of hippocampal regions CA3 and CA1 in matching entorhinal input with retrieval of associations between objects and context: theoretical comment on Lee et al. (2005). *Behav. Neurosci.* 119, 342–345.

Hauber, W., and Sommer, S. (2009). Prefrontostriatal circuitry regulates effort-related decision making. *Cereb. Cortex* 19, 2240–2247.

Heimer, L., Zahm, D. S., Churchill, L., Kalivas, P. W., and Wohltmann, C. (1991). Specificity in the projection patterns of accumbal core and shell inthe rat. *Neuroscience* 41, 89–125.

Herbert, M., Eppinger, B., and Kray, J. (2011). Younger but not older adults benefit from salient feedback during learning. *Front. Psychol.* 2:171. doi: 10.3389/fpsyg.2011.00171

Holden, H. M., Hoebel, C., Loftis, K., and Gilbert, P. E. (2012). Spatial pattern separation in cognitively normal young and older adults. *Hippocampus.* doi: 10.1002/hipo. 22017. [Epub ahead of print].

Humphries, M. D., and Prescott, T. J. (2010). The ventral basal ganglia, a selection mechanism at the cross- roads of space, strategy, and reward. *Prog. Neurobiol.* 90, 385–417.

Ito, R., Robbins, T. W., Pennartz, C. M., and Everitt, B. J. (2008). Functional interaction between the hippocam- pus and nucleus accumbens shell is necessary for the acquisition of appetitive spatial context condition- ing. *J. Neurosci.* 28, 6950–6959.

Jeffery, K. J., Anderson, M. I., Hayman, R., and Chakraborty, S. (2004). A proposed architecture for the neu- ral representation of spatial con- text. *Neurosci. Biobehav. Rev.* 28, 201–218.

Kaasinen, V., Vilkman, H., Hietala, J., Nagren, K., Helenius, H., Olsson, H., Farde, L., and Rinne, J. (2000). Age-related dopamine D2/D3 receptor loss in extrastriatal regions of the human brain. *Neurobiol. Aging* 21, 683–688.

Kalivas, P. W., Churchill, L., and Klitenick, M. A. (1993). GABA and enkephalin projection from the nucleus accumbens and ventral pal- lidum to the ventral tegmental area. *Neuroscience* 57, 1047–1060.

Kennedy, P. J., and Shapiro, M. L. (2004). Retrieving memories via internal context requires the hippocampus. *J. Neurosci.* 24, 6979–6985.

Lacy, J. W., Yassa, M. A., Stark, S. M., Muftuler, L. T., and Stark, C. E. (2011). Distinct pattern sep- aration related transfer functions in human CA3/dentate and CA1 revealedusinghigh-resolutionfMRI and variable mnemonic similarity. *Learn. Mem.* 18, 15–18.

Lavoie, A. M., and Mizumori, S. J. (1994). Spatial, movement- and reward-sensitive discharge by medial ventral striatum neurons of rats.*Brain Res.* 638, 157–168.

Lee, I., Yoganarasimha, D., Rao, G., and Knierim, J. J. (2004). Comparison of population coherence of place cells in hippocampal subfields CA1 and CA3. *Nature* 430, 456–459.

Legault, M., and Wise, R. A. (2001). Novelty-evoked elevations of nucleus accumbens dopamine: dependence on impulse flow from the ventral subiculum and glu- tamatergic neurotransmission in the ventral tegmental area. *Eur. J. Neurosci.* 13, 819–828.

Leutgeb, S., Leutgeb, J. K., Treves, A.,Moser, M. B., and Moser, E. I. (2004). Distinct ensemble codes in hippocampal areas CA3 and CA1. *Science* 305, 1295–1298.

Lisman, J. E., and Grace, A. A. (2005). The hippocampal-VTA loop: con- trolling the entry of information into long-term memory. *Neuron* 46, 703–713.

Luo, A. H., Tahsili-Fahadan, P., Wise, R. A., Lupica, C. R., and Aston-Jones, G. (2011). Linking context with reward: a functional circuit from hippocampal CA3 to ven- tral tegmental area. *Science* 333, 353–357.

Maldonado-Irizarry, C. S., and Kelley, A. E. (1995). Excitatory amino acid receptors within nucleus accum- bens subregions differentially medi- ate spatial learning in the rat. *Behav. Pharmacol.* 6, 527–539.

Markus, E. J., Barnes, C. A., McNaughton, B. L., Gladden, V. L., and Skaggs, W. E. (1994). Spatial information content and reliability of hippocampal CA1 neurons: effects of visual input. *Hippocampus* 4, 410–421. Marr, D. (1971). Simple memory: a the- ory for archicortex. *Philos. Trans. R. Soc. Lond. B Biol. Sci.* 262, 23–81.

Martig, A. K., Jones, G. L., Smith,K. E., and Mizumori, S. J. (2009). Context dependent effects of ventral tegmental area inactivation on spa- tial working memory. *Behav. Brain Res.* 203, 316–320.

Martig, A. K., and Mizumori, S. J. (2011a). Ventral tegmental area and substantia nigra neural correlates of spatial learning. *Learn. Mem.* 18, 260–271.

Martig, A. K., and Mizumori, S. J. (2011b). Ventral tegmental area dis- ruption selectively affects CA1/CA2 but not CA3 place fields dur- ing a differential reward work- ing memory task. *Hippocampus* 21, 172–184.

Matsumoto, M., and Hikosaka, O. (2007). Lateral habenula as a source of negative reward signals in dopamine neurons. *Nature* 447, 1111–1115.

McClure, S. M., Berns, G. S., and Montague, P. R. (2003). Temporal prediction errors in a passive learn- ing task activate human striatum. *Neuron* 38, 339–346.

McEchron, M. D., and Disterhoft, J. (1999). Hippocampal encoding of non-spatial trace conditioning. *Hippocampus* 9, 385–396.

McNaughton, B. L., and Morris, R. M. (1987). Hippocampal synap- tic enhancement and information storage within a distributed mem- ory system. *Trends Neurosci.* 10, 408–415.

Mell, T., Heekeren, H. R., Marschner, A., Wartenburger, I., Villringer, A., and Reischies, F. M. (2005). Effect of aging on stimulus-reward associ- ation learning. *Neuropsychologia* 43, 554–563.

Miyashita, T., Kubik, S., Haghighi, N., Steward, O., and Guzowski, J. F. (2009). Rapid activation of plasticity-associated gene transcrip- tion in hippocampal neurons pro- vides a mechanism for encoding of one-trial experience. *J. Neurosci.* 29, 898–906.

Mizumori, S. J., Lavoie, A. M., and Kalyani, A. (1996). Redistribution of spatial representation in the hip- pocampus of aged rats perform- ing a spatial memory task. *Behav. Neurosci.* 110, 1006–1016.

Mizumori, S. J., Ragozzino, K. E., Cooper, B. G., and Leutgeb, S. (1999). Hippocampal representa- tional organization and spatial con- text.

*Hippocampus* 9, 444–451.

Mizumori, S. J., Smith, D. M., and Puryear, C. B. (2007a). Hippocampal and neocortical interactions during context dis- crimination: electrophysiological evidence from the rat. *Hippocampus* 17, 851–862.

Mizumori, S. J. Y., Smith, D. M., and Puryear, C. B. (2007b). "Mnemonic contributions of hippocampal place cells," in *Neurobiology of Learning and Memory*, eds J. L. Martinez and R. P. Kesner (New York, NY: Academic Press), 155–189.

Mizumori, S. J. Y. (ed.). (2008). *A Context for Hippocampal Place Cells During Learning*. New York, NY: Oxford University Press.

Mizumori, S. J., Yeshenko, O., Gill, K. M., and Davis, D. M. (2004). Parallel processing across neural systems: implications for a multiple memory system hypothesis. *Neurobiol. Learn. Mem.* 82, 278–298.

Mogenson, G. J., Jones, D. L., and Yim, C. Y. (1980). From motiva- tion to action: functional interface between the limbic system and the motor system. *Prog. Neurobiol.* 14, 69–97.

Mozley, L. H., Gur, R. C., Mozley, P. D., and Gur, R. E. (2001). Striatal dopamine transporters and cogni- tive functioning in healthy men and women. *Am. J. Psychiatry* 158, 1492–1499.

Muller, R. U., and Kubie, J. L. (1987). The effects of changes in the environment on the spatial firing of hippocampal complex-spike cells. *J. Neurosci.* 7, 1951–1968.

Nadel, L. (2008). "The Hippocampus and Context Revisited," in *Hippo- campal Place Fields: Relevance to Learning and Memory*, ed S. J. Y. Mizumori (New York, NY: Oxford University Press), 3–15.

Nadel, L., and Payne, J. D. (2002). "The hippocampus, wayfinding and episodic memory," in *The Neural Basis of Navigation: Evidence from Single Cell Recording*, ed P. E. Sharp (MA: Kluwer Academic Publication).

Nadel, L., and Wilner, J. (1980). Context and conditioning: a place for space. *Physiol. Psychol.* 8, 218–228.

Nakazawa, K., Sun, L. D., Quirk, M. C., Rondi-Reig, L., Wilson, M. A., and Tonegawa, S. (2003). Hippocampal CA3 NMDA receptors are cru- cial for memory acquisition of one-time experience. *Neuron* 38, 305–315.

Nieuwenhuis, S., Ridderinkhof, K. R., Talsma, D., Coles, M. G., Holroyd, C. B., Kok, A., and Van Der Molen, M. W. (2002). A computational account of altered error process- ing in older age: dopamine and the error-related negativity. *Cogn. Affect. Behav. Neurosci.* 2, 19–36.

Nobre, A. C., Coull, J. T., Frith, C. D., and Mesulam, M. M. (1999). Orbitofrontal cortex is activated during breaches of expectation in tasks of visual attention. *Nat. Neurosci.* 2, 11–12.

O'Keefe, J. (1976). Place units in the hippocampus of the freely moving rat. *Exp. Neurol.* 51, 78–109.

O'Keefe, J., and Burgess, N. (1996). Geometric determinants of the place fields of hippocampal neurons. *Nature* 381, 425–428.

O'Keefe, J., and Conway, D. H. (1978). Hippocampal place units in the freely moving rat: why they fire where they fire. *Exp. Brain Res.* 31, 573–590.

O'Keefe, J., and Dostrovsky, J. (1971). The hippocampus as a spatial map. Preliminary evidence from unit activity in the freely-moving rat. *Brain Res.* 34, 171–175.

O'Keefe, J., and Nadel, L. (1978). *The Hippocampus as a Cognitive Map*. Oxford, UK: Oxford University Press.

O'Reilly, R. C., and McClelland, J. L. (1994). Hippocampal conjunc- tive encoding, storage, and recall: avoiding a trade-off. *Hippocampus* 4, 661–682.

Oler, J. A., and Markus, E. J. (2000). Age-related deficits in the abil- ity to encode contextual change: a place cell analysis. *Hippocampus* 10, 338–350.

Olton, D. S., Branch, M., and Best, P. J. (1978). Spatial correlates of hippocampal unit activity. *Exp. Neurol.* 58, 387–409.

Pearce, J. M., and Hall, G. (1980). A model for Pavlovian learning: variations in the effectiveness of conditioned but not of uncondi- tioned stimuli. *Psychol. Rev.* 87, 532–552.

Pennartz, C. M., Berke, J. D., Graybiel, A. M., Ito, R., Lansink, C. S., Van Der Meer, M., Redish, A. D., Smith, K. S., and Voorn, P. (2009). Corticostriatal interactions during learning, memory processing, and decision making. *J. Neurosci.* 29, 12831–12838.

Pennartz, C. M., Ito, R., Verschure, P. F., Battaglia, F. P., and Robbins, T. W. (2011). The hippocampal- striatal axis in learning, prediction and goal-directed behavior. *Trends Neurosci.* 34, 548–559.

Penner, M. R., and Mizumori, S. J. (2012). Neural systems analysis of decision making during goal- directed navigation. *Prog. Neurobiol.* 96, 96–135.

Penner, M. R., Roth, T. L., Chawla, M. K., Hoang, L. T., Roth, E. D., Lubin, F. D., Sweatt, J. D., Worley, P. F., and Barnes, C. A. (2011). Age- related changes in Arc transcription and DNA methylation within the hippocampus. *Neurobiol. Aging* 32, 2198–2210.

Pezze, M. A., and Feldon, J. (2004). Mesolimbic dopaminergic path ways in fear conditioning. *Prog. Neurobiol.* 74, 301–320.

Pezze, M. A., Heidbreder, C. A., Feldon, J., and Murphy, C. A. (2001). Selective responding of nucleus accumbens core and shell dopamine to aversively conditioned contextual and discrete stimuli. *Neuroscience* 108, 91–102.

Puryear, C. B., Kim, M. J., and Mizumori, S. J. (2010). Conjunctive encoding of movement and reward by ventral tegmental area neurons in the freely navigating rodent. *Behav. Neurosci.* 124, 234–247.

Puryear, C. B., and Mizumori, S. J. (2008). Reward prediction error sig- nals by reticular formation neurons. *Learn. Mem.* 15, 895–898.

Ranck, J. B. Jr. (1973). Studies on single neurons in dorsal hippocam- pal formation and septum in unre- strained rats. I. Behavioral correlates and firing repertoires. *Exp. Neurol.* 41, 461–531.

Rangel, A., Camerer, C., and Montague, P. R. (2008). A framework for study- ing the neurobiology of value-based decision making. *Nat. Rev. Neurosci.* 9, 545–556.

Redgrave, P., and Gurney, K. (2006). The short-latency dopamine sig- nal: a role in discovering novel actions? *Nat. Rev. Neurosci.* 7, 967–975.

Rescorla, R. A., and Wagner, A. R. (eds). (1972). *A Theory of Pavlovian Conditioning: Variations in the Effectiveness of Reinforcement and Nonreinforcement*. New York, NY: Appleton Century Crofts.

Roesch, M. R., Calu, D. J., and Schoenbaum, G. (2007). Dopamine neurons encode the better option in rats deciding between differently delayed or sized rewards. *Nat. Neurosci.* 10, 1615–1624.

Rosenzweig, E. S., and Barnes, C. A. (2003). Impact of aging on hippocampal function: plasticity, network dynamics, and cognition. *Prog. Neurobiol.* 69, 143–179.

Rossato, J. I., Bevilaqua, L. R., Izquierdo, I., Medina, J. H., and Cammarota, M. (2009). Dopamine controls persistence of long-term memory storage. *Science* 325, 1017–1020.

Samanez-Larkin, G. R., Gibbs, S. E., Khanna, K., Nielsen, L., Carstensen, L. L., and Knutson, B. (2007). Anticipation of monetary gain but not loss in healthy older adults. *Nat. Neurosci.* 10, 787–791.

Samsonovich, A., and McNaughton, B. L. (1997). Path integration and cognitive mapping in a continu- ous attractor neural network model. *J. Neurosci.* 17, 5900–5920.

Sargolini, F., Florian, C., Oliverio, A., Mele, A., and Roullet, P. (2003). Differential involvement of NMDA and AMPA receptors within the nucleus accumbens in consolida- tion of information necessary for place navigation and guidance strat- egy of mice. *Learn. Mem.* 10, 285–292.

Satoh, T., Nakai, S., Sato, T., and Kimura, M. (2003). Correlated cod- ing of motivation and outcome of decision by dopamine neurons. *J. Neurosci.* 23, 9913–9923.

Save, E., Nerad, L., and Poucet, B. (2000). Contribution of multiple sensory information to place field stability in hippocampal place cells. *Hippocampus* 10, 64–76.

Schott, B. H., Niehaus, L., Wittmann, C., Schütze, H., Seidenbecher, I., Heinze, H. J., and Düzel, E. (2007). Ageing and early-stage

Parkinson's disease affect separa- ble neural mechanisms of mesolim- bic reward processing. *Brain* 130, 2412–2424.

Schultz, W., Dayan, P., and Montague, P. R. (1997). A neural substrate of prediction and reward. *Science* 275, 1593–1599.

Schultz, W., and Dickinson, A. (2000). Neuronal coding of prediction errors. *Annu. Rev. Neurosci.* 23, 473–500.

Schultz, W., Preuschoff, K., Camerer, C., Hsu, M., Fiorillo, C. D., Tobler, P. N., and Bossaerts, P. (2008). Explicit neural signals reflecting reward uncertainty. *Philos. Trans. R. Soc. Lond. B Biol. Sci.* 363, 3801–3811.

Seamans, J. K., and Phillips, A. G. (1994). Selective memory impair- ments produced by transient lidocaine-induced lesions of the nucleus accumbens in rats. *Behav. Neurosci.* 108, 456–468.

Setlow, B., and McGaugh, J. L. (1998). Sulpiride infused into the nucleus accumbens posttraining impairs memory of spatial water maze training. *Behav. Neurosci.* 112, 603–610.

Shen, J., Barnes, C. A., McNaughton, B. L., Skaggs, W. E., and Weaver, K. L. (1997). The effect of aging on experience-dependent plasticity of hippocampal place cells. *J. Neurosci.* 17, 6769–6782.

Small, S. A., Chawla, M. K., Buonocore, M., Rapp, P. R., and Barnes, C. A. (2004). Imaging correlates of brain function in monkeys and rats isolates a hippocampal subregion differentially vulnerable to aging. *Proc. Natl. Acad. Sci. U.S.A.* 101, 7181–7186.

Smith, D. M., and Mizumori, S. J. (2006a). Hippocampal place cells, context, and episodic memory. *Hippocampus* 16, 716–729.

Smith, D. M., and Mizumori, S. J. (2006b). Learning-related develop- ment of context-specific neuronal responses to places and events: the hippocampal role in context pro- cessing. *J. Neurosci.* 26,3154–3163.

Smith, K. S., Berridge, K. C., and Aldridge, J. W. (2011). Disentangling pleasure from incentive salience and learning signals in brain reward circuitry. *Proc. Natl. Acad. Sci. U.S.A.* 108, E255–E264.

Smith-Roe, S. L., Sadeghian, K., and Kelley, A. E. (1999). Spatial learning and performance in the radial arm maze is impaired after N-methyl- D-aspartate (NMDA) receptor blockade in striatal subregions. *Behav. Neurosci.* 113, 703–717.

Stark, S. M., Yassa, M. A., and Stark, C. E. (2010). Individual differences in spatial pattern separation per- formance associated with healthy aging in humans. *Learn. Mem.* 17, 284–288.

Sutton, R., and Barto, A. (1998). *Reinforcement Learning: An Intro- duction.* Cambridge, UK: MIT Press. Sutton, R. S. (1988). Learning to predict by the methods of temporal differences. *Mach. Learn.* 3,9–44.

Tanila, H., Shapiro, M., Gallagher, M., and Eichenbaum, H. (1997). Brain aging: changes in the nature of information coding by the hippocampus. *J. Neurosci.* 17, 5155–5166.

Tobler, P.N., O'Doherty, J. P., Dolan, R. J., and Schultz, W. (2006). Human neural learning depends on reward prediction errors in the block- ing paradigm. *J. Neurophysiol.* 95, 301–310.

Tse, D., Langston, R. F., Kakeyama, M., Bethus, I., Spooner, P. A., Wood, E. R., Witter, M. P., and Morris, R. G. (2007). Schemas and memory con- solidation. *Science* 316,76–82.

Vazdarjanova, A., and Guzowski, J. F. (2004). Differences in hippocam- pal neuronal population responses to modifications of an environmen- tal context: evidence for distinct, yet complementary, functions of CA3 and CA1 ensembles. *J. Neurosci.* 24, 6489–6496.

Volkow, N. D., Gur, R. C., Wang, G. J., Fowler, J. S., Moberg, P. J., Ding, Y. S., Hitzemann, R., Smith, G., and Logan, J. (1998a). Association between decline in brain dopamine activity with age and cognitive and motor impairment in healthy individuals. *Am. J. Psychiatry* 155, 344–349.

Volkow, N. D., Wang, G. J., Fowler, J. S., Ding, Y. S., Gur, R. C., Gatley, J., Logan, J., Moberg, P. J., Hitzemann, R., Smith, G., and Pappas, N. (1998b). Parallel loss of presynaptic and postsynaptic dopamine mark- ersinnormalaging. *Ann. Neurol.* 44, 143–147.

Volkow, N. D., Wang, G. J., Fowler, J. S., Logan, J., Gatley, S. J., Macgregor, R. R., Schlyer, D. J., Hitzemann, R., and Wolf, A. P. (1996). Measuring age-related changes in dopamine D2 receptors with 11C-raclopride and 18F-N-methylspiroperidol. *Psychiatry Res.* 67,11–16.

Voorn, P., Vanderschuren, L. J., Groenewegen, H. J., Robbins, T. W., and Pennartz, C. M. (2004). Putting a spin on the dorsal-ventral divide of the striatum. *Trends Neurosci.* 27, 468–474.

Wang, Y., Chan, G. L., Holden, J. E., Dobko, T., Mak, E., Schulzer, M., Huser, J. M., Snow, B. J., Ruth, T.., Calne, D. B., and Stoessl, A. J. (1998). Age-dependent decline of dopamine D1 receptors in human brain: a PET study. *Synapse* 30, 56–61.

Wiener, S. I. (1996). Spatial, behavioral and sensory correlates of hippocam- pal CA1 complex spike cell activity: implications for information pro- cessing functions. *Prog. Neurobiol.* 49,335–361.

Wikenheiser, A. M., and Redish, A. D. (2011). Changes in reward contingency modulate the trial- to-trial variability of hippocampal place cells. *J. Neurophysiol.* 106, 589–598.

Wilson, I. A., Gallagher, M., Eichenbaum, H., and Tanila, H. (2006). Neurocognitive aging: prior memories hinder new hippocampal encoding. *Trends Neurosci.* 29, 662–670.

Wilson, I. A., Ikonen, S., Gallagher, M., Eichenbaum, H., and Tanila, H. (2005). Age-associated alterations of hippocampal place cells are sub- region specific. *J. Neurosci.* 25, 6877–6886.

Wilson, I. A., Ikonen, S., Gureviciene, I., McMahan, R. W., Gallagher, M., Eichenbaum, H., and Tanila, H. (2004). Cognitive aging and the hip- pocampus: how old rats represent new environments. *J. Neurosci.* 24, 3870–3878.

Wilson, I. A., Ikonen, S., McMahan, W., Gallagher, M., Eichenbaum, H., and Tanila, H. (2003). Place cell rigidity correlates with impaired spatial learning in aged rats. *Neurobiol. Aging* 24,297–305.

Yacubian, J., Glascher, J., Schroeder,., Sommer, T., Braus, D. F., and Buchel, C. (2006). Dissociable sys- tems for gain- and loss-related value predictions and errors of prediction in the human brain. *J. Neurosci.* 26, 9530–9537.

Yang, C. R., and Mogenson, G. J. (1987). Hippocampal signal trans- mission to the pedunculopontine nucleus and its regulation by dopamine D2 receptors in the nucleus accumbens: an electrophys- iological and behavioural study. *Neuroscience* 23, 1041–1055.

Yassa, M. A., Lacy, J. W., Stark, S. M., Albert, M. S., Gallagher, M., and Stark, C. E. (2011a). Pattern separation deficits associated with increased hippocampal CA3 and dentate gyrus activity in nonde- mented older adults. Hippocampus 21, 968–979.

Yassa, M. A., Mattfeld, A. T., Stark, M., and Stark, C. E. (2011b). Age-related memory deficits linked to circuit-specific dis- ruptions in the hippocampus. Proc. Natl. Acad. Sci. U.S.A. 108, 8873–8878.

Yassa, M. A., and Stark, C. E. (2011). Pattern separation in the hip- pocampus. Trends Neurosci. 34, 515–525.

Young, B. J., Fox, G. D., and Eichenbaum, H. (1994). Correlates of hippocampal complex-spike cell activity in rats performing a non- spatial radial maze task. J. Neurosci. 14, 6553–6563.

Zamarian, L., Sinz, H., Bonatti, E., Gamboz, N., and Delazer, M. (2008). Normal aging affects decisions under ambiguity, but not decisions under risk. Neuropsychology 22, 645–657.

Zweifel, L. S., Parker, J. G., Lobb, C. J., Rainwater, A., Wall, V. Z., Fadok, J. P., Darvas, M., Kim, M. J., Mizumori, S. J., Paladini, C. A., Phillips, P. E., and Palmiter, R. D. (2009). Disruption of NMDAR-dependent burst firing by dopamine neurons provides selective assessment of phasic dopamine dependent behavior. Proc. Natl. Acad. Sci. U.S.A. 106, 7281–7288.

# 19

# Aging specifically impairs switching to an allocentric navigational strategy

**Mathew A. Harris**[1,2]*, **Jan M. Wiener**[3] **and Thomas Wolbers**[1,2,4]

[1] Centre for Cognitive and Neural Systems, University of Edinburgh, Edinburgh, UK
[2] Centre for Cognitive Ageing and Cognitive Epidemiology, University of Edinburgh, Edinburgh, UK
[3] Psychology Research Centre, Bournemouth University, Poole, UK
[4] German Center for Neurodegenerative Diseases, Otto-von-Guericke University, Magdeburg, Germany

**Edited by:**
*Emma R. Wood, University of Edinburgh, UK*

**Reviewed by:**
*Weimin Mou, University of Alberta, Canada*
*Hugo Spiers, University College London, UK*

***Correspondence:**
*Mathew A. Harris, Centre for Cognitive and Neural Systems, University of Edinburgh, 1 George Square, Edinburgh, EH8 9JZ, UK.*
*e-mail: m.a.harris-2@sms.ed.ac.uk*

Navigation abilities decline with age, partly due to deficits in numerous component processes. Impaired switching between these various processes (i.e., switching navigational strategies) is also likely to contribute to age-related navigational impairments. We tested young and old participants on a virtual plus maze task (VPM), expecting older participants to exhibit a specific strategy switching deficit, despite unimpaired learning of allocentric (place) and egocentric (response) strategies following reversals within each strategy. Our initial results suggested that older participants performed worse during place trial blocks but not response trial blocks, as well as in trial blocks following a strategy switch but not those following a reversal. However, we then separated trial blocks by both strategy and change type, revealing that these initial results were due to a more specific deficit in switching to the place strategy. Place reversals and switches to response, as well as response reversals, were unaffected. We argue that this specific "switch-to-place" deficit could account for apparent impairments in both navigational strategy switching and allocentric processing and contributes more generally to age-related decline in navigation.

**Keywords: aging, spatial navigation, strategy switching, allocentric processing, virtual reality, plus maze**

## INTRODUCTION

Cognitive faculties deteriorate in both normal aging and dementia, and navigation abilities may be among those most severely affected. Brain areas associated with navigation, including the hippocampus and entorhinal cortex, show more extensive degradation in aging and dementia than other brain regions (Driscoll et al., 2003; Du et al., 2003, 2006), and show reduced functional activation during navigation with age (Moffat et al., 2006). Furthermore, some research has confirmed that aging does impair navigational processes specifically dependent on these areas, such as cognitive mapping (Moffat and Resnick, 2002; Iaria et al., 2009) and path integration (Allen et al., 2004; Mahmood et al., 2009; Harris and Wolbers, 2012). These navigational processes are in turn dependent on a range of more fundamental processes (memory, perception, attention, movement control, etc.) also affected by aging. Some aspects of navigation, such as retracing a learned route, seem less susceptible to aging (Jansen et al., 2010), and as many complex navigational processes decline with structural changes such as hippocampal atrophy (Nedelska et al., 2012), older people may be forced to rely on these intact simpler mechanisms (Wiener et al., submitted). However, there are still further aspects of navigation that may be affected by aging but have not yet been well explored. For example, in everyday navigation we do not usually rely solely on any single navigational process; instead we must constantly switch between various different navigational strategies, such as following a familiar route and heading towards a visible landmark. We argue that this strategy switching is fundamentally important to navigation and that a deficit may contribute heavily to navigation impairments observed in aging.

According to the noradrenaline (NA) hypothesis, strategy switching is coordinated by the prefrontal cortex (PFC) and mediated by the locus coeruleus-noradrenaline (LCNA) system in response to changes in reward contingency, monitored by the anterior cingulate cortex (ACC) and orbitofrontal cortex (OFC; Aston-Jones and Cohen, 2005). The locus coeruleus (LC) operates in two modes; high phasic-low tonic, which promotes focused single task performance, and high tonic-low phasic, which promotes behavioral flexibility, such as strategy switching (Aston-Jones and Cohen, 2005; Bouret and Sara, 2005). The LC shows extensive degradation in aging (Mouton et al., 1994; Manaye et al., 1995; Grudzien et al., 2007) and NA shows signs of depletion or dysregulation (Luine et al., 1990; Li et al., 2001; Allard et al., 2011), suggesting that we may see an impairment in strategy switching in aging. Animal research has provided some support for the NA hypothesis. For example, Tait et al. (2007) tested rats on an attentional set shifting task that involves locating a reward based on one of two strategies. Following a lesion to the dorsal noradrenergic bundle (one of the LC's two main efferent fiber bundles), rats were impaired at switching between the two strategies compared to controls. Set shifting impairments have also been observed in aged mice (Young et al., 2010; Tanaka et al., 2011), monkeys (Moore et al., 2003; Hara et al., 2012), and humans (Ashendorf and McCaffrey, 2008; Gamboz et al., 2009), demonstrating that aging and noradrenergic depletion at least have similar effects on strategy switching.

In navigation, numerous strategies are required in order to utilize a range of cues that are inconsistently available, as well as to operate on smaller and larger scales. These various strategies can be discriminated by reference frame, with some operating in relation to the body's changing orientation (egocentric), and others in relation to a static external coordinate system (allocentric). For example, using environmental cues to work out how to get to a known location relies on allocentric processing, while following a known route encoded as a series of turns depends on egocentric processing. Allocentric strategies have been demonstrated to depend on the hippocampus (O'Keefe, 1990; Hartley et al., 2003; Compton, 2004; Bohbot et al., 2007), while egocentric strategies have been associated with the caudate nucleus (Cook and Kesner, 1988; Iaria et al., 2003; Postle and D'Esposito, 2003). Hippocampal and caudal grey matter are negatively correlated, suggesting that these two areas operate in competition (Bohbot et al., 2007). It is thought that the PFC determines which of these parallel systems guides behavior (Doeller et al., 2008), supposedly as mediated by the ACC, OFC, and LCNA system, as above.

The plus maze task has been used extensively to study the use of allocentric and egocentric strategies in rats (Ragozzino, 2007; Rich and Shapiro, 2007). The task involves starting from one of two opposing arms of a plus-shaped maze and locating a reward at one of the two remaining arms. Which arm is rewarded depends on the current strategy (as well as the current start arm, which is pseudorandomised). Sometimes the subject is rewarded for finishing in a specific place, i.e., the east or west arm of the maze; at other times simply for a particular response, i.e., turning left or turning right. The task can therefore be used to study switches and reversals, much like the attentional set-shifting task, but in a navigational context. Several studies (Ragozzino et al., 1999; Rich and Shapiro, 2007; Young and Shapiro, 2009) have demonstrated impaired strategy switching, but unaffected reversals, following inactivation of regions of the medial PFC, which is both comparable to findings of studies using the attentional set shifting task, and consistent with the NA hypothesis. However, while some studies have used virtual mazes to assess spontaneous use of allocentric and egocentric strategies (Iaria et al., 2003; Bohbot et al., 2007), to our knowledge, there has not yet been any research into navigational strategy switching using human subjects.

We therefore set out to explore the effects of aging on navigational strategy switching in humans. We tested normal healthy young and old adults on a virtual version of the plus maze task. While the task is computerized, it is the same as the standard plus maze task in other respects, and still requires use of the same allocentric place-based and egocentric response-based strategies. We expected older people to exhibit a specific strategy switching impairment; performing worse than younger participants in blocks following a strategy switch, but not in those following a reversal, and not due to impaired learning of either strategy.

## MATERIALS AND METHODS

### PARTICIPANTS

Eighteen (10 female) young participants (20–29 years, mean 22.22 years) and 20 (11 female) old participants (60–84 years, mean 68.6 years) were recruited from existing databases of volunteers within the local communities of Edinburgh and Bournemouth. Most therefore had previous experience of participating in research. All participants had normal or corrected-to-normal vision and no known cognitive deficits or neurological disorders.

### PROCEDURE

Participants provided information on their age, gender, and computer experience, before completing two computerized navigation tasks on a standard desktop computer with a 24″ widescreen monitor. In addition to age and gender information, participants were asked to rate their own experience of computers and of computer games on a nine-point scale from very inexperienced to very experienced. The first computer task, a spatial working memory task, was designed to assess memory for routes and places, as well as reward sensitivity. The second was the virtual plus maze task (VPM), designed to assess switching between different navigational strategies, such as egocentric response-based strategies and allocentric place-based strategies. Participants were made fully aware of these details of the experimental procedure, and all provided informed consent before participating. This study was approved by ethics committees at both the University of Edinburgh and Bournemouth University, and conformed to the Code of Ethics and Conduct of the British Psychological Society.

### SPATIAL WORKING MEMORY TASK

This task served as a control task, designed to assess the working memory processes underlying performance at the main task; primarily place recall and route recall. Place recall trials were set in a virtual environment consisting of an open field surrounded by mountain scenery, with six identical landmarks arranged in a central circle. Participants were automatically moved to three of the six landmarks, returned to the origin and reoriented, then asked to revisit the same three landmarks in any order. Route recall trials were set in a grid like maze shrouded in fog to restrict visibility. Participants were first directed along a route through five junctions by arrows appearing at each one, then asked to retrace the same route without directions. An additional aspect of this task assessed sensitivity to the reward signal used in the main task. This signal would be the only feedback participants would receive in the main task, so it was important that they were able to monitor it. Throughout place and route encoding phases, the signal (a yellow ball) would sometimes appear at a landmark or junction. While revisiting the landmarks and retracing the routes, participants also had to indicate whether or not a ball had appeared at each location. The task included 10 place recall trials and 10 route recall trials, alternating between the two types.

### VIRTUAL PLUS MAZE TASK

Our computerized adaptation of the plus maze task (**Figure 1**) allowed us to easily administer it to human subjects within a virtual environment. The environment consisted of a grass-textured ground plane, surrounded by continuous mountain scenery, with a central plus maze composed of curbed paths and transparent walls. The continuous mountain scenery provided visual cues from which participants could infer their orientation, without including localized landmarks that could be used as beacons. In

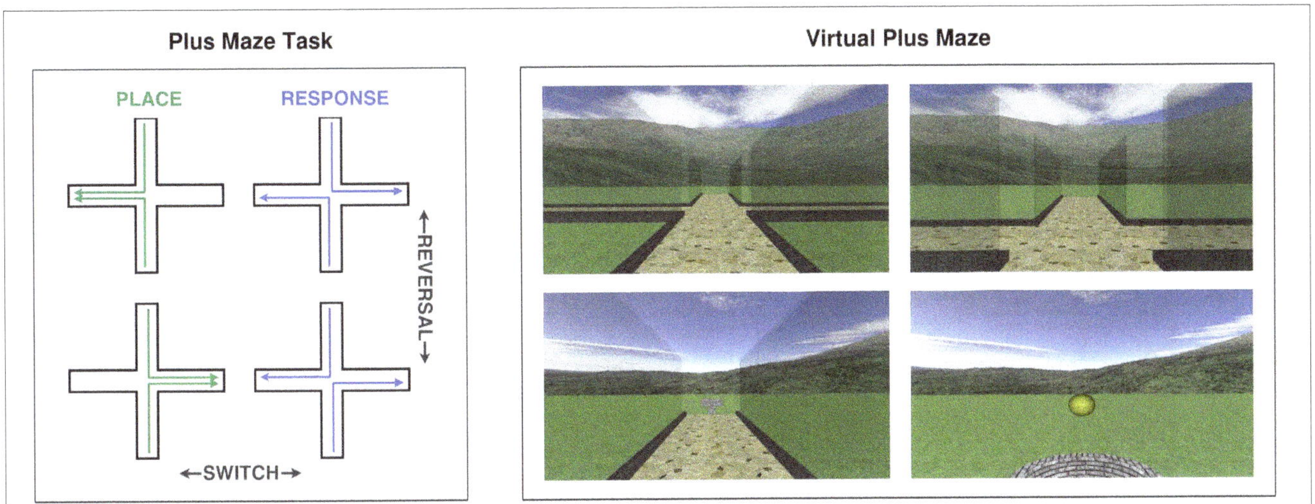


**FIGURE 1 | Left:** Diagrammatic representation of the plus maze task, illustrating place and response strategies, and switch and reversal change types. **Right:** Screen images captured during the virtual plus maze task, at the start point, at the junction before turning, at the junction after turning and at the goal (showing a reward).

each trial, participants started from one of two opposing start arms (in a pseudorandomised order), approached the central junction, and decided within 3 s whether to turn left or right in order to find a reward at one of the other two goal arms. A yellow ball emerged from the well at the end of the goal arm as a reward signal if the correct choice was made. Participants were rewarded either for going to the correct place (i.e., east or west, regardless of required response), or for making the correct response (i.e., left or right, regardless of heading). Between blocks of 20 trials, either a switch, a reversal or no change occurred. Switches changed the rewarded strategy from place to response, or vice versa. Reversals retained the same strategy, but changed the rewarded place or response, e.g., from east to west, or from left to right. These changes were made less predictable by the inclusion of no changes between some blocks. Participants completed a total of 320 trials, incorporating five switches and five reversals. This included three switches in one direction and two in the other, as well as three reversals for one strategy and two for the other, depending on the starting strategy, which was alternated and counterbalanced within each age group.

### DATA ANALYSIS

Data analysis was performed in Matlab (Mathworks, Natick, MA). Computer experience information was combined to produce a single score. Spatial working memory task data were reduced to three scores for place recall (total correct places visited), route recall (total correct turns made), and reward sensitivity (total rewards remembered). VPM performance was assessed in terms of the number of correct trials, the number of blocks for which the strategy was learned, and the number of trials for which the learned strategy was stable. Data from blocks following no change were merged with data for the previous block. One young female participant was excluded as an outlier, as she performed more than two standard deviations below the group mean in terms of overall number of trials correct. We then used mixed model ANOVAs and $t$-tests to assess differences between age groups in numbers of trials correct, blocks learned and stable trials. $p$-values were adjusted correct for multiple comparisons according to the Bonferroni method. We also performed stepwise regression analyses to assess the contribution of age, gender, computer use, and spatial working memory task performance to measures of VPM performance.

Learning was analyzed using a Bayesian estimation procedure developed by Smith and colleagues (Smith et al., 2004, 2005, 2007), together with WinBUGs (Lunn et al., 2000) and the "matbugs" Matlab function. This approach can be used to estimate, at each time point throughout a series of trials, the likelihood of responses to all subsequent trials being correct, based on observed performance data. The point at which the lower 95% confidence interval of this estimation first exceeds and remains above the chance probability of a correct response for each individual trial (50% in this experiment) corresponds to acquisition of the reward contingency. We used this to identify whether or not the strategy was learned for each block and, if so, for how many trials the learned strategy was stable, i.e., the number of trials after the point of acquisition.

## RESULTS

Older participants performed worse at the VPM in terms of overall performance, measured as the total number of trials correct ($t_{35} = 3.052, p = 0.002$), strategy learning, in terms of the total number of blocks learned ($t_{35} = 3.301, p = 0.001$), and learning speed, as indicated by the number of trials for which the learned strategy remained stable ($t_{35} = 3.107, p = 0.002$; **Figure 2**). They also reported a significantly lower level of computer experience ($t_{33} = 3.705, p < 0.001$) and performed worse at the spatial working memory task in terms of place recall ($t_{35} = 4.701, p < 0.001$) and reward sensitivity ($t_{35} = 3.596, p < 0.001$), although not route recall ($t_{35} = 0.381, p = 0.353$). We performed stepwise

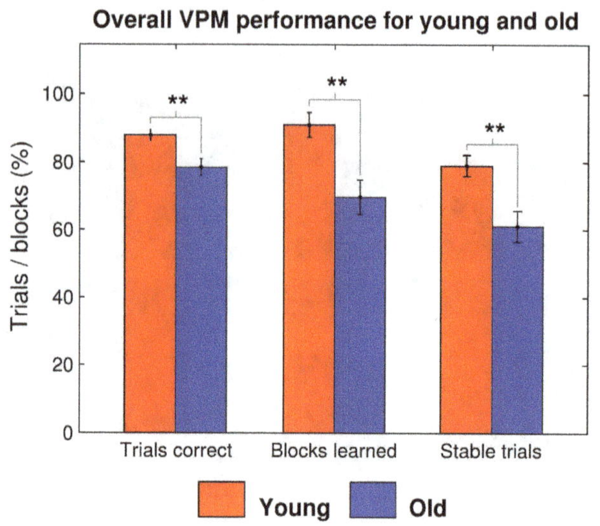


**FIGURE 2 | Overall virtual plus maze task performance, as measured by the mean percentage of trials correct, blocks learned, and stable trials for young (red) and old (blue) participants.** Significant group differences are indicated at the *0.05, **0.01, and ***0.001 levels.

regression analyses to check for factors that predicted VPM performance, which confirmed that age was a significant predictor in terms of overall trials correct ($\beta = 9.673$, $p = 0.004$), blocks learned ($\beta = 22.222$, $p = 0.002$), and stable trials ($\beta = 18.295$, $p = 0.003$). However, none of the potential control variables (gender, computer use, place recall, route recall, and reward sensitivity) were retained in the models as significant predictors of any of the measures of VPM performance (**Tables 1–3**). Further stepwise regression analyses for each age group separately (excluding age as a predictor) maintained that none of the potential control variables were significant predictors for any measure of VPM performance. These variables were therefore not considered in further analyses.

To explore the root of the age-related deficit in VPM performance, we split the data by block type for further analyses. We first used One-Way repeated measures ANOVAs to check for learning effects across blocks of each strategy type for each age group, but found no main effect of block order on performance (young place: $F_{(85, 4)} = 0.790$, $p = 0.535$; young response: $F_{(85, 4)} = 0.401$, $p = 0.808$; old place: $F_{(94, 4)} = 0.828$, $p = 0.511$; and old response: $F_{(94, 4)} = 0.826$, $p = 0.512$), allowing us to average performance across blocks of the same type. We then performed Two-Way mixed ANOVAs with age group as a between-groups factor and block strategy as a within-subjects factor, assigning data from place and response blocks to separate conditions. These demonstrated a significant main effect of both age (trials correct: $F_{(35, 1)} = 9.356$, $p = 0.004$; blocks learned: $F_{(35, 1)} = 11.929$, $p = 0.001$; and stable trials: $F_{(35, 1)} = 9.689$, $p = 0.004$) and strategy (trials correct: $F_{(35, 1)} = 6.450$, $p = 0.016$; blocks learned: $F_{(35, 1)} = 10.678$, $p = 0.002$; and stable trials: $F_{(35, 1)} = 7.149$, $p = 0.011$) on all three measures of VPM performance, as well as significant interactions between the two (trials correct: $F_{(35, 1)} = 6.709$, $p = 0.014$; blocks learned: $F_{(35, 1)} = 8.133$, $p = 0.007$; and stable trials: $F_{(35, 1)} = 7.293$, $p = 0.011$). *Post-hoc* tests revealed that older people performed worse specifically during place blocks (trials correct: $t_{35} = 3.189$, $p_B = 0.003$; blocks learned: $t_{35} = 3.485$, $p_B = 0.002$; and stable trials: $t_{35} = 3.287$, $p_B = 0.002$; **Figure 3**), accounting for the main effects of age and strategy, as well as for the interaction between them. This seems to suggest that older people may exhibit an allocentric strategy deficit.

However, we then performed further ANOVAs with change type as the within-subjects factor, including data for blocks following switches and blocks following reversals in separate conditions. Data from blocks following unlearned blocks had to be excluded, as, even if that block was learned, it may not have necessitated a strategy switch or reversal. Data from the first block was also excluded as it of course preceded all changes. These gave similar results, again demonstrating a

**Table 1 | Results of stepwise regression analysis predicting trials correct, with significant predictors (age group) highlighted in blue.**

| | | Trials correct | | |
|---|---|---|---|---|
| **Predictor** | **β** | **SE** | **In** | ***p*** |
| Age group | −9.673 | 3.089 | Yes | 0.004 |
| Gender | 3.921 | 3.126 | No | 0.219 |
| Computer use | −0.391 | 0.742 | No | 0.602 |
| Place recall | −0.009 | 0.385 | No | 0.981 |
| Route recall | 0.358 | 0.239 | No | 0.144 |
| Reward sensitivity | 0.510 | 0.301 | No | 0.100 |

**Table 2 | Results of stepwise regression analysis predicting blocks learned, with significant predictors (age group) highlighted in blue.**

| | | Blocks learned | | |
|---|---|---|---|---|
| **Predictor** | **β** | **SE** | **In** | ***p*** |
| Age group | −22.222 | 6.521 | Yes | 0.002 |
| Gender | 7.460 | 6.628 | No | 0.269 |
| Computer use | −1.168 | 1.560 | No | 0.460 |
| Place recall | −0.523 | 0.807 | No | 0.521 |
| Route recall | 0.801 | 0.503 | No | 0.121 |
| Reward sensitivity | 0.897 | 0.644 | No | 0.174 |

**Table 3 | Results of stepwise regression analysis predicting stable trials, with significant predictors (age group) highlighted in blue.**

| | | Stable trials | | |
|---|---|---|---|---|
| **Predictor** | **β** | **SE** | **In** | ***p*** |
| Age group | −18.295 | 5.738 | Yes | 0.003 |
| Gender | 7.032 | 5.814 | No | 0.235 |
| Computer use | −0.558 | 1.381 | No | 0.689 |
| Place recall | −0.241 | 0.714 | No | 0.738 |
| Route recall | 0.731 | 0.441 | No | 0.107 |
| Reward sensitivity | 0.981 | 0.557 | No | 0.088 |

significant main effect of age (trials correct: $F_{(35, 1)} = 8.083$, $p = 0.007$; blocks learned: $F_{(35, 1)} = 9.790$, $p = 0.004$; and stable trials: $F_{(35, 1)} = 8.441$, $p = 0.006$), and also a significant main effect of change type (trials correct: $F_{(35, 1)} = 23.112$, $p < 0.001$; blocks learned: $F_{(35, 1)} = 20.976$, $p < 0.001$; and stable trials: $F_{(35, 1)} = 26.915$, $p < 0.001$) and a significant age by change type interaction (trials correct: $F_{(35, 1)} = 5.074$, $p = 0.031$; blocks learned: $F_{(35, 1)} = 7.277$, $p = 0.011$; and stable trials: $F_{(35, 1)} = 6.638$, $p = 0.014$) for all three dependent variables. *Post-hoc* tests revealed that older people performed worse specifically for blocks following strategy switches (trials correct: $t_{35} = 2.667$, $p_B = 0.012$; blocks learned: $t_{35} = 3.043$, $p_B = 0.004$; and stable trials: $t_{35} = 2.878$, $p_B = 0.007$; **Figure 4**), accounting for the effects of age and change type and the interaction between them. This seems to suggest that older people are impaired at strategy switching, rather than simply at employing allocentric strategies.

Taken together, these results suggest that either older people exhibit two separate general deficits in allocentric strategy use and strategy switching, which both contribute to impaired VPM performance, or they exhibit a more specific deficit in switching to an allocentric strategy. We assessed these two hypotheses by separating the data into four block types; those following a switch to the place strategy (S2P), those following a switch to response (S2R), those after a reversal of place (RP) and those after a reversal of response (RR). Further mixed ANOVAs with block type as the within-subjects factor revealed a significant main effect of age (trials correct: $F_{(35, 1)} = 8.949$, $p = 0.005$; blocks learned: $F_{(35, 3)} = 9.486$, $p = 0.004$; and stable trials: $F_{(35, 3)} = 8.177$, $p = 0.007$) and block type (trials

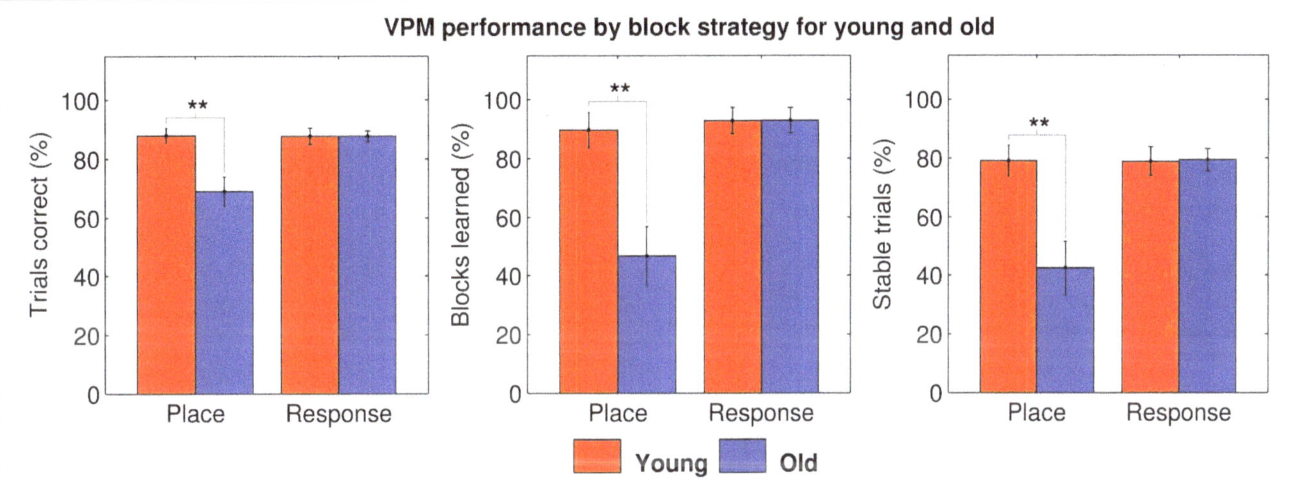


**FIGURE 3 | VPM performance in terms of trials correct (left), blocks learned (middle), and stable trials (right) during place and response blocks for young (red) and old (blue) participants.** Significant group differences are indicated at the *0.05, **0.01, and ***0.001 levels following Bonferroni correction.

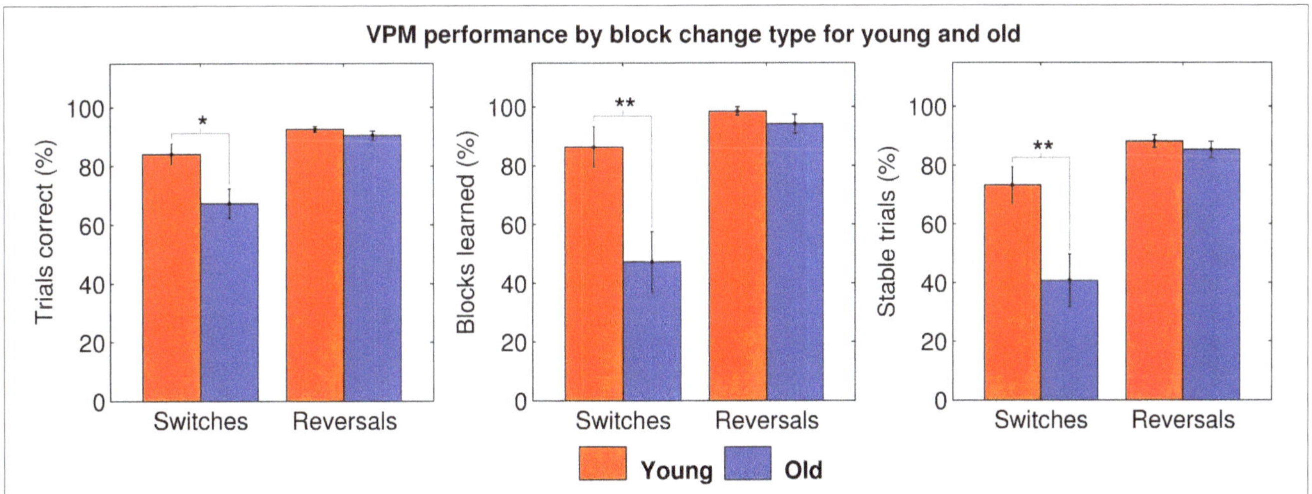


**FIGURE 4 | VPM performance in terms of trials correct (left), blocks learned (middle), and stable trials (right) during blocks following switches and reversals for young (red) and old (blue) participants, excluding data from first blocks and blocks following unlearned blocks.** Significant group differences are indicated at the *0.05, **0.01, and ***0.001 levels following Bonferroni correction.

correct: $F_{(35, 1)} = 9.762$, $p < 0.001$; blocks learned: $F_{(35, 3)} = 9.927$, $p < 0.001$; and stable trials: $F_{(35, 3)} = 9.755$, $p < 0.001$) as well as a significant interaction between the two (trials correct: $F_{(105, 3)} = 5.702$, $p = 0.001$; blocks learned: $F_{(105, 3)} = 6.773$, $p < 0.001$; and stable trials: $F_{(105, 3)} = 5.570$, $p = 0.001$). *Post-hoc* tests clarified that this was due to a more specific deficit in switching to place blocks (trials correct: $t_{33} = 2.895$, $p_B = 0.013$; blocks learned: $t_{33} = 3.634$, $p_B = 0.002$; and stable trials: $t_{33} = 3.192$, $p_B = 0.006$; **Figure 5**) among the older participants.

In an effort to understand why older participants failed to learn the place strategy following a switch, we explored the use of alternative strategies during unlearned blocks. For this analysis we simply associated each block with a particular strategy-direction combination if the participant responded in accordance with it significantly more than expected by chance ($p < 0.001$). As shown in **Figure 6**, while older participants often simply did not acquire any strategy, for the majority of the time they employed an incorrect strategy. Interestingly, the older participants used an incorrect place strategy just as often as an incorrect response strategy, providing evidence that they were able to use a place strategy just as well, despite the deficit in switching to this strategy (switch-to-place deficit). The older group also exhibited perseverative errors (continuing to use the strategy from the block preceding a change) in less than one third of blocks in which they used an incorrect strategy, suggesting that, in most cases, failure to learn the correct strategy was not simply due to failure to detect a change in reward contingency. There was very little incidence of regressive errors (changing back to the strategy used before the block preceding a change). Where other types of error were made, older participants again used both incorrect place and response strategies, suggesting that they were not simply reverting to a preferred response strategy.

We also assessed response times, but while the older participants generally took significantly longer to respond ($t_{35} = 3.159$, $p = 0.003$), this difference was consistent across all block types (switch to place: $t_{35} = 2.721$, $p_B = 0.040$; switch to response: $t_{35} = 2.984$, $p_B = 0.021$; RP: $t_{35} = 3.315$, $p_B = 0.009$; and RR: $t_{35} = 2.577$, $p_B = 0.057$). This suggests that the difference in response time was not related to differences in overall performance or the switch-to-place deficit reported above. A difference in response times could have affected performance due to the limited time (3 s) that participants had to respond, but very few participants from either group ever took longer than this to respond, and there was no significant difference between groups in the number of trials to which a response was not provided in time ($t_{35} = 0.920$, $p = 0.364$). Interestingly, response times did not increase significantly following a switch or reversal ($t_{35} = 0.971, p = 0.335$).

## DISCUSSION

We demonstrated aging-impaired navigation using a VPM, with older participants responding correctly for significantly fewer trials, stably acquiring the correct strategy for significantly fewer blocks, and maintaining a stable strategy for significantly fewer trials. As expected, this impairment was related to decreased ability—as measured by numbers of trials correct, blocks learned and stable trials—to switch between navigational strategies, despite intact ability to perform reversals within strategies. However, further investigation revealed that this deficit was more specific than expected, applying only to switching in one direction; to the place strategy. There was a significant age difference in trials correct, blocks learned, and stable trials for place blocks following a switch, but none for post-switch response blocks, or for blocks of either strategy following a reversal. This specific effect also produced an apparent age difference in performance during place blocks but not response blocks, in contrast to our original hypothesis. We also explored the behavior of older participants

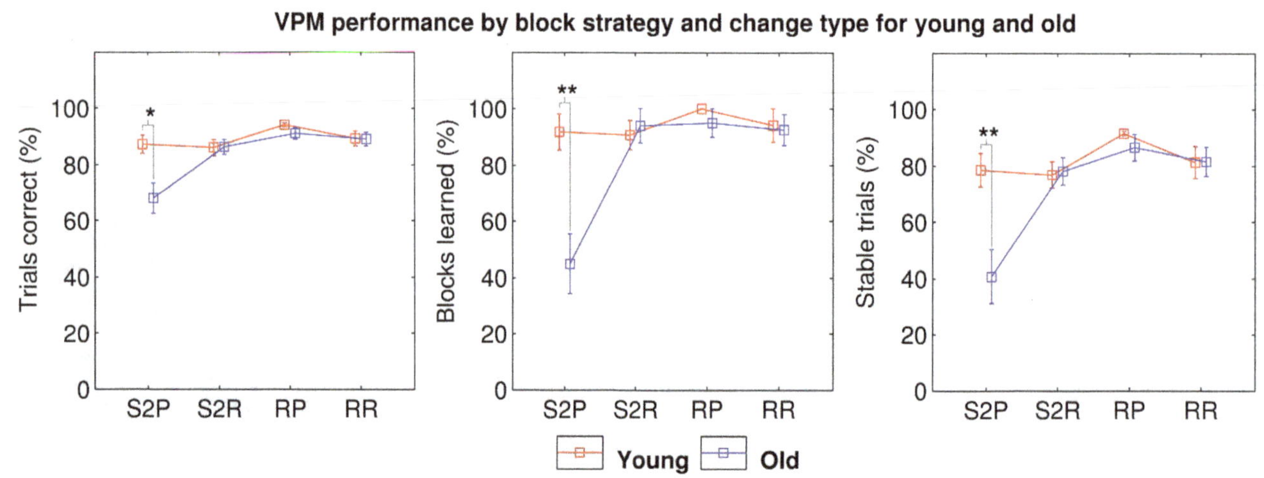


**FIGURE 5 | VPM performance in terms of trials correct (left), blocks learned (middle), and stable trials (right) during blocks following switches to the place strategy (S2P), switches to the response strategy (S2R), reversals of place (RP), and reversals of response (RR) for young (red) and old (blue) participants, excluding data from first blocks and blocks following unlearned blocks.** Significant differences are indicated at the *0.05, **0.01, and ***0.001 levels following Bonferroni correction.

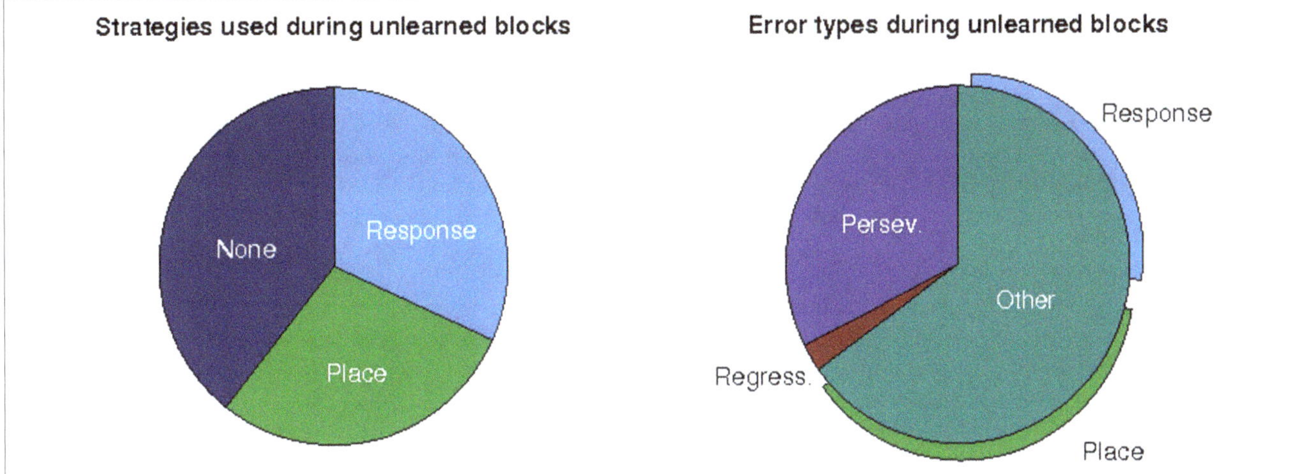


**FIGURE 6 | Left:** Strategies used during unlearned blocks as a proportion of all unlearned blocks for old participants. **Right:** Error types made during unlearned blocks as a proportion of all unlearned blocks in which an incorrect strategy was used for old participants.

during unlearned blocks, finding that while they often failed to acquire any strategy, they more often used an incorrect strategy, and that this was not usually attributable to perseverative or regressive error types.

Our initial results appeared to provide evidence of an age-related strategy switching deficit, as hypothesized and as found previously using set-shifting tasks (Moore et al., 2003; Gamboz et al., 2009; Young et al., 2010). Such a deficit can be interpreted in terms of the NA hypothesis of strategy switching (Aston-Jones and Cohen, 2005; Bouret and Sara, 2005), as LCNA dysfunction is observed in aging (Mouton et al., 1994; Li et al., 2001; Grudzien et al., 2007) and has been shown to impair strategy switching (Tait et al., 2007). During unlearned blocks, older participants did not usually exhibit perseverative errors, suggesting that any switching deficit would result from a failure of the LCNA system and PFC to engage a new strategy, rather than a failure of the ACC/OFC to detect a change in reward, or of the LCNA system to disengage the old strategy.

However, while we hypothesized a general strategy switching deficit, we found that the older participants did not exhibit an impairment in switching from the place to the response strategy. We also found an age difference in performance during place blocks, which may have indicated an allocentric processing deficit, as demonstrated previously in older animals (Frick et al., 1995; Kikusui et al., 1999; Begega et al., 2001). But similarly, this did not apply to place blocks following a reversal, and therefore did not suggest a general allocentric processing deficit. Instead, we found that these effects could both be attributed to a single specific impairment in switching to the place strategy. We believe this is the first study to identify this specific impairment, but we propose that previous findings interpreted as evidence of a general strategy switching deficit may actually relate to this more specific deficit. Furthermore, impaired switching to allocentric processing is likely to affect navigation in general, and may account for previous findings of age-related decline in allocentric navigation performance.

A strategy switching deficit could be attributed to LCNA or PFC dysfunction (Aston-Jones and Cohen, 2005; Bouret and Sara, 2005), whereas an allocentric processing deficit would most likely be attributed to hippocampal atrophy (Driscoll et al., 2003; Du et al., 2003, 2006). However, the cohort of older participants used in this study appear to have retained normal functionality of the areas of PFC and hippocampus responsible for co-ordinating switching and allocentric navigation, respectively. The specific switch-to-place deficit observed may instead stem from a functional difference somewhere between these two systems in the network involved in guiding navigation. We speculate that the interaction between hippocampus and PFC may be compromised in the older participants. In this case, when a response strategy is no longer rewarded, a switch would still be initiated by the LCNA system and the hippocampal place strategy would still be available to switch to, but the PFC would fail to select the place strategy as the best to use, perhaps due to reduced weighting of inputs from the hippocampus. If the weighting of caudal inputs is retained, then switches to response should be unaffected. Similarly, once a place strategy has been selected, although this will be more difficult, use of the strategy and performance of reversals should also remain unimpaired. There is some existing evidence of a change in the functional connectivity between the hippocampus and PFC in aging and dementia (Grady et al., 2003; Wang et al., 2006; Bai et al., 2009).

Reduced hippocampal-prefrontal connectivity could also account for other aspects of navigational aging, such as a preference among older people for egocentric strategies (Rodgers et al., 2012; Wiener et al., 2012). We recently demonstrated that this preference persists even when an allocentric strategy would be more beneficial to task performance (Wiener et al., submitted). This may result from older people's inability to switch to an allocentric strategy, due in turn to reduced hippocampal-prefrontal connectivity. Alternatively, reduced hippocampal-prefrontal connectivity could effect this strategy preference directly. In this case, the egocentric preference may contribute to the switch-to-place deficit. In the present study, older participants may have found it easier to switch to the response strategy due to their egocentric strategy preference, thus masking the effects of a more general switching deficit on their switch-to-response performance. Unfortunately, this behavioral data does not allow us to easily discern whether the effects were due solely to an age difference in functional hippocampus-PFC connectivity underlying the switch-to-place deficit, nor whether there was additional dysregulation of the LCNA system, corresponding to a more general deficit in strategy switching in combination with an egocentric strategy preference. Further investigation using neuroimaging is necessary to confirm the functional, morphological, or structural changes responsible for the behavioral age differences reported here.

In summary, we have demonstrated a specific age-related deficit in switching to an allocentric navigational strategy, while both switching to an egocentric strategy and reversals within strategies were unaffected. This deficit is unlikely to result from diminished allocentric processing functionality of the hippocampus, as older participants were still able to use a place strategy, and sometimes did so even when incorrect. It is also unlikely to stem from an impairment in reward monitoring in the ACC or OFC, as most errors made by older participants were not perseverative. Instead, we propose that the deficit corresponds to a failure to engage the place strategy due to decreased functional connectivity between the hippocampus and PFC. Dysregulation in the LCNA system may also contribute to this deficit, either in combination with a preference for egocentric strategies, or simply because the hippocampus-PFC connection could be affected by noradrenergic input from LC. Whatever the underlying cause, the specific switch-to-place deficit may explain more general impairments in navigational strategy switching and allocentric processing that have been observed previously, and is likely to contribute to the age-related decline of navigation ability in general.

## ACKNOWLEDGMENTS

This study was funded by the University of Edinburgh, Bournemouth University, and the Biotechnology and Biological Sciences Research Council. Thanks also to Richard West and Cathy Spain for help with data collection, and to Anne Smith for assistance with running the learning analysis.

## REFERENCES

Allard, S., Gosein, V., Cuello, A. C., and Ribeiro-da-Silva, A. (2011). Changes with aging in the dopamin- ergic and noradrenergic innervation of rat neocortex. *Neurobiol. Aging* 32, 2244–2253.

Allen, G. L., Kirasic, K. C., and Rashotte, M. A. (2004). Aging and path integration skill: kinesthetic and vestibular contributions to wayfinding. *Percept. Psychophys.* 66, 170–179.

Ashendorf, L., and McCaffrey, R. J. (2008). Exploring age-related decline on the Wisconsin Card Sorting Test. *Clin. Neuropsychol.* 22, 262–272.

Aston-Jones, G., and Cohen, J. D. (2005). An integrative theory of locus coeruleus-norepinephrine function: adaptive gain and optimal performance. *Annu. Rev. Neurosci.* 28,403–450.

Bai, F., Zhang, Z., Watson, D. R., Yu, H., Shi, Y., Yuan, Y., et al. (2009). Abnormal functional connectivity of the hippocampus during episodic memory retrieval processing net- work of amnestic mild cognitive impairment. *Biol. Psychiatry* 65, 951–958.

Begega, A., Cienfuegos, S., Rubio, S., Santin, J. L., Miranda, R., and Arias, J. L. (2001). Effectsofageingonallo- centric and egocentric strategies in the Wistar rat. *Behav. Processes* 53, 75–85.

Bohbot, V. D., Lerch, J., Thorndycraft, B., Iaria, G., and Zijdenbos, A. P. (2007). Gray matter differences cor- relate with spontaneous strategies in a human virtual navigation task. *J. Neurosci.* 27, 10078–10083.

Bouret, S., and Sara, S. J. (2005). Network reset: a simplified over- arching theory of locus coeruleus noradrenaline function. *Trends Neurosci.* 28, 574–582.

Compton, D. M. (2004). Behavior strategy learning in the rat: effects of lesions in the dorsal striatum or dor- sal hippocampus. *Behav. Processes* 67,335–342.

Cook, D., and Kesner, R. P. (1988). Caudate nucleus and memory for egocentic localization. *Behav. Neural Biol.* 49, 332–343.

Doeller, C. F., King, J. A., and Burgess, N. (2008). Parallel striatal and hippocampal systems for landmarks and boundaries in spatial memory. *Proc. Natl. Acad. Sci. U.S.A.* 105, 5915–5920.

Driscoll, I., Hamilton, D. A., Petropoulos, H., Yeo, R. A., Brooks, W. M., Baumgartner, R. M., et al. (2003). The aging hippocampus: cognitive, biochemical and struc- tural findings. *Cereb. Cortex* 13, 1344–1351.

Du, A., Schuff, N., Chao, L. L., Kornak,., Jagust, W. J., Kramer, J. H., et al. (2006). Age effects on atrophy rates of entorhinal cortex and hippocam- pus. *Neurobiol. Aging* 27, 733–740.

Du, A., Schuff, N., Zhu, X. P., Jagust, W. J., Miller, B. L., Reed, B. R., et al. (2003). Atrophy rates of entorhi- nal cortex in AD and normal aging. *Neurology* 60, 481–486.

Frick, K. M., Baxter, M. G., Markowska, A. L., Olton, D. S., and Price, D. L. (1995). Age-related spatial reference and working memory deficits assessed in the water maze. *Neurobiol. Aging* 16, 149–160.

Gamboz, N., Borella, E., and Brandimonte, M. A. (2009). The role of switching, inhibition and working memory in older adults' performance in the Wisconsin Card Sorting Test. *Neuropsychol. Dev. Cogn. B Aging Neuropsychol. Cogn.* 16, 260–284.

Grady, C. L., McIntosh, A. R., and Craik, F. I. (2003). Age-related dif- ferences in the functional connec- tivity of the hippocampus during memory encoding. *Hippocampus* 13, 572–586.

Grudzien, A., Shaw, P., Weintraub, S., Bigio, E., Mash, D. C., and Mesulam, M. M. (2007). Locus coeruleus neurofibrillary degen- eration in aging, mild cognitive impairment and early Alzheimer's disease. *Neurobiol. Aging* 28, 327–335.

Hara, Y., Rapp, P. R., and Morrison, J. H. (2012). Neurological and morphological bases of cognitive declineinagedrhesusmonkeys. *Age (Dordr.)* 34, 1051–1073.

Harris, M. A., and Wolbers, T. (2012). Ageing effects on path integra- tion and landmark navigation. *Hippocampus* 22, 1770–1780.

Hartley, T., Maguire, E. A., Spiers, H. J., and Burgess, N. (2003). The well-worn route and the path less traveled: distinct neural bases of route following and wayfinding in humans. *Neuron* 37, 877–888.

Iaria, G., Palermo, L., Committeri, G., and Barton, J. J. (2009). Age dif- ferences in the formation and use of cognitive maps. *Behav. Brain Res.* 196, 187–191.

Iaria, G., Petrides, M., Dagher, A., Pike, B., and Bohbot, V. D. (2003). Cognitive strategies dependent on the hippocampus and caudate nucleus in human navigation: vari- ability and change with practice. *J. Neurosci.* 23, 5945–5952.

Jansen, P., Schmelter, A., and Heil, M. (2010). Spatial knowledge acquisi- tion in younger and elderly adults: a study in a virtual environment. *Exp. Psychol.* 57, 54–60.

Kikusui, T., Tonohiro, T., and Kaneko, T. (1999). Age-related working memory deficits in the allocentric place discrimination task: pos- sible involvement in cholinergic dysfunction. *Neurobiol. Aging* 20, 629–636.

Li, S., Lindenberger, U., and Sikstrom, S. (2001). Aging cognition: from neuromodulation to representation. *Trends Cogn. Sci.* 5, 479–486.

Luine, V., Bowling, D., and Hearns, M. (1990). Spatial memory deficits in aged rats: contributions of monoaminergic systems. *Brain Res.* 537, 271–278.

Lunn, D. J., Thomas, A., Best, N., and Spiegelhalter, D. (2000). WinBUGS - a Bayesian modelling framework: concepts, structure, and extensibility. *Stat. Comput.* 10, 325–337.

Mahmood, O., Adamo, D., Briceno, E., and Moffat, S. D. (2009). Age differences in visual path integration. *Behav. Brain Res.* 205, 88–95.

Manaye, K. F., McIntire, D. D., Mann, D. M., and German, D. C. (1995). Locus coeruleus cell loss in the aging human brain: a non-random pro- cess. *J. Comp. Neurol.* 358, 79–87.

Moffat, S. D., Elkins, W., and Resnick, S. M. (2006). Age differences in the neural systems supporting human allocentric spatial navigation. *Neurobiol. Aging* 27, 965–972.

Moffat, S. D., and Resnick, S. M. (2002). Effects of age on virtual environ- ment place navigation and allo- centric cognitive mapping. *Behav. Neurosci.* 116, 851–859.

Moore, T. L., Killiany, R. J., Herndon, J. G., Rosene, D. L., and Moss, M. B. (2003). Impairment in abstrac- tion and set shifting in aged rhe- sus monkeys. *Neurobiol. Aging* 24, 125–134.

Mouton, P. R., Pakkenberg, B., Gundersen, H. J. G., and Price, D. L. (1994). Absoulte number and size of pigmented locus coeruleus neurons in young and aged individuals.

*J. Chem. Neuroanat.* 7, 185–190. Nedelska, Z., Andel, R., Laczó, J., Vlcek,., Horinek, D., Lisy, J., et al. (2012). Spatial navigation impairment is proportional to right hippocampal volume. *Proc. Natl. Acad. Sci. U.S.A.* 109, 2590–2594.

O'Keefe, J. (1990). A computational theory of the hippocampal cognitive map. *Prog. Brain Res.* 83, 301–312.

Postle, B. R., and D'Esposito, M. (2003). Spatial working memory activity of the caudate nucleus is sensitive to frame of reference. *Cogn. Affect. Behav. Neurosci.* 3, 133–144.

Ragozzino, M. E. (2007). The contribu- tion of the medial prefrontal cortex, orbitofrontal cortex, and dorsome- dial striatum to behavioural flex- ibility. *Ann. N.Y. Acad. Sci.* 1121, 355–375.

Ragozzino, M. E., Detrick, S., and Kesner, R. P. (1999). Involvement of the prelimbic-infralimbic areas of the rodent prefrontal cortex in flex- ibility for place and response learn- ing. *J. Neurosci.* 19, 4585–4594.

Rich, E. L., and Shapiro, M. L. (2007). Prelimbic/infralimbic inactivation impairs memory for multiple task switches, but not flexible selection of familiar tasks. *J. Neurosci.* 27, 4747–4755.

Rodgers, M. K., Sindone, J. A. III., and Moffat, S. D. (2012). Effects of age on navigation strategy. *Neurobiol. Aging* 33, 202.e15–202.e22.

Smith, A. C., Frank, L. M., Wirth, S., Yanike, M., Hu, D., Kubota, Y.,et al. (2004). Dynamic analysis of learning in behavioral experiments. *J. Neurosci.* 24, 447–461.

Smith, A. C., Stefani, M. R., Moghaddam, B., and Brown, E. N. (2005). Analysis and design of behavioral experiments to characterize population learning. *J. Neurophysiol.* 93, 1776–1792. Smith, A. C., Wirth, A., Suzuki, W., and Brown, E. N. (2007). Bayesian analysis of interleaved learning and response bias in behavioral experiments. *J. Neurophysiol.* 97, 2516–2524.

Tanaka, S., Young, J. W., Gresack, J. E., Geyer, M. A., and Risbrough, V. B. (2011). Factor analysis of attentional set-shifting performance in young and aged mice. *Behav. Brain Funct.* 7, 33.1–33.9.

Tait, D. S., Brown, V. J., Farovik, A., Theobald, D. E., Dalley, J. W., and Robbins, T. W. (2007). Lesions of the dorsal noradrenergic bun- dle impair attentional set-shifting in the rat. *Eur. J. Neurosci.* 25, 3719–3724.

Wang, L., Zang, Y., He, Y., Liang, M., Zhang, X., Tian, L., et al. (2006). Changes in hippocampal connectiv- ityintheearlystagesofAlzheimer's disease: evidence from resting state fMRI. *Neuroimage* 31, 496–504.

Wiener, J. M., Kmecova, H., and de Condappa, O. (2012). Route repetition and route retrac- ing: effects of cognitive aging. *Front. Aging Neurosci.* 4:7. doi: 10.3389/fnagi.2012.00007

Young, J. J., and Shapiro, M. L. (2009). Double dissociation and hierarchical organization of strat- egy switches and reversals in the r, PFC. *Behav. Neurosci.* 123, 1028–1035.

Young, J. W., Powell, S. B., Geyer, M. A., Jeste, D. V., and Risbrough, V. B. (2010). The mouse attentional- set-shifting task: a method for assaying successful cognitive ageing? *Cogn. Affect. Behav. Neurosci.* 10, 243–251.

# 20

# Spatial navigation—a unique window into physiological and pathological aging

***Ivana Gazova*[1,2]*, Kamil Vlcek*[2,3], *Jan Laczó*[1,2], *Zuzana Nedelska*[1,2], *Eva Hyncicova*[1], *Ivana Mokrisova*[1], *Katerina Sheardova*[2] *and Jakub Hort*[1,2]**

[1] *Department of Neurology, Memory Disorders Clinic, 2nd Faculty of Medicine, Charles University in Prague and University Hospital Motol, Prague 5, Czech Republic*

[2] *International Clinical Research Center and St. Anne's University Hospital Brno, Brno, Czech Republic*

[3] *Department of Neurophysiology of Memory, Institute of Physiology Academy of Sciences of the Czech Republic v.v.i., Prague, Czech Republic*

***Edited by:***
*Thomas Wolbers, University of Edinburgh, UK*

***Reviewed by:***
*Jacques Micheau, University of Bordeaux 1, France*
*Jose-Vicente Lafuente, University of Basque Country, Spain*

****Correspondence:***
*Ivana Gazova, Department of Neurology, Memory Disorders Clinic, 2nd Faculty of Medicine, Charles University in Prague and University Hospital Motol, V Uvalu 84, Prague 5, 150 06, Czech Republic.*
*e-mail: ivana.gazova1@gmail.com*

Spatial navigation is a skill of determining and maintaining a trajectory from one place to another. Mild progressive decline of spatial navigation develops gradually during the course of physiological ageing. Nevertheless, severe spatial navigation deficit can be the first sign of incipient Alzheimer's disease (AD), occurring in the stage of mild cognitive impairment (MCI), preceding the development of a full blown dementia. Patients with amnestic MCI, especially those with the hippocampal type of amnestic syndrome, are at very high risk of AD. These patients present with the same pattern of spatial navigation impairment as do the patients with mild AD. Spatial navigation testing of elderly as well as computer tests developed for routine clinical use thus represents a possibility for further investigation of this cognitive domain, but most of all, an opportunity for making early diagnosis of AD.

**Keywords: spatial navigation, physiological ageing, pathological ageing, mild cognitive impairment, Alzheimer's disease, allocentric navigation, egocentric navigation**

## INTRODUCTION

Spatial navigation is the ability to determine and maintain a route from one place to another (Gallistel, 1990). It consists of phylogenetically old cognitive functions allowing animals and humans to remember important locations and their mutual relations as well as their relation to the organism itself. Spatial navigation deficits are frequently observed in older population with a significant influence on the quality of life. Spatial navigation difficulties can represent the first sign of Alzheimer's disease (AD) development. The recent trend of spatial navigation research relies on tests translated from animal experiments, e.g., the human analog of the Morris Water Maze (MWM), used for clinical examination of people at risk of AD. In this article we summarize findings on spatial navigation changes in the physiological and pathological ageing and their practical significance for the early diagnosis of AD. As many neuropsychological tools still evoke controversies regarding the accuracy of detecting AD in its predementia stages, it is important to design a battery of tests, including spatial navigation testing for improving early diagnosis of AD.

## PHYSIOLOGICAL AND PATHOLOGICAL AGEING

Physiological ageing is associated with structural and functional changes, mainly in the prefrontal cortex (Cabeza et al., 1997; Resnick et al., 2003) and to a lesser extent in the hippocampus (Jack et al., 1998; Grady et al., 1999), these are mirrored by changes in cognitive functions. Age-related changes in cognition include mild decline in attention, executive functions, working memory, and free memory recall, while other functions such as visuospatial functions, language, and semantic memory remain generally preserved for a long time (Park, 2000).

Pathological ageing is caused by underlying vascular or neurodegenerative diseases leading gradually to a dementia syndrome, where AD is the most common cause. The hallmark of AD is medial temporal lobe (MTL) atrophy including the hippocampus and the enthorinal cortex (Jack et al., 1997). Some recent studies on patients with AD suggested that atrophy is unequally distributed even within the hippocampus being most pronounced in the CA1 subfield compared to hippocampal atrophy pattern in normal ageing, where the CA1 subfield is relatively spared (Frisoni et al., 2008; Mueller and Weiner, 2009). The CA1 atrophy in patients with mild cognitive impairment (MCI) can even predict conversion to dementia due to AD (Chételat et al., 2008; Devanand et al., 2012). Besides the MTL structures, the precuneus was shown to be impaired very early even in presymptomatic AD (Scahill et al., 2002). With the disease progression, structures beyond MTL including lateral temporal, parietal and frontal cortices become affected (Braak and Braak, 1991). The first clinical sign of AD is usually the insidious onset of episodic memory impairment caused by neuropathological changes in MTL. Early in the course of the disease, memory impairment is followed by executive dysfunction together with impairment of working memory and attention. Later on, other cognitive domains including praxis, visuo-constructive skills, and language become affected, which reflects the spreading of the pathology further to the neocortex (Kertesz et al., 1986; Baudic et al., 2006). Proceeding cognitive impairment leads to a decline in every day functional abilities, which constitutes an important criterion for the diagnosis of the dementia syndrome.

In recent years, increasing attention has been paid to the mild end of the cognitive spectrum encompassing a transient zone between the normal ageing and dementia, caused most frequently by AD. This transitional zone has been described by the term MCI (Petersen et al., 1999). The concept of MCI refers to a group of individuals who have some cognitive impairment yet of insufficient severity to constitute dementia due to a very slight degree of functional impairment. The individuals with MCI form a heterogeneous group. Those with memory impairment (amnesia) present amnestic MCI (aMCI), those with the non-memory domain impairment (i.e., executive functions, language, and visuo-spatial skills) present non-amnestic MCI (naMCI) (Petersen et al., 2001). Further sub-classification of both MCI subtypes is based on the number of affected cognitive domains. Isolated memory impairment represents aMCI single domain (aMCIsd), similarly, single non-memory domain impairment represents naMCI single domain (naMCIsd). Impairment in additional domains to these two subtypes assigns to aMCI multiple domain (aMCImd), or naMCI multiple domain (naMCImd). Individuals with aMCI subtype have a high risk of AD development; while those with naMCI subtype have a higher probability of progressing to non-AD dementias such as dementia with Lewy bodies, frontotemporal or vascular dementia. The risk of progression from MCI to dementia, particularly to AD, is not uniform and varies across epidemiological studies (Tierney et al., 1996; Petersen et al., 1999; Morris et al., 2001). The average rate of conversion is estimated to 12% per year (Petersen and Morris, 2003). In contrast, in healthy elderly subjects the rate of conversion to dementia is about 1–2% per year (Petersen et al., 1999).

Although aMCI patients represent at-risk population for AD development, this population is somewhat heterogeneous as it encompasses also individuals who will never progress to dementia. Lately, much effort is spent to identify the high risk patients with underlying AD pathology already in this prodromal (predementia) stage of the disease. For identification of prodromal AD patients, a combination of neuropsychological tests with various biomarkers is used. These include structural and functional neuroimaging, focused on the hippocampus and related structures (Small et al., 1999; Visser et al., 1999; Desikan et al., 2010), magnetic resonance spectroscopy (Modrego et al., 2011), cerebrospinal fluid assessment of amyloid-β peptide, tau and phosphorylated tau proteins (Hulstaert et al., 1999; Shaw et al., 2009), and amyloid labeling PET ligands (Resnick et al., 2010). Among neuropsychological tools, specific memory tests play an important role for identification of memory profile characteristic for AD that is present already in the predementia stages (Sarazin et al., 2007)—"amnestic syndrome of the hippocampal type" (Dubois and Albert, 2004). This syndrome forms a clinical core of the revised research diagnostic criteria for AD (Dubois et al., 2007) and is characterized by decreased memory recall despite controlled encoding and using of facilitation retrieval techniques (cueing or recognition) (Dubois, 2000). The MCI individuals with amnestic syndrome of the hippocampal type (HaMCI), compared to those with the amnestic syndrome of the non-hippocampal type (NHaMCI), form the major at-risk subgroup of MCI population (Sarazin et al., 2007) for the development of dementia due to AD. Although the tests designed to detect hippocampal amnestic syndrome (Grober et al., 1988) were shown to reflect atrophy of the hippocampus, especially its CA1 subfield (Sarazin et al., 2010), it still remains controversial, whether these tests are superior to other tests for the detection of early stage dementia (de Jager et al., 2010; Carlesimo et al., 2011). The uncertainty about the usefulness of cued recall as a diagnostic tool for MCI and AD is expressed also in the National Institute on Aging and the Alzheimer's Association guidelines (Albert et al., 2011; McKhann et al., 2011), which take into account symptoms of patients with predominant parietal atrophy.

Recent studies indicate that there is a promising chance that, spatial navigation tests reflecting MTL damage may identify patients with AD already in the prodromal stages (Laczó et al., 2009).

## SPATIAL NAVIGATION STRATEGIES AND ITS MORPHOLOGICAL CORRELATES

While navigating through the environment, people can use two basic navigation strategies associated with distinct internal representations of space. The egocentric navigation is body-centered strategy that utilizes distances and directions to or from individual landmarks with respect to the subject's body position. The allocentric navigation is a world-centered strategy using information about distances and angles between different locations in the environment independent of the position of the subject.

Animal research yielded valuable information about the role of MTL in the processes of spatial navigation (O'Keefe and Dostrovsky, 1971; O'Keefe and Nadel, 1978; Morris et al., 1982). A key structure of the allocentric navigation is the hippocampus, especially its CA1 subfield (Brun et al., 2008). In 1971 O'Keefe and Dostrovsky discovered specific place-firing cells in the hippocampus of the rat (O'Keefe and Dostrovsky, 1971). These findings supported the theory of a cognitive map (Tolman, 1948) and the dissociation between the egocentric and allocentric navigation strategies. Experiments in the MWM demonstrated spatial navigation impairment in the rats after hippocampal lesion (Morris et al., 1982). Hippocampus is crucial for consolidation, encoding, and long term storage of spatial information (Squire, 1992). The association of hippocampus with allocentric navigation in humans has been demonstrated in various studies in real-space and virtual environments (Maguire et al., 1998; Astur et al., 2002). In one study, Holdstock et al. (2000) tested patient (YR) with selective bilateral hippocampal lesion for recall of visuospatial information and found that YR was more impaired at recalling allocentric than egocentric information. More specifically, right CA1 hippocampal subfield seems to be involved in encoding of allocentric spatial information in humans (Suthana et al., 2009). There is evidence that egocentric information is processed outside of the hippocampal system (O'Keefe and Nadel, 1978), in the parietal cortex including precuneus and the caudate nucleus (Mountcastle et al., 1975; Maguire et al., 1998). Lesions of the right posterior parietal cortex are characterized by an egocentric orientation deficit (Kase et al., 1977; Levine et al., 1985; Stark et al., 1996).

## SPATIAL NAVIGATION IMPAIRMENT IN PHYSIOLOGICAL AND PATHOLOGICAL AGEING

Spatial navigation has been thoroughly studied in animal models. Navigational tasks based on the models of MWM (Morris, 1981) were used in testing rats of different age (Ingram, 1988; McLay et al., 1999; Begega et al., 2001). Results of these studies suggested age-related deficit of navigational abilities in aged rodents and inspired translational research of spatial navigation in humans. Studies in different environments compared healthy elderly persons with younger adults. Significant deficits in learning a route through a hospital lobby was described in participants 60 years and older, with a tendency to be impaired even in participants in their 50s (Barrash, 1994). Several studies suggested that elderly people have lower cognitive capacity limits in temporospatial processing. In one experiment using series of slides of unfamiliar neighborhood, elderly adults recalled landmarks by their saliency and non-spatial associations rather than by their spatial relationships (Lipman, 1991). However, many other studies emphasized deficits specifically in spatial configuration memory and in place navigation in aged population. Wilkniss et al. (1997) let participants undergo navigational tasks in university building and found that older persons made more errors than their younger counterparts in temporal ordering of landmarks, in recalling the learned route, and in using the learned map in navigation. These deficits suggest a lower ability to use a configural spatial representation to navigate. Another study showed navigational difficulties of healthy elderly while driving a car leading to avoidance of unfamiliar places and routes and thus limiting their mobility (Burns, 1999). Human analog of the MWM was developed in an effort to transform navigational tasks into laboratory conditions. It was employed in a study that demonstrated impairment in acquisition and use of the cognitive map of the maze in the group of elderly participants (Newman and Kaszniak, 2000). Moffat and Resnick (2002) were among the first authors implementing the use of virtual reality in testing of spatial navigation. They compared performance of elderly and younger individuals in the virtual analog of MWM and found deficit of place learning using room-geometry cues in the group of older participants. Furthermore, they suggested that allocentric impairment may contribute to age-related deficit of spatial navigation. This hypothesis was later supported by the study of Iaria and colleagues, according to which the older participants are less effective in forming and using the cognitive maps of an environment (Iaria et al., 2009). A recent study examined age-related differences in strategy preference and found a shift toward egocentric navigation strategy in older participants, which may reflect an adaptation mechanism for the hippocampal dysfunction (Rodgers et al., 2012). Studies correlating hippocampal volume with spatial navigation performance in cognitively healthy elderly provided however contradicting results, with some of them documenting positive correlation (Driscoll et al., 2003; Head and Isom, 2010) and other reporting no association (Moffat et al., 2006; Nedelska et al., 2012).

Spatial navigation impairment occurs early in AD (Monacelli et al., 2003; Pai and Jacobs, 2004); reports about spatial deficits such as getting lost in familiar places and other can in many cases lead to diagnosis of dementia (Klein et al., 1999). The combination of visual perception and memory deficits is probably the mostly defining factor of spatial disorientation in patients with AD (Henderson et al., 1989), where both allocentric and egocentric navigation strategies are impaired (Hort et al., 2007; Weniger et al., 2011). According to several studies, these general spatial deficits in AD seem to be linked mainly to impairment of visual motion processing (Kavcic et al., 2006). Nevertheless, spatial navigation impairment can be detected even before the development of the full blown dementia syndrome, in the stage of MCI (Mapstone et al., 2003; delpolyi et al., 2007; Hort et al., 2007; Laczó et al., 2011). Given that aMCI is associated with a higher risk of progression to AD, the current research of spatial navigation has focused on this group of patients. A visuospatial subtype of aMCI with impaired radial motion perception indicating spatial perception deficit was identified in one of the first studies in this field (Mapstone et al., 2003). Spatial navigation impairment was documented in aMCI patients performing a route-learning task in the hospital lobby (delpolyi et al., 2007). In this study, the patients, who made at least one error on the road, did not differ in neuropsychological tests from those with no errors on the road, but they had lower right MTL and posterior parietal cortex volumes that probably underlie spatial navigation deficit. Temporal order spatial memory was recently suggested as another cognitive marker of AD and aMCI (Bellassen et al., 2012). Remembering a sequence of three turns in a simple maze distinguished well between AD, healthy older subjects, and group of patients with frontotemporal lobe degeneration. Spatial navigation impairment is present even in patients with isolated memory deficit aMCIsd (Hort et al., 2007). The patients with aMCIsd tested in the real-space human version of the MWM had an isolated impairment of allocentric navigation, suggesting spatial memory impairment due to MTL dysfunction. On the other hand, the patients with aMCImd had more general spatial navigation impairment in both, allocentric and egocentric strategies, indicating that structures beyond MTL, presumably the parietal cortex, are affected in this group (Hort et al., 2007). Consistent with these findings patients with aMCI were impaired in both egocentric and allocentric strategies in a study using virtual reality environment, where right precuneus volume was associated with egocentric navigation performance (Weniger et al., 2011). Further study examined spatial navigation in a real-space human version of MWM and found more profound spatial navigation deficit in the HaMCI group in comparison to the NHaMCI group, especially in allocentric navigation, which corresponds with the probable hippocampal dysfunction (Laczó et al., 2009). In addition, the HaMCI group resembled the AD group in spatial navigation performance thus indicating that spatial navigation deficit in the HaMCI may be the first sign of incipient AD. In the same vein, in another study using real-space human analogy of MWM (Nedelska et al., 2012), right hippocampal volume in aMCI and AD patients was associated with an allocentric navigation performance. Thus testing of the allocentric navigation, targeting hippocampus and its CA1 subfield (Suthana et al., 2009), and egocentric navigation, focusing more on posterior parietal cortex and precuneus, could be a useful method of recognizing the aMCI patients at higher risk of AD.

Virtual analogs can probably substitute the real space environment in estimating the navigational deficits of MCI and AD patients, as implied by two recent studies. In an experiment consisting of learning a route through a hospital lobby and of a follow-up spatial tests series, strong correlation was found across all subject groups between the total spatial score from the real hospital lobby and the total score from its virtual analog (Cushman et al., 2008). Similarly, high correlation was found in another study between scores in a real-space human version of MWM and its virtual 2D analog on a computer monitor representing the circular space as from above (Laczó et al., 2012). These results suggest that computer analogs of real space tests can yield measures of broad applicability to early detection of navigational impairment in MCI or AD.

## CONCLUSION

In the course of physiological ageing, there is a selective mild decline of spatial navigation. Particularly allocentric navigation is impaired, which may be a consequence of the age-related deficits in mediotemporal functioning observed in the elderly. AD is associated with the development of characteristic pathological changes in the brain, especially in the hippocampus and its CA1 subfield, that further spread to parietal cortex, including precuneus, and other areas as the disease progresses. The severe spatial navigation deficits demonstrated in patients in early stage of AD are caused by both hippocampal and parietal dysfunction. Those spatial navigation deficits can be detected even in the stage of MCI patients with amnestic syndrome of hippocampal types, who are at the highest risk of AD development, and who manifest with the spatial navigation deficit similar to that in AD. Therefore, spatial navigation testing could become a reliable tool of identifying patients in the prodromal stages of AD, before the development of dementia syndrome (Vlcek, 2011). Adding spatial navigation tests to neuropsychological batteries will increase the diagnostic accuracy and early detection of patients with AD in the predementia stages. Given that real-space testing is technically difficult, new methods of testing are being developed. 2D computer tests and virtual reality environments appear to be promising areas for extension of spatial navigation testing to the routine clinical use.

## ACKNOWLEDGMENT

This work was supported by Grant Agency of the Czech Republic Grants 309/09/1053 and 309/09/0286; European Regional Development Fund—Project FNUSA-ICRC (No. CZ.1.05/1.1.00/02.0123); Internal Grant Agency of the Ministry of Health of the Czech Republic Grant NT11225-4; Ministry of Education, Youth and Sports of the Czech Republic Grants 1M0517 and LC554, and research project AV0Z50110509, Grant Agency of Charles University in Prague (No. 2120145) and Institutional Support of Laboratory Research Grant No. 2/2012 (699002).

## REFERENCES

Albert, M. S., DeKosky, S. T., Dickson, D., Dubois, B., Feldman, H. H., Fox, N. C., Gamst, A., Holtzman, D. M., Jagust, W. J., Petersen, R. C., Snyder, P. J., Carrillo, M. C., Thies, B., and Phelps, C. H. (2011). The diagnosis of mild cognitive impairment due to Alzheimer's disease: recommen- dations from the National Institute on Aging-Alzheimer's Association workgroups on diagnostic guide- lines for Alzheimer's disease. *Alzheimers Dement.* 7, 270–279.

Astur, R. S., Taylor, L. B., Mamelak, A. N., Philpott, L., and Sutherland, R. J. (2002). Humans with hippocampus damage display severe spatial mem- ory impairments in a virtual Morris water task. *Behav. Brain Res.* 132, 77–84.

Barrash, J. (1994). Age-related decline in route learning ability. *Dev. Neuropsychol.* 10, 189–201.

Baudic, S., Barba, G. D., Thibaudet, M. C., Smagghe, A., Remy, P., and Traykov, L. (2006). Executive func- tion deficits in early Alzheimer's disease and their relations with episodic memory. *Arch. Clin. Neuropsychol.* 21, 15–21.

Begega, A., Cienfuegos, S., Rubio, S., Santín, J. L., Miranda, R., and Arias, J. L. (2001). Effects of ageing on allocentric and egocentric spatial strategies in the Wistar rat. *Behav. Processes* 53, 75–85.

Bellassen, V., Iglói, K., de Souza, L. C., Dubois, B., and Rondi-Reig, L. (2012). Temporal order memory assessed during spatiotemporal nav- igation as a behavioral cognitive marker for differential Alzheimer's disease diagnosis. *J. Neurosci.* 32, 1942–1952.

Braak, H., and Braak, E. (1991). Neuropathological staging of Alzheimer-related changes. *Acta Neuropathol.* 82, 239–259.

Brun, V. H., Leutgeb, S., Wu, H. Q., Schwarcz, R., Witter, M. P., Moser, E. I., and Moser, M. B. (2008). Impaired spatial representation in CA1 after lesion of direct input from entorhinal cortex. *Neuron* 57, 290–302.

Burns, P. C. (1999). Navigation and the mobility of older drivers. *J. Gerontol. B Psychol. Sci. Soc. Sci.* 54, 49–55.

Cabeza, R., Grady, C. L., Nyberg, L., McIntosh, A. R., Tulving, E., Kapur, S., Jennings, J. M., Houle, S., and Craik, F. I. (1997). Age-related dif- ferences in neural activity during memory encoding and retrieval: a positron emission tomography study. *J. Neurosci.* 17, 391–400.

Carlesimo, G. A., Perri, R., and Caltagirone, C. (2011). Category cued recall following controlled encoding as a neuropsychological tool in the diagnosis of Alzheimer's disease: a review of the evidence. *Neuropsychol. Rev.* 21, 54–65.

Chételat, G., Fouquet, M., Kalpouzos, G., Denghien, I., De la Sayette, V., Viader, F., Mézenge, F., Landeau, B., Baron, J. C., Eustache, F., and Desgranges, B. (2008). Three- dimensional surface mapping of hippocampal atrophy progression from MCI to AD and over normal aging as assessed using voxel-based morphometry. *Neuropsychologia* 46, 1721–1731.

Cushman, L. A., Stein, K., and Duffy, C. J. (2008). Detecting naviga- tional deficits in cognitive aging and Alzheimer disease using virtual real- ity. *Neurology* 71, 888–895.

deIpolyi, A. R., Rankin, K. P., Mucke, L., Miller, B. L., and Gorno-Tempini, M. L. (2007). Spatial cognition and the human navigation network in AD and MCI. *Neurology* 69, 986–997.

de Jager, C. A., Honey, T. E., Birks, J., and Wilcock, G. K. (2010). Retrospective evaluation of revised criteria for the diagnosis of Alzheimer's disease using a cohort with post-mortem diagnosis. *Int. J. Geriatr. Psychiatry* 25, 988–997.

Desikan, R. S., Sabuncu, M. R., Schmansky, N. J., Reuter, M., Cabral, H. J., Hess, C. P., Weiner, M. W., Biffi, A., Anderson, C. D., Rosand, J., Salat, D. H., Kemper, T. L., Dale, A. M., Sperling, R. A., and Fischl, B. (2010). Alzheimer's disease neuroimaging initiative. Selective disruption of the cerebral neocortex in Alzheimer's disease. *PLoS ONE* 5:e12853. doi: 10.1371/ journal. pone.0012853

Devanand, D. P., Bansal, R., Liu, J., Hao, X., Pradhaban, G., and Peterson, B. S. (2012). MRI hip- pocampal and entorhinal cortex mapping in predicting conversion to Alzheimer's disease. *Neuroimage* 60, 1622–1629.

Driscoll, I., Hamilton, D. A., Petropoulos, H., Yeo, R. A., Brooks, W. M., Baumgartner, R. N., and Sutherland, R. J. (2003). The aging hippocampus: cognitive, biochemical and structural findings. *Cereb. Cortex* 13, 1344–1351.

Dubois, B. (2000). 'Prodromal Alzheimer's disease': a more useful concept than mild cognitive impairment? *Curr. Opin. Neurol.* 13, 367–369.

Dubois, B., and Albert, M. L. (2004). Amnestic MCI or prodromal Alzheimer's disease? *Lancet Neurol.* 3, 246–248.

Dubois, B., Feldman, H. H., Jacova, C., Dekosky, S. T., Barberger-Gateau, P., Cummings, J., Delacourte, A., Galasko, D., Gauthier, S., Jicha, G., Meguro, K., O'brien, J., Pasquier, F., Robert, P., Rossor, M., Salloway, S., Stern, Y., Visser, P. J., and Scheltens, P. (2007). Research crite- ria for the diagnosis of Alzheimer's disease: revising the NINCDS- ADRDA criteria. *Lancet Neurol.* 6, 734–746.

Frisoni, G. B., Ganzola, R., Canu, E., Rüb, U., Pizzini, F. B., Alessandrini, F., Zoccatelli, G., Beltramello, A., Caltagirone, C., and Thompson, P. M. (2008). Mapping local hip- pocampal changes in Alzheimer's disease and normal ageing with MRI at 3 Tesla. *Brain* 131, 3266–3276.

Gallistel, C. R. (1990). *The Orga- nization of Learning.* Cambridge, MA: MIT Press.

Grady, C. L., McIntosh, A. R., Rajah, M. N., Beig, S., and Craik, F. I. (1999). The effects of age on the neural cor- relates of episodic encoding. *Cereb. Cortex* 9, 805–814.

Grober, E., Buschke, H., Crystal, H., Bang, S., and Dresner, R. (1988).

Screening for dementia by memory testing. *Neurology* 38, 900–903.

Head, D., and Isom, M. (2010). Age effects on wayfinding and route learning skills. *Behav. Brain Res.* 209, 49–58.

Henderson, V. W., Mack, W., and Williams, B. W. (1989). Spatial dis- orientation in Alzheimer's disease. *Arch. Neurol.* 46, 391–394.

Holdstock, J. S., Mayes, A. R., Cezayirli, E., Isaac, C. L., Aggleton, J. P., and Roberts, N. (2000). A com- parison of egocentric and allocen- tric spatial memory in a patient with selective hippocampal damage. *Neuropsychologia* 38, 410–425.

Hort, J., Laczó, J., Vyhnálek, M., Bojar, M., Bures, J., and Vlcek, K. (2007). Spatial navigation deficit in amnestic mild cognitive impair- ment. *Proc. Natl. Acad. Sci. U.S.A.* 104, 4042–4047.

Hulstaert, F., Blennow, K., Ivanoiu, A., Schoonderwaldt, H. C., Riemenschneider, M., De Deyn, P. P., Bancher, C., Cras, P., Wiltfang, J., Mehta, P. D., Iqbal, K., Pottel, H., Vanmechelen, E., and Vanderstichele, H. (1999). Improved discrimination of AD patients using beta-amyloid(1-42) and tau levels in CSF. *Neurology* 52, 1555–1562.

Iaria, G., Palermo, L., Committeri, G., and Barton, J. (2009). Age differ- ences in the formation and use of cognitive maps. *Behav. Brain Res.* 196, 187–191.

Ingram, D. K. (1988). Complex maze learning in rodents as a model of age-related memory impairment. *Neurobiol. Aging* 9, 475–485.

Jack, C. R. Jr., Petersen, R. C., Xu, Y. C., O'Brien, P. C., Smith, G. E., Ivnik, R. J., Tangalos, E. G., and Kokmen, E. (1998). Rate of medial temporal lobe atrophy in typical aging and Alzheimer's disease. *Neurology* 51, 993–999.

Jack, C. R. Jr., Petersen, R. C., Xu, Y. C., Waring, S. C., O'Brien, P. C., Tangalos, E. G., Smith, G. E., Ivnik, R. J., and Kokmen, E. (1997). Medial temporal atrophy on MRI in nor- mal aging and very mild Alzheimer's disease. *Neurology* 49, 786–794.

Kase, C. S., Troncoso, J. F., Court, J. E., Tapia, J. F., and Mohr, J. P. (1977). Global spatial disori- entation. Clinico-pathologic corre- lations. *J. Neurol. Sci.* 34, 267–278.

Kavcic, V., Fernandez, R., Logan, D., and Duffy, C. J. (2006). Neurophysiological and per- ceptual correlates of navigational impairment in Alzheimer's disease. *Brain* 129, 736–746.

Kertesz, A., Appell, J., and Fisman, M. (1986). The dissolution of lan- guage in Alzheimer's disease. *Can. J. Neurol. Sci.* 13, 415–418.

Klein, D. A., Steinberg, M., Galik, E., Steele, C., Sheppard, J. M., Warren, A., Rosenblatt, A., and Lyketsos, C. G. (1999). Wandering behaviour in community-residing persons with dementia. *Int. J. Geriatr. Psychiatry* 14, 272–279.

Laczó, J., Andel, R., Vlèek, K., Macoška, V., Vyhnálek, M., Tolar, M., and Bojar, M. (2011). Spatial navigation and APOE in amnestic mild cogni- tive impairment. *Neurodegener. Dis.* 8, 169–177.

Laczó, J., Andel, R., Vyhnalek, M., Vlcek, K., Magerova, H., Varjassyova, A., Nedelska, Z., Gazova, I., Bojar, M., Sheardova, K., and Hort, J. (2012). From morris water maze to computer tests in the prediction of Alzheimer's disease. *Neurodegener. Dis.* 10, 153–157.

Laczó, J., Vlček, K., Vyhnálek, M., Vajnerová, O., Ort, M., Holmerová, I., Tolar, M., Anděl, R., Bojar, M., and Hort, J. (2009). Spatial nav- igation testing discriminates two types of amnestic mild cognitive imairment. *Behav. Brain Res.* 202, 252–259.

Levine, D. N., Warach, J., and Farah, M. (1985). Two visual systems in men- tal imagery: dissociation of "what" and "where" in imagery disorders due to bilateral posterior cerebral lesions. *Neurology* 35, 1010–1018.

Lipman, P. D. (1991). Age and exposure differences in acquisition of route information. *Psychol. Aging* 6, 128–133.

Maguire, E. A., Burgess, N., Donnett, J. G., Frackowiak, R. S., Frith, C. D., and O'Keefe, J. (1998). Knowing where and getting there: a human navigation network. *Science* 280, 921–924.

Mapstone, M., Steffenella, T. M., and Duffy, C. J. (2003). A visuospatial variant of mild cognitive impair- ment: getting lost between aging and AD. *Neurology* 60, 802–808.

McKhann, G. M., Knopman, D. S., Chertkow, H., Hyman, B. T., Jack, C. R. Jr., Kawas, C. H., Klunk, W. E., Koroshetz, W. J., Manly, J. J., Mayeux, R., Mohs, R. C., Morris, J. C., Rossor, M. N., Scheltens, P., Carrillo, M. C., Thies, B., Weintraub, S., and Phelps, C. H. (2011). The diagnosis of dementia due to Alzheimer's disease: rec- ommendations from the National Institute on Aging-Alzheimer's Association workgroups on diag- nostic guidelines for Alzheimer's disease. *Alzheimers Dement.* 7, 263–269.

McLay, R. N., Freeman, S. M., Harlan, R. E., Kastin, A. J., and Zadina, J. E. (1999). Tests used to assess the cognitive abilities of aged rats: their relation to each other and to hippocampal morphology and neu- rotrophin expression. *Gerontology* 45, 143–155.

Modrego, P. J., Fayed, N., and Sarasa, M. (2011). Magnetic resonance spectroscopy in the prediction of early conversion from amnestic mild cognitive impairment to dementia: a prospective cohort study. *BMJ Open* 1, e000007.

Moffat, S. D., Kennedy, K. M., Rodrigue, K. M., and Raz, N. (2006). Extrahippocampal contri- butions to age differences in human spatial navigation. *Cereb. Cortex* 17, 1274–1282.

Moffat, S. D., and Resnick, S. M. (2002). Effects of age on virtual environ- ment place navigation and allo- centric cognitive mapping. *Behav. Neurosci.* 116, 851–859.

Monacelli, A. M., Cushman, L. A., Kavcic, V., and Duffy, C. J. (2003). Spatial disorientation in Alzheimer's disease: the remem- brance of things passed. *Neurology* 61, 1491–1497.

Morris, G. M. (1981). Spatial local- ization does not require the pres- ence of local cues. *Learn. Motiv.* 12, 239–260.

Morris, R. G., Garrud, P., Rawlins, J. N., and O'Keefe, J. (1982). Place navigation impaired in rats with hippocampal lesions. *Nature* 297, 681–683.

Morris, J. C., Storandt, M., Miller, J. P., McKeel, D. W., Price, J. L., Rubin, E. H., and Berg, L. (2001). Mild cognitive impairment repre- sents early-stage Alzheimer disease. *Arch. Neurol.* 58, 397–405.

Mountcastle, V. B., Lynch, J. C., Georgopoulos, A., Sakata, H., and Acuna, C. (1975). Posterior parietal association cortex of the monkey: command functions for operations within extrapersonal space. *J. Neurophysiol.* 38, 871–908.

Mueller, S. G., and Weiner, M. W. (2009). Selective effect of age, Apo e4, and Alzheimer's disease on hippocampal subfields. *Hippocampus* 19, 558–564.

Nedelska, Z., Andel, R., Laczó, J., Vlcek, K., Horinek, D., Lisy, J., Sheardova, K., Bures, J., and Hort, J. (2012). Spatial navigation impairment is proportional to right hippocampal volume. *Proc. Natl. Acad. Sci. U.S.A.* 109, 2590–2594.

Newman, M. C., and Kaszniak, A. W. (2000). Spatial memory and aging: performance on a human analog of the Morris water maze task. *Aging Neuropsychol. Cogn.* 7, 86–93.

O'Keefe, J., and Dostrovsky, J. (1971). The hippocampus as a spatial map. Preliminary evidence from unit activity in the freely-moving rat. *Brain Res.* 34, 171–175.

O'Keefe, J., and Nadel, L. (1978). *The Hippocampus as A Cognitive Map.* Oxford: Clarendon.

Pai, M. C., and Jacobs, W. J. (2004). Topographical disorientation in community-residing patients with Alzheimer's disease. *Int. J. Geriatr. Psychiatry* 19, 250–255.

Park, D. C. (2000). "Basic mechanisms accounting for age-related decline in cognitive functions," in *Cognitive Ageing. A Primer,* eds D. C. Park and N. Schwarz (Philadelphia, PA: Psychology), 3–21.

Petersen, R. C., Doody, R., Kurz, A., Mohs, R. C., Morris, J. C., Rabins, P. V., Ritchie, K., Rossor, M., Thal, L., and Winblad, B. (2001). Current concepts in mild cogni- tive impairment. *Arch. Neurol.* 58, 1985–1992.

Petersen, R. C., and Morris, J. C. (2003). "Clinical features," in *Mild Cognitive Impairment: Aging to Alzheimer's Disease,* ed. R. C. Petersen (New York, NY: Oxford University Press, Inc.), 15–40.

Petersen, R. C., Smith, G. E., Waring, S. C., Ivnik, R. J., Tangalos, E. G., and Kokmen, E. (1999). Mild cogni- tive impairment: clinical character- ization and outcome. *Arch. Neurol.* 56, 303–308.

Resnick, S. M., Pham, D. L., Kraut, M. A., Zonderman, A. B., and Davatzikos, C. (2003). Longitudinal magnetic resonance imaging studies of older adults: a shrinking brain. *J. Neurosci.* 23, 3295–3301.

Resnick, S. M., Sojkova, J., Zhou, Y., An, Y., Ye, W., Holt, D. P., Dannals, R. F., Mathis, C. A., Klunk, W. E., Ferrucci, L., Kraut, M. A., and Wong, D. F. (2010). Longitudinal cognitive decline is associated with fibrillar amyloid-beta mea- sured by [11C]PiB. *Neurology* 74, 807–815.

Rodgers, M. K., Sindone, J. A. III., and Moffat, S. D. (2012). Effects of age on navigation strategy. *Neurobiol. Aging* 33, 202.e15–22.

Sarazin, M., Berr, C., De Rotrou, J., Fabrigoule, C., Pasquier, F., Legrain, S., Michel, B., Puel, M., Volteau, M., Touchon, J., Verny, M., and Dubois, B. (2007). Amnestic syn- drome of the medial temporal type identifies prodromal AD: a longitudinal study. *Neurology* 69, 1859–1867.

Sarazin, M., Chauviré, V., Gerardin, E., Colliot, O., Kinkingnéhun, S., de Souza, L. C., Hugonot-Diener, L., Garnero, L., Lehéricy, S., Chupin, M., and Dubois, B. (2010). The amnestic syndrome of hippocam- pal type in Alzheimer's disease: an MRI study. *J. Alzheimers Dis.* 22, 285–294.

Scahill, R. I., Schott, J. M., Stevens, J. M., Rossor, M. N., and Fox, N. C. (2002). Mapping the evo- lution of regional atrophy in Alzheimer's disease: unbiased anal- ysis of fluid-registered serial MRI. *Proc. Natl. Acad. Sci. U.S.A.* 99, 4703–4707.

Shaw, L., Vanderstichele, H., Knapik- Czajka, M., Clark, C., Aisen, P., Petersen, R. C., Blennow, K., Soares, H., Simon, A., Lewczuk, P., Dean, R., Siemers, E., Potter, W., Lee, V. M., and Trojanowski, J. Q. (2009). Alzheimer's disease neuroimag- ing initiative. Cerebrospinal fluid biomarker signature in

Alzheimer's disease neuroimaging initiative subjects. *Ann. Neurol.* 65, 403–413.

Small, S. A., Perera, G. M., DeLaPaz, R., Mayeux, R., and Stern, Y. (1999). Differential regional dysfunction of the hippocampal formation among elderly with memory decline and Alzheimer's disease. *Ann. Neurol.* 45, 466–472.

Squire, L. R. (1992). Memory and the hippocampus: a synthesis from findings with rats, monkeys and humans. *Psychol. Rev.* 99, 195–231.

Stark, M., Coslett, H. B., and Saffran, E. M. (1996). Impairment of an egocentric map of locations: impli- cations for perception and action. *Cogn. Neuropsychol.* 13, 481–524.

Suthana, N. A., Ekstrom, A. D., Moshirvaziri, S., Knowlton, B., and Bookheimer, S. Y. (2009). Human hippocampal CA1 involvement during allocentric encoding of spatial information. *J. Neurosci.* 29, 10512–10519.

Tierney, M. C., Szalai, J. P., Snow, W. G., Fisher, R. H., Nores, A., Nadon, G., Dunn, E., and St. George-Hyslop, P. H. (1996). Prediction of probable Alzheimer's disease in memory- impaired patients: a prospective longitudinal study. *Neurology* 46, 661–665.

Tolman, E. C. (1948). Cognitive maps in rats and men. *Psychol. Rev.* 56, 144–155.

Visser, P. J., Scheltens, P., Verhey, F. R., Schmand, B., Launer, L. J., Jolles, J., and Jonker, C. (1999). Medial temporal lobe atrophy and mem- ory dysfunction as predictors for dementia in subjects with mild cog- nitive impairment. *J. Neurol.* 246, 477–485.

Vlcek, K. (2011). "Spatial naviga- tion impairment in healthy aging and Alzheimer's disease," in *The Clinical Spectrum of Alzheimer's Disease. The Charge toward Comprehensive Diagnostic and Therapeutic Strategies,* ed. S. De La Monte (Rijeka, Croatia: Intech), 75–100.

Weniger, G., Ruhleder, M., Lange, C., Wolf, S., and Irle, E. (2011). Egocentric and allocentric memory as assessed by virtual reality in indi- viduals with amnestic mild cogni- tive impairment. *Neuropsychologia* 49, 518–527.

Wilkniss, S. M., Jones, M. G., Korol, D. L., Gold, P. E., and Manning, C. A. (1997). Age-related differences in an ecologically based study of route learning. *Psychol. Aging* 12, 372–375.

# 21

# Age differences in virtual environment and real world path integration

**Diane E. Adamo[1,2], Emily M. Briceño[3], Joseph A. Sindone[4], Neil B. Alexander[5] and Scott D. Moffat[6]***

[1] *Eugene Applebaum College of Pharmacy and Health Sciences, Wayne State University, Detroit, MI, USA*
[2] *Institute of Gerontology, Wayne State University, Detroit, MI, USA*
[3] *Department of Psychology, Wayne State University, Detroit, MI, USA*
[4] *Department of Linguistics, University of Michigan, Ann Arbor, MI, USA*
[5] *Mobility Research Center, Geriatrics Center and Division of Geriatric Medicine, University of Michigan Hospitals and Veterans Affairs Ann Arbor Health Care System Geriatric Research Education and Clinical Center, Ann Arbor, MI, USA*
[6] *School of Psychology, Georgia Institute of Technology, Atlanta, GA, USA*

**Edited by:**
*Thomas Wolbers, German Center for Neurodegenerative Diseases (DZNE), Germany*

**Reviewed by:**
*Mark May, Helmut-Schmidt University Hamburg, Germany*
*Mathew A. Harris, University of Edinburgh, UK*

***Correspondence:**
*Scott D. Moffat, School of Psychology, Georgia Institute of Technology, J. S. Coon Bldg., 654 Cherry Street, Atlanta, GA 30332-0170, USA.*
*e-mail: scott.moffat@psych.gatech.edu*

Accurate path integration (PI) requires the integration of visual, proprioceptive, and vestibular self-motion cues and age effects associated with alterations in processing information from these systems may contribute to declines in PI abilities. The present study investigated age-related differences in PI in conditions that varied as a function of available sources of sensory information. Twenty-two healthy, young ($23.8 \pm 3.0$ years) and 16 older ($70.1 \pm 6.4$ years) adults participated in distance reproduction and triangle completion tasks (TCTs) performed in a virtual environment (VE) and two "real world" conditions: guided walking and wheelchair propulsion. For walking and wheelchair propulsion conditions, participants wore a blindfold and wore noise-blocking headphones and were guided through the workspace by the experimenter. For the VE condition, participants viewed self-motion information on a computer monitor and used a joystick to navigate through the environment. For TCTs, older compared to younger individuals showed greater errors in rotation estimations performed in the wheelchair condition, and for rotation and distance estimations in the VE condition. Distance reproduction tasks (DRTs), in contrast, did not show any age effects. These findings demonstrate that age differences in PI vary as a function of the available sources of information and by the complexity of outbound pathway.

**Keywords: aging, Alzheimer's disease, hippocampus, navigation, path integration, spatial memory**

## INTRODUCTION

An important aspect of spatial navigation is path integration (PI) (Mittelstaedt and Mittelstaedt, 1982; Cheng and Spetch, 1998), which refers to the ability to monitor one's position in space using self-motion cues derived from visual (linear and radial optic flow), vestibular (translational and rotational accelerations), and/or proprioception (feedback from muscles, tendons, and joints). Optic flow refers to the processing of the flow of visual information resulting from movement of the observer. Decline in the ability to process optic flow has been linked with declines in navigation abilities observed with early onset of Alzheimer's disease (delpolyi et al., 2007). Vestibular cues derived from sensory receptors in the middle ear (utricle, saccule, and semicircular canals) detect differences in linear and angular accelerations. Detecting changes in the speed of translation (distance-specific) and rotation (direction-specific relative to global spatial coordinates) contribute to updating spatial information used in PI tasks. Support for the importance of vestibular information in PI is evidenced by the observation that labyrinthine-defective human subjects have difficulty estimating and reproducing the length of a path or a previously seen target (Glasauer et al., 1994, 1999). Proprioception provides information about body and limb position awareness and is used to mediate one's conscious perception of movement (Goodwin et al., 1972; McCloskey, 1978; Gandevia et al., 1992) and encode body movements in space (Chance et al., 1998; Mittelstaedt and Mittelstaedt, 2001). Thus, these primary sensory systems all contribute significantly to the ability to navigate one's environment.

Studies on ants (Cheng et al., 2009), bees (Frisch, 1967), and, particularly, rodents (Mittelstaedt and Mittelstaedt, 1982; Etienne et al., 1988) show that when eliminating visual and olfactory cues (Etienne et al., 1986) animals are able to use PI effectively (Mittelstaedt and Mittelstaedt, 1982; Jeffery et al., 1997). Although sensory-specific contributions to PI vary within species, bees rely on optic flow (Srinivasan et al., 2000) and ants determine distance through proprioceptors (Wohlgemuth et al., 2001). In rats, recordings from anterior thalamic head-direction cells show that vestibular and visual movement cues, along with motor efferent information (Zugaro et al., 2001) work interactively to determine the directional frame of reference during PI tasks (Sharp et al., 1995; Blair and Sharp, 1996).

Although specific procedures employed to evaluate *human* PI vary, paradigms typically restrict participants to a subset of self-motion cues (visual, vestibular, and proprioceptive) in order to evaluate the relative contribution of sensory input (Loomis et al., 1993; Chance et al., 1998; Philbeck et al., 2008). To restrict individuals to proprioceptive and vestibular information, participants typically wear a blindfold and noise-blocking headphones and are then required to reproduce movements through which they were transported. Individuals may be moved along a single linear distance and be asked to return to the origin by reproducing the distance they traveled by moving in the opposite direction. In contrast, triangle completion tasks (TCTs) are more complicated in that participants may be moved along two legs of a triangle and then when reaching the end of the second leg of the triangle, must rotate and return to the origin without assistance. In this task, spatial components associated with angles turned and distances traveled must be successfully integrated in order to approximate the return to the origin.

Healthy young adults are fairly accurate when reproducing distances and angular rotations (Mittelstaedt and Mittelstaedt, 1982, 2001; Israel and Berthoz, 1989; Glasauer et al., 1994; Israel et al., 1995; Ivanenko et al., 1997; Marlinsky, 1999). In addition, Wiener et al. (2011) showed that head orientation assists with deriving a homing vector for locomotion tasks performed in the absence of visual and auditory information. However, when required to combine linear and rotational displacements simultaneously (as in TCTs), healthy young adults demonstrate greater difficulty with the task, with errors mainly driven by the rotation component of the movement (Loomis et al., 1993; Marlinsky, 1999). Further, the contribution of motor-efferent signals derived from self-movements cannot be ignored as a source of information contributing to PI abilities (Mittelstaedt and Mittelstaedt, 2001).

Despite numerous demonstrations of age-related declines in navigation in both human (Moffat and Resnick, 2002; Driscoll et al., 2005; Cushman et al., 2008; Rodgers et al., 2012) and non-human (Ingram, 1988; McLay et al., 1999) species, few studies have investigated possible age differences in PI. Allen et al. (2004) found that older adults performed similarly to young adults when returning to the origin of a triangle under guided walking conditions. However, when performing this same task following passive conveyance in a wheelchair, older individuals showed greater errors than young individuals, suggesting that performance is related to the amount of sensory information available. That is, age differences are minimized when both proprioceptive and vestibular perceptual signals are available. In a study designed to examine age-differences in visual PI, Mahmood et al. (2009) found that older compared to younger adults had greater difficulty in a TCT presented on a computer. Similar age effects in PI were observed by Harris and Wolbers (2012) using a virtual environment (VE).

Although age-related declines in PI have been demonstrated in one real-world and two VE studies, the extent to which each of the sources of sensory information contribute to these differences is not known as no study has investigated all three sensory systems in the same participants. This is critical as each sensory system known to contribute to PI, shows some age-related decline (Adamo et al., 2007, 2009; Horning and Gorman, 2007; Kulmala et al., 2008). Understanding the contribution of sensory-specific information to PI abilities may contribute to improving interventions to offset age-associated declines in wayfinding abilities that rely on the integration of sensory specific information (Loomis et al., 1993; Chance et al., 1998; Philbeck et al., 2008) and cognitive functions (Davis et al., 2008). Therefore, the present study investigated the relative contribution of three sources of sensory information to age-related differences in PI. The contribution of various sources of sensory information to PI was investigated by providing conditions that reduced a source of sensory information. For blindfolded/auditory blocking walking conditions self-motion cues were derived primarily from proprioceptive and vestibular cues. Motor efferent information is also available. For blindfolded/auditory blocking wheelchair propulsion conditions self-motion cues were primarily derived from vestibular cues since they were seated in a wheelchair and only performed active movements when operating the joystick during return paths. During VE conditions, self-motion cues were derived from optic flow and there were no visual landmark or cues available. Passive viewing was completed before individuals used a joystick to complete return paths. For outbound paths, sensory information was specific to each condition. In the wheelchair and VE conditions return paths required the use of a joystick to complete task requirements. The focus of this study investigated PI abilities derived specifically from self-movement cues.

## METHODS

Thirty-eight, right handed, young ($n = 22$, 10 female, mean age $= 23.8 \pm 3.0$ years) and older ($n = 16$, 11 female, mean age $= 70.1 \pm 6.4$ years) adults participated in this study. Participants were free from any neurological or musculoskeletal conditions that may have impaired performance and scored >28/30 on the Mini Mental State Exam (MMSE) (Folstein et al., 1975). Visual acuity was 20/40 or higher for all individuals. Participants were recruited from the Metropolitan Detroit/Ann Arbor area and Wayne State University. Informed consent approved by the Institutional Review Board at the University of Michigan and the Human Investigation Committee at Wayne State University was completed before each testing session.

### SCREENING TOOLS AND ASSESSMENTS

Vision and mobility assessments were administered to all participants. Tests for contrast sensitivity (Mars Letter Contrast Sensitivity Test) and color vision (Ishihara Color Plates Test) ensured that any potential visual deficits would not interfere with their ability to perform the VE condition. The Timed Up and Go task (Podsiadlo and Richardson, 1991) assessed safe walking ability. To determine whether the participants experienced any symptoms of motion sickness following performance of the tasks in the VE, the 16-item Nausea Symptom Questionnaire was administered.

### EXPERIMENTAL SET-UP

Two real world conditions and one VE condition were used to assess PI abilities. The real world conditions consisted of guided walking and wheelchair propulsion and took place in a human research laboratory that was $12.2 \times 9.1$ m. For both real world conditions, participants wore a halo structure on their head. This consisted of a rigid plastic structure that was placed on the head in a position parallel to the ground. The halo was embedded with eight equally distributed reflective markers (Light Emitting Diodes, LEDs) that were connected with a thin cable and then to a transmitter. The transmitter powered the reflective markers, and the position of the reflective markers embedded in the halo was recorded by four Optotrak Certus™ position sensors (cameras) placed in the testing volume. The reflective markers tracked whole body movements.

For the walking condition, a gait belt worn by the participant and lightly grasped by the experimenter was used to steer the participants through the distances traveled and angles turned during the walking task. Participants also wore noise-reducing earphones and a blindfold to suppress auditory and visual information. Comfortable walking shoes were worn.

For the wheelchair condition, participants were comfortably seated in an IMC Heartway Rumba S HP with a Dynamic DL 5.2i armrest control unit mounted on the right side of the chair. Individuals moved a joystick device with their right hand to execute forward, backward, and turning movements while seated in the chair.

The VE condition was administered using a modified version of Unreal Tournament 2003 and the software package Unreal Editor 3.0 (Epic Games, Inc.). In a dimly lit room, participants were seated 23″ away from an 18″ flat screen LCD monitor. Seat height was adjusted so that the eyes were level with the midpoint of the computer monitor. A Thrustmaster Top Gun Fox 2 Pro joystick mounted on top of a 27 5/8th in. platform was placed on the right side of the individual. The VE condition consisted of passively viewing a movement trajectory on a computer monitor, then maneuvering a joystick when responding to the requirements of the active portion of the task (see below).

#### EXPERIMENTAL PROCEDURES

Following completion of screening tools, participants performed PI tasks in the following order: walking, wheelchair propulsion, and VE. The VE was presented last because of concerns that motion sickness or dizziness induced by VE navigation may affect performance on the real world tasks and may increase risk for falls in the blindfolded walking condition. For each condition, two tasks were performed that consisted of: (1) rotating and returning to the origin of a triangle and (2) reproducing a linear distance traveled.

#### REAL WORLD-TRIANGLE COMPLETION AND DISTANCE REPRODUCTION TASKS

The TCT involved passive motion of two linear distances separated by one angular rotation. For real-world walking, participants were guided along the first leg of a triangle and brought to a complete stop. The experimenter then rotated and guided participants through the second leg of the triangle. After stopping at the end of the second leg, participants were signaled to rotate and walk to the origin. For real world wheelchair propulsion, participants were seated in the chair and the experimenter guided the movement of the wheelchair by standing behind it and reaching forward to activate the joystick. The experimenter followed a path outlined on the floor that indicated the precise distance required to travel and angle to turn. For return paths, participants either walked (walking condition) or propelled their wheelchair (wheelchair condition) back to the origin (see **Figures 1A,B**, respectively). After their position was recorded, they were moved away from their end position and briefly removed the blindfold in order to allow them to re-orient to the environment. This reduced the potential desire to remove the blindfold at unscheduled moments during subsequent trials when they may perceive some confusion about their location. Triangles were counterbalanced according to the length of the leg and angle turned. The length of the first and second leg ranged from 1.2 to 5.5 m and the turning angle was either 36 or 104°. The starting position for each triangle was varied.

In the distance reproduction task (DRT), participants were guided through a linear displacement of 3.0, 6.1, and 9.1 m. When they came to a complete stop, participants were then rotated toward the origin and signaled to travel back to the starting position. After their end position was recorded, participants were escorted away from the end position before briefly removing the blindfold as indicated above. The starting position varied for each distance.

In order to ensure the experimenter provided a similar walking and wheelchair propulsion velocity for young and older individuals, a sub analysis of movements was analyzed. The walking speed for the experimenter was 0.78 m/sec and 0.69 m/sec, for young and older participants, respectively, and these differences were not statistically significant ($p = 0.45$). Likewise, the movement speed for the experimenter when pushing the wheelchair was 0.65 m/sec for younger individuals and 0.56 m/sec for older individuals. These differences were not statistically significant ($p = 0.17$). Similar velocities (0.6 m/sec) were used by the experimenter during walking and wheelchair propulsion conditions in the Allen et al. (2004) study.

#### VIRTUAL ENVIRONMENT-TRIANGLE COMPLETION AND DISTANCE REPRODUCTION TASKS

When performing the TCT and DRT in the VE, participants first passively viewed motion of the linear path for the DRTs and then the outbound paths, separated by a rotation for the TCTs (see **Figure 1C**). Speeds of movement during passive viewing were matched for both the TCT and DRT.

Three DRTs (3.0, 6.1, and 9.1 m) and six TCTs were completed each condition (walk, wheelchair, and VE). One additional practice trial preceded two test trials for each condition × task combination (see **Table 1** for details about the triangles).

#### PRACTICE SESSION

For real world conditions, participants were familiarized with the testing environment by performing specified movements in the testing area. For the walking condition, individuals were guided through the movement by the experimenter, first without, then while wearing the gait belt, blindfold, and noise blocking earphones. The experimenter explained to the participants that a tap on the shoulder would be used to indicate reference movement onset and movement termination. When the reference movement distance was completed, participants were rotated and then instructed to reproduce the distance traveled or to return to

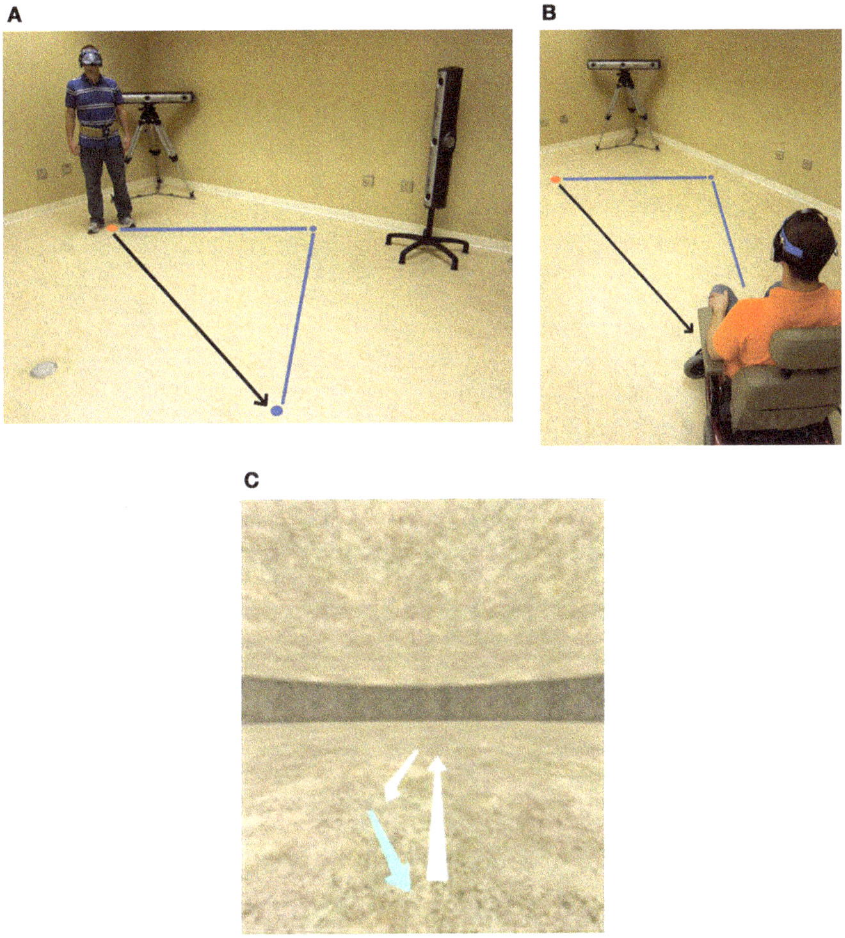

**FIGURE 1 | Schematic of experimental setup: participants wore noise reducing headphones and a blindfold during guided walking (A) and wheelchair propulsion (B) conditions.** Data were collected from reflective markers placed on a halo structure worn on the head of the participant. VE condition consisted of passively viewing a movement trajectory on a computer monitor **(C)** then moving a joystick when responding to the active portion of the task. Guided movements (lighter shaded lines) and participants movements (darker shaded lines) are shown on the schematic.

**Table 1 | Six triangles were presented to the participants.**

| | T1 | T2 | T3 | T4 | T5 | T6 |
|---|---|---|---|---|---|---|
| Leg 1 (m) | 1.2 | 5.5 | 2.4 | 1.8 | 2.4 | 5.5 |
| Turning angle (degree) | 36 | 36 | 36 | 104 | 104 | 104 |
| Leg 2 (m) | 1.8 | 2.4 | 5.5 | 1.2 | 5.5 | 2.4 |

*The distance of the first and second leg and turning angle were counterbalanced across triangles. Triangles performed in the VE were scaled identically.*

the origin of the triangle. Two practice trials were performed to ensure individuals understood the instructions.

For the wheelchair condition, participants were seated in the wheelchair and were requested to travel in a straight line and maneuver around cones placed equidistance apart on the floor by moving the joystick located on the armrest of the wheelchair. Following this, the experimenter propelled the participant through the testing environment. This was done first with and then without the participant wearing the blindfold and noise blocking earphones. Likewise, the experimenter explained that a tap on the shoulder would be used to indicate reference movement onset and movement termination. Additional time (approximating 15 min) was provided to practice this task when compared to that needed to practice walking tasks, in order to allow the individual to become comfortable using the controls.

A practice session was also provided prior to participating in the VE condition. Participants viewed a cubic room that contained landmarks. They first were provided with instruction on the use of the joystick and then used the joystick to move freely around the room. When participants demonstrated competence with the use of the joystick in moving freely around the room, competency with joystick control was verified by completing a speed task. The speed task consisted of traveling through a long and circuitous virtual hallway; participants were required to travel through the hallway in 120 s or less to verify joystick competence.

### TESTING SESSION

For real world conditions, the experimenter guided the participants through the testing paths, and then tapped them on the shoulder to signal when it was time to reproduce the distance traveled or return to the origin of the triangle. When individuals moved beyond the detectable range of the positions sensors, distance and angular measurements of end positions were taken with a measuring tape and goniometer. Trials were also terminated if safety was a risk (for example, if bumping into a wall was imminent). For the VE condition, participants first passively viewed motion of a linear distance in a long hallway, and then were asked to use a joystick to travel the same distance they previously viewed. Speeds of movement during passive and active viewing were deliberately mismatched to prevent participants from using a simple time-counting strategy to perform reproductions. Participants were informed of this mismatch and told explicitly not to use time estimation to reproduce the distances and that attempting to do so would be futile.

### DATA COLLECTION

For real world conditions, movement data were recorded from the Optotrak Certus™ motion capture system. Movement data detected from at least three active markers on the halo were used to calculate a centroid using Matlab software that, in turn, provided a single trajectory corresponding to each person's movements. When movements were beyond the detectable range of the position sensors, floor measurements were taken. Movement data for the VE condition were collected within Unreal Tournament 2003. Data collected for all conditions were processed using customized Labview software.

### DATA ANALYSIS

In order to evaluate the error across different distances, the relative error was calculated for each condition (walk, wheelchair, and VE) and task (DRT, TCT) combination.

The relative distance error for DRT and TCT was calculated as a proportion of the distance traveled relative to the required distance, (Relative distance error = |*dactual* – *d*required|/*d*required). The relative rotation error for TCT was calculated as a proportion of the angle turned relative to the required rotation, (Relative rotation error = |*ractual* – *r*required|/*r*required). Age differences for assessments and control measures were reported as means ± SD.

## RESULTS

Independent sample *t*-tests showed no statistically significant differences for MMSE scores (29.0 ± 1.2 and 28.5 ± 1.4) years of education (15.6 ± 1.9 and 15.0 ± 2.0), motion sickness symptoms or fatigue between young and old groups ($p > 0.05$), respectively. In addition, there were no statistically significant differences between young and older individuals for visual screening and walking assessments or reports of motion sickness post-participation in the VE condition (*p*'s > 0.05) (see **Table 2**).

**Table 2 | Mean (SD) for screening assessments in young and older adults.**

| | Young | Older | *P*-values |
|---|---|---|---|
| MMSE | 29.0 (1.2) | 28.5 (1.4) | 0.13 |
| Education (years) | 15.6 (1.9) | 15.0 (2.0) | 0.41 |
| Motion Sickness | 2.1 (1.7) | 1.9 (1.9) | 0.48 |
| Fatigue | 0.27 (0.45) | 0.38 (0.50) | 0.51 |
| Fatigue (% reporting 0/1)* | 72.7/27.3 | 62.5/37.5 | 0.50 |
| Contrast sensitivity | 1.7 (0.04) | 1.7 (0.06) | 0.23 |
| Ishihara color-blindness | 20.2 (1.0) | 20.4 (0.8) | 0.58 |
| TUG (s) | 8.4 (1.7) | 9.1 (2.3) | 0.23 |
| Speed test (s) | 93.3 (3.2) | 100.4 (5.7) | 0.08 |

*Independent t-tests were conducted with the exception of chi square test *.*

### RELATIVE ERROR FOR TRIANGLE COMPLETION TASKS

Analyses of the TC tasks involved decomposing the error as a function of the required linear distance traveled and angle turned to understand how each individual component contributed to overall performance. A repeated measures ANOVA was conducted to test for main and interaction effects for condition (walk, wheelchair, and VE) and triangle (1–6) with age as the between subjects factor and relative distance error and relative rotation error as dependent variables.

There was a significant main effect for age [$F_{(1, 36)} = 6.8, p < 0.05$] with older adults showing greater errors than young adults and a significant main effect for condition [$F_{(2, 72)} = 22.8, p < 0.0001$] with greater errors found in the VE condition when compared to the wheelchair; and in the wheelchair condition when compared to the walking condition. There were no significant main effects of triangle [$F_{(5, 180)} = 1.1$. $p > 0.05$], thus triangle was collapsed across conditions for subsequent comparisons and no significant main effects for gender [$F_{(1, 36)} = 0.22, p > 0.05$]. A significant two-way age x condition interaction [$F_{(2, 72)} = 7.6, p < 0.01$] indicated that age differences were specific to condition tested.

Pairwise comparisons based on estimated marginal means determined that older individuals, mean (SE); 47.8 (4.1) generated greater relative distance errors ($p < 0.05$) than younger individuals mean (SE); 35.4 (3.6) in the VE condition. For rotation estimations, older individuals generated greater errors in the wheelchair ($p < 0.05$) and VE ($p < 0.01$) conditions mean (SE); 29.1 (3.2), 51.9 (4.1), respectively when compared to younger individuals mean (SE); 18.8 (2.8), 24.1 (3.5), respectively (see **Figures 2A,B**).

In young individuals, relative rotation error was greater in the VE 35.4 (3.6) than walking mean (SE); 27.9 (3.8) condition ($p < 0.05$) and in the wheelchair mean (SE); 30.6 (2.0) than walking condition, showing a tendency toward statistical significance ($p = 0.06$). There were no significant differences between conditions for relative distance error. However, for older individuals, relative distance error was greater in the VE mean (SE); 47.9 (4.1) than walking mean (SE); 31.7 (4.3) condition ($p < 0.01$) and in the VE mean (SE); 47.9 (4.1) than wheelchair mean (SE); 33.3 (2.3) condition ($p < 0.01$). Greater relative rotation error was found in the VE mean (SE); 51.9 (4.1) compared to the wheelchair mean (SE); 29.1 (3.2), condition ($p < 0.01$) and in the VE compared to the walking mean (SE); 17.4 (2.9) condition ($p < 0.01$).

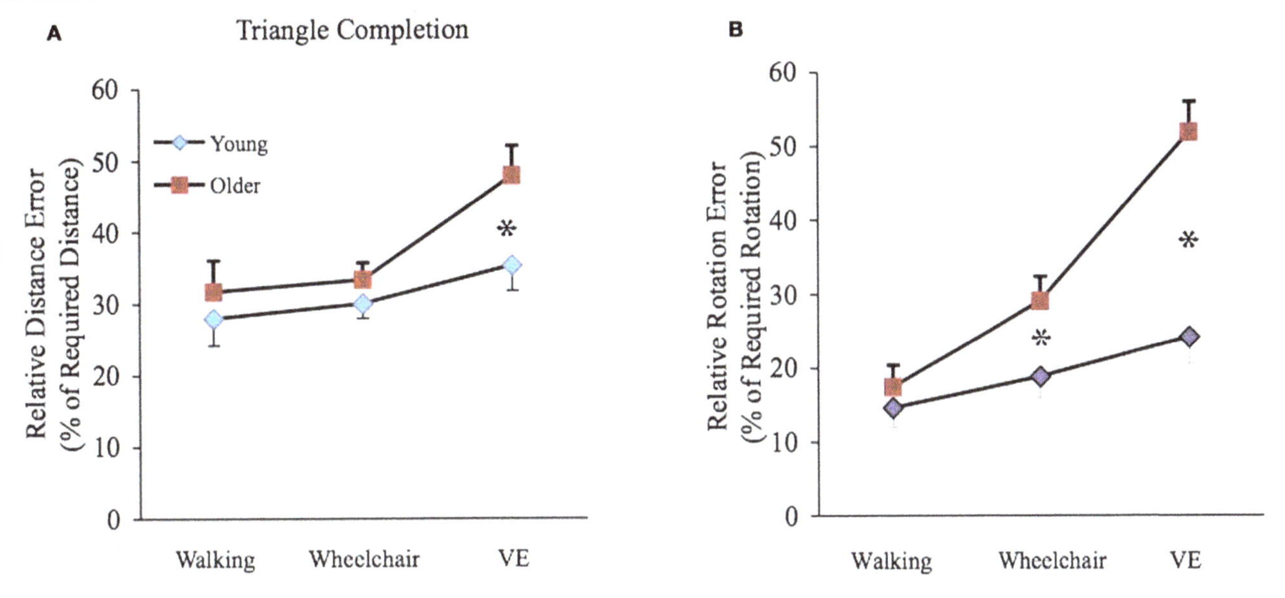


**FIGURE 2 | (A)** Mean (± SE) relative distance error (RDE) for young (filled diamond) and older (filled square) participants. Age differences were significant in the VE condition (*$p < 0.05$). **(B)** Mean (± SE) relative rotation error (RRE) for young (filled diamond) and older (filled square) participants. Age differences were significant in the wheelchair (*$p < 0.05$) and VE (*$p < 0.01$) conditions.

Likewise, greater error was found in the wheelchair than walking condition ($p < 0.01$).

### RELATIVE ERROR FOR DISTANCE REPRODUCTION TASKS

A repeated measures ANOVA with age group as the between subjects factor and condition (walk, chair, and VE) and distance traveled (3.0, 6.1, and 9.1 m) as within-subject factors showed a main effect for condition [$F_{(2, 74)} = 15.0$, $p < 0.01$] and relative distance error as dependent variable. There were no significant main effects for age [$F_{(1, 36)} = 0.28$, $p > 0.05$] or distance traveled [$F_{(2, 72)} = 0.1$, $p > 0.05$]. Pairwise comparisons based on estimated marginal means showed that relative distance error was greater in the VE mean (SE); 22.6 (2.3) than wheelchair mean (SE); 20.8 (1.9) and walking mean (SE); 12.3 (2.0) conditions ($p$'s $< 0.05$) (see **Figure 3**).

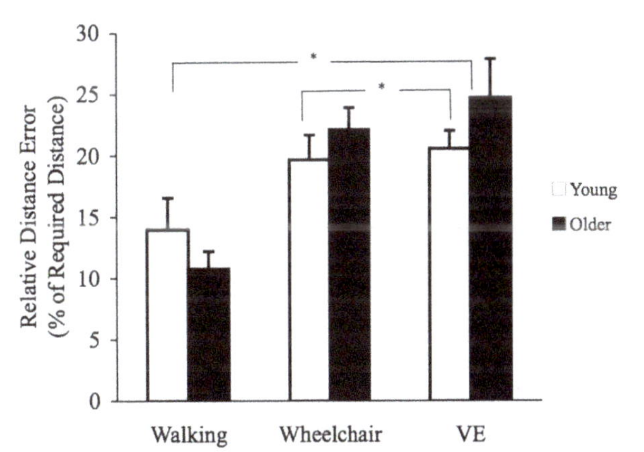


**FIGURE 3 | Mean (± SE) relative distance error (RDE) for young (open) and older (filled) participants.** Conditions differences were found between VE and wheelchair; VE and walking conditions (*$p$'s $< 0.05$).

## DISCUSSION

Findings from this study showed that age differences in PI abilities were related to the availability of sensory information and task type (DRT, TCT). For DR tasks, older and younger individuals performed in a similar manner showing greater relative error in the VE than wheelchair condition, and in the wheelchair than walking condition. For TC tasks, older individuals were significantly further away from the origin than their younger counterparts for all conditions. When decomposing return to origin errors as a function of rotation and distance estimations, older individuals generated significantly greater rotation estimation errors in the wheelchair and VE conditions, and greater distance and rotation estimation errors in the VE condition when compared to young individuals.

### TRIANGLE COMPLETION TASKS

In the present study, there were larger errors when completing the TCT tasks in the VE than in real-world environments. This indicates that participants performed better at PI when they were blindfolded but allowed movement than when they were allowed vision but remained still. In support of this observation, previous work has found that proprioceptive/efferent sources of information have been shown to improve performance of a visually based VE task (Chance et al., 1998; Sun et al., 2004).

Indeed, locomotion was shown to enhance encoding of optic flow information used in VE TCT (Philbeck et al., 2001; Kearns et al., 2002) suggesting that the availability of vestibular and proprioceptive sensory information contributes to successful updating of movements (Loomis et al., 1993; Philbeck et al., 2008). In addition, Sun et al. (2004) showed that participants who remained stationary while viewing optic flow from a VE head mounted display performed less well in a TCT than subjects who walked or were transported in a wheelchair while viewing optic flow from a VE display. These findings suggest that optic flow by itself does not induce automatic updating of heading direction in a manner similar to that provided by vestibular and proprioception (Loomis et al., 2002). Our results are consistent with this interpretation.

When decomposing the relative contribution of rotation and distance estimations to TCT errors in the VE, greater errors were found for all rotation estimations across all triangles in older than young individuals. Similar errors in rotation were found for older individuals in other studies (Mahmood et al., 2009; Harris and Wolbers, 2012). Mahmood et al. (2009) showed that estimating the absolute rotation of a PI task contributed significantly to the overall error. However, Harris and Wolbers (2012) reported that rotation error was largely due to under rotating.

Further, the age effects found in the VE may be related to age-related differences in the processing of visual motion, especially optic flow (Atchley et al., 1998). Indeed, processing of self-motion cues is related to higher order processing (Wolbers et al., 2007) which may be vulnerable with aging. Kavcic et al. (2011) showed that older individuals required higher thresholds for detecting optic flow than younger individuals. In their study, participants were asked to judge which field on the visual display (left or right) was moving faster than the other. Older individuals required faster movements in opposing directions to distinguish differences in movement speed. However, this is in contrast to findings from others (Atchley et al., 1998; Billino et al., 2008a) who found optic flow detection to be unaffected by age suggesting that processing visual information is context-dependent and may be explained by differences in methodologies used to test for detection thresholds (Billino et al., 2008b). Indeed, Mossio et al. (2008) found estimating distances traveled in VE tasks when using optic flow were highly dependent on the strategy used by the participant and specific features associated with the presentation of visual information, such as texture regularity and depth cues, for example.

Allen et al. (2004) found no age difference in TCT in the walking condition. However, they found significant age differences in the same task following passive conveyance in the wheelchair, which they concluded, was largely the result of errors in estimating rotation. These findings are similar to the present results showing that the type of available sensory information distinguishes age differences in PI.

Tasks performed in the wheelchair condition restrict visual and proprioceptive feedback, forcing participants to rely on vestibular input. This finding is compatible with the observation that older individuals have greater difficulty using vestibular information when visual information is not available (Deshpande and Patla, 2007) and when there is decreased sensitivity of proprioceptors (Deshpande and Patla, 2007). In addition, as pointed out by Agrawal et al. (2009) degeneration of the vestibular system (Johnsson, 1971) may not be compensated for by proprioceptive information in older adults.

Vestibular and proprioceptive information also is critical for PI in animals (Mittelstaedt and Mittelstaedt, 1982; Etienne et al., 1988) Animals with vestibular damage showed declines in navigation when landmark cues were absent (Cohen, 2000; Stackman and Herbert, 2002), a finding which parallels the observation that labyrinthine-defective human subjects have difficulty estimating and reproducing the length of a path or a previously seen target (Glasauer et al., 1994, 1999).

### DISTANCE REPRODUCTION TASKS

Previous studies have shown that young individuals can accurately estimate path length following passive translation (Israel and Berthoz, 1989) and guided walking (Glasauer et al., 1994, 2002; Klatzky et al., 1990). However, no previous study has compared age differences in distance estimations across three different perceptual conditions.

In the present study, the DRT showed no age differences in performance, and both younger and older adults showed a similar magnitude of errors as a function of condition (VE>W/C>Walk). Our lack of age-differences in DRT is somewhat at odds with Mahmood et al. (2009) who showed that older individuals were less accurate in reproducing long (but not short) distances than younger individuals. However, there were substantial differences between studies in both the speed of movements and the distances traveled. In the Mahmood et al. (2009) study, distances ranged from 22.9 to 140.2 virtual m, and the speed of movement averaged 11.2 m/sec, which comes closer to replicating traveling by a motorized vehicle. Similarly, movement speeds were faster in the Harris and Wolbers (2012) study compared to the present study, which may explain a lack of age differences. In the present study, the VE speeds averaged 0.9 m/sec and distances traveled average 5.8 m. This suggests that when optic flow information is presented at slower speeds and/or over shorter distances, performance may improve in older adults resulting in negligible age differences for DRTs.

This investigation of age-related differences in PI abilities is limited by its relatively small sample size and cross sectional design, offering comparisons between older and young adults at a single time point. Indeed, longitudinal studies may offer a better representation of PI abilities when increasing age may be accompanied by declines in sensorimotor and cognitive function. In addition, the age range of the older adults (70.1 ± 6.4 years), health status and screening scores (MMSE scores > 28/30) indicate an active, healthy cohort, the results of which may not translate to a more at-risk population. Another potential limitation to the study was the lack of counterbalancing of task order. The VE condition was presented last to all participants leading to a possible confounding with subject fatigue that could potentially differ by age group. However, the fact that younger and older participants did not differ in fatigue at the end of the study suggests that this lack of counterbalancing likely played a minimal role in the age-differences observed.

We also acknowledge that factors other than sensory differences between conditions could contribute to the age differences observed herein. Among these additional factors may be age difference in working and episodic memory or spatial cognition and spatial imagery, age differences in interfacing with unfamiliar technological devices or possibly other factors that were not measured in the present study.

In sum, specific age and condition effects found in the present study may be explained with reference to the availability of sensory information (visual, proprioceptive, and vestibular). Findings from this study could be used to target interventions at reducing wayfinding difficulties in older adults. In addition, the paradigm used in this study is sensitive to detecting small changes in performance and future research may indicate its potential to serve as an indicator to track the onset and progression of dementia over time.

## ACKNOWLEDGMENTS

Del Harder Research Award, Detroit Medical Center, Detroit, Michigan awarded to Diane E. Adamo. Special thanks to Bernard Martin for assistance with design of the data analysis software.

## REFERENCES

Adamo, D. E., Alexander, N. B., and Brown, S. H. (2009). The influence of age and physical activity on upper limb proprioceptive ability. *J. Aging Phys. Act.* 17,272–293.

Adamo, D. E., Martin, B. J., and Brown, S. H. (2007). Age-related differences in upper limb proprioceptive acuity. *Percept. Mot. Skills* 104, 1297–1309.

Agrawal, Y., Carey, J. P., Della Santina, C. C., Schubert, M. C., and Minor, L. B. (2009). Disorders of bal- ance and vestibular function in US adults: data from the National Health and Nutrition Examination Survey, 2001–2004. *Arch. Intern. Med.* 169, 938–944.

Allen, G. L., Kirasic, K. C., Rashotte, M. A., and Haun, D. B. (2004). Aging and path integration skill: kines- thetic and vestibular contributions to wayfinding. *Percept. Psychophys.* 66,170–179.

Atchley, P., Andersen, G. J., and Wuestefeld, A. P. (1998). Cooperativity, priming, and 3- D surface detection from optic flow. *Percept. Psychophys.* 60, 981–992.

Billino, J., Bremmer, F., and Gegenfurtner, K. R. (2008a). Differential aging of motion pro- cessing mechanisms: evidence against general perceptual decline. *Vision Res.* 48, 1254–1261.

Billino, J., Bremmer, F., and Gegenfurtner, K. R. (2008b). Motion processing at low light levels: differential effects on the perception of specific motion types. *J. Vis.* 8, 14.1–14.10.

Blair, H. T., and Sharp, P. E. (1996). Visual and vestibular influences on head-direction cells in the anterior thalamus of the rat. *Behav. Neurosci.* 110, 643–660.

Chance, S. S., Gaunet, F., Beall, A. C., and Loomis, J. M. (1998). Locomotion mode affects the updating of objects encoountered during travel: the contribution of vestibular and proprioceptive inputs to path integration. *Presence* 7,168–178.

Cheng, K., Narendra, A., Sommer, S., and Wehner, R. (2009). Traveling in clutter: navigation in the Central Australian desert ant Melophorus bagoti. *Behav. Processes* 80, 261–268.

Cheng, K., and Spetch, M. (1998). *Mechanisms of Landmark Use in Mammals and Birds*. New York, NY: Oxford University Press, 1–17.

Cohen, H. S. (2000). Vestibular disor- ders and impaired path integration along a linear trajectory. *J. Vestib. Res.* 10,7–15.

Cushman, L. A., Stein, K., and Duffy, C. J. (2008). Detecting naviga- tional deficits in cognitive aging and Alzheimer disease using virtual reality. *Neurology* 71, 888–895.

Davis, R. L., Therrien, B. A., and West, M. A. (2008). Cue condi- tions and Wayfinding in Older and Younger Women. *GeroNurse Res.* 1, 252–263.

delpolyi, A. R., Rankin, K. P., Mucke, L., Miller, B. L., and Gorno-Tempini, M. L. (2007). Spatial cognition and the human navigation network in AD and MCI. *Neurology* 69, 986–997.

Deshpande, N., and Patla, A. E. (2007). Visual-vestibular interaction during goal directed locomotion: effects of aging and blurring vision. *Exp. Brain Res.* 176,43–53.

Driscoll, I., Hamilton, D. A., Yeo, R. A., Brooks, W. M., and Sutherland, R. J. (2005). Virtual navigation in humans: the impact of age, sex, and hormones on place learning. *Horm. Behav.* 47, 326–335.

Etienne, A. S., Maurer, R., and Saucy, F. (1988). Limitations in the assess- ment of path dependent informa- tion. *Behavior* 106, 81–111.

Etienne, A. S., Maurer, R., Saucy, F., and Teroni, E. (1986). Short-distance homing in golden hamster after a passive outward journey. *Anim. Behav.* 34, 696–715.

Folstein, M. F., Folstein, S. E., and Mchugh, P. R. (1975). "Mini-mental state". A practical method for grad- ing the cognitive state of patients for the clinician. *J. Psychiatr. Res.* 12, 189–198.

Frisch, K. V. (1967). *The Dance Language and Orientation of Bees*. Cambridge: Harvard University Press.

Gandevia, S. C., McCloskey, D. I., and Burke, D. (1992). Kinaesthetic sig- nals and muscle contraction. *Trends Neurosci.* 15,62–65.

Glasauer, S., Amorim, M. A., Viaud Delmon, I., and Berthoz, A. (2002). Differential effects of labyrinthine dysfunction on distance and direc- tion during blindfolded walking of a triangular path. *Exp. Brain Res.* 145, 489–497.

Glasauer, S., Amorim, M. A., Vitte, E., and Berthoz, A. (1994). Goal- directed linear locomotion in nor- mal and labyrinthine-defective sub- jects. *Exp. Brain Res.* 98, 323–335.

Glasauer, S., Dieterich, M., and Brandt, T. (1999). Simulation of patholog- ical ocular counter-roll and skew- torsion by a 3-D mathematical model. *Neuroreport* 10, 1843–1848.

Goodwin, G. M., McCloskey, D. I., and Matthews, P. B. (1972). Proprioceptive illusions induced by muscle vibration: contribution by muscle spindles to perception? *Science* 175, 1382–1384.

Harris, M. A., and Wolbers, T. (2012). Ageing effects on path integra- tion and landmark navigation. *Hippocampus* 22, 1770–1780.

Horning, E., and Gorman, S. (2007). Vestibular rehabilitation decreases fall risk and improves gaze stabil- ity for an older individual with unilateral vestibular hypofunc- tion. *J. Geriatr. Phys. Ther.* 30, 121–127.

Ingram, D. K. (1988). Complex maze learning in rodents as a model of age-related memory impairment. *Neurobiol. Aging* 9, 475–485.

Israel, I., and Berthoz, A. (1989). Contribution of the otoliths to the calculation of linear displacement. *J. Neurophysiol.* 62, 247–263.

Israel, I., Sievering, D., and Koenig, E. (1995). Self-rotation estimate about the vertical axis. *Acta Otolaryngol.* 115, 3–8.

Ivanenko, Y., Grasso, R., Israel, I., and Berthoz, A. (1997). Spatial orienta- tion in humans: perception of angu- lar whole-body displacements in two-dimensional trajectories. *Exp. Brain Res.* 117, 419–427.

Jeffery, K. J., Donnett, J. G., Burgess, N., and O'Keefe, J. M. (1997). Directional control of hippocampal place fields. *Exp. Brain Res.* 117, 131–142.

Johnsson, L. G. (1971). Degenerative changes and anomalies of the vestibular system in man. *Laryngoscope* 81, 1682–1694.

Kavcic, V., Vaughn, W., and Duffy, C. J. (2011). Distinct visual motion pro- cessing impairments in aging and Alzheimer's disease. *Vision Res.* 51, 386–395.

Kearns, M. J., Warren, W. H., Duchon, A. P., and Tarr, M. J. (2002). Path integration from optic flow and body senses in a homing task. *Perception* 31, 349–374.

Klatzky, R. L., Loomis, J. M., Golledge, R. G., Cicinelli, J. G., Doherty, S., and Pellegrino, J. W. (1990). Acquisition of route and survey knowledge in the absence of vision. *J. Mot. Behav.* 22, 19–43.

Kulmala, J., Era, P., Tormakangas, T., Parssinen, O., Rantanen, T., and Heikkinen, E. (2008). Visual acuity and mortality in older people and factors on the pathway. *Ophthalmic Epidemiol.* 15, 128–134.

Loomis, J. M., Klatzky, R. L., Golledge, R. G., Cicinelli, J. G., Pellegrino, J. W., and Fry, P. A. (1993). Nonvisual navigation by blind and sighted: assessment of path integration ability. *J. Exp. Psychol. Gen.* 122, 73–91.

Loomis, J. M., Philbeck, J. W., and Zahorik, P. (2002). Dissociation between location and shape in visual space. *J. Exp. Psychol. Hum. Percept. Perform.* 28, 1202–1212.

Mahmood, O., Adamo, D., Briceno, E., and Moffat, S. D. (2009). Age differences in visual path integration. *Behav. Brain Res.* 205, 88–95.

Marlinsky, V. V. (1999). Vestibular and vestibulo-proprioceptive perception of motion in the horizontal plane in blindfolded man–III. Route infer- ence. *Neuroscience* 90, 403–411.

McCloskey, D. I. (1978). Kinesthetic sensibility. *Physiol. Rev.* 58, 763–820.

McLay, R. N., Freeman, S. M., Harlan, R. E., Kastin, A. J., and Zadina, J. E. (1999). Tests used to assess the cognitive abilities of aged rats: their relation to each other and to hippocampal morphology and neu- rotrophin expression. *Gerontology* 45, 143–155.

Mittelstaedt, H., and Mittelstaedt, M. L. (1982). "Homing in path inte- gration," in *Avian Navigation*, eds F. Papi and H. G. Wallraff (New York, NY: Springer), 290–297.

Mittelstaedt, M. L., and Mittelstaedt, H. (2001). Idiothetic naviga- tion in humans: estimation of path length. *Exp. Brain Res.* 139, 318–332.

Moffat, S. D., and Resnick, S. M. (2002). Effects of age on virtual environment place navigation and allocentric cognitive map- ping. *Behav. Neurosci.* 116, 851–859.

Mossio, M., Vidal, M., and Berthoz, A. (2008). Traveled distances: new insights into the role of optic flow. *Vision Res.* 48, 289–303.

Philbeck, J. W., Behrmann, M., and Loomis, J. M. (2001). Updating of locations during whole-body rota- tions in patients with hemispa- tial neglect. *Cogn. Affect. Behav. Neurosci.* 1, 330–343.

Philbeck, J. W., Woods, A. J., Arthur, J., and Todd, J. (2008). Progressive locomotor recalibration during blind walking. *Percept. Psychophys.* 70, 1459–1470.

Podsiadlo, D., and Richardson, S. (1991). The timed "Up and Go": a test of basic functional mobility for frail elderly persons. *J. Am. Geriatr. Soc.* 39, 142–148.

Rodgers, M. K., Sindone, J. A. 3rd., and Moffat, S. D. (2012). Effects of age on navigation strategy. *Neurobiol. Aging* 33, 202.e215–202.e222.

Sharp, P. E., Blair, H. T., Etkin, D., and Tzanetos, D. B. (1995). Influences of vestibular and visual motion information on the spa- tial firing patterns of hippocam- pal place cells. *J. Neurosci.* 15, 173–189.

Srinivasan, M. V., Zhang, S., Altwein, M., and Tautz, J. (2000). Honeybee navigation: nature and calibration of the "odometer." *Science* 287, 851–853.

Stackman, R. W., and Herbert, A. M. (2002). Rats with lesions of the vestibular system require a visual landmark for spatial navigation. *Behav. Brain Res.* 128, 27–40.

Sun, H. J., Campos, J. L., Young, M., Chan, G. S., and Ellard, C. G. (2004). The contributions of static visual cues, nonvisual cues, and optic flow in distance estimation. *Perception* 33, 49–65.

Wiener, J. M., Berthoz, A., and Wolbers, T. (2011). Dissociable cognitive mechanisms underlying human path integration. *Exp. Brain Res.* 208, 61–71.

Wohlgemuth, S., Ronacher, B., and Wehner, R. (2001). Ant odometry in the third dimension. *Nature* 411, 795–798.

Wolbers, T., Wiener, J. M., Mallot, H. A., and Buchel, C. (2007). Differential recruitment of the hip- pocampus, medial prefrontal cor- tex, and the human motion complex during path integration in humans. *J. Neurosci.* 27, 9408–9416.

Zugaro, M., Tabuchi, E., Fouquier, C., Berthoz, A., and Wiener, S. (2001). Active locomotion increases peak firing rates of anterodorsal thalamic head direction cells. *J. Neruophysiol.* 86, 692–702.

# 22

# Wading pools, fading memories—place navigation in transgenic mouse models of Alzheimer's disease

***Heikki Tanila* ***

*A. I. Virtanen Institute, University of Eastern Finland, Kuopio, Finland*

**Edited by:**
*Emma R. Wood, University of Edinburgh, UK*

**Reviewed by:**
*Kathy R. Magnusson, Oregon State University, USA*
*Ashok Kumar, University of Florida, USA*

***Correspondence:**
*Heikki Tanila, Professor in Molecular Neurobiology, A. I. Virtanen Institute, University of Eastern Finland, P. O. Box 1627, Neulaniementie 2, 70211 Kuopio, Finland.*
*e-mail: heikki.tanila@uef.fi*

The Morris swim navigation task ("water maze") has been a primary research tool to assess hippocampal-dependent spatial learning and memory in rodents for three decades. Originally developed for rats, its application to mouse studies has been a tedious process, but nowadays there are more studies performed with the Morris swim task in mice than in rats. The task has proved to be particularly useful in demonstrating age-related memory impairment in transgenic mouse models of Alzheimer's disease (AD). This review focuses on task details that are most relevant for its application to mouse studies in general and characteristic patterns of impaired performance in Alzheimer model mice as compared with rodents sustaining hippocampal lesions.

**Keywords: spatial memory, amyloid-beta, amyloid precursor protein, presenilin-1, tau**

## INTRODUCTION

Exactly 30 years ago Richard Morris and colleagues published in an article in Nature on a novel behavioral task for place navigation in rats and demonstrated the sensitivity of the task for hippocampal lesions (Morris et al., 1982). Since then the task has been known as the "Morris water maze" and been employed in thousands of published studies worldwide. Originally meant to be a test for rats, which are good swimmers by nature, it also has been successfully applied more and more often to memory testing in mice, which are innately strictly terrestrial animals. To acknowledge the important three decade milestone of this task, this review aims at giving a critical overview of applications of Morris water maze in testing mouse models of the most important memory disorder of mankind, Alzheimer's disease (AD).

## IMPORTANT TECHNICAL DETAILS IN THE TASK

In fact, the name "water maze" is a misnomer in the strictest meaning of the word, because the task is performed in an open wading pool and not in a labyrinth-like series of pathways. In particular, since one of the earliest modifications of the swim task was to place a walled radial maze inside the wading pool, resulting in a true water maze [usually called a "radial-arm water maze"; (Buresová et al., 1985)], it would be more appropriate to call the original task the "Morris swim navigation task" or simply as the "Morris swim task," as will be done in this review. The test environment consists of a wading pool with a diameter of 120–200 cm and a movable submerged platform, which can vary from 10 to 15 cm in diameter, based on animal size. The submerged platform has to be placed close enough to the surface so that a swimming animal will not be able to swim over it without noticing the platform. Several tricks have been used to make sure that the platform really is hidden from the animal. The original trick was to use milk powder to make the water opaque. Because of the bacterial growth this is not an ideal solution, and has been replaced by inorganic white pigment. Another strategy is to avoid any additives in the water by making both the pool and the platform of matt black plastic and provide the room lighting so that light reflects from the water surface. This approach gives a beautiful contrast for video tracking with a white albino rat, but is much less optimal for the most common mouse strain used in place navigation studies, the C57BL/6 mouse. Having marked black mice with a piece of white adhesive tape for years, our lab eventually decided to use a pool made of white plastic and a transparent plastic platform, which combination eventually proved to work. Even though numerous published studies have only utilized a stopwatch to measure the escape latency as a measure of learning in the Morris swim task, this is not acceptable, because of the lack of control for the swimming speed. A good-quality video tracking system is a must for a proper task monitoring. Besides providing a measure of the swim path length for speed calculation, it also yields several other parameters that help identify the strategy and nature of memory impairment of the animal, such as the mean distance from the wall or from the platform, and occupancy near the platform location in the probe trial without the presence of the platform itself.

The standard swim navigation task consists of 3–8 acquisition trials for 3–5 days, with the platform kept in a fixed location. The last trial of the last day is usually a probe trial, without the platform, to see the eventual search bias of the animal. Ideally, the animal would swim in small circles tightly around the former platform location to indicate that it has an established memory of the location. The probe trial can be delayed to or replicated on the next day to reveal more long-term retention of the memory for the specific location. Some details in the task design are fundamentally important for the desired specificity for hippocampal function. First, the starting positions have to vary to make the task performance dependent on true navigation and not egocentric response learning. If a constant start position is used, the task performance will no longer be impaired by hippocampal lesion (Eichenbaum et al., 1990). Second, the environment must provide multiple prominent cues for triangulation. On the other hand, a single cue may not be too prominent, because it will easily attract the animal as a beacon. Especially for mice, this prominent cue is the experimenter him- or herself! A not uncommon error for the experimenter is to anticipate picking up the animal and moving toward the platform at the end of the trial, thus providing a strong cue leading to the target. Besides the probe trial for search bias, the original task design also included another control trial, a visible platform variant of the task. Normal performance in this version, with the platform above the water surface or marked with a pole and flag, should imply that the animal is motivated to climb onto the platform, able to master the motor task requirements, and has normal vision. However, with respect to exclusion of visual impairment, the ability to use the visual platform task as a control has been questioned (Lindner et al., 1997). Rats with hippocampal lesions show initial impairment also in the visual platform task (Morris et al., 1982). So the true value of adding this version is somewhat in doubt. More importantly, it makes a big difference whether visual platform task is run before or after the hidden platform task. If run before in the usual way with curtains around the pool to eliminate all distal cues, it encourages the animal to ignore the distal landmarks, which in the next phase become fundamentally important. This task protocol may thus discourage the use of true navigation strategy and favor the development of alternate search strategies, which eventually show up as poor performance in the probe task. Therefore, it would be recommended to run the visible platform task after the hidden platform version or skip that altogether.

## THE TASK IS APPLICABLE TO MICE AFTER ALL

Initial experiences in applying the Morris swim navigation task to mice were so discouraging that it was long speculated that mice, as strictly terrestrial animals, are not capable of learning the task at all. For instance, one hallmark study that directly compared place learning between C57Bl/6 mice and Long–Evans rats showed mice to be inferior learners in the Morris swim task, even though their performance was equal to rats on a dry radial-arm maze (Whishaw and Tomie, 1996). The authors attributed the inferior performance of mice in the swim task to the better adaptation of rats to swimming. However, there are a number of less well known factors that may account for the poor performance of mice in the Morris swim task even to a greater extent than the simple motor aspect of swimming.

The first important difference in cognitive abilities between mice and rats are robust differences between mouse strains in their learning ability (see Kennard and Woodruff-Pak, 2011 for a recent review). This is a general problem in using mice in cognitive tasks, but especially pronounced in the Morris swim task, because there are strain differences not only in spatial memory *per se*, but also in visual acuity and the learning pattern (Kennard and Woodruff-Pak, 2011). In fact, one reason why the C57BL/6, among all laboratory mouse strains, has become the most widely used strain in cognitive testing derives from its good performance in place learning tasks, including the Morris swim task (Owen et al., 1997). This mouse strain is also suitable for aging studies, showing impairment in spatial memory between 12 and 24 months of age according to various studies. In contrast, FVB, 129/Sv, and DBA strains, which are often found in genetically engineered hybrid lines, are clearly inferior in spatial learning as measured in the Morris swim task (Kennard and Woodruff-Pak, 2011).

One severe problem with mice, as compared to rats, is that many mice actually avoid the escape platform. If they find it accidentally, they may jump off and continue swimming. This may be partly related to the common habit of picking up mice with a net, which they experience as highly aversive. Furthermore, as worse swimmers than rats, mice occasionally have difficulties in climbing onto the platform. An established solution in mouse pool testing is to give them an extra day of pretraining in an alley that leads to the platform. A second and still largely unsolved problem is that mice often do not display a clear search bias in the probe task. One obvious problem in early studies was the downscaling of the pool size in order to correspond to the difference in body sizes between the rat and the mouse. The use of a pool with a diameter as small as 80–90 cm resulted in mice swimming in large circles, but maintaining the appropriate distance from the pool wall. Enlarging the pool to almost the same size as used for rats seemed to solve the problem, but only partially. The fundamental problem seems to be that the mice do not develop the habit of swimming in small circles around the presumed platform location in the probe trials like the rats do. Rather, they make a quick search of the presumed location of the platform, and as soon as they fail to find it, they return to the start location or begin to swim toward the experimenter in the hope of getting picked up (**Figure 1**). Therefore, the most commonly used occupancy-based parameters for assessing spatial memory, such as "time in the target quadrant" or "time in the vicinity of the platform," do not reveal as clear a search bias as corresponding parameters in rats. A recent systematic study comparing the power of various parameters to assess search bias in mice came to the conclusion that the best parameter to assess spatial memory in the Morris swim task is

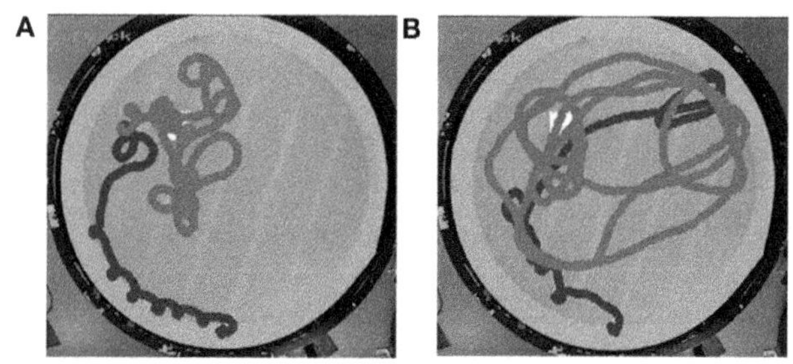


**FIGURE 1 | It is unusual for mice to demonstrate the ideal search pattern in the probe test (A).** Instead, they usually make one approach to the correct former platform position. As soon as they fail to find the platform, they switch to a wider search pattern, but still show some preference to the original target area **(B)**. Black trace: first 20 s, gray trace: following 40 s. The white square indicates the original platform location. Pool diameter 120 cm.

the mean distance to the former platform location (Maei et al., 2009).

Finally, the small body size and especially the thin layer of subcutaneous fat, as compared to rats, render mice susceptible to hypothermia during prolonged exposure to the pool water, which is kept close to room temperature for practical reasons and to ensure sufficient motivation to escape from the water. In the first systematic study on this topic, we found to our great surprise that the regular five daily swims in 20°C water with 30 s between the trials was enough to cause up to 9°C drop in the rectal temperature (Iivonen et al., 2003). The decline in core temperature was accompanied by slowing of the swimming speed. Moreover, the effect was dependent on the sex and genotype of the mice; females were more susceptible to hypothermia than males and transgenic mice carrying Alzheimer-associated APP and PS1 mutations were more vulnerable than their non-transgenic littermates, because of a smaller body weight. Raising the water temperature from 20 to 24°C only partially alleviated the hypothermia. However, increasing the inter-trial interval from 30 s to 13 min removed the net cooling effect of five trials on the core temperature and swimming speed. It is nowadays a common practice to allow mice enough time to warm up between the swims and to assist with external heating devices. Nonetheless, vulnerability to hypothermia is a serious limitation in experimental planning. For instance, in the context of aging studies, a long line of evidence suggests that training distributed over several days is less sensitive to age-related place learning impairment than massed trials (see Foster, 2012 for review). One quite common procedure with aged rats is to give eight trials on one day followed by a probe test 24 h later. This would be very difficult to adapt to mice, which on the one hand would require more trials than rats to attain the same spatial bias and on the other hand would not tolerate the unavoidable hypothermia induced by such massive water exposure.

## MORRIS SWIM TASK HAS BECOME A GOLD STANDARD TEST FOR MEMORY IN AD MOUSE MODELS

Notwithstanding all the above mentioned precautions, the Morris swim navigation task has become the gold standard in demonstrating spatial memory impairment in mouse models of AD. In contrast to large differences between various transgenic AD model mice in several common memory tests, such as fear conditioning or object recognition, all established AD model mice show deficits in the Morris swim task as they age. In addition, the impairment is highly reproducible. We have tested about 3000 APP/PS1 transgenic mice in the Morris swim task during the past 10 years, and have never failed to see an impairment in a test group of transgenic mice, as compared to their wild-type littermates, provided that the mice were past a critical age. Using the terminology for assessing animal models of human disease, one can say that the Morris swim navigation task has *face validity*, because one of the most prominent everyday problems of AD patients is easily getting lost outside their home environment. The test can be considered to have *construct validity*, since transgenic mouse models of AD, whether carrying single APP mutation, combined APP + PS1 mutation, or tau mutation, all display age-related impairment in the task performance (**Table 1**). Finally, the task has *predictive validity*, because all AD drugs in clinical use at present (rivastigmine, galantamine, donepezil, memantine) show a beneficial effect in the Morris swim task in various mouse models (Sweeney et al., 1988; Minkeviciene et al., 2004; Van Dam et al., 2005, 2008).

## DIFFERENT NATURE OF IMPAIRED TASK PERFORMANCE BETWEEN AD MODEL MICE AND RODENTS WITH HIPPOCAMPAL LESIONS

There are some important differences in the spatial learning deficit in the Morris swim task between transgenic AD model

**Table 1 | Summary of genetic mouse models of Alzheimer's disease with reported impairment in the Morris swim navigation task.**

| Transgene | Mouse line | Onset age (months) | References |
|---|---|---|---|
| **APP** | | | |
| huAPP751 | APP751 | <12 | Moran et al., 1995 |
| APP-CTF | APPC100 | 10 | Berger-Sweeney et al., 1999 |
| APPswe | APP23 | 3 | Van Dam et al., 2003 |
| APPswe | Tg2576 | 6 | Westerman et al., 2002 |
| APPswe,ind | TgCRND8 | 3 | Chishti et al., 2001 |
| APPind | PDAPP | <13 | Daumas et al., 2008 |
| APPswe,ind | J20 | 6–7 | Palop et al., 2003 |
| **APP + PS1** | | | |
| APPswe/PS1 (M146L) | APP/PS1 (M146L) | 6–8 | Trinchese et al., 2004 |
| APPswe/PS1(A246E) | APP/PS1(A246E) | 11–12 | Puoliväli et al., 2002 |
| APPswe/PS1dE9 | APdE9 | 10–14 | Minkeviciene et al., 2008 |
| **APP + PS1 + tau** | | | |
| APPswe/PS1(M146V)/tauP301L | 3xTg-AD | 4 | Billings et al., 2005 |
| **Tau** | | | |
| P301L tau | Tg4510 | 1.3 | Santacruz et al., 2005 |
| G272V and P301S tau | THY-Tau22 | 3–10 | Schindowski et al., 2006 |

*The onset age for the impairment is indicated.*

mice (at least in APP transgenics that have been studied the most) and rodents with hippocampal lesions. First, the learning deficit in transgenic mice is never as severe as in animals with hippocampal lesions, and the transgenic mice are usually able to learn the task if allowed some extra training. In this regard, APP transgenic mice closely resemble aged rats (Foster, 2012). Notably, these statements are largely based on comparison between published studies, since few studies have compared the outcome of an experimental lesion with the pathological changes induced by a genetic manipulation. One demonstrative example is our study from 10 years ago, in which we compared the effects of the APP/PS1 transgenic background and fimbria-fornix transection (FFX) on spatial learning in the Morris swim task in C57BL/6 mice (Liu et al., 2002). While the FFX mice showed practically no improvement during five days, APP/PS1 mice showed a clear learning curve, albeit a slower task acquisition than wild-type littermates. A second difference between transgenic APP mice and animals with hippocampal lesions is in the number of cognitive processes affected. When we compared learning within and between daily sessions, a clear dissociation emerged between APP/PS1 and FFX mice. Whereas FFX mice were impaired in both within and between session learning, APP/PS1 mice showed robust learning within a session, but seemed to forget most of what they learned by the next morning (Liu et al., 2002). This "saw-tooth" learning curve in the Morris swim task is also a common finding in aged rats (Foster, 2012). A parsimonious explanation of this difference is that the hippocampus is necessary for navigation (triangulation based on external landmarks and self-motion) in real time, as well as for episodic encoding and memory consolidation. In contrast, accumulation of amyloid-β in the hippocampus interferes only with the long-term memory formation. The susceptibility of APP transgenic mice for faster forgetting of spatial information has been confirmed in at least two other mouse models in later studies (Billings et al., 2005; Daumas et al., 2008). The third difference is that long escape latencies at an early stage of task acquisition in APP transgenic mice are largely due to strong thigmotaxis, which is a prominent feature in genetically modified mice in the Morris swim task in general (Lipp and Wolfer, 1998). This is illustrated in **Figure 2**, which shows parallel learning curves for 12-month-old APdE9 and wild-type littermate male mice in terms of escape latency (**Figure 2A**), path length (**Figure 2B**), and time spent in the wall zone (**Figure 2C**). On top of strong thigmotaxis, APdE9 mice also show poor search bias in the probe test (**Figure 2D**). Without any doubt the Morris swim task is a complex one and involves many cognitive processes at the same time, such as general adaptation to the stressful situation, abandoning of an ineffective tendency to search for an escape in the pool wall, locating the submerged platform based on distal landmarks, and finally encoding that information to long-term memory. A human analogy may be to give the task of delivering a package by bike to a remotely known address in a city to a person who has never ridden a bike before. The learning process involves the motor aspect of bike riding, learning how to cope with busy traffic, and finally, by

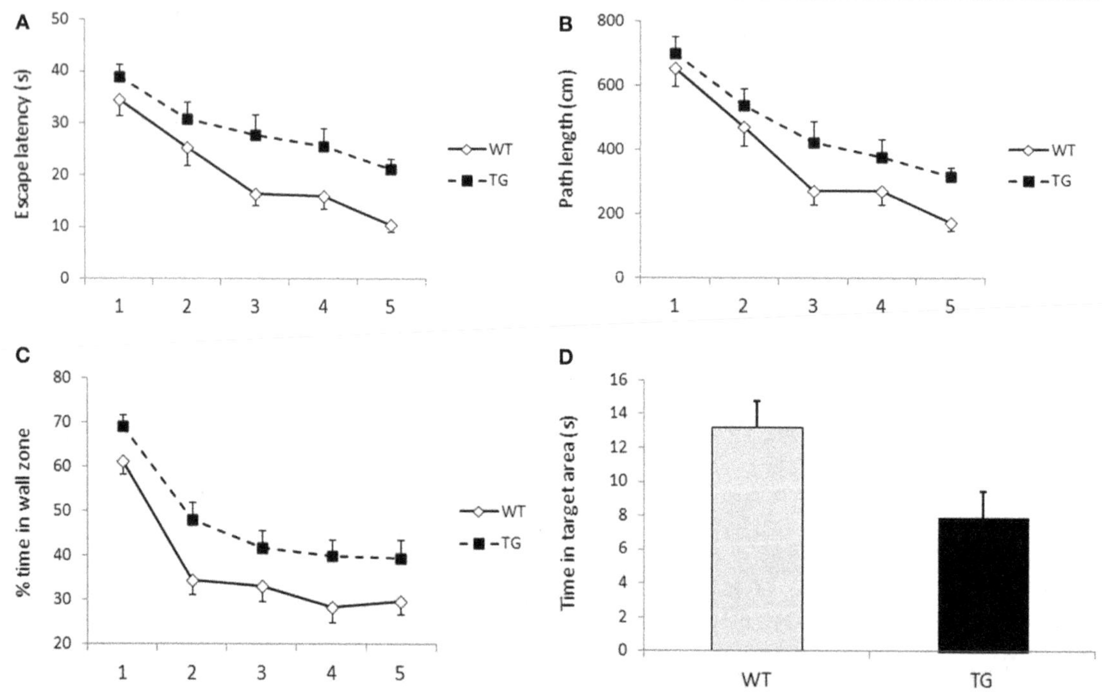


**FIGURE 2 | (A)** Escape latency over five days of Morris swim task acquisition in 12-month-old male APPSwe/PS1dE9 (tg, $n = 13$) mice and their wild-type littermates (WT, $n = 15$). Genotype difference was significant ($p = 0.001$, ANOVA with repeated measures). Group means and SEMs are shown. **(B)** Corresponding plot for path length ($p = 0.01$, ANOVA with repeated measures). **(C)** Thigmotaxis, in terms of % time in the most peripheral 1/3 of the pool area, showed a similar time course as escape latency and path length ($p = 0.001$, ANOVA with repeated measures). **(D)** The genotypes also differ in the time spent in the former platform area (diameter 30 cm) during the probe test on the last trial of day 5 ($p = 0.03$, Student's *t*-test).

trial and error, to remember successful and unsuccessful routes to the destination in a complex city map. In fact, it may be the feature of the Morris swim task to draw on several parallel cognitive processes that explains its sensitivity to demonstrating cognitive impairment in AD model mice. It is likely that several cognitive processes are compromised in APP transgenic mice due to synaptic pathology involving both the hippocampus and neocortex.

## WHICH BRAIN PATHOLOGY ACCOUNTS FOR THE SPATIAL LEARNING IMPAIRMENT IN AD MICE?

What then is the pathological feature in AD model mice which accounts for the impaired task acquisition and development of search bias in the Morris swim task? An important feature of all established APP transgenic mouse models is that very young mice (~2 months) are indistinguishable from their wild-type littermates in the task performance. Because the APP transgene is translated to protein already during a late embryonic stage, normal performance in young transgenic mice implies that the behavioral deficit is not due to a developmental abnormality, but rather to age-related neurodegeneration. The same conclusion can be drawn from conditional mutant tau expressing mice (Santacruz et al., 2005). An obvious candidate accounting for the behavioral deficit is amyloid plaque formation. However, the available literature does not support a direct relationship between amyloid plaque formation and spatial memory deficit. Namely, the time course between amyloid plaque formation and the onset of spatial memory deficit varies greatly between different APP transgenic mouse lines. As exemplified in **Figure 3**, some mouse lines show memory impairment before the first amyloid plaques can be found in a neuropathological examination, while in some other mouse lines these two events can co-occur, and in some other lines, memory impairment may follow amyloid plaque formation by several months.

The poor correlation between amyloid plaque load in postmortem examination and performance in cognitive tests is also a well-established finding in human studies (Nagy et al., 1995).

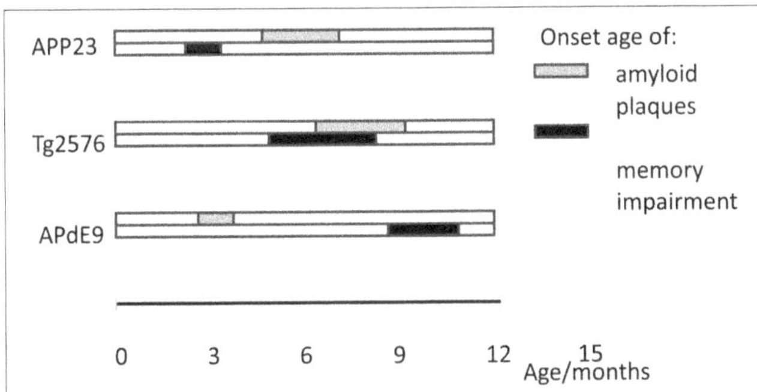


**FIGURE 3 | Timeline of amyloid plaque deposition vs. memory impairment in the Morris swim task in three different APP transgenic mouse lines: APP23 (APPswe under Thy-1 promoter, Van Dam et al., 2003), Tg2576 (APPswe under hamster PrP promoter, Kawarabayashi et al., 2001; Westerman et al., 2002), and APdE9 (APPswe and deletion of exon 9 of presenilin-1 under mouse PrP, Garcia-Alloza et al., 2006; Minkeviciene et al., 2008).**

However, it is possible that these different mouse lines exhibit different harmful effects induced by Aβ formation. For instance, memory deficits before plaque formation may model the impact of soluble Aβ oligomeric species, whereas memory deficits after plaque formation may model the impact of inflammatory mediators around the plaques. An issue that has attracted little attention so far is whether the exact nature of impaired performance in such a complex task as Morris swim navigation also differs between those mouse lines that show early vs. late memory impairment with regard to the appearance of amyloid plaques. Similarly, the correlation between insoluble intracellular tau deposits and impaired Morris swim task performance is not straightforward. Turning off the inducible P301L tau mutant transgene restores the task performance, but if done at a later time point than tau aggregation begins, tau aggregates continue to accumulate in the brain (Santacruz et al., 2005). This finding implies that also for tau aggregates, the soluble species may be the most harmful ones for memory formation.

## POTENTIAL AND LIMITATIONS OF THE MORRIS SWIM TASK IN EXPERIMENTAL AD RESEARCH

As with any test, the Morris swim task has its limitations. It is often criticized for being too stressful for the animals (Kennard and Woodruff-Pak, 2011). This is unavoidable, but the stress level can be reduced by proper pretraining and the use of testing schemes that allow sufficient time for mice to recover between trials. The concern about stressfulness, however, is outweighed by the guaranteed motivation for mice to perform a cognitive task for several days in a row without strict food restriction, which by itself may interfere with the disease process. Another serious limitation is that the classic version of the task is basically a once-a-lifetime learning experience. We have tried to test the same APdE9 mice at a young age before AD pathology and a second time around 12 months of age. Despite several intervening months, the mice show very rapid initial task learning. On the other hand, repeated testing has been successfully applied when mice are trained to criterion using one platform position and then introduced to a new task with a novel platform position repeatedly (Chen et al., 2000). However, this approach is quite tedious and is not well-suited for testing a large number of mice at two different age points. For this purpose, the radial-arm water maze may be a more appropriate solution (Alamed et al., 2006). Nevertheless, because of its established role as the gold standard memory test and the accumulated reference material over the years, the classic Morris swim navigation task is likely to prevail for years as a central tool in the cognitive assessment of AD model mice, both in studies delving into the disease pathogenesis and studies on the efficacy of new therapeutic interventions. Therefore, knowledge about its use potential and pitfalls should be available in all laboratories working on cognitive assessment of AD model mice.

## ACKNOWLEDGMENTS

Supported by EU 7th Framework program grant HEALTH-F2-2007-201159. I wish to thank Susanna Kemppainen for technical assistance in the manuscript preparation.

## REFERENCES


Alamed, J., Wilcock, D. M., Diamond, D. M., Gordon, M. N., and Morgan, D. (2006). Two-day radial-arm water maze learning and mem- ory task; robust resolution of amyloid-related memory deficits in transgenic mice. *Nat. Protoc.* 1, 1671–1679.

Berger-Sweeney, J., McPhie, D. L., Arters, J. A., Greenan, J., Oster- Granite, M. L., and Neve, R. L. (1999). Impairments in learning and memory accompanied by neurodegeneration in mice trans- genic for the carboxyl-terminus of the amyloid precursor protein. *Brain Res. Mol. Brain Res.* 66, 150–162.

Billings, L. M., Oddo, S., Green, K. N., McGaugh, J. L., and LaFerla, F. M. (2005). Intraneuronal Abeta causes the onset of early Alzheimer's disease-related cognitive deficits in transgenic mice. *Neuron* 45, 675–688.

Buresová, O., Bures, J., Oitzl, M. S., and Zahálka, A. (1985). Radial maze in the water tank: an aver- sively motivated spatial working memory task. *Physiol. Behav.* 34, 1003–1005.

Chen, G., Chen, K. S., Knox, J., Inglis, J., Bernard, A., Martin, S. J., Justice, A., McConlogue, L., Games, D., Freedman, S. B., and Morris, R. G. (2000). A learning deficit related to age and beta- amyloid plaques in a mouse model of Alzheimer's disease. *Nature* 408, 975–979.

Chishti, M. A., Yang, D. S., Janus, C., Phinney, A. L., Horne, P., Pearson, J., Strome, R., Zuker, N., Loukides, J., French, J., Turner, S., Lozza, G., Grilli, M., Kunicki, S., Morissette, C., Paquette, J., Gervais, F., Bergeron, C., Fraser, P. E., Carlson, G. A., George-Hyslop, P. S., and Westaway, D. (2001). Early- onset amyloid deposition and cog- nitive deficits in transgenic mice expressing a double mutant form of amyloid precursor protein 695. *J. Biol. Chem.* 27, 21562–21570.

Daumas, S., Sandin, J., Chen, K. S., Kobayashi, D., Tulloch, J., Martin, S. J., Games, D., and Morris, R. G. (2008). Faster forgetting contributes to impaired spatial memory in the PDAPP mouse: deficit in memory retrieval asso- ciated with increased sensitivity to interference? *Learn. Mem.* 15, 625–632.

Eichenbaum, H., Stewart, C., and Morris, R. G. (1990). Hippocampal representation in place learning. *J. Neurosci.* 10, 3531–3542.

Foster, T. C. (2012). Dissecting the age-related decline on spatial learn- ing and memory tasks in rodent models: N-methyl-D-aspartate receptors and voltage-dependent $Ca^{2+}$ channels in senescent synap- tic plasticity. *Prog. Neurobiol.* 96, 283–303.

Garcia-Alloza, M., Robbins, E. M., Zhang-Nunes, S. X., Purcell, S. M., Betensky, R. A., Raju, S., Prada, C., Greenberg, S. M., Bacskai, B. J., and Frosch, M. P. (2006). Characterization of amyloid depo- sition in the APPswe/PS1dE9 mouse model of Alzheimer disease. *Neurobiol. Dis.* 24, 516–524.

Iivonen, H., Nurminen, L., Harri, M., Tanila, H., and Puoliväli, J. (2003). Hypothermia in mice tested in Morris water maze. *Behav. Brain Res.* 141, 207–213.

Kawarabayashi, T., Younkin, L. H., Saido, T. C., Shoji, M., Ashe, K. H., and Younkin, S. G. (2001). Age-dependent changes in brain, CSF, and plasma amyloid (beta) protein in the Tg2576 transgenic mouse model of Alzheimer's disease. *J. Neurosci.* 21, 372–381.

Kennard, J. A., and Woodruff-Pak, D. S. (2011). Age sensitivity of behav- ioral tests and brain substrates of normal aging in mice. *Front. Aging Neurosci.* 3:9. doi: 10.3389/fnagi. 2011.00009

Lindner, M. D., Plone, M. A., Schallert, T., and Emerich, D. F. (1997). Blind rats are not profoundly impaired in the reference memory Morris water maze and cannot be clearly dis- criminated from rats with cogni- tive deficits in the cued platform task. *Brain Res. Cogn. Brain Res.* 5, 329–333.

Lipp, H. P., and Wolfer, D. P. (1998). Genetically modified mice and cog- nition. *Curr. Opin. Neurobiol.* 8, 272–280.

Liu, L., Ikonen, S., Heikkinen, T., Heikkilä, M., Puoliväli, J., van Groen, T., and Tanila, H. (2002). Effects of fimbria-fornix lesion and amyloid pathology on spatial learning and memory in transgenic APP+PS1 mice. *Behav. Brain Res.* 134, 433–445.

Maei, H. R., Zaslavsky, K., Teixeira, C. M., and Frankland, P. W. (2009). What is the most sensitive measure of water maze probe test performance? *Front. Integr. Neurosci.* 3:4.doi:10.3389/neuro.07. 004.2009

Minkeviciene, R., Banerjee, P., and Tanila, H. (2004). Memantine improves spatial learning in a transgenic mouse model of Alzheimer's disease. *J. Pharmacol. Exp. Ther.* 311, 677–682.

Minkeviciene, R., Ihalainen, J., Malm, T., Matilainen, O., Keksa- Goldsteine, V., Goldsteins, G., Iivonen, H., Leguit, N., Glennon, J., Koistinaho, J., Banerjee, P., and Tanila, H. (2008). Age-related decrease in stimulated glutamate release and vesicular glutamate transporters in APP/PS1 transgenic and wild-type mice. *J. Neurochem.* 105, 584–594.

Moran, P. M., Higgins, L. S., Cordell, B., and Moser, P. C. (1995). Age-related learning deficits in transgenic mice expressing the 751-amino acid iso- form of human beta-amyloid pre- cursor protein. *Proc. Natl. Acad. Sci. U.S.A.* 92, 5341–5345.

Morris, R. G., Garrud, P., Rawlins, J. N., and O'Keefe, J. (1982). Place navigation impaired in rats with hippocampal lesions. *Nature* 297, 681–683.

Nagy, Z., Esiri, M. M., Jobst, K. A., Morris, J. H., King, E. M., McDonald, B., Litchfield, S., Smith, A., Barnetson, L., and Smith, A. D. (1995). Relative roles of plaques and tangles in the dementia of Alzheimer's disease: correlations using three sets of neuropathological criteria. *Dementia* 6, 21–31.

Owen, E. H., Logue, S. F., Rasmussen, D. L., and Wehner, J. M. (1997). Assessment of learning by the Morris water task and fear con- ditioning in inbred mouse strains and F1 hybrids: implications of genetic background for single gene mutations and quantitative trait loci analyses. *Neuroscience* 80, 1087–1099.

Palop, J. J., Jones, B., Kekonius, L., Chin, J., Yu, G. Q., Raber, J., Masliah, E., and Mucke, L. (2003). Neuronal depletion of calcium- dependent proteins in the dentate gyrus is tightly linked to Alzheimer's disease-related cognitive deficits. *Proc. Natl. Acad. Sci. U.S.A.* 100, 9572–9577.

Puoliväli, J., Wang, J., Heikkinen, T., Heikkilä, M., Tapiola, T., van Groen, T., and Tanila, H. (2002). Hippocampal A beta 42 levels correlate with spatial memory deficit in APP and PS1 double transgenic mice. *Neurobiol. Dis.* 9, 339–347.

Santacruz, K., Lewis, J., Spires, T., Paulson, J., Kotilinek, L., Ingelsson, M., Guimaraes, A., DeTure, M., Ramsden, M., McGowan, E., Forster, C., Yue, M., Orne, J., Janus, C., Mariash, A., Kuskowski, M., Hyman, B., Hutton, M., and Ashe, K. H. (2005). Tau suppression in a neurodegenerative mouse model improves memory function. *Science* 309, 476–481.

Schindowski, K., Bretteville, A., Leroy, K., Bégard, S., Brion, J. P., Hamdane, M., and Buée, L. (2006). Alzheimer's disease-like tau neu- ropathology leads to memory deficits and loss of functional synapses in a novel mutated tau transgenic mouse without any motor deficits. *Am. J. Pathol.* 169, 599–616.

Sweeney, J. E., Höhmann, C. F., Moran, T. H., and Coyle, J. T. (1988). A long-acting cholinesterase inhibitor reverses spatial memory deficits in mice. *Pharmacol. Biochem. Behav.* 31, 141–147.

Trinchese, F., Liu, S., Battaglia, F., Walter, S., Mathews, P. M., and Arancio, O. (2004). Progressive age- related development of Alzheimer- like pathology in APP/PS1 mice. *Ann. Neurol.* 55, 801–814.

Van Dam, D., Abramowski, D., Staufenbiel, M., and De Deyn, P. P. (2005). Symptomatic effect of donepezil, rivastigmine, galan- tamine and memantine on cognitive deficits in the APP23 model. *Psychopharmacology (Berl.)* 180, 177–190.

Van Dam, D., Coen, K., and De Deyn, P. P. (2008). Cognitive evaluation of disease-modifying efficacy of donepezil in the APP23 mouse model for Alzheimer's disease. *Psychopharmacology (Berl.)* 197, 37–43.

Van Dam, D., D'Hooge, R., Staufenbiel, M., Van Ginneken, C., Van Meir, F., and De Deyn, P. P. (2003). Age-dependent cognitive decline in the APP23 model precedes amy- loid deposition. *Eur. J. Neurosci.* 17, 388–396.

Westerman, M. A., Cooper-Blacketer, D., Mariash, A., Kotilinek, L., Kawarabayashi, T., Younkin, L. H., Carlson, G. A., Younkin, S. G., and Ashe, K. H. (2002). The relation- ship between Abeta and memory in the Tg2576 mouse model of Alzheimer's disease. *J. Neurosci.* 22, 1858–1867.

# 23

# Less efficient pattern separation may contribute to age-related spatial memory deficits

**Heather M. Holden[1] and Paul E. Gilbert[1,2]***

[1] Department of Psychology, San Diego State University, San Diego, CA, USA
[2] San Diego State University, University of California San Diego Joint Doctoral Program in Clinical Psychology, San Diego, CA, USA

**Edited by:**
Emma R. Wood, University of Edinburgh, UK

**Reviewed by:**
Junming Wang, University of Mississippi Medical Center, USA
Ashok Kumar, University of Florida, USA

***Correspondence:**
Paul E. Gilbert, San Diego State University, University of California San Diego Joint Doctoral Program in Clinical Psychology, 6363 Alvarado Court, Suite 103, San Diego, CA 92120, USA.
e-mail: pgilbert@sciences.sdsu.edu

Spatial memory deficits have been well-documented in older adults and may serve as an early indicator of mild cognitive impairment (MCI) or Alzheimer's disease (AD) in some individuals. Pattern separation is a critical mechanism for reducing potential interference among similar memory representations to enhance memory accuracy. A small but growing literature indicates that spatial pattern separation may become less efficient as a result of normal aging, possibly due to age-related changes in subregions of the hippocampus. This decreased efficiency in spatial pattern separation may be a critical processing deficit that could be a contributing factor to spatial memory deficits and episodic memory impairment associated with aging. The present paper will review recently published studies in humans, non-human primates, and rodents that have examined age-related changes in spatial pattern separation. The potential basic science, translational, and clinical implications from these studies are discussed to illustrate the need for future research to further examine the relationship between spatial pattern separation and brain changes associated with aging and neurodegenerative disease.

**Keywords: hippocampus, dentate gyrus, aging, spatial memory, interference, pattern separation**

## SPATIAL MEMORY DECLINE IN AGING

In the United States, Alzheimer's disease (AD) is the most common cause of dementia in older adults and accounts for 60–80% of dementia cases (Alzheimer's Association, 2012). In the year 2012, an estimated 5.4 million Americans will be diagnosed with AD, however, this number is projected to increase to 11–16 million by 2050 (Alzheimer's Association, 2012). As a result of the aging "baby boom" generation and increasing longevity in the US population, the disease is a growing public health concern with costs estimated to reach $200 billion in 2012. Although a number of risk factors for AD have been discussed (e.g., diagnosis of mild cognitive impairment (MCI), family history of AD, apolipoprotein epsilon E4 allele), one of the most well-documented risk factors for the disease is increasing age (Kamboh, 2004). Therefore, a major aim of recent research has focused on identifying early indicators of cognitive dysfunction in older adults.

A variety of cognitive functions may be affected in older adults, however, one of the most commonly reported deficits associated with aging is memory loss. Although not all memory domains are equally affected by aging (e.g., source vs. item memory), some domains such as spatial memory appear to be particularly sensitive to age-related change. Age-related spatial memory decline has been well-documented in both humans (reviewed by Iachini et al., 2009) and animal models (reviewed by Sharma et al., 2010). Spatial memory deficits also have been well-documented in older adults diagnosed with AD (Sahakian et al., 1988; Kessels et al., 2005) or mild cognitive impairment (MCI: Alescio-Lautier et al., 2007; deIpolyi et al., 2007; Hort et al., 2007). Some evidence suggests that spatial memory deficits even may serve as an early indicator of AD (Buccione et al., 2007; deIpolyi et al., 2007; Hort et al., 2007). Age-related spatial memory deficits may result from changes in a variety of brain regions including the hippocampus, temporal lobes, and the frontal-parietal network (Iachini et al., 2009). In particular, spatial memory decline associated with aging has been suggested to result from age-related changes in the hippocampus across species (reviewed by Barnes, 1988). However, it is only recently that studies have begun to examine how age-related changes in particular subregions of the hippocampus may affect specific mnemonic processes. One such process is spatial pattern separation, a mechanism that may be essential for the accurate formation and retrieval of spatial memories. Less efficient spatial pattern separation in older humans and animals may contribute to impairments in spatial memory, particularly in situations when spatial interference is high.

## PATTERN SEPARATION

Pattern separation is a mechanism for separating partially overlapping patterns of activation so that one pattern may be retrieved as separate from other similar patterns. A pattern separation mechanism may be critical for reducing potential interference among similar memory representations to enhance memory accuracy (Gilbert and Brushfield, 2009). A number of models have suggested that the hippocampus supports pattern separation (Marr, 1971; McNaughton and Nadel, 1990; O'Reilly and McClelland, 1994; Shapiro and Olton, 1994; Rolls and Kesner, 2006; Kesner, 2007; Myers and Scharfman, 2009; Rolls, 2010). In particular, the dentate gyrus (DG) and CA3 subregions of the hippocampus have been shown to play a critical role in pattern separation in animal models using electrophysiological methods (McNaughton et al., 1989; Tanila, 1999; Leutgeb et al., 2007), neurotoxin-induced lesions (Gilbert et al., 2001; Lee et al., 2005; Gilbert and Kesner, 2006; Goodrich-Hunsaker et al., 2008; McTighe et al., 2009; Morris et al., 2012), and genetic manipulations (Kubik et al., 2007; McHugh et al., 2007). In addition, studies using high-resolution functional magnetic resonance imaging (fMRI) have shown that the human hippocampus (Kirwan and Stark, 2007), and specifically the DG/CA3 subregions (Bakker et al., 2008; Lacy et al., 2011), are active during pattern separation tasks (also see reviews by Carr et al., 2010; Yassa and Stark, 2011b).

## AGE-RELATED CHANGES IN THE BRAIN

Aging has been shown to result in gray matter and white matter changes in a variety of brain regions (Allen et al., 2005; Ziegler et al., 2008; Driscoll et al., 2009; Kennedy and Raz, 2009), including the hippocampus (Good et al., 2001; Allen et al., 2005; Driscoll and Sutherland, 2005; Raz et al., 2005; Walhovd et al., 2010). Longitudinal studies have reported that non-demented older adults show decreased volume in the hippocampus and parahippocampal cortices (Driscoll et al., 2009). However, hippocampal volume has been reported to decrease at a faster rate than other medial temporal lobe structures (Raz et al., 2004). Longitudinal changes in hippocampal volume have been shown to be the primary determinant of memory decline (Mungas et al., 2005; Kramer et al., 2007). fMRI signal intensity has been shown to decline in all hippocampal subregions in older adults (Small et al., 2002). However, the DG subregion may be particularly susceptible to age-related changes in both humans (Small et al., 2002) and animal models (Small et al., 2004; Patrylo and Williamson, 2007). In addition, significant age-related changes have been documented in the perforant pathway in both humans (Yassa et al., 2011a) and animal models (Geinisman et al., 1992). This diminished input from the entorhinal cortex to the DG also may impact connections to the CA3 subregion and this reduction in connectivity was shown to reliably predict spatial learning deficits in old rats (Smith et al., 2000).

## PATTERN SEPARATION AND AGING

There is a small but growing literature suggesting that pattern separation may be adversely affected by aging. Wilson et al. (2006) proposed a model to account for age-related susceptibility to interference. This model suggests that age-related changes in the DG subregion of the hippocampus may result in less efficient pattern separation due to an impaired ability to reduce similarity among new input patterns. Furthermore, age-related changes in the hippocampus strengthen the autoassociative network of the CA3 subregion that supports pattern completion, a mechanism that allows a complete representation of stored information to be retrieved using partial cues. These age-related changes may cause the CA3 subregion of the hippocampus to become entrenched in pattern completion at the expense of processing new information and pattern separation. As further evidence for this hypothesis, a recent study by Yassa et al. (2011a) reported that reduced pattern separation activity in the DG/CA3 regions of aged humans was linked to structural changes in the perforant pathway. The changes were suggested to weaken the processing of novel information while strengthening the processing of stored information. Shing et al. (2011) report that increased false alarm rates in older adults when performing an episodic memory task may be linked to CA3–4/DG volume, which may reflect individual age-related differences in maintaining a pattern separation-pattern completion equilibrium.

Given the well-documented role of the DG in supporting pattern separation and the potential susceptibility of this region to age-related change, recent behavioral studies have begun to examine pattern separation in older humans. Using a continuous recognition paradigm developed by Kirwan and Stark (2007), Toner et al. (2009) reported that non-demented older adults are impaired on a pattern separation task for visual object information. A subsequent fMRI study supported these findings and additionally demonstrated increased age-related activity in the DG and CA3 subregions when pattern separation demands were high on a visual object task (Yassa et al., 2010a).

## SPATIAL PATTERN SEPARATION IN OLDER HUMANS

Recent studies also have begun to examine spatial pattern separation deficits in older adults. A study by Stark et al. (2010) reported that spatial pattern separation is impaired in a subset of older adults. Participants studied unique pairs of pictures and later were asked to identify whether the pictures were both in the same location as before or whether one of the pictures was in a different location. In the *same* condition, neither of the pictures in a pair was moved. In the three *different* conditions (close, medium, far) the location of one of the pictures in a pair was moved by varying both the distance and the angle from the original location. Older adults were separated into an *aged impaired* group and *aged unimpaired* group, based on standardized word learning task performance. Analyses revealed performance deficits on the *close, medium,* and *far* trials for the *aged impaired* group relative to both the *aged unimpaired* and young groups. Therefore, the findings suggest that spatial pattern separation may be impaired in a subset of older adults.

A subsequent study by Holden et al. (2012) examined the ability of cognitively normal young and older adults to perform a spatial memory task involving varying degrees of spatial interference to assess spatial pattern separation. During the sample phase of each trial, a circle appeared briefly on a computer screen. The participant was instructed to remember the location of the circle. During the choice phase, two circles were displayed simultaneously and the participant was asked to indicate which circle was in the same location as the sample phase circle. The two choice phase circles were separated by one of four possible spatial separations across trials: 0, 0.5, 1.0, and 1.5 cm. Smaller separations are likely to create increased overlap among memory representations, which may result in heightened interference and a greater need for pattern separation. Consistent with this hypothesis, the performance of both young and older adults increased as a function of increased spatial separation. However, young adults outperformed older adults, suggesting that spatial pattern separation may be less efficient in older adults. In an attempt to replicate the findings of Stark et al. (2010), the older adult group was separated into *older impaired* and *older unimpaired* groups based on performance on a standardized delayed word recall measure. Consistent with Stark et al. (2010), the *older impaired* group was significantly impaired relative to both the *older unimpaired* and young groups.

## SPATIAL PATTERN SEPARATION IN OLDER ANIMALS

Kubo-Kawai and Kawai (2007) conducted a study in aged monkeys that is similar in nature to the two aforementioned studies conducted in older humans. This study tested young and older monkeys on a delay non-match-to-position task involving manipulations of the spatial distance between two locations. During the sample phase, a plate was positioned to cover a baited food well along a single row of four food wells. The animal displaced the plate to receive a reward. During the choice phase, an identical plate was positioned to cover the unbaited sample phase well (incorrect choice) and a second identical plate was positioned to cover a different baited food well in one of the three remaining locations (correct choice). The distance between the two choice phase plates was manipulated across trials and included separations of 12, 24, and 36 cm. The data showed that the ability of both young and older monkeys to choose the correct plate improved as a function of increased spatial separation between the two plates during the choice phase. However, no age-related differences in performance were detected across separations. In a second experiment, the sample phase followed the same procedure described for the previous experiment. However, on the choice phase, two rows of food wells were used. The plate covering the unbaited sample phase food well (incorrect choice) was located on one row, whereas the plate covering the new location was positioned to cover a baited food well (correct choice) on a different row of wells. Spatial separations of 15, 25.6, and 37.1 cm were used to separate the plates across choice phase trials. The data revealed that older monkeys were impaired relative to young monkeys across all three separations, with the largest group differences found on trials involving the closest 15 cm separation. One could speculate that smaller separations were likely to create increased overlap among memory representations, which may result in heightened interference and a greater need for pattern separation. Although this study was not designed or interpreted by the authors to assess pattern separation, these findings in aged monkeys are in accordance with the findings from the studies involving older humans.

A recent study from our lab (Gracian et al., unpublished observations) provides further behavioral evidence that spatial pattern separation may be impaired in aged animals. Young and old rats were trained on a radial eight-arm maze to discriminate between a rewarded arm and a non-rewarded arm that were either adjacent to one another (high spatial interference) or separated by a distance of two arm positions (low spatial interference). Performance on this task recently was shown to be dependent on the DG hippocampal subregion (Morris et al., 2012). Gracian et al. showed that young and old rats committed similar numbers of errors in the separated condition. However, in the adjacent condition, old rats committed significantly more errors compared to young rats. The results suggest that decreased spatial pattern separation in aged rats may impair performance on the adjacent condition, which involved greater spatial interference among distal cues. However, performance increased in the separated condition when there was less overlap among distal cues and less need for pattern separation.

A recently published study by Marrone et al. (2011) provides further neurobiological insight into how age-related changes in the DG may affect pattern separation and spatial memory. In this study, young and aged rats were allowed to explore either: (1) the same environment on two occasions or (2) one environment followed by a different environment. A marker of cellular activity (zif268/egr1) was used to examine granule cell activity during exploration of the environments. Older animals were found to recruit distinct populations of granule cells during exploration of the same environment on two different occasions, which the authors interpret to be an indication of greater pattern separation. However, when the aged animals visited different environments, the reliability of repeated zif268 expression in young and aged animals was comparable, thus the age-related increase in pattern separation was no longer apparent. The study also found that increased pattern separation in the similar contexts was correlated with a reduced ability of older animals to disambiguate similar contexts during a sequential spatial recognition task. The authors conclude that spatial memory performance in aged animals is most impaired in situations where interference is increased, presumably due to decreased pattern separation. Collectively, the aforementioned studies offer evidence that spatial pattern separation may become less efficient as a result of aging.

## IMPLICATIONS

Age-related memory decline has been suggested to stem from subregion-specific epigenetic and transcriptional changes in the hippocampus (Penner et al., 2010). For example, neurogenesis is reduced in aged animals (Kuhn et al., 1996) and is related to decreased hippocampal volume and impaired performance on hippocampal-dependent tasks (Driscoll et al., 2006). These newborn neurons may be involved in mnemonic processes particularly dependent on the DG subregion, such as pattern separation (Clelland et al., 2009; Aimone et al., 2010, 2011; Creer et al., 2010; Deng et al., 2010; Sahay et al., 2011), whereas older DG cells may contribute to pattern completion (Nakashiba et al., 2012). Sahay et al. (2011) suggest that interventions that increase neurogenesis during adulthood may have clinical implications for reversing age-related impairments in pattern separation and associated DG dysfunction. Therefore, the development of behavioral tasks sensitive to age-related changes in spatial pattern separation may have implications for future studies of neurogenesis.

Age-related changes in spatial pattern separation also may contribute to episodic memory deficits, which have been well-documented in older adults (Rand-Giovannetti et al., 2006) and are a prominent feature of AD that may be detectable several years before disease onset (Bondi et al., 1999). Episodic memory also is impaired in non-demented older adults who are at risk for AD based on genetics (Saunders et al., 1993) or a diagnosis of MCI (Hodges et al., 2006). One key feature of episodic memory that differentiates it from other types of memory is that the elements of an episodic memory must be associated into a context to demarcate the episode in space and time. In addition, a pattern separation mechanism may be necessary to separate the elements of different episodic memories to avoid interference (Gilbert et al., 2001). It is possible that less efficient spatial pattern separation in older adults may result in poorer memory due to increased interference among the spatial components of episodic memories. The identification of a key mnemonic processing deficit in pattern separation may result in behavioral interventions that structure daily living tasks to mitigate interference in the spatial domain and potentially improve spatial and episodic memory in older adults.

Normal and pathological aging may have differential effects on hippocampal subregions. The DG subregion may be particularly susceptible to age-related changes in humans, however, there may be less impact on pyramidal cells in the CA subregions (Small et al., 2002). In contrast, the CA subregions may be more vulnerable to pathological changes associated with AD (Braak and Braak, 1996; West et al., 2000; Price et al., 2001; Apostolova et al., 2010). As mentioned previously, a primary goal in AD research is to identify risk factors and preclinical markers of the disease in older adults. Given the differential effects of normal aging and AD on the various subregions of the hippocampus, tasks that are sensitive to dysfunction in particular subregions, such as measures of pattern separation, may help to differentiate between cognitive impairment associated with normal aging and pathological changes associated with AD. In support of this idea, a recent study by Yassa et al. (2010b) reported that individuals with amnestic MCI show impairments compared to healthy older adults on an object recognition memory task that taxes pattern separation. In addition, structural and functional changes were observed in the DG/CA3 hippocampal subregions of these individuals.

## CONCLUSIONS

In conclusion, spatial memory deficits have been well-documented in older adults and may serve as an early indicator of MCI or AD in some individuals. The operation of a pattern separation mechanism may be critical for reducing interference among similar memory representations to enhance memory accuracy. Evidence suggests that brain regions critical to pattern separation, including the DG and CA3 hippocampal subregions, may be particularly susceptible to adverse age-related changes. A small but growing literature indicates that spatial pattern separation may become less efficient as a result of normal aging. This decreased efficiency in pattern separation may contribute to spatial memory deficits and episodic memory impairment associated with aging. Based on the aforementioned studies, it is clear that additional research is needed to examine the relationship between spatial pattern separation and brain changes associated with aging and neurodegenerative disease.

## ACKNOWLEDGMENTS

A portion of the research reviewed in the paper was supported by a National Institutes of Health Grant (#AG034202) from the National Institute on Aging awarded to Paul E. Gilbert.

## REFERENCES

Aimone, J. B., Deng, W., and Gage, F.H. (2010). Adult neurogenesis: integrating theories and separat- ing functions. *Trends Cogn. Sci.* 14, 325–337.

Aimone, J. B., Deng, W., and Gage, F. H. (2011). Resolving new memories: a critical look at the dentate gyrus, adult neurogenesis, and pattern separation. *Neuron* 70, 589–596.

Alescio-Lautier, B., Michel, B. F., Herrera, C., Elahmadi, A., Chambon, C., Touzet, C., and Paban, V. (2007). Visual and visu- ospatial short-term memory in mild cognitive impairment and Alzheimer disease: role of attention. *Neuropsychologia* 45, 1948–1960.

Allen, J. S., Bruss, J., Brown, C. K., and Damasio, H. (2005). Normal neuroanatomical variation due to age: the major lobes and a parcellation of the temporal region. *Neurobiol. Aging* 26, 1245–1260.

Alzheimer's Association. (2012). Alzheimer's Association report: 2012 Alzheimer's disease facts and figures. *Alzheimers Dement.* 8, 131–168.

Apostolova, L. G., Hwang, K. S., Andrawis, J. P., Green, A. E., Babakchanian, S., Morra, J. H., Cummings, J. L., Toga, A. W., Trojanowski, J. Q., Shaw, L. M., Jack, C. R. Jr., Petersen, R. C., Aisen, P. S., Jagust, W. J., Koeppe, R. A., Mathis, C. A., Weiner, M. W., and Thompson, P. M., Alzheimer's Disease Neuroimaging Initiative. (2010). 3D PIB and CSF biomarker associations with hippocam- pal atrophy in ADNI subjects. *Neurobiol. Aging* 31, 1284–1303.

Bakker, A., Kirwan, C. B., Miller, M., and Stark, C. E. (2008). Pattern sep- aration in the human hippocampal CA3 and dentate gyrus. *Science* 319, 1640–1642.

Barnes, C. A. (1988). Aging and the physiology of spatial memory. *Neurobiol. Aging* 9, 563–568.

Bondi, M. W., Salmon, D. P., Galasko, D., Thomas, R. G., and Thal, L. J. (1999). Neuropsychological func- tion and apolipoprotein E geno- type in the preclinical detection of Alzheimer's disease. *Psychol. Aging* 14, 295–303.

Braak, H., and Braak, E. (1996). Development of Alzheimer-related neurofibrillary changes in the neo- cortex inversely recapitulates corti- cal myelogenesis. *Acta Neuropathol.* 92, 197–201.

Buccione, I., Perri, R., Carlesimo, G. A., Fadda, L., Serra, L., Scalmana, S., and Caltagirone, C. (2007). Cognitive and behavioural pre- dictors of progression rates in Alzheimer's disease. *Eur. J. Neurol.* 14, 440–446.

Carr, V. A., Rissman, J., and Wagner, A. D. (2010). Imaging the human medial temporal lobe with high- resolution fMRI. *Neuron* 65, 298–308.

Clelland, C. D., Choi, M., Romberg, C., Clemenson, G. D. Jr., Fragniere, A., Tyers, P., Jessberger, S., Saksida, L. M., Barker, R. A., Gage, F. H., and Bussey, T. J. (2009). A functional role for adult hippocampal neuro- genesis in spatial pattern separation. *Science* 325, 210–213.

Creer, D. J., Romberg, C., Saksida, L. M., van Praag, H., and Bussey, T. J. (2010). Running enhances spa- tial pattern separation in mice. *Proc. Natl. Acad. Sci. U.S.A.* 107, 2367–2372.

delpolyi, A. R., Rankin, K. P., Mucke, L., Miller, B. L., and Gorno-Tempini, M. L. (2007). Spatial cognition and the human navigation network in AD and MCI. *Neurology* 69, 986–997.

Deng, W., Aimone, J. B., and Gage, F. H. (2010). New neurons and new memories: how does adult hip- pocampal neurogenesis affect learn- ingand memory? *Nat. Rev. Neurosci.* 11, 339–350.

Driscoll, I., Davatzikos, C., An, Y., Wu, X., Shen, D., Kraut, M., and Resnick, S. M. (2009). Longitudinal pattern of regional brain volume change dif- ferentiates normal aging from MCI. *Neurology* 72, 1906–1913.

Driscoll, I., Howard, S. R., Monfils, M. H., Tomanek, B., Brooks, W. M., and Sutherland, R. J. (2006). The aging hippocampus: a multi-level analysisinthe rat. *Neuroscience* 139, 1173–1185.

Driscoll, I., and Sutherland, R. J. (2005). The aging hippocampus: navigating between rat and human experiments. *Rev. Neurosci.* 16, 87–121.

Geinisman, Y., deToledo-Morrell, L., Morrell, F., Persina, I. S., and Rossi, M. (1992). Age-related loss of axospinous synapses formed by two afferent systems in the rat den- tate gyrus as revealed by the unbi- ased stereological dissector tech- nique. *Hippocampus* 2, 437–444.

Gilbert, P. E., Kesner, R. P., and Lee, I. (2001). Dissociating hippocam- pal subregions: double dissociation between dentate gyrus and CA1. *Hippocampus* 11, 626–636.

Gilbert, P. E., and Brushfield, A. M. (2009). The role of the CA3 hippocampal subregion in spa- tial memory: a process oriented behavioral assessment. *Prog. Neuropsychopharmacol. Biol. Psychiatry* 33, 774–781.

Gilbert, P. E., and Kesner, R. P. (2006). The role of the dorsal CA3 hippocampal subregion in spa- tial working memory and pattern separation. *Behav. Brain Res.* 169, 142–149.

Good, C. D., Johnsrude, I. S., Ashburner, J., Henson, R. N., Friston, K. J., and Frackowiak, R. S. (2001). A voxel-based morphome- tric study of ageing in 465 normal adult human brains. *Neuroimage* 14, 21–36.

Goodrich-Hunsaker, N. J., Hunsaker, M. R., and Kesner, R. P. (2008). The interactions and dissociations of the dorsal hippocampus subre- gions: how the dentate gyrus, CA3, and CA1 process spatial informa- tion. *Behav. Neurosci.* 122, 16–26.

Hodges, J. R., Erzinclioglu, S., and Patterson, K. (2006). Evolution of cognitive deficits and conversion to dementia in patients with mild cog- nitive impairment: a very-long-term follow-up study. *Dement. Geriatr. Cogn. Disord.* 21, 380–391.

Holden, H. M., Hoebel, C., Loftis, K., and Gilbert, P. E. (2012). Spatial pattern separation in cognitively normal young and older adults. *Hippocampus*. doi: 10.1002/hipo.22017. [Epub ahead of print].

Hort, J., Laczó, J., Vyhnálek, M., Bojar, M., Bures, J., and Vlcek, K. (2007). Spatial navigation deficit in amnestic mild cognitive impair- ment. *Proc. Natl. Acad. Sci. U.S.A.* 104, 4042–4047.

Iachini, I., Iavarone, A., Senese, V. P., Ruotolo, F., and Ruggiero, G. (2009). Visuospatial memory in healthy elderly, AD and MCI: a review. *Curr. Aging Sci.* 2, 43–59.

Kamboh, M. I. (2004). Molecular genetics of late-onset Alzheimer's disease. *Ann. Hum. Genet.* 68, 381–404.

Kennedy, K. M., and Raz, N. (2009). Aging white matter and cogni- tion: differential effects of regional variations in diffusion properties on memory, executive functions, and speed. *Neuropsychologia* 47, 916–927.

Kesner, R. P. (2007). A behavioral analysis of dentate gyrus function. *Prog. Brain Res.* 163, 567–576.

Kessels, R. P., Boekhorst, S. T., and Postma, A. (2005). The contribu- tion of implicit and explicit memory to the effects of errorless learning: a comparison between young and older adults. *J. Int. Neuropsychol. Soc.* 11, 144–151.

Kirwan, C. B., and Stark, C. E. (2007). Overcoming interference: an fMRI investigation of pattern separation in the medial temporal lobe. *Learn. Mem.* 14, 625–633.

Kramer, J. H., Mungas, D., Reed, B. R., Wetzel, M. E., Burnett, M. M., Miller, B. L., Weiner, M. W., and Chui, H. C. (2007). Longitudinal MRI and cognitive change in healthy elderly. *Neuropsychology* 21, 412–418.

Kubik, S., Miyashita, T., and Guzowski, J. F. (2007). Using immediate-early genes to map hippocampal subre- gional functions. *Learn. Mem.* 14, 758–770.

Kubo-Kawai, N., and Kawai, N. (2007). Interference effects by spatial prox- imity and age-related declines in spatial memory by Japanese mon- keys (*Macaca fuscata*): deficits in the combined use of multiple spatial cues. *J. Comp. Psychol.* 121, 189–197. Kuhn, H. G., Dickinson-Anson, H., and Gage, F. H. (1996). Neurogenesis in the dentate gyrus of the adult rat: age-related decrease of neuronal progenitor proliferation. *J. Neurosci.* 16, 2027–2033.

Lacy, J. W., Yassa, M. A., Stark, S. M., Muftuler, L. T., and Stark, C. E. (2011). Distinct pattern sep- aration related transfer functions in human CA3/dentate and CA1 revealed using high-resolution fMRI and variable mnemonic similarity. *Learn. Mem.* 18, 15–18.

Lee, I., Jerman, T. S., and Kesner, R. P. (2005). Disruption of delayed memory for a sequence of spatial locations following CA1- or CA3- lesions of the dorsal hippocam- pus. *Neurobiol. Learn. Mem.* 84, 138–147.

Leutgeb, J. K., Leutgeb, S., Moser, M. B., and Moser, E. I. (2007). Pattern separation in the dentate gyrus and CA3 of the hippocampus. *Science* 315, 961–966.

Marr, D. (1971). Simple memory: a theory for archicortex. *Proc. R. Soc. Lond. B Biol. Sci.* 262, 23–81.

Marrone, D. F., Adams, A. A., and Satvat, E. (2011). Increased pat- tern separation in the aged fas- cia dentata. *Neurobiol Aging* 32, 2317.e23–e32.

McHugh, T. J., Jones, M. W., Quinn, J. J., Balthasar, N., Coppari, R., Elmquist, J. K., Lowell, B. B., Fanselow, M. S., Wilson, M. A., and Tonegawa, S. (2007). Dentate gyrus NMDA receptors mediate rapid pat- tern separation in the hippocampal network. *Science* 317, 94–99.

McNaughton, B. L., Barnes, C. A., Meltzer, J., and Sutherland, R. J. (1989). Hippocampal granule cells are necessary for nor- mal spatial learning but not for spatially-selective pyramidal cell discharge. *Exp. Brain Res.* 76, 485–496.

McNaughton, B. L., and Nadel, L. (1990). "Hebb-Marr networks and the neurobiological representation of action in space," in *Neuroscience and Connectionist Theory*, eds M. A. Gluck and D. E. Rumelhart (Hillsdale, NJ: Erlbaum), 1–63.

McTighe, S. M., Mar, A. C., Romberg, C., Bussey, T. J., and Saksida, L. M. (2009). A new touchscreen test of pattern separation: effect of hip- pocampal lesions. *Neuroreport* 20, 881–885.

Morris, A. M., Churchwell, J. C., Kesner, R. P., and Gilbert, P. E. (2012). Selective lesions of the den- tate gyrus produce disruptions in place learning for adjacent spatial locations. *Neurobiol. Learn. Mem.* 97, 326–331.

Mungas, D., Harvey, D., Reed, B. R., Jagust, W. J., DeCarli, C., Beckett, L., Mack, W. J., Kramer, J. H., Weiner, M. W., Schuff, N., and Chui, H. C. (2005). Longitudinal volumetric MRI change and rate of cognitive decline. *Neurology* 65, 565–571.

Myers, C. E., and Scharfman, H. E. (2009). A role for hilar cells in pattern separation in the dentate gyrus: a computational approach. *Hippocampus* 19, 321–337.

Nakashiba, T., Cushman, J. D., Pelkey, A., Renaudineau, S., Buhl, D. L., McHugh, T. J., Barrera, V. R., Chittajallu, R., Iwamoto, K. S., McBain, C. J., Fanselow, M. S., and Tonegawa, S. (2012). Young dentate granule cells mediate pattern sep- aration, whereas old granule cells facilitate pattern completion. *Cell* 149, 188–201.

O'Reilly, R. C., and McClelland, J. (1994). Hippocampal conjunc- tive encoding, storage, and recall: avoiding a trade-off. *Hippocampus* 4, 661–682.

Patrylo, P. R., and Williamson, A. (2007). The effects of aging on den- tate circuitry and function. *Prog. Brain Res.* 163, 679–696.

Penner, M. R., Roth, T. I., Chawla, K., Hoang, L. T., Roth, E. D., Lubin, F. D., Sweatt, J. D., Worley,

P. F., and Barnes, C. A. (2010). Age related changes in Arc transcription and DNA methylation within the hippocampus. *Neurobiol. Aging* 32, 2198–2210.

Price, J. L., Ko, A. I., Wade, M. J., Tsou, S. K., McKeel, D. W., and Morris, J. C. (2001). Neuron number in the entorhinal cortex and CA1 in preclinical Alzheimer disease. *Arch. Neurol.* 58, 1395–1402.

Rand-Giovannetti, E., Chua, E. F., Driscoll, A. E., Schacter, D. L., Albert, M. S., and Sperling, R. A. (2006). Hippocampal and neocortical activation during repetitive encoding in older persons. *Neurobiol. Aging* 27, 173–182.

Raz, N., Gunning-Dixon, F., Head, D., Rodrigue, K. M., Williamson, A., and Acker, J. D. (2004). Aging, sex- ual dimorphism, and hemispheric asymmetry of the cerebral cortex: replicability of regional differences in volume. *Neurobiol. Aging* 25, 377–396.

Raz, N., Lindenberger, U., Rodrigue, K. M., Kennedy, K. M., Head, D., Williamson, A., Dahle, C., Gerstorf, D., and Acker, J. D. (2005). Regional brain changes in aging healthy adults: general trends, individual differences and modifiers. *Cereb. Cortex* 15, 1676–1689.

Rolls, E. T. (2010). A computational theory of episodic memory forma- tion in the hippocampus. *Behav. Brain Res.* 215, 180–196.

Rolls, E. T., and Kesner, R. P. (2006). A computational theory of hippocam- pal function, and empirical tests of the theory. *Prog. Neurobiol.* 79, 1–48.

Sahakian, B. J., Morris, R. G., Evenden, J. L., Heald, A., Levy, R., Philpot, M., and Robbins, T. W. (1988). A com- parative study of visuospatial mem- ory and learning in Alzheimer-type dementia and Parkinson's disease. *Brain* 111, 695–718.

Sahay, A., Wilson, D. A., and Hen, R. (2011). Pattern separation: a com- mon function for new neurons in hippocampus and olfactory bulb. *Neuron* 70, 582–588.

Saunders, A. M., Strittmatter, W. J., Schmechel, D., George-Hyslop, P. H., Pericak-Vance, M. A., Joo, S. H., Rosi, B. L., Gusella, J. F., Crapper- MacLachlan, D. R., Alberts, M. J., Hulette, C., Crain, B., Goldgaber, D., and Roses, A. D. (1993). Association of apolipoprotein E alleles epsilon 4 with late-onset familial and spo- radic Alzheimer's disease. *Neurology* 43, 1467–1472.

Shapiro, M. L., and Olton, D. S. (1994). "Hippocampal Function and Interference," in *Memory Systems*, eds D. L. Schacter and E. Tulving (London: MIT), 141–146.

Sharma, S., Rakoczy, S., and Brown- Borg, H. (2010). Assessment of spa- tial memory in mice. *Life Sci.* 87, 521–536.

Shing, Y. L., Rodrigue, K. M., Kennedy, K. M., Fandakova, Y., Bodammer, N., Werkle-Bergner, M., Lindenberger, U., and Raz, N. (2011). Hippocampal subfield volumes: age, vascular risk, and correlation with associative mem- ory. *Front. Aging Neurosci.* 3:2. doi: 10.3389/fnagi.2011.00002

Small, S. A., Chawla, M. K., Buonocore, M., Rapp, P. R., and Barnes, C. A. (2004). Imaging correlates of brain function in monkeys and rats isolates a hippocampal subregion differentially vulnerable to aging. *Proc. Natl. Acad. Sci. U.S.A.* 101, 7181–7186.

Small, S. A., Tsai, W. Y., DeLaPaz, R., Mayeux, R., and Stern, Y. (2002). Imaging hippocampal function across the human life span: is memory decline normal or not? *Ann. Neurol.* 51, 290–295.

Smith, T. D., Adams, M. M., Gallagher, M., Morrison, J. H., and Rapp, P. R. (2000). Circuit-specific alterations in hippocampal synaptophysin immunoreactivity predict spatial learning impairment in aged rats. *J. Neurosci.* 20, 6587–6593.

Stark, S. M., Yassa, M. A., and Stark, C. E. (2010). Individual differences in spatial pattern separation per- formance associated with healthy aging in humans. *Learn. Mem.* 17, 284–288.

Tanila, H. (1999). Hippocampal place cells can develop distinct representations of two visually iden- tical environments. *Hippocampus* 9, 235–246.

Toner, C. K., Pirogovsky, E., Kirwan, C. B., and Gilbert, P. E. (2009). Visual object pattern separation deficits in nondemented older adults. *Learn. Mem.* 16, 338–342.

Walhovd, K. B., Fjell, A. M., Dale, A. M., McEvoy, L. K., Brewer, J., Karow, D. S., Salmon, D. P., and Fennema-Notestine, C., Alzheimer's Disease Neuorimaging Initiative. (2010). Multi-modal imaging predicts memory performances in normal aging and cognitive decline. *Neurobiol. Aging* 31, 1107–1112.

West, M. J., Kawas, C. H., Martin, L. J., and Troncoso, J. C. (2000). The CA1 region of the human hippocam- pus is a hot spot in Alzheimer's disease. *Ann. N.Y. Acad. Sci.* 908, 255–259.

Wilson, I. A., Gallagher, M., Eichenbaum, H., and Tanila, H. (2006). Neurocognitive aging: prior memories hinder new hippocampal encoding. *Trends Neurosci.* 29, 662–670.

Yassa, M. A., Lacy, J. W., Stark, S. M., Albert, M. S., Gallagher, M., and Stark, C. E. (2010a). Pattern separation deficits associated with increased hippocampal CA3 and dentate gyrus activity in nonde- mented older adults. *Hippocampus* 21,968–979.

Yassa, M. A., Mattfeld, A. T., Stark, S. M., and Stark, C. E. (2011a). Age-related memory deficits linked to circuit-specific disruptions in the hippocampus. *Proc. Natl. Acad. Sci. U.S.A.* 108, 8873–8878.

Yassa, M. A., Stark, S. M., Bakker, A., Albert, M. S., Gallagher, M., and Stark, C. E. (2010b). High- resolution structural and functional MRI of hippocampal CA3 and den- tate gyrus in patients with amnes- tic Mild Cognitive Impairment. *Neuroimage* 51, 1242–1252.

Yassa, M. A., and Stark, C. E. (2011b). Pattern separation in the hip- pocampus. *Trends. Neurosci.* 34, 515–525.

Ziegler, D. A., Piguet, O., Salat, D. H., Prince, K., Connally, E., and Corkin, S. (2008). Cognition in healthy aging is related to regional white matter integrity, but not cortical thickness. *Neurobiol. Aging* 31, 1912–1926.

24

# Local amplification of glucocorticoids in the aging brain and impaired spatial memory

**_Joyce L. W. Yau* and Jonathan R. Seckl_**

*Centre for Cognitive Ageing and Cognitive Epidemiology and Endocrinology Unit, Centre for Cardiovascular Science, The Queen's Medical Research Institute, University of Edinburgh, Edinburgh, UK*

***Edited by:***
*Emma R. Wood, University of Edinburgh, UK*

***Reviewed by:***
*Jacques Micheau, University of Bordeaux 1, France*
*Eric Blalock, University of Kentucky, USA*

***Correspondence:***
*Joyce L. W. Yau, Queen's Medical Research Institute, 47 Little France Crescent, Edinburgh, EH16 4TJ, UK.*
*e-mail: joyce.yau@ed.ac.uk*

The hippocampus is a prime target for glucocorticoids (GCs) and a brain structure particularly vulnerable to aging. Prolonged exposure to excess GCs compromises hippocampal electrophysiology, structure, and function. Blood GC levels tend to increase with aging and correlate with impaired spatial memory in aging rodents and humans. The magnitude of GC action within tissues depends not only on levels of steroid hormone that enter the cells from the periphery and the density of intracellular receptors but also on the local metabolism of GCs by 11β-hydroxysteroid dehydrogenases (11β-HSD). The predominant isozyme in the adult brain, 11β-HSD1, locally regenerates active GCs from inert 11-keto forms thus amplifying GC levels within specific target cells including in the hippocampus and cortex. Aging associates with elevated hippocampal and neocortical 11β-HSD1 and impaired spatial learning while deficiency of 11β-HSD1 in knockout (KO) mice prevents the emergence of cognitive decline with age. Furthermore, short-term pharmacological inhibition of 11β-HSD1 in already aged mice reverses spatial memory impairments. Here, we review research findings that support a key role for GCs with special emphasis on their intracellular regulation by 11β-HSD1 in the emergence of spatial memory deficits with aging, and discuss the use of 11β-HSD1 inhibitors as a promising novel treatment in ameliorating/improving age-related memory impairments.

**Keywords: corticosterone, cortisol, watermaze, hippocampus, 11β-HSD1, neurosteroids, CYP7B1**

## INTRODUCTION

Cognitive decline is a key feature of aging but significant impairments of learning and memory are not inevitable or strictly linked to chronological age. Marked inter-individual variability exists, ranging from almost no decline through mild impairments to frank dementia. This phenomenon has been described in several species including rodents and humans but the mechanisms underlying the individual differences remain poorly understood. One important mechanistic hypothesis is that variations in hypothalamic-pituitary-adrenal (HPA) activity and consequent exposure to glucocorticoids (GCs; cortisol in humans, corticosterone in rodents) during life may contribute to the inter-individual differences in cognitive decline in animals and humans.

The adrenal cortex synthesizes GCs and these steroid hormones are released directly into the peripheral circulation following stimulation of the HPA axis in response to external (stress) and internal (circadian) cues. Collectively, GCs released in coordination with the rapidly acting sympathetic-adrenomedullary system, help an organism respond to "stressors" or threats to homeostasis by mobilizing energy stores, suppressing nonessential physiological processes (e.g., reproduction, digestion) and initiating behavioral responses. Circulating GC levels are normally tightly regulated by negative feedback inhibition upon the HPA axis where GCs act back on the hypothalamus and pituitary glucocorticoid receptors (GRs) (to suppress CRH and ACTH production) to terminate its own release. GC feedback also occurs in higher centers such as the hippocampus and cingulate cortex.

GCs readily enter the brain, a major target for GC action (McEwen et al., 1968). Here GCs bind to classical nuclear (hormone) receptors to regulate the transcription of specific genes, either by direct binding of receptor homodimers to DNA (Datson et al., 2001) or via protein-protein interactions with other transcription factors such as fos and Jun-1 (Heck et al., 1994; Hayashi et al., 2004). Through activation of their intracellular receptors, GCs affect a wide range of processes including altering neurotransmission, electrophysiological activity, cellular metabolism, and structure, as well as neuronal division, maturation, and death.

### CORTICOSTEROID RECEPTORS

Two types of corticosteroid receptors exist, the type I high affinity mineralocorticoid receptors (MR) and type II lower affinity GRs (Reul and de Kloet, 1985). Although sharing almost identical DNA-binding domains, MR and GR can exert distinct cellular functions as the genes they bind to show little overlap (Datson et al., 2001). GRs are widely distributed throughout the brain in most neurons and glia. GRs have a lower affinity for physiological GCs and only become substantially activated as hormone levels rise following stress. MR is expressed in neurons only and has a more restricted distribution with high expression confined particularly to the hippocampus (**Figure 1**), and septum. MRs having a 10-fold higher affinity for physiological

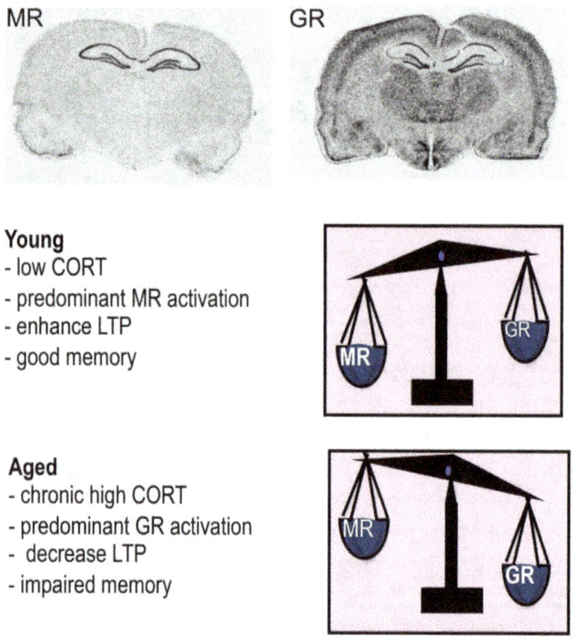


**FIGURE 1 | Mineralocorticoid receptor (MR) and glucocorticoid receptor (GR) mRNA expression in rat brain.** The high affinity MR is predominantly occupied under low corticosterone (CORT) levels typically observed in young animals under basal conditions and this leads to enhanced LTP and good memory. When CORT levels rises such as in aging, MR is fully occupied and the excess GCs now occupy more GR so the balance of receptors activated is now predominantly GR which decreases LTP and impairs memory.

corticosteroids (GCs and the mineralocorticoid aldosterone) are extensively occupied under basal conditions when hormone levels are low (Reul and de Kloet, 1985; McEwen et al., 1986).

In addition to the delayed genomic effects via intracellular MR and GR, it has become evident from recent work that GCs also affect brain function through rapid non-genomic membrane-associated mechanisms (Groeneweg et al., 2011) (**Figure 2**). The latter mode of action explains the rapid (minutes) effects of GCs on the excitability and activation of neurons in several brain regions (e.g., hypothalamus, hippocampus, amygdala, and prefrontal cortex) and provides a physiological basis for rapid effects on behavior (de Kloet et al., 2008). A membrane-localized form of MR appears to mediate the rapid GC signaling in the hippocampus (Karst et al., 2005). However, not all rapid GC effects occur via MRs with some [e.g., increase in spine density of hippocampal neurons (Komatsuzaki et al., 2005)] depending on membrane-located GRs rather than MRs and others [e.g., long-term potentiation (LTP) induction (Wiegert et al., 2006), NMDA-dependent neurotoxicity (Xiao et al., 2010)] occurring independent of MR or GR but mediated possibly through as yet unidentified membrane-localized receptors.

## BLOOD GLUCOCORTICOID LEVELS

Short term increases in GC levels are normally adaptive and beneficial but prolonged exposure to elevated GC levels such as during chronic stress or as a consequence of failure or impairment of negative feedback control of GC secretion (e.g., Cushing's syndrome, major depression) will lead to excessive GC responses and to pathology in the periphery (e.g., diabetes, hypertension, osteoporosis, central obesity) and CNS (e.g., depression, impaired learning, and memory). Cushing's syndrome patients with hyper-secretion of cortisol show reduced hippocampal volume and impaired performance on hippocampal learning tasks (Starkman et al., 1992). Notably, successful treatment to correct the excessive secretion of GCs reverses the pathology including hippocampal structural recovery and the restoration, to some extent, of mood, learning, and memory (Starkman et al., 1999). Conversely, severely reduced GC levels, as in Addison's disease, also result in pathology and cognitive impairments (Tytherleigh et al., 2004) and are treated with lifelong corticosteroid replacement. Thus both too little and too much GCs can have detrimental effects on memory, emphasizing the crucial need to maintain optimal levels of GCs for health and survival.

## GLUCOCORTICOIDS AND HIPPOCAMPUS-DEPENDENT MEMORY

GCs via binding to abundant MRs and GRs in the hippocampus control the excitability of neuronal networks that underlie learning and memory processes. While not the focus of this review, it is worth noting that other brain areas rich in GRs such as the basolateral amygdala (BLA) and prefrontal cortex, which controls emotional and working memory respectively, interacts with the hippocampus to modulate cognitive function (Roozendaal and McGaugh, 1997, 2011). An efficient interplay between activation of MR and GR appears essential for maximal learning. The two receptors have different roles in learning as evident from rodent studies, especially in the watermaze using antagonists of MR and GR at the various phases of spatial learning (Oitzl and de Kloet, 1992); MRs have a major role in behavioral reactivity toward stimuli while GRs are involved in consolidating learned information. Furthermore, the ratio of occupation and presumably activation of MR/GR appears to determine whether GCs improve or impair memory (de Kloet et al., 1999). Thus, optimal enhanced memory occurs when GC levels are mildly elevated such that most MRs and only some GRs are activated (i.e., increased MR/GR ratio) but impaired memory results when circulating GC levels are greatly increased such as found in some aging individuals (i.e., low MR/GR ratio) (Kim and Diamond, 2002; Tytherleigh et al., 2004; Herbert et al., 2006) (**Figure 1**). Indeed, circulating basal (nadir) GC levels do not always increase as a function of chronological age with only a proportion of individuals showing increasingly high GC levels with advancing age while some show levels within the young normal range (Lupien et al., 1994).

## MR AND GR ACTIVATION

Whether the consequence of the receptor activation is positive or negative for memory depend largely on the context of the situation/event to be remembered, the timing and the magnitude of the increased GC levels (de Kloet et al., 1999; Joels et al., 2006). Acute stress or increased GC levels occurring around the time of learning and within the context of the event to be remembered enhances memory consolidation. In contrast, they impair memory if occurring either before or a considerable time

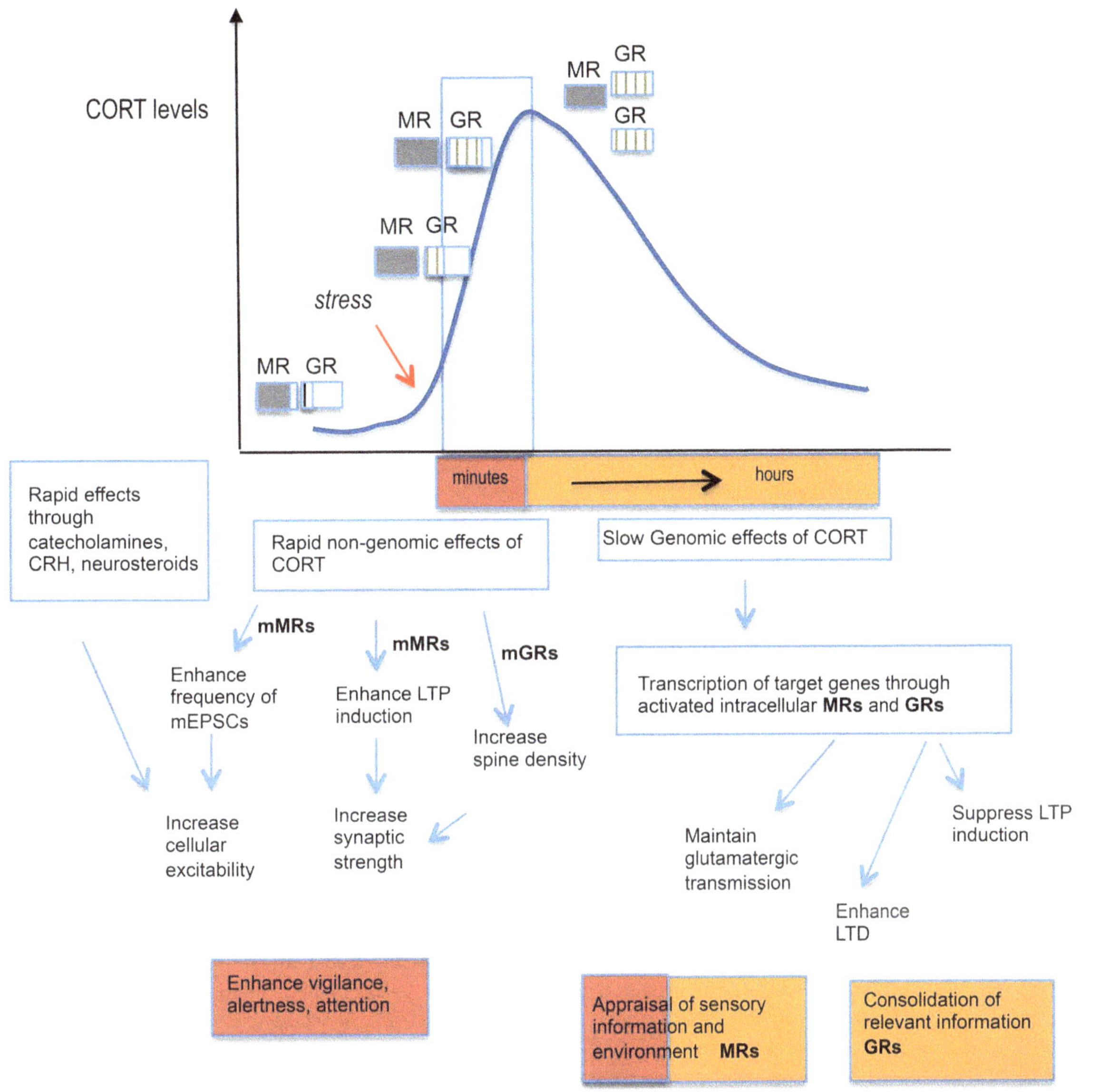


**FIGURE 2 | Schematic diagram showing stress hormone effects: from cellular responses to behavior.** Activation of the HPA axis by stress leads to a rapid rise in circulating corticosterone (CORT) levels which starts to fully occupy MR and increasingly occupy GRs. The varying level of occupancy of MRs and GRs are represented by extent of shading or lines within the boxes. The CORT levels normally return to baseline levels by 2 h through negative feedback regulation upon the HPA axis. The initial rapid effects of CORT via activation of membrane-located MRs enhance LTP induction and enhance miniature excitatory postsynaptic currents in the hippocampus while membrane-located GRs appear to increase neuronal spine density. Together with other stress hormones released such as the catecholamines (noradrenaline and adrenaline) and corticotropin-releasing hormone (CRH), which also strengthen synaptic transmission in the hippocampus, these rapid events contribute to enhanced vigilance, alertness, and attention. The slower genomic effects of CORT through activation of intracellular MRs and GRs and the transcription of target genes, leads to the maintenance of glutamatergic transmission via MRs and suppression of LTP induction but enhanced LTD via GRs in the hippocampus. MRs and GRs contributes to different aspects of cognitive processing with MR activation responsible for the appraisal of sensory information and environmental cues, while GRs are important for the consolidation of events/information in memory.

after the learning task (Quervain et al., 1998; Cazakoff et al., 2010). Evidence, mainly from animal studies, suggests that GCs preferentially enhances memory consolidation of emotionally arousing experiences (Roozendaal et al., 2006). Animal learning tasks, including the Morris watermaze and radial arm maze for spatial memory training, are designed to be generally affectively arousing because they require motivation to elicit changes in behavior. Even learning tasks that include no rewarding or aversive stimulation, such as the object recognition task, induces modest novelty-induced stress or arousal during training (Okuda et al., 2004). GCs released during learning appear essential for establishing enduring memories (De Kloet et al., 1998). Thus, small increases in GCs enhance hippocampus-mediated learning and memory while larger, prolonged elevations impair memory (Lupien and McEwen, 1997; Kim and Diamond, 2002). This follows the inverted U-shaped dose-response relationship between GC levels and effects on hippocampal LTP, an electrophysiological phenomenon associated with synaptic strengthening which is one of the major cellular mechanisms underlying learning and memory. Low moderate GC levels occupy predominantly high affinity MR which increases LTP and memory, while high GC levels occupy the lower affinity GR (in addition to MR) and impair LTP and memory (Pavlides et al., 1995, 1996; Kim and Diamond, 2002; Kim et al., 2007). One recent study supports the inverted-U-shaped relationship between intrinsic stress intensity (i.e., increased endogenous GCs induced by factors associated with the learning task, in this case water temperature) and spatial memory in the radial arm watermaze. Thus, rats trained at 19°C made fewer errors than rats trained at either more (16°C) or less (25°C) stressful conditions (Salehi et al., 2010).

### THE AGING HIPPOCAMPUS

The hippocampus not only plays a central role in the processing of spatial and contextual information (Morris et al., 1982; Moser et al., 1995) but also exerts an inhibitory influence over HPA function (Jacobson and Sapolsky, 1991). With its high density of MRs and GRs, the hippocampus is also particularly sensitive to the deleterious actions of chronic GC excess, potentiating neurotoxicity, dendritic atrophy, and perhaps even neuronal loss (Sapolsky, 1987). The idea that excess GCs could promote aging of the hippocampus was first established over 30 years ago following a study that showed a positive correlation between hippocampal aging (astrocyte reactivity as a marker of neuronal damage) and plasma levels of corticosterone in aging rats (Landfield et al., 1978). While only a few studies have shown high GC levels or stress actually cause hippocampal neuron loss (Uno et al., 1989; Sousa et al., 1998), much evidence support chronic stress (or high GCs) causing hippocampal atrophy (Watanabe et al., 1992; Magarinos and McEwen, 1995).

In humans, including those with Cushing's disease, Alzheimer's disease, depression, and normal aging, higher cortisol levels have been associated with poorer memory and hippocampal shrinkage/neuronal loss (De Leon et al., 1988; Wolkowitz et al., 1990; Newcomer et al., 1994; Mitchell and Dening, 1996; Lupien et al., 1998; Karlamangla et al., 2005; MacLullich et al., 2005). Moreover, increased HPA activity, as a consequence of impaired HPA axis negative feedback control, has been hypothesized to contribute to the decline in cognitive function, including deficits on spatial tasks with aging (Ohta, 1981; Lupien et al., 1998; McEwen et al., 1999). In support, the extent of age-related cognitive impairments in rodents and humans correlates with increased HPA activity (Issa et al., 1990; Meaney et al., 1995; Yau et al., 1995; Lupien et al., 1996, 1998). Aging rodents also show difficulty with hippocampus-dependent tasks that require a spatial mapping strategy; acquisition deficits have been reported in spatial information processing tests including Barnes hole-board task, radial arm mazes, and Morris watermaze (Ingram et al., 1981; Barnes and McNaughton, 1985; Gage et al., 1989; Issa et al., 1990; Gallagher et al., 1993; Yau et al., 1994, 1995).

### GLUCOCORTICOIDS AND OTHER BRAIN SITES

Although GCs act on the hippocampus to modulate the formation of new memories, it also acts at other sites, notably the amygdala and prefrontal cortex, which functionally interact. Thus, GC effects on hippocampal LTP and memory can be blocked by lesions to the BLA (Roozendaal and McGaugh, 1997; Kim et al., 2001) and much evidence supports a role of the BLA via emotional arousal-induced noradrenergic activation and GR actions in the modulation of memory consolidation and working memory (Roozendaal and McGaugh, 2011). Given that amygdala function is affected by aging (Iidaka et al., 2002; Charles et al., 2003), it might be expected that fear conditioning would also be disrupted with aging and hence influence hippocampal memory deficits. However, age-related impairments in spatial memory appear not to be influenced by emotional and contextual memories, which tend to be preserved with aging (Comblain et al., 2004; Gould and Feiro, 2005; May et al., 2005; Bergado et al., 2011; Broster et al., 2012).

## GLUCOCORTICOIDS AND INTER-INDIVIDUAL DIFFERENCES IN SPATIAL MEMORY

### AGED RATS

As a group, aged rats show impaired spatial learning. However, there are substantial inter-individual differences in performance (Yau et al., 1995). This increased variation in aged rats allows subdivision into categories (cognitively-unimpaired, cognitively-impaired) in the watermaze according to their latency to find the submerged platform on the last days of training relative to the mean latency of young controls (Issa et al., 1990; Tombaugh et al., 2002) or to a learning index score computed from probe trials (during retraction of the platform to the bottom of the pool during 30 s of 90 s trials) (Gallagher et al., 1993; Wilson et al., 2004; Robitsek et al., 2008). Aged rats have also been subdivided into impaired and unimpaired categories according to their spatial memory performance in a Y-maze two-trial spatial recognition task where the mean value of the percentage of visits in the novel arm of impaired rats were not different from chance values (Vallee et al., 1997). We typically find approximately ~20–25% of aged Lister hooded rat cohorts differ significantly (>2.5 SD) from young controls in the watermaze (escape latency and probe times) and another ~20–25% not significantly different (<0.5 SD) from young controls (**Figure 3**). It is the cognitively impaired groups that selectively show elevated plasma corticosterone levels (Issa et al., 1990; Yau et al., 1995), and reduced hippocampal corticosteroid receptor density (Issa et al., 1990; Yau et al., 1995) compared to both young and similarly aged cognitively unimpaired rats (Issa et al., 1990). While aged rats with watermaze performances not significantly different from young rats have been sub-classed as "cognitively unimpaired," it is important to note that they are not cognitively the same as young rats. Indeed, we found that aged Lister hooded rats, categorized as unimpaired by their performance in the conventional spatial memory watermaze task, were impaired in a more cognitively demanding delayed matching-to-place paradigm spatial memory watermaze task (Steele and Morris, 1999) when compared to young controls (Yau and Seckl, unpublished).

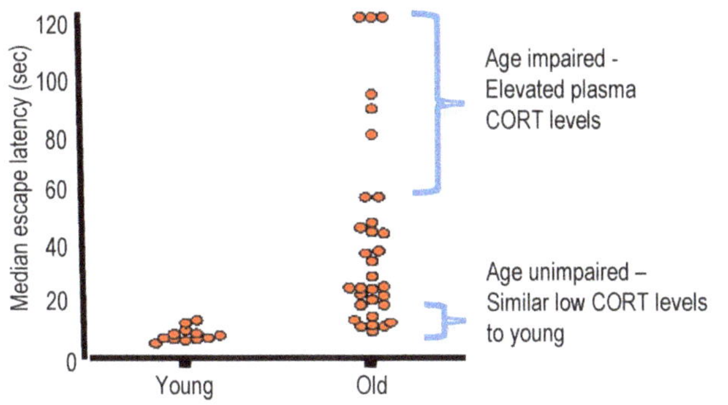


**FIGURE 3 | Aged Lister hooded rats show inter-individual differences in spatial learning in the watermaze.** 24 months old male Lister hooded rats show impaired spatial learning and memory in the watermaze as a group compared to 6 months old controls. However, individual performances taking the median of the escape latencies (4 trials/day) for the last 2 days of training shows a large spread of learning abilities for aged rats. Plasma corticosterone (CORT) levels in the aged rats correlated negatively with spatial memory with impaired aged rats showing increased CORT while unimpaired aged rats had lower CORT similar to young controls (Based on Yau et al., 1995, with permission from Elsevier).

## AGED MICE

Aged mice also show impaired spatial memory in the watermaze (Verbitsky et al., 2004; Pawlowski et al., 2009) and increased plasma CORT levels (Yau et al., 2001, 2007; Holmes et al., 2010) such that higher CORT levels correlates with impaired learning in the watermaze (Yau et al., 2001). However, in contrast to aged rats, subdividing aged mice cohorts into cognitively aged-impaired and aged-unimpaired groups is less clear-cut with large variations in performance found even in young controls (Pawlowski et al., 2009). Mice in general take longer to train in the watermaze than rats and show less consistent performance with some aged mice tending to float rather than swim. The Y-maze spatial recognition task, in contrast to the watermaze, is an ethologically relevant test based on the rodent's innate curiosity to explore novel areas and presents no negative or positive reinforcers and little stress for the rodents. When spatial memory was tested in the Y-maze using a 2 h inter-trial interval, young C57BL/6J mice can still remember the novel arm (exploring it more than the other two arms) while aged mice were overall impaired as a group (not distinguishing the novel arm between the three arms). As in the watermaze, inter-individual differences in Y-maze spatial memory performances exist in aged mice, but with a smaller percentage of aged mice "unimpaired" (<20%) while the majority were "impaired" (Yau and Seckl, unpublished).

## GLUCOCORTICOIDS AND MAINTAINENCE OF SPATIAL MEMORY WITH AGING

In rats, manipulations which keep GC levels low throughout life, such as postnatal handling during the first two weeks of life (which permanently increases hippocampal expression of GR, thus improving HPA axis negative feedback to reduce circulating GC levels), denser maternal care (licking and arched back nursing of her offspring), or adrenalectomy at middle age with low dose corticosterone replacement, prevent later hippocampal morphological changes and spatial memory deficits with aging (Landfield et al., 1981; Meaney et al., 1988). Although such manipulations are probably not clinically utilizable, they suggest that pharmacological treatments to increase GR density in the adult hippocampus may reduce GC levels long-term and ameliorate or prevent the emergence of spatial memory impairments with aging. One potent long-term regulator of MR and GR in the hippocampus is serotonin; this neurotransmitter directly increases GR in primary neuronal cultures and *in vivo* following postnatal handling of rat pups (Mitchell et al., 1990; Meaney et al., 1994; Lai et al., 2003) while lesions of the serotonergic pathway reduces hippocampal MR and GR (Yau et al., 1997). Antidepressants, which amongst other effects, increases serotonin levels, increase hippocampal GR density, improve HPA feedback regulation and thus reduce GC levels in adult rats and mice (Reul et al., 1993; Montkowski et al., 1995; Barden, 1996). Chronic (2 months) treatment of aged Lister hooded rats with amitriptyline, however, did not prevent spatial memory impairments but treatment of young (8 months) animals improved spatial memory, reduced plasma corticosterone levels, and increased hippocampal MR mRNA expression (Yau et al., 1995). Since hippocampal MR enhances LTP (Pavlides et al., 1994) and has a positive influence on memory while central MR blockade impairs spatial memory in adult rats (Yau et al., 1999), the antidepressant induced increase in hippocampal MR may, in part, underlie the better spatial memory in the young rats. Aged rats may lack the plasticity for antidepressants to be effective at enhancing memory later in life. In support, earlier treatment with antidepressants from middle age (for 6 months) improved HPA negative feedback (Rowe et al., 1997) and reduced the emergence of spatial memory impairments in a cohort of aged rats (Yau et al., 2002).

## TISSUE SELECTIVE REGULATION OF GLUCOCORTICOID EXPOSURE

While many studies have measured blood GC levels and correlated this to GC actions within tissues of interest, the principal determinant of GC action is the level of hormone inside the cell. The magnitude of intracellular GC action has long been thought to be determined by the concentration of active hormone in the circulation [modulated by hormone binding to plasma proteins, mainly corticosteroid binding globulin (CBG)] and the density of intracellular receptors in target tissues. However, during the past two decades, enzymic pre-receptor metabolism of GCs by 11β-hydroxysteroid dehydrogenases (11β-HSDs) has emerged as a key mechanism for tissue specific control of active GC levels (Seckl, 1997). 11β-HSDs are microsomal (endoplasmic reticulum) enzymes which catalyse the interconversion of active GCs (corticosterone in rodents, cortisol in humans) and inert 11-keto forms [11-dehydrocorticosterone (11-DHC), cortisone]. They thus, potently regulate steroid access to receptors within specific tissues (Seckl, 1997).

### 11β-HYDROXYSTEROID DEHYDROGENASE TYPE 1

11β-HSD1 is the predominant isoform in the adult rodent and human brain, where it is widely distributed with particularly high expression in the hippocampus, cerebellum, and cortex in both neurons and glia cells (Moisan et al., 1990; Sandeep et al., 2004). 11β-HSD2 whilst highly expressed in the fetal CNS until mid-gestation, in the adult brain is restricted to the nucleus of the solitary tract (NTS) in mice and this plus a few other scattered brain stem and diencephalic nuclei in rats. 11β-HSD2 acts as a dehydrogenase to inactivate GCs before they can bind to receptors. It is best noted for its role to exclude GCs from otherwise non-selective MRs in the distal nephron, thus allowing aldosterone selectivity. 11β-HSD1 in contrast functions as a 11β-reductase (regenerating active GCs from inert 11-DHC) in intact cells, thus locally "amplifying" GC levels within brain cells as well as in liver, adipose tissue, immune system cells etc (**Figure 4**). This direction of action, far from protecting neurons against GC excess, would be anticipated to increase local intraneuronal GC levels, potentiating their effects including toxicity. Consistent with this hypothesis, *in vitro* otherwise inert 11-DHC potentiates kainate neurotoxicity in hippocampal cells in culture, as a consequence of its conversion to active corticosterone by 11β-HSD1 expressed in the neurons, an effect lost in the presence of an 11β-HSD inhibitor (Rajan et al., 1996). The importance of such regeneration of GCs within cells *in vivo* was shown in mice homozygous for targeted disruption of the 11β-HSD1 gene (Kotelevtsev et al., 1997). 11β-HSD1 appears to be the only 11β-reductase, at least in mice, since knockout (KO) animals cannot convert 11-DHC to active corticosterone and showed evidence of reduced tissue GC actions (e.g., resist hyperglycaemia induced by obesity or stress) (Kotelevtsev et al., 1997). So are there brain effects of 11β-HSD1 deficiency?

#### 11β-HSD1 AND HPA AXIS ACTIVITY

Expression of 11β-HSD1 in brain sites (prefrontal cortex, hippocampus, hypothalamus) and pituitary that underpin negative feedback actions of GCs suggests that this enzyme may influence HPA axis activity. In order to maintain tissue GC levels in feedback sites that normally express 11β-HSD1, higher levels of plasma GCs would be predicted to result as a consequence of loss of local production of active GCs at these sites. Indeed mice lacking 11β-HSD1 on the 129/MF1 strain showed evidence of reduced HPA axis feedback sensitivity (elevated nadir levels of plasma corticosterone, enlarged adrenal glands, and exaggerated GC response to an acute stressor) (Harris et al., 2001). However,

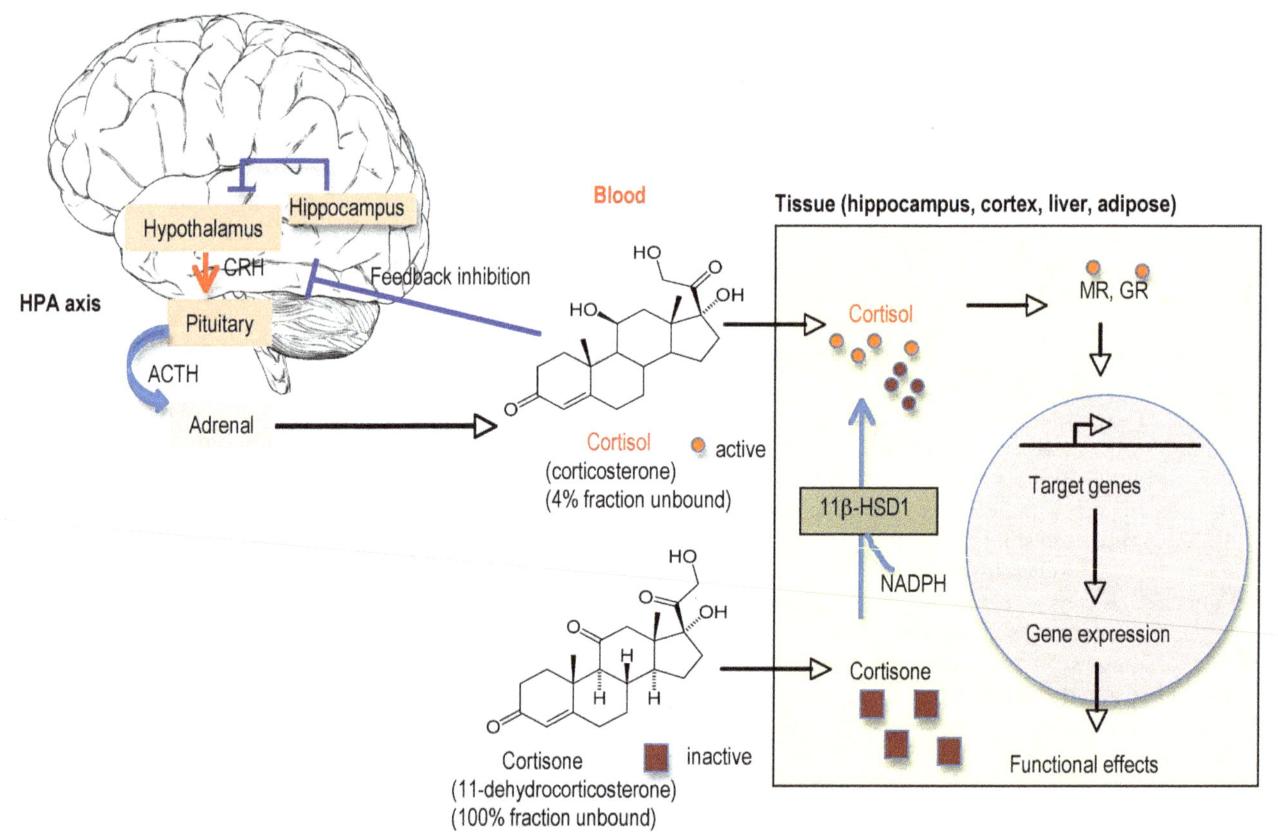


**FIGURE 4 | Regulation of glucocorticoid (GC) levels in blood and tissues.** Circulating GC levels are tightly regulated by negative feedback inhibition at the hypothalamic-pituitary-adrenal (HPA) axis. Active GCs (cortisol in humans, corticosterone in rodents) circulate mostly bound to CBG (corticosteroid binding globulin) such that only ~4% are free to enter tissues. The inactive GCs (cortisone, 11-dehydrocorticosterone) the products of 11β-HSD2 metabolism mainly in kidney, circulates unbound to plasma proteins so all are available to enter tissues. Once inside the cell, there is another level of control by the presence of 11β-HSD1 (found in specific cells in the adult brain such as in hippocampus and cortex and other tissues such as liver and adipose). 11β-HSD1 regenerates active GCs from their inactive forms thereby effectively amplifying intracellular GC levels before they bind to MR and/or GR (depending on brain region). The activated receptors then translocate into the nucleus to activate the transcription of target genes.

the effects of 11ß-HSD1 deficiency on HPA axis activity were lost when the mice were bred onto another genetic background strain. Thus, 11β-HSD1 KO mice congenic on a C57BL/6J background show normal nadir plasma corticosterone levels and efficient negative feedback regulation thought to be due to compensatory increased GR expression in the hippocampus and paraventricular nucleus of the hypothalamus (Carter et al., 2009). Activation of the HPA axis is therefore not an inevitable consequence of 11β-HSD1 deficiency or inhibition. The genetic background appears crucial in governing the HPA axis response to 11β-HSD1 deficiency or inhibition.

## IMPLICATIONS OF 11β-HSD1 FUNCTION IN THE AGING BRAIN

If 11β-HSD1 locally regenerates active GCs thus amplifying GC action within specific cells *in vivo*, this direction of enzyme activity would be anticipated to impair spatial memory in the aging brain when there is the additional contribution of increased "free" unbound GCs from the periphery in individuals with elevated blood GC levels. Indeed, a lack of the enzyme in the aged brain appears beneficial to memory processes as shown in 11β-HSD1 KO mice (Yau et al., 2001). Thus, aged 11β-HSD1 KO mice congenic on the 129 strain, despite modestly elevated plasma corticosterone levels throughout life, show ameliorated GC-related learning impairments in the watermaze (Yau et al., 2001). *This is the opposite of what would be anticipated if only circulating corticosterone levels were taken into consideration.* Hippocampal tissue corticosterone levels measured *ex-vivo* were significantly lower in aged 11β-HSD1 KO mice than aged controls (Yau et al., 2001, 2011), supporting the important role the enzyme plays in determining the levels of GCs within cells and thus their action.

### AGED 11β-HSD1 KNOCKOUT MICE

Different genetic background mouse strains can exhibit marked differences in learning and memory (Owen et al., 1997). The original 11β-HSD1 KO mice generated on the 129 Ola background learnt a cued version of a watermaze task (Yau et al., 2001), but had difficulty learning the classical task. Subsequently, aged 11β-HSD1 KO mice congenic on the C57BL/6J background, the strain of choice in many behavioral tests, also showed an improved cognitive phenotype resisting the spatial memory impairments observed in many aged control mice, this time observed in the standard reference memory watermaze and also Y-maze spatial recognition tasks (Yau et al., 2007). Even a 50% reduction in 11β-HSD1 in heterozygous 11β-HSD1 KOs is enough to prevent age-related spatial memory impairments (Sooy et al., 2010).

### INCREASED HIPPOCAMPAL 11β-HSD1 AND IMPAIRED SPATIAL MEMORY

Aged C57BL/6J mice showed increased 11β-HSD1 expression in the cortex (layer V) and CA3 cells of the hippocampus compared to young controls. Moreover, hippocampal and cortical 11β-HSD1 mRNA levels correlate with impaired spatial learning in the watermaze (Holmes et al., 2010). The selective increase of 11β-HSD1 in the CA3 subregion of the memory-impaired hippocampus may be of functional significance since it is the CA3 cells that undergo dendritic atrophy following chronic restraint stress or corticosterone injections (Magarinos and McEwen, 1995), both of which impair spatial memory (Luine et al., 1994; Conrad et al., 1996; Wright and Conrad, 2005; Hoffman et al., 2011). CA3 appears crucial for memory acquisition and consolidation in the watermaze (Florian and Roullet, 2004). Furthermore, CA3 cells selectively fail to rapidly encode new spatial information in memory-impaired aged rats (Wilson et al., 2005). This suggests that the implied increase of GC levels driven by variable overexpression of 11β-HSD1 in CA3 of aged mice may be a major contributor to the spatial memory deficits with aging. The mechanisms underlying the upregulation of 11β-HSD1 in CA3 and cortex of aged mice are unknown. GCs and stress elevate hippocampal 11β-HSD1 in young animals affording a possible feed-forward system to amplify GC action (Low et al., 1994). Consistent with increased 11β-HSD1 levels in the hippocampus impairing memory with aging, transgenic mice overexpressing 11β-HSD1 in the forebrain under the CAMIIK promoter resulting in 50% increase in the hippocampus, developed premature memory impairments with deficits in hippocampus-dependent learning tasks (watermaze spatial reference memory and passive avoidance memory) at 18 months (Holmes et al., 2010).

## HIPPOCAMPAL PLASTICITY AND AGING

### LTP AND LTD

In the absence of hippocampal neuron loss, age-related spatial learning deficits in rats may be the result of more subtle changes in synaptic structure or function (Rapp and Gallagher, 1996; Smith et al., 2000). Consistent with this idea, impaired hippocampal synaptic plasticity, specifically LTP in aged rats relates to individual differences in spatial learning ability (Deupree et al., 1991; Bach et al., 1999). Indeed, LTP induced in the CA1 region using theta-frequency stimulation (5 Hz) was selectively impaired in hippocampal slices from a subpopulation of aged rats that had previously shown poor spatial learning in the water maze (Tombaugh et al., 2002). Elevated corticosterone levels (presumably occupying both MR and GR) also impairs Primed Burst Potentiation (PBP), a low threshold form of LTP, in the hippocampal CA1 in the rat, while low levels of corticosterone (that would occupy mostly MRs) facilitates PBP (Diamond et al., 1992). Although the involvement of other hormones and/or brain regions may also play a role, high levels of corticosterone directly impairs hippocampal synaptic potentiation (Alfarez et al., 2002). In addition, induction of long-term depression (LTD), which in contrast to LTP weakens rather than strengthens synaptic contacts by repeated stimulation (Bear and Malenka, 1994), is enhanced by high corticosterone levels (Coussens et al., 1997) and during aging (Norris et al., 1996, 1998).

### PRIMED BURST POTENTIATION

Primed burst stimulation induces lower potentiation in the hippocampus of young animals compared to the LTP induction protocol (Diamond et al., 1994, 1996; Alfarez et al., 2002), but few reports have shown this reliably in aged animals (Moore et al., 1993). We found very little PBP (a single

200 Hz stimulus followed 180 ms later by a burst of four stimuli at 200 Hz) in hippocampal slices from either 25 months old 11β-HSD1 KO or age matched controls. However, LTP induced with a single 100 Hz tetanus, was increased in hippocampal slices from aged 11β-HSD1 KO mice compared to aged-matched C57BL/6J controls (Yau et al., 2007). Thus, an increase in LTP in the hippocampus of aged 11β-HSD1 KO mice may, in part, underlie their retention of spatial memory with age.

## GLUCOCORTICOIDS, NEUROGENESIS, AND AGING

Adult neurogenesis, the generation of new neurons via mitotic cell division, occurs in the dendate gyrus of the hippocampus throughout life. Although the full functional significance of these new neurons is not fully understood, there is increasing evidence to support the notion that these newborn neurons can mature, form synapses, integrate with the local circuitry, and are involved in hippocampus-dependent learning (Lemaire et al., 2012; Marin-Burgin and Schinder, 2012). Of relevance to aging, high levels of GCs or stress reduce neurogenesis (Czeh et al., 2002; Wong and Herbert, 2006). Indeed, neurogenesis is substantially reduced with aging in rodents (Seki and Arai, 1995; Kuhn et al., 1996) and this may be in part related to increased GC levels since within a cohort of aged rats, those with the highest GC levels had the lowest levels of neurogenesis (Montaron et al., 2006). Furthermore, when aged rats were subdivided into aged unimpaired and aged impaired according to their spatial learning abilities (the top and bottom 30% of the population), cell proliferation in the granule cell layer of the dentate gyrus correlated with spatial memory performances (Drapeau et al., 2003). However, when neurogenesis was examined in the aged 11β-HSD1 KO, there was no significant difference compared to aged C57BL/6J controls, although an increase in neurogenesis was observed in young 11β-HSD1 KO mice (Yau et al., 2007). This suggests that the maintained spatial memory in the aged 11β-HSD1 KO mice is not a consequence of increased neurogenesis and that reduced intrahippocampal GCs is insufficient to overcome the other factors linked with aging (e.g., decreased serotonin) that regulate neurogenesis.

## 11β-HSD1 INHIBITORS AND MAINTENANCE OF SPATIAL MEMORY WITH AGING

Since aged mice with complete or partial 11β-HSD1 deficiency throughout life are protected from spatial memory impairments (Yau et al., 2007; Sooy et al., 2010), inhibiting 11β-HSD1 activity might benefit cognitive function in the aging brain. The big question is can short-term pharmacological inhibition of 11β-HSD1 have memory-enhancing effects in aged rodents and humans? *In vivo* studies in humans are hampered by the non-selectivity of the originally available liquorice-based inhibitors. Carbenoxolone, an old drug formerly used clinically to treat peptic ulcers, inhibits both 11β-HSD1 and 11β-HSD2. This may not matter in the adult brain as the predominant isozyme is 11β-HSD1. Initial small exploratory studies, albeit randomized, double-blind, and placebo-controlled in healthy elderly men and middle-aged patients with type 2 diabetes (52–75 years) showed that carbenoxolone improved aspects of cognitive function (verbal fluency and verbal memory) after 4–6 weeks treatment (Sandeep et al., 2004). Note that amilioride was also given to prevent renal mineralocorticoid excess and hence hypertension. This gave the first indication that inhibition of 11β-HSD1 (assuming the effects were centrally mediated) may be a promising new approach to prevent/ameliorate cognitive decline in humans.

### SELECTIVE 11β-HSD1 INHIBITION

Selective 11β-HSD1 inhibitors that can cross the blood brain barrier have recently been developed (Webster et al., 2007). Two weeks peripheral treatment with a CNS active selective 11β-HSD1 inhibitor (UE1961) in aged C57BL/6J mice improved spatial memory in the Y-maze compared to vehicle treated age-matched controls (Sooy et al., 2010). Moreover, intracerebroventricular administration of another selective 11β-HSD1 inhibitor (UE2316) for 2 weeks also reversed spatial memory impairments in aged C57BL/6J mice confirming mediation by brain 11β-HSD1 inhibition (Yau et al., unpublished). Thus, spatial memory impairments in aged mice are not always a consequence of irreversible brain structural changes and the effects of the inhibitor are most likely the consequence of reduced intracellular GC levels during spatial learning and recall. Previous studies have shown that it is the consequence of increased GCs as a result of hippocampal structural changes (e.g., chronic stress-induced dendritic atrophy) impairing HPA axis feedback that has the more important influence on spatial memory performance since such impairments can be prevented on the day of testing by blocking GC synthesis (Roozendaal et al., 2001; Wright et al., 2006).

### OTHER POTENTIAL EFFECTS OF 11β-HSD1 INHIBITORS

Depending on the duration of treatment, selective 11β-HSD1 inhibitors may result in resistance of target tissues to GCs, including HPA axis regulatory centers of the brain and pituitary. This could lead to compensatory activation of the HPA axis in an attempt to compensate for the GC deficiency in negative feedback loci expressing 11β-HSD1 in a similar manner to that observed in 11β-HSD1 KO mice on the 129 genetic background (Harris et al., 2001). A hyperactive HPA axis would lead not only to excess plasma cortisol, but perhaps also to excess mineralocorticoid precursors (corticosterone and deoxycorticosterone) and androgens, all of which may manifest as unwanted side effects, such as hypertension and hirsutism/hyperandrogenization in women. The degree of HPA axis activation may depend on the genetic background of the individual, as in mice, as well as the levels of 11β-HSD1 in these tissues, which may differ under various environmental conditions (e.g., with stress, diet, aging). There is also the question of whether inhibition of 11β-HSD1 will affect other types of memory other than spatial memory in cognitively impaired aged individuals. In particular, emotional and fear associated memories, involving the basolateral amygdala, are known to be enhanced with increased GCs (Roozendaal and McGaugh, 2011). Hence, 11β-HSD1 inhibitors may compromise the strength of such memories but whether this is the case remains to be determined.

## MAINTENANCE OF SPATIAL MEMORY WITH AGING VIA PREDOMINANT MR ACTIVATION

Impaired spatial memory in aged C57BL/6J mice correlates with higher plasma GCs which are thought to activate the lower affinity GR. Indeed central blockade of GR (but not MR) for 2 weeks reversed the impaired spatial memory in aged C57BL/6J mice in the Y-maze (Yau et al., 2011). This again suggests that the impaired memory in aged C57BL/6J mice is not a direct consequence of irreversible structural changes. The improved spatial memory in aged 11β-HSD1 KO mice has been proposed to occur via reduced intracellular GC levels altering the balance of receptor activation in favor of MR activation. In support, central blockade of MR but not GR in aged 11β-HSD1 KO mice reversed their improved spatial memory phenotype such that they were now impaired in the Y-maze (Yau et al., 2011). Therefore, decreasing GR/increasing MR activation appears effective at preventing spatial memory impairments even in already aged mice. Reducing GC action by altering the receptor balance from predominant GR activation to predominant MR activation may be achieved by the use of selective 11β-HSD1 inhibitors or GR antagonists. Long-term treatment with GR antagonists in humans, however, may potentially cause compensatory activation of the HPA axis to overcome the blockade thus producing generalized GC resistance (Bamberger and Chrousos, 1995). While the use of selective 11β-HSD1 inhibitors causes compensatory activation of the HPA axis simply to accommodate the reduced regeneration of GCs, elevation of cortisol levels was not observed with carbenoxolone in elderly humans (Sandeep et al., 2004) or with selective 11β-HSD1 inhibitors in clinical trials (Rosenstock et al., 2010). Similarly, corticosterone levels were not increased in aged C57BL/6J mice treated short-term with a selective 11β-HSD1 inhibitor (Sooy et al., 2010).

### LINKS BETWEEN COGNITION AND GLUCOSE METABOLISM

GCs play a role in the regulation of peripheral glucose mobilization and metabolism. Much less is known about the effects of GCs on glucose metabolism in brain tissues. GCs inhibit glucose utilization in the hippocampus (Sapolsky, 1986). Adrenalectomy decreases serum glucose levels and increases hippocampal glucose utilization (Kadekaro et al., 1988). While exogenously administered GCs adversely affect human memory consolidation and recall (Newcomer et al., 1994), glucose improves memory performance in normal elderly individuals (Hall et al., 1989) and in subjects with probable Alzheimer's disease (Craft et al., 1993). Studies in rodents suggest that hyperglycemia and high-fat diets adversely affect hippocampal function (Kamal et al., 2000; Molteni et al., 2002). In humans, hyperglycemia associate with decline in cognitive function with aging (Convit et al., 2003). Since 11β-HSD1 KO mice lack the enzyme in all tissues, it is possible that the cognitive protection in aged 11β-HSD1 KO mice may reflect, in part, their improved metabolic profiles (Kotelevtsev et al., 1997; Morton et al., 2001), rather than solely the direct effects of enzyme deficiency in the brain. However, aged 11β-HSD1 KO mice show no significant difference in glucose tolerance compared to age-matched controls (Yau et al., 2007). Moreover, the 11β-HSD inhibitor carbenoxolone improved cognitive function in aged humans without altering plasma glucose levels (Sandeep et al., 2004). Thus, the implication is that direct CNS effects of 11β-HSD1 deficiency or inhibition are more likely responsible for the observed improved cognitive function.

## HIPPOCAMPAL GENE EXPRESSION ASSOCIATED WITH 11β-HSD1 DEFICIENCY AND MAINTENANCE OF SPATIAL MEMORY WITH AGING

To further our understanding of how GC action affects age-related memory performance, it will be important to determine the downstream genes/pathways activated by hippocampal MR and GRs that leads to the impaired and improved spatial memory of aged mice with and without 11β-HSD1. Several studies have examined hippocampal gene expression changes associated with age-related cognitive decline in rats and mice (Burger et al., 2007; Rowe et al., 2007; Pawlowski et al., 2009). Using microarrays, many hippocampal genes were found to be altered with aging regardless of cognitive status. Down-regulated genes in rat hippocampus are involved in mitochrondrial function, cell signaling, neural plasticity, and synaptic function whereas up-regulated genes underpin inflammation, glial structure, cholesterol transport, and lipid/protein degradation. Genes selectively downregulated in spatial memory impaired aged rats characterized in the watermaze and culled soon after training include a number of immediate early genes (IEGs) such as *Arc and Zif268* (also called *Egr-1* and *NGFI-A*) and glucose ultilization/insulin signaling genes such as *Irs1, GcK,* and *Insr* (Rowe et al., 2007). *Zif268,* is thought to activate the transcription of genes essential for hippocampus-dependent long-term memory (Jones et al., 2001). Reduced resting levels of *Zif268* mRNA in the CA1 hippocampal area of aged rats with impaired spatial learning have been observed by microarray analysis and in situ hybridization histochemistry (Yau et al., 1996; Blalock et al., 2003). Whether the selective alterations in gene transcription in cognitively impaired but not unimpaired aged animals is related to their HPA activity and hence circulating GC levels is not known. Hippocampal gene expression microarrays and proteomic approaches in behaviorally defined aged mice including aged 11β-HSD1 KO mice and animals given selective 11β-HSD1 inhibitors may indicate new drug targets for the enhancement of memory in the aged individual.

## NEUROSTEROIDS, CYP7B1, AND SPATIAL MEMORY WITH AGING

Recent studies have revealed additional substrates for 11β-HSD1. These include additional functions in the metabolism of neurosteroids such as dehydroepiandrosterone (DHEA) and pregnenolone, metabolism of 7-oxysterols, as well as in the detoxification of various xenobiotics (Odermatt and Nashev, 2010). Neurosteroids have long been implicated to play an important role in the modulation of spatial learning and memory processes (Vallee et al., 2001). Circulating levels of DHEA derive from the adrenal cortex and decline significantly with aging in humans and this parallels cognitive decline (Orentreich et al., 1992). In rodents there is very little DHEA in brain because they lack adrenal expression of the enzyme cyp17α that converts pregnenolone to DHEA (Le Goascogne et al., 1991) though there may be limited local CNS synthesis (Liu et al., 2009). However, high levels of its precursor pregnenolone have been measured in the hippocampus of young rats and this declines with aging correlating with spatial memory impairments (Vallee et al., 1997). Pregnenolone, DHEA, and related 3β-hydroxysteroids are 7α-hydroxylated in brain by the cytochrome P450-7B1 (CYP7B1) enzyme into their bioactive steroid metabolites (Rose et al., 1997). High levels of CYP7B1 is expressed in the hippocampus and enzyme activity is selectively decreased in aged rats with impaired spatial memory but not in aged cognitively unimpaired rats (Yau et al., 2006). In the memory-impaired aged rats, central administration of an active product, 7α-hydroxypregnenolone, reversed the spatial memory deficits and improved memory in a radial arm watermaze memory task thus effectively overcoming reduced CYP7B1 activity in the aged brain (Yau et al., 2006). It has recently been proposed that the products of CYP7B1, 7α-hydroxypregnenolone, and 7α-hydroxyDHEA, may exert anti-GC effects in target tissues by competing with 11-keto GCs for access to 11β-HSD1, thus attenuating regeneration of active GCs (Muller et al., 2006a). Thus, 11β-HSD1, in addition to its known role in reactivating GCs within target cells, has also been shown to carry out the inter-conversion of 7α-hydroxyDHEA into 7β-hydroxyDHEA, at least *in vitro* (Muller et al., 2006b) (**Figure 5**). Enzyme kinetic data from yeast-expressed human 11β-HSD1 implies that the 7-hydroxysteroid substrates are preferred to cortisone. Hence in tissues, 7-hydroxysteroid substrates may act like endogenous "inhibitors" of 11β-HSD1, reducing their regeneration of active GCs. This adds another level of potential fine tuning of GC action within specific target CNS cells but whether this occurs *in vivo* under normal or pathological conditions is not known.

## CONCLUSIONS

The local amplification of GC action in the brain by 11β-HSD1 plays a pivotal role in the emergence of spatial learning impairments with aging. Evidence over the past decade has confirmed that while elevated plasma GCs correlate with impaired spatial learning with aging, it is the level of active GCs within specific brain cells regulated by 11β-HSD1 that appears essential for the control of spatial memory in the aged animal. Importantly, whereas treatments to lower blood GC levels need to be maintained long-term to ameliorate spatial memory deficits in aged rats, lowering GC levels inside cells expressing the enzyme by selective 11β-HSD1 inhibitors requires only short-term treatment and can reverse spatial memory deficits in already aged mice. Whether this is the case in humans remains to be tested. The data also show that spatial memory deficits in aged rodents are not necessarily irreversible due to structural changes but appear to be regulated in the short-term by intracellular GC actions activating MR and GR to regulate the transcription of target genes that influence memory formation. Future investigations to determine

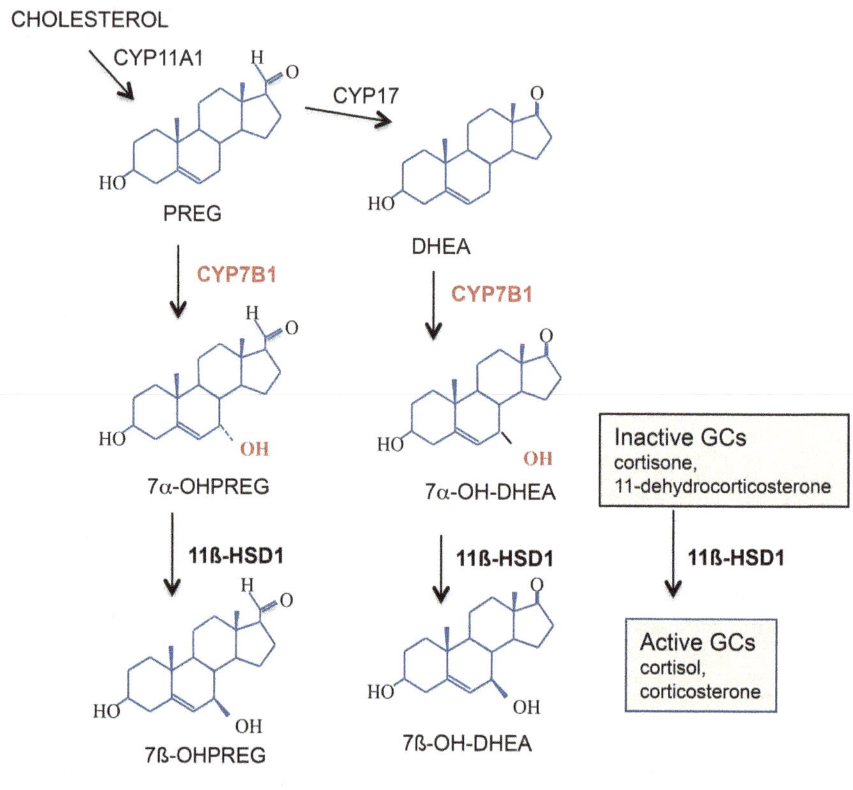


**FIGURE 5 | 7α-Hydroxylated steroids are also substrates for 11β-HSD1.** Both 11β-HSD1 and CYP7B1 are expressed in the rodent and human hippocampus. CYP7B1 7α-hydroxylates pregnenolone (PREG) and dehydroepiandrosterone (DHEA) into their more active 7α-hydroxylated metabolites which are also substrates for 11β-HSD1. If levels of these 7α-hydroxylated metabolites within specific cells become high enough, they may compete with the inactive GCs for 11β-HSD1 and effectively act as endogenous "inhibitors" of 11β-HSD1 amplification of intracellular GC action.

the mechanisms whereby 11β-HSD1 in the brain is upregulated by aging and the downstream pathways following predominant brain MR activation in aged 11β-HSD1 KO mice will be crucial in the understanding of how GCs maintain or impair hippocampus-dependent spatial learning and memory with aging. Whether or not this approach is of utility in pathological brain aging, such as Alzheimer's disease and other dementias, remains to be determined, but of substantial interest.

## ACKNOWLEDGMENTS

The authors' work was supported by project grants from The Wellcome Trust, BBSRC, MRC, and fellowships (Joyce L. W. Yau) from Alzheimer's Research UK and RCUK. The authors are members of The University of Edinburgh Centre for Cognitive Ageing and Cognitive Epidemiology, part of the cross council Lifelong Health and Wellbeing Initiative. Funding from the BBSRC, EPSRC, ESRC, and MRC is gratefully acknowledged.

## REFERENCES


Alfarez, D. N., Wiegert, O., Joels, M., and Krugers, H. J. (2002). Corticosterone and stress reduce synaptic potentiation in mouse hippocampal slices with mild stimulation. *Neuroscience* 115, 1119–1126.

Bach, M. E., Barad, M., Son, H., Zhuo, M., Lu, Y. F., Shih, R., Mansuy, I., Hawkins, R. D., and Kandel, E. R. (1999). Age-related defects in spatial memory are correlated with defects in the late phase of hippocam- pal long-term potentiation *in vitro* and are attenuated by drugs that enhance the cAMP signaling path- way. *Proc. Natl. Acad. Sci. U.S.A.* 96, 5280–5285.

Bamberger, C. M., and Chrousos, G. P. (1995). The glucocorticoid receptor and RU486 in man. *Ann. N.Y. Acad. Sci.* 761, 296–310.

Barden, N. (1996). Modulation of glucocorticoid receptor gene expression by antidepressant drugs. *Pharmacopsychiatry* 29, 12–22.

Barnes, C. A., and McNaughton, B. L. (1985). An age comparison of the rates of acquisition and forgetting of spatial information in relation to long-term enhancement of hip- pocampalsynapses. *Behav. Neurosci.* 99, 1040–1048.

Bear, M. F., and Malenka, R. C. (1994). Synaptic plasticity: LTP and LTD. *Curr. Opin. Neurobiol.* 4, 389–399.

Bergado, J. A., Almaguer, W., Rojas, Y., Capdevila, V., and Frey, J. U. (2011). Spatial and emotional mem- ory in aged rats: a behavioral- statistical analysis. *Neuroscience* 172, 256–269.

Blalock, E. M., Chen, K. C., Sharrow, K., Herman, J. P., Porter, N. M., Foster, T. C., and Landfield, P. W. (2003). Gene microarrays in hippocampal aging: statis- tical profiling identifies novel processes correlated with cogni- tive impairment. *J. Neurosci.* 23, 3807–3819.

Broster, L. S., Blonder, L. X., and Jiang, Y. (2012). Does emotional memory enhancement assist the memory- impaired? *Front. Aging Neurosci.* 4:2. doi: 10.3389/fnagi.2012.00002

Burger, C., Lopez, M. C., Feller, J. A., Baker, H. V., Muzyczka, N., and Mandel, R. J. (2007). Changes in transcription within the CA1 field of the hippocampus are asso- ciated with age-related spatial learn- ing impairments. *Neurobiol. Learn. Mem.* 87, 21–41.

Carter, R. N., Paterson, J. M., Tworowska, U., Stenvers, D. J., Mullins, J. J., Seckl, J. R., and Holmes, M. C. (2009). Hypo thalamic-pituitary-adrenal axis abnormalities in response to deletion of 11beta-HSD1 is strain- dependent. *J. Neuroendocrinol.* 21, 879–887.

Cazakoff, B. N., Johnson, K. J., and Howland, J. G. (2010). Converging effects of acute stress on spatial and recognition memory in rodents: a review of recent behavioural and pharmacological findings. *Prog. Neuropsychopharmacol. Biol. Psychiatry* 34, 733–741.

Charles, S. T., Mather, M., and Carstensen, L. L. (2003). Aging and emotional memory: the forgettable nature of negative images for older adults. *J. Exp. Psychol. Gen.* 132, 310–324.

Comblain, C., D'Argembeau, A., Van der Linden, M., and Aldenhoff, L. (2004). The effect of ageing on the recollection of emotional and neutral pictures. *Memory* 12, 673–684.

Conrad, C. D., Galea, L. A., Kuroda, Y., and McEwen, B. S. (1996). Chronic stress impairs rat spa- tial memory on the Y maze, and this effect is blocked by tianeptine pretreatment. *Behav. Neurosci.* 110, 1321–1334.

Convit, A., Wolf, O. T., Tarshish, C., and de Leon, M. J. (2003). Reduced glucose tolerance is associated with poor memory performance and hippocampal atrophy among normal elderly. *Proc. Natl. Acad. Sci. U.S.A.* 100, 2019–2022.

Coussens, C. M., Kerr, D. S., and Abraham, W. C. (1997). Glucocorticoid receptor activation lowers the threshold for NMDA- receptor-dependent homosynaptic long-term depression in the hip- pocampus through activation of voltage-dependent calcium channels. *J. Neurophysiol.* 78, 1–9.

Craft, S., Dagogo-Jack, S. E., Wiethop, B. V., Murphy, C., Nevins, R. T., Fleischman, S., Rice, V., Newcomer, J. W., and Cryer, P. E. (1993). Effects of hyperglycaemia on mem- ory and hormone levels in dementia of the Alzheimer type: a longitu- dinal study. *Behav. Neurosci.* 107, 926–940.

Czeh, B., Welt, T., Fischer, A. K., Erhardt, A., Schmitt, W., Muller, M. B., Toschi, N., Fuchs, E., and Keck, M. E. (2002). Chronic psy- chosocial stress and concomitant repetitive transcranial magnetic stimulation: effects on stress hor- mone levels and adult hippocampal neurogenesis. *Biol. Psychiatry* 52, 1057–1065.

Datson, N. A., van der Perk, J., de Kloet, E. R., and Vreugdenhil, E. (2001). Identification of corticosteroid-responsive genes in rat hippocampus using serial analysis of gene expression. *Eur. J. Neurosci.* 14, 675–689.

de Kloet, E. R., Karst, H., and Joels, M. (2008). Corticosteroid hormones in the central stress response: quick- and-slow. *Front. Neuroendocrinol.* 29, 268–272.

de Kloet, E. R., Oitzl, M. S., and Joels, M. (1999). Stress and cog- nition: are corticosteroids good or bad guys? *Trends Neurosci.* 22, 422–426.

De Kloet, E. R., Vreugdenhil, E., Oitzl, M. S., and Joels, M. (1998). Brain corticosteroid receptor balance in health and disease. *Endocr. Rev.* 19, 269–301.

De Leon, M. J., McRae, T., Tsai, J. R., George, A. E., Marcus, L., Freedman, M., Wolf, A. P., and McEwen, B. S. (1988). Abnormal cortisol response in Alzheimer's disease linked to hippocampal atrophy. *Lancet* 2, 391–392.

Deupree, D. L., Turner, D. A., and Watters, C. L. (1991). Spatial per- formance correlates with *in vitro* potentiation in young and aged Fischer 344 rats. *Brain Res.* 554, 1–9. Diamond, D. M., Bennett, M. C., Fleshner, M., and Rose, G. M. (1992). Inverted-U relationship between the level of peripheral corticosterone and the magnitude of hippocampal primed burst potentiation. *Hippocampus* 2, 421–430.

Diamond, D. M., Fleshner, M., Ingersoll, N., and Rose, G. M. (1996). Psychological stress impairs spatial working memory: relevance to electrophysiological studies of hippocampal function. *Behav. Neurosci.* 110, 661–672.

Diamond, D. M., Fleshner, M., and Rose, G. M. (1994). Psychological stress repeatedly blocks hippocam- pal primed burst potentiation in behaving rats. *Behav. Brain Res.* 62, 1–9.

Drapeau, E., Mayo, W., Aurousseau, C., Le Moal, M., Piazza, P. V., and Abrous, D. N. (2003). Spatial memory performances of aged rats in the water maze predict lev- els of hippocampal neurogenesis. *Proc. Natl. Acad. Sci. U.S.A.* 100, 14385–14390.

Florian, C., and Roullet, P. (2004). Hippocampal CA3-region is crucial for acquisition and memory con- solidation in Morris water maze task in mice. *Behav. Brain Res.* 154, 365–374.

Gage, F. H., Dunnett, S. B., and Bjorklund, A. (1989). Age-related impairments in spatial memory are independent of those in sensori- motor skills. *Neurobiol. Aging* 10, 347–352.

Gallagher, M., Burwell, R., and Burchinal, M. (1993). Severity of spatial learning impairment in aging: development of a learning index for performance in the Morris water maze. *Behav. Neurosci.* 107, 618–626.

Gould, T. J., and Feiro, O. R. (2005). Age-related deficits in the retention of memories for cued fear condi- tioning are reversed by galantamine treatment. *Behav. Brain Res.* 165, 160–171.

Groeneweg, F. L., Karst, H., de Kloet, R., and Joels, M. (2011). Rapid non-genomic effects of corticos- teroids and their role in the central stress response. *J. Endocrinol.* 209, 153–167.

Hall, J. L., Gonder-Frederick, L. A., Chewning, W. W., Silveira, J., and Gold, P. E. (1989). Glucose enhancement of performance on memory tests in young and aged humans. *Neuropsychologia* 27, 1129–1138.

Harris, H. J., Kotelevtsev, Y., Mullins, J. J., Seckl, J. R., and Holmes, M. C. (2001). Intracellular regeneration of glucocorticoids by 11ß-HSD-1 plays a key role in regulation of the HPA axis: analysis of 11ß-HSD- 1 deficient mice. *Endocrinology* 142, 114–120.

Hayashi, R., Wada, H., Ito, K., and Adcock, I. M. (2004). Effects of glu- cocorticoids on gene transcription. *Eur. J. Pharmacol.* 500, 51–62.

Heck, S., Kullmann, M., Gast, A., Ponta, H., Rahmsdorf, H. J., Herrlich, P., and Cato, A. C. (1994). A dis- tinct modulating domain in gluco- corticoid receptor monomers in the repression of activity of the tran- scription factor AP-1. *EMBO J.* 13, 4087–4095.

Herbert, J., Goodyer, I. M., Grossman, A. B., Hastings, M. H., de Kloet, E. R., Lightman, S. L., Lupien, S. J., Roozendaal, B., and Seckl, J. R. (2006). Do corticosteroids damage the brain? *J. Neuroendocrinol.* 18, 393–411.

Hoffman, A. N., Krigbaum, A., Ortiz, J. B., Mika, A., Hutchinson, K. M., Bimonte-Nelson, H. A., and Conrad, C. D. (2011). Recovery after chronic stress within spa- tial reference and working mem- ory domains: correspondence with hippocampal morphology. *Eur. J. Neurosci.* 34, 1023–1030.

Holmes, M. C., Carter, R. N., Noble, J., Chitnis, S., Dutia, A., Paterson, J. M., Mullins, J. J., Seckl, J. R., and Yau, J. L. (2010). 11beta- hydroxysteroid dehydrogenase type 1 expression is increased in the aged mouse hippocampus and parietal cortex and causes mem- ory impairments. *J. Neurosci.* 30, 6916–6920.

Iidaka, T., Okada, T., Murata, T., Omori, M., Kosaka, H., Sadato, N., and Yonekura, Y. (2002). Age- related differences in the medial temporal lobe responses to emo- tional faces as revealed by fMRI. *Hippocampus* 12, 352–362.

Ingram, D. K., London, E. D., and Goodrick, C. L. (1981). Age and neurochemical correlates of radial maze performance in rats. *Neurobiol. Aging* 2, 41–47.

Issa, A. M., Rowe, W., Gauthier, S., and Meaney, M. J. (1990). Hypo thalamic-pituitary-adrenal activity in aged, cognitively impaired and cognitively unimpaired rats. *J. Neurosci.* 10, 3247–3254.

Jacobson, L., and Sapolsky, R. (1991). The role of the hippocampus in feedback regulation of the hypo thalamic-pituitary-adrenal axis. *Endocr. Rev.* 12, 118–134.

Joels, M., Pu, Z., Wiegert, O., Oitzl, M. S., and Krugers, H. J. (2006). Learning under stress: how does it work? *Trends Cogn. Sci.* 10, 152–158.

Jones, M. W., Errington, M. L., French, P. J., Fine, A., Bliss, T. V., Garel, S., Charnay, P., Bozon, B., Laroche, S., and Davis, S. (2001). A requirement for the immediate early gene Zif268 in the expression of late LTP and long-term memories. *Nat. Neurosci.* 4, 289–296.

Kadekaro, M., Ito, M., and Gross, P. M. (1988). Local cerebral glu- cose utilization is increased in acutely adrenalectomized rats. *Neuroendocrinology* 47, 329–334.

Kamal, A., Biessels, G. J., Duis, S. E., and Gispen, W. H. (2000). Learning and hippocampal synaptic plas- ticity in streptozotocin-diabetic rats: interaction of diabetes and ageing. *Diabetologia* 43, 500–506.

Karlamangla, A. S., Singer, B. H., Chodosh, J., McEwen, B. S., and Seeman, T. E. (2005). Urinary cortisol excretion as a predictor of incident cognitive impairment. *Neurobiol. Aging* 26(Suppl. 1), 80–84.

Karst, H., Berger, S., Turiault, M., Tronche, F., Schutz, G., and Joels, M. (2005). Mineralocorticoid recep- tors are indispensable for nonge- nomic modulation of hippocampal glutamate transmission by corticos- terone. *Proc. Nat. Acad. Sci. U.S.A.* 102, 19204–19207.

Kim, J. J., and Diamond, D. M. (2002). The stressed hippocampus, synaptic plasticity and lost memories. *Nat. Rev.* 3, 453–462.

Kim, J. J., Lee, H. J., Han, J. S., and Packard, M. G. (2001). Amygdala is critical for stress-induced mod- ulation of hippocampal long-term potentiation and learning. *J. Neurosci.* 21, 5222–5228.

Kim, J. J., Lee, H. J., Welday, A. C., Song, E., Cho, J., Sharp, P. E., Jung, M. W., and Blair, H. T. (2007). Stress- induced alterations in hippocam- pal plasticity, place cells, and spatial memory. *Proc. Nat. Acad. Sci. U.S.A.* 104, 18297–18302.

Komatsuzaki, Y., Murakami, G., Tsurugizawa, T., Mukai, H., Tanabe, N., Mitsuhashi, K., Kawata, M., Kimoto, T., Ooishi, Y., and Kawato, S. (2005). Rapid spinogenesis of pyramidal neurons induced by acti- vation of glucocorticoid receptors in adult male rat hippocampus. *Biochem. Biophys. Res. Commun.* 335, 1002–1007.

Kotelevtsev, Y., Holmes, M. C., Burchell, A., Houston, P. M., Schmoll, D., Jamieson, P., Best, R., Brown, R., Edwards, C. R. W., Seckl, R., and Mullins, J. J. (1997). 11ß- Hydroxysteroid dehydrogenase type 1 knockout mice show attenuated glucocorticoid-inducible responses and resist hyperglycemia on obesity or stress. *Proc. Natl. Acad. Sci. U.S.A.* 94, 14924–14929.

Kuhn, H. G., Dickinson-Anson, H., and Gage, F. H. (1996). Neurogenesis in the dentate gyrus of the adult rat: age-related decrease of neuronal progenitor proliferation. *J. Neurosci.* 16, 2027–2033.

Lai, M., McCormick, J. A., Chapman, E., Kelly, P. A., Seckl, J. R., and Yau, J. L. (2003). Differential reg- ulation of corticosteroid receptors by monoamine neurotransmitters and antidepressant drugs in primary hippocampal culture. *Neuroscience* 118, 975–984.

Landfield, P., Waymire, J., and Lynch, G. (1978). Hippocampal aging and adrenocorticoids: a quan- titative correlation. *Science* 202, 1098–1102.

Landfield, P. W., Baskin, R. K., and Pitler, T. A. (1981). Brain aging cor- relates: retardation by hormonal- pharmacological treatments. *Science* 214, 581–584.

Le Goascogne, C., Sananes, N., Gouezou, M., Takemori, S., Kominami, S., Baulieu, E. E., and Robel, P. (1991). Immunoreactive cytochrome P-450(17 alpha) in rat and guinea-pig gonads, adrenal glands and brain. *J. Reprod. Fertil.* 93, 609–622.

Lemaire, V., Tronel, S., Montaron, M. F., Fabre, A., Dugast, E., and Abrous, D. N. (2012). Long-lasting plasticity of hippocampal adult- born neurons. *J. Neurosci.* 32, 3101–3108.

Liu, Y., Pocivavsek, A., and Papadopoulos, V. (2009). Dehydroepiandrosterone formation is independent of cytochrome P450 17alpha-hydroxylase/17, 20 lyase activity in the mouse brain. *J. Steroid Biochem. Mol. Biol.* 115, 86–90.

Low, S. C., Moisan, M.-P., Edwards, C. R. W., and Seckl, J. R. (1994). Glucocorticoids and chronic stress up-regulate 11ß-hydroxysteroid dehydrogenase activity and gene expression in the hip- pocampus. *J. Neuroendocrinol.* 6, 285–290.

Luine, V., Villegas, M., Martinez, C., and McEwen, B. S. (1994). Repeated stress causes reversible impairments of spatial memory performance. *Brain Res.* 639, 167–170.

Lupien, S., Lecours, A. R., Lussier, I., Schwartz, G., Nair, N., and Meaney, M. J. (1994). Basal cortisol- levels and cognitive deficits in human aging. *J. Neurosci.* 14, 2893–2903.

Lupien, S., Lecours, A. R., Schwartz, G., Sharma, S., Hauger, R. L., Meaney, M. J., and Nair, N. (1996). Longitudinal-study of basal cortisol-levels in healthy elderly subjects - evidence for subgroups. *Neurobiol. Aging* 17, 95–105.

Lupien, S. J., de Leon, M., de Santi, S., Convit, A., Tarshish, C., Nair, N. P. V., Thakur, M., McEwen, B. S., Hauger, R. L., and Meaney, M. J. (1998). Cortisol levels during human aging predict hippocampal atrophy and mem- ory deficits. *Nat. Neurosci.* 1, 69–73.

Lupien, S. J., and McEwen, B. S. (1997). The acute effects of corticosteroids on cognition: integration of animal and human model studies. *Brain Res. Rev.* 24, 1–27.

MacLullich, A. M., Deary, I. J., Starr, J. M., Ferguson, K. J., Wardlaw, J. M., and Seckl, J. R. (2005). Plasma cortisol levels, brain volumes and cognition in healthy elderly men. *Psychoneuroendocrinology* 30, 505–515.

Magarinos, A. M., and McEwen, B. S. (1995). Stress-induced atrophy of apical dendrites of hippocampal CA3c neurons: involvement of glu- cocorticoid secretion and excitatory amino acid receptors. *Neuroscience* 69, 89–98.

Marin-Burgin, A., and Schinder, A. F. (2012). Requirement of adult- born neurons for hippocampus- dependent learning. *Behav. Brain Res.* 227, 391–399.

May, C. P., Rahhal, T., Berry, E. M., and Leighton, E. A. (2005). Aging, source memory, and emotion. *Psychol. Aging* 20, 571–578.

McEwen, B. S., DeKloet, E. R., and Rostene, W. (1986). Adrenal steroid receptors and action in the ner- vous system. *Physiol. Rev.* 66, 1121–1188.

McEwen, B. S., de Leon, M. J., Lupien, S. J., and Meaney, M. J. (1999). Corticosteroids, the aging brain and cognition. *Trends Endocrinol. Metab.* 10, 92–96.

McEwen, B., Weiss, J., and Schwartz, L. (1968). Selective retention of corticosterone by limbic struc- tures in the rat brain. *Nature* 220, 911–912.

Meaney, M. J., Aitken, D. H., van Berkel, C., Bhatnagar, S., and Sapolsky, R. M. (1988). Effect of neonatal handling on age-related impairments associated with the hippocampus. *Science* 239, 766–768.

Meaney, M. J., Diorio, J., Francis, D., Larocque, S., Odonnell, D., Smythe, J. W., Sharma, S., and Tannenbaum, B. (1994). Environmental-regulation of the development of glucocorticoid receptor systems in the rat forebrain the role of serotonin. *Ann. N.Y. Acad. Sci.* 746, 260–274.

Meaney, M. J., Odonnell, D., Rowe, W., Tannenbaum, B., Steverman, A., Walker, M., Nair, N., and Lupien, S. (1995). Individual-differences in hypothalamic-pituitary-adrenal activity in later life and hip- pocampal aging. *Exp. Gerontol.* 30, 229–251.

Mitchell, A. J., and Dening, T. R.(1996). Depression-related cog- nitive impairment: possibilities for its pharmacological treatment. *J. Affect. Disord.* 36, 79–87. Mitchell, J. B., Rowe, W., Boksa, P., and Meaney, M. (1990). Serotonin regulates type II corticosteroid receptor binding in hippocam- pal cell cultures. *J. Neurosci.* 10, 1745–1752.

Moisan, M.-P., Seckl, J. R., and Edwards, C. R. W. (1990). 11ß-hydroxysteroid dehydrogenase bioactivity and messenger RNA expression in rat forebrain: localization in hypothalamus, hippocampus and cortex. *Endocrinology* 127, 1450–1455.

Molteni, R., Barnard, R. J., Ying, Z., Roberts, C. K., and Gomez-Pinilla, F. (2002). A high-fat, refined sugar diet reduces hippocam- pal brain-derived neurotrophic factor, neuronal plasticity, and learning. *Neuroscience* 112, 803–814.

Montaron, M. F., Drapeau, E., Dupret, D., Kitchener, P., Aurousseau, C., Le Moal, M., Piazza, P. V., and Abrous, D. N. (2006). Lifelong corticosterone level determines age-related decline in neurogenesis and memory. *Neurobiol. Aging* 27, 645–654.

Montkowski, A., Barden, N., Wotjak, C., Stec, I., Ganster, J., Meaney, M., Engelmann, M., Reul, J., Landgraf, R., and Holsboer, F. (1995). Long-term antidepressant treatment reduces behavioural deficits in transgenic mice with impaired glucocorticoid receptor function. *J. Neuroendocrinol.* 7, 841–845.

Moore, C. I., Browning, M. D., and Rose, G. M. (1993). Hippocampal plasticity induced by primed burst, but not long-term potentiation, stimulation is impaired in area CA1 of aged Fischer 344 rats. *Hippocampus* 3, 57–66.

Morris, R. G. M., Garrud, P., Rawline, J. N. P., and O'Keefe, J. (1982). Place navigation is impaired in rats with hippocampal lesions. *Nature* 297, 681–683.

Morton, N. M., Holmes, M. C., Fievet, C., Staels, B., Tailleux, A., Mullins, J. J., and Seckl, J. R. (2001). Improved lipid and lipoprotein profile, hepatic insulin sensitivity, and glucose tolerance in 11beta- hydroxysteroid dehydrogenase type 1 null mice. *J. Biol. Chem.* 276, 41293–41300.

Moser, M. B., Moser, E. I., Forrest, E., Andersen, P., and Morris, R. (1995). Spatial learning with a min- islab in the dorsal hippocampus. *Proc. Nat. Acad. Sci. U.S.A.* 92, 9697–9701.

Muller, C., Hennebert, O., and Morfin, R. (2006a). The native anti- glucocorticoid paradigm. *J. Steroid Biochem. Mol. Biol.* 100, 95–105.

Muller, C., Pompon, D., Urban, P., and Morfin, R. (2006b). Inter-conversion of 7alpha- and 7beta-hydroxy- dehydroepiandrosterone by the human 11beta-hydroxysteroid dehydrogenase type 1. *J. Steroid Biochem. Mol. Biol.* 99, 215–222.

Newcomer, J. W., Craft, S., Hershey, T., Askins, K., and Bardgett, M. E. (1994). Glucocorticoid-induced impairment in declarative mem- ory performance in adult humans. *J. Neurosci.* 14, 2047–2053.

Norris, C. M., Korol, D. L., and Foster, T. C. (1996). Increased susceptibility to induction of long-term depres- sion and long-term potentiation reversal during aging. *J. Neurosci.* 16, 5382–5392.

Norris, C. M., Halpain, S., and Foster, T. C. (1998). Reversal of age- related alterations in synaptic plasticity by blockade of L-type Ca2+ channels. *J. Neurosci.* 18, 3171–3179.

Odermatt, A., and Nashev, L. G. (2010). The glucocorticoid-activating enzyme 11beta-hydroxysteroid dehydrogenase type 1 has broad substrate specificity: physiological and toxicological considerations. *J. Steroid Biochem. Mol. Biol.* 119, 1–13.

Ohta, R. J. (1981). Spatial problem solv- ing: the response selection tenden- cies of young and elderly adults. *Exp. Aging Res.* 7, 81–84.

Oitzl, M. S., and de Kloet, E. R. (1992). Selective corticosteroid antagonists modulate specific aspects of spa- tial orientation learning. *Behav. Neurosci.* 106, 62–71.

Okuda, S., Roozendaal, B., and McGaugh, J. L. (2004). Glucocorticoid effects on object recognition memory require training-associated emotional arousal. *Proc. Nat. Acad. Sci. U.S.A.* 101, 853–858.

Orentreich, N., Brind, J. L., Vogelman, J. H., Andres, R., and Baldwin, H. (1992). Long-term longitudinal measurements of plasma dehy- droepiandrosterone sulphate in normal men. *J. Clin. Endocrinol. Metab.* 75, 1002–1004.

Owen, E. H., Logue, S. F., Rasmussen, D. L., and Wehner, J. M. (1997). Assessment of learning by the Morris water task and fear con- ditioning in inbred mouse strains and F1 hybrids: implications of genetic background for single gene mutations and quantitative trait loci analyses. *Neuroscience* 80, 1087–1099.

Pavlides, C., Kimura, A., Magarinos, A.-M., and McEwen, B. S. (1994). Type I adrenal steroid receptors prolong hippocampal long-term potentiation. *Neuroreport* 5, 2673–2677.

Pavlides, C., Ogawa, S., Kimura, A., and McEwen, B. S. (1996). Role of adrenal steroid mineralocorti- coid and glucocorticoid receptors in long-term potentiation in the CA1 field of hippocampal slices. *Brain Res.* 738, 229–235.

Pavlides, C., Watanabe, Y., Magarinos, A. M., and McEwen, B. S. (1995). Opposing roles of type I and type II adrenal steroid recep- tors in hippocampal long-term potentiation. *Neuroscience* 68, 387–394.

Pawlowski, T. L., Bellush, L. L., Wright, A. W., Walker, J. P., Colvin, R. A., and Huentelman, M. J. (2009). Hippocampal gene expression changes during age-related cog- nitive decline. *Brain Res.* 1256, 101–110.

Quervain, D. J.-F., Roozendaal, B., and McGaugh, J. L. (1998). Stress and glucocorticoids impair retrieval of long-term spatial memory. *Nature* 394, 787–790.

Rajan, V., Edwards, C. R. W., and Seckl, J. R. (1996). 11ß-hydroxysteroid dehydrogenase in cultured hip- pocampal cells reactivates inert 11-dehydrocorticosterone, potenti- ating neurotoxicity. *J. Neurosci.* 16, 65–70.

Rapp, P. R., and Gallagher, M. (1996). Preserved neuron number in the hippocampus of aged rats with spatial learning deficits. *Proc. Natl. Acad. Sci. U.S.A.* 93, 9926–9930.

Reul, J. M. H. M., and de Kloet, E. R. (1985). Two receptor systems for corticosterone in rat brain: microdissection and differential occupation. *Endocrinology* 117, 2505–2511.

Reul, J. M. H. M., Stec, I., Söder, M., and Holsboer, F. (1993). Chronic treatment of rats with the antide- pressant amitriptyline attenuates the activity of the hypothalamic- pituitary-adrenocortical system. *Endocrinology* 133, 312–320.

Robitsek, R. J., Fortin, N. J., Koh, M. T., Gallagher, M., and Eichenbaum, H. (2008). Cognitive aging: a common decline of episodic recollection and spatial memory in rats. *J. Neurosci.* 28, 8945–8954.

Roozendaal, B., and McGaugh, J. L. (1997). Basolateral amygdala lesions block the memory-enhancing effect of glucocorticoid administration in the dorsal hippocampus of rats. *Eur. J. Neurosci.* 9, 76–83.

Roozendaal, B., and McGaugh, J. L. (2011). Memory modu- lation. *Behav. Neurosci.* 125, 797–824.

Roozendaal, B., Okuda, S., Van der Zee, E. A., and McGaugh, J. L. (2006). Glucocorticoid enhancement of memory requires arousal- induced noradrenergic activation in the basolateral amygdala. *Proc. Natl. Acad. Sci. U.S.A.* 103, 6741–6746.

Roozendaal, B., Phillips, R. G., Power, A. E., Brooke, S. M., Sapolsky, R. M., and McGaugh, J. L. (2001). Memory retrieval impairment induced by hippocampal CA3 lesions is blocked by adrenocorti- cal suppression. *Nat. Neurosci.* 4, 1169–1171.

Rose, K. A., Stapleton, G., Dott, K., Kieny, M. P., Best, R., Schwarz, M., Russell, D. W., Björkhem, I., Seckl, J., and Lathe, R. (1997). Cyp7b, a novel brain cytochrome P450, catalyzes the synthesis of neurosteroids 7a-hydroxy dehy- droepiandrosterone and 7a-hydroxy pregnenolone. *Proc. Natl. Acad. Sci. U.S.A.* 94, 4925–4930.

Rosenstock, J., Banarer, S., Fonseca, V. A., Inzucchi, S. E., Sun, W., Yao, W., Hollis, G., Flores, R., Levy, R., Williams, W. V., Seckl, J. R., and Huber, R. (2010). The 11-beta-hydroxysteroid dehydroge- nase type 1 inhibitor INCB13739 improves hyperglycemia in patients with type 2 diabetes inade- quately controlled by metformin monotherapy. *Diabetes Care* 33, 1516–1522.

Rowe, W. B., Blalock, E. M., Chen, K. C., Kadish, I., Wang, D., Barrett, J. E., Thibault, O., Porter, N. M., Rose, G. M., and Landfield, P. W. (2007). Hippocampal expres- sion analyses reveal selective association of immediate-early, neuroenergetic, and myelinogenic pathways with cognitive impair- ment in aged rats. *J. Neurosci.* 27, 3098–3110.

Rowe, W., Steverman, A., Walker, M., Sharma, S., Barden, N., Seckl, J. R., and Meaney, M. J. (1997). Antidepressants restore hypothalamic-pituitary- adrenal feedback function in aged, cognitively-impaired rats. *Neurobiol. Aging* 18, 527–533.

Salehi, B., Cordero, M. I., and Sandi, C. (2010). Learning under stress: the inverted-U-shape function revisited. *Learn. Mem.* 17, 522–530.

Sandeep, T. C., Yau, J. L., MacLullich, A. M., Noble, J., Deary, I. J., Walker, B. R., and Seckl, J. R. (2004). 11Beta-hydroxysteroid dehydrogenase inhibition improves cognitive function in healthy elderly men and type 2 diabetics. *Proc. Natl. Acad. Sci. U.S.A.* 101, 6734–6739.

Sapolsky, R. M. (1986). Glucocorticoid toxicity in the hippocampus: reversal by supplementation with brain fuels. *J. Neurosci.* 2, 2240–2247.

Sapolsky, R. M. (1987). Glucocorticoids and hippocampal damage. *Trends Neurol. Sci.* 10, 346–349.

Seckl, J. R. (1997). 11ß-hydroxysteroid dehydrogenase in the brain: a novel regulator of glucocorticoid action? *Front. Neuroendocrinol.* 18, 49–99.

Seki, T., and Arai, Y. (1995). Age-related production of new granule cells in the adult dentate gyrus. *Neuroreport* 6, 2479–2482.

Smith, T. D., Adams, M. M., Gallagher, M., Morrison, J. H., and Rapp, P. R. (2000). Circuit-specific alterations in hippocampal synap- tophysin immunoreactivity predict spatial learning impairment in aged rats. *J. Neurosci.* 20, 6587–6593.

Sooy, K., Webster, S. P., Noble, J., Binnie, M., Walker, B. R., Secki, J. R., and Yau, J. L. W. (2010). Partial deficiency or short-term inhibition of 11β-hydroxysteroid dehydroge- nase type 1 improves cognitive func- tion in ageing mice. *J. Neurosci.* 30, 13867–13872.

Sousa, N., Almeida, O. F., Holsboer, F., Paula-Barbosa, M. M., and Madeira, M. D. (1998). Maintenance of hippocampal cell numbers in young and aged rats submitted to chronic unpredictable stress. Comparison with the effects of corticosterone treatment. *Stress* 2, 237–249.

Starkman, M. N., Gebarski, S. S., Berent, S., and Schteingart, D. E. (1992). Hippocampal formation volume, memory dysfunction and cortisol levels in patients with Cushing's syndrome. *Biol. Psychiatry* 32, 756–765.

Starkman, M. N., Giordani, B., Gebarski, S. S., Berent, S., Schork, M. A., and Schteingart, D. E. (1999). Decrease in cortisol reverses human hippocampal atrophy fol- lowing treatment of Cushing's disease. *Biol. Psychiatry* 46, 1595–1602.

Steele, R. J., and Morris, R. G. (1999). Delay-dependent impairment of a matching-to-place task with chronic and intrahippocampal infusion of the NMDA- antagonist D-AP5. *Hippocampus* 9, 118–136.

Tombaugh, G. C., Rowe, W. B., Chow, A. R., Michael, T. H., and Rose, G. M. (2002). Theta-frequency synaptic potentiation in CA1 *in vitro* distinguishes cognitively impaired from unimpaired aged Fischer 344 rats. *J. Neurosci.* 22, 9932–9940.

Tytherleigh, M. Y., Vedhara, K., and Lightman, S. L. (2004). Mineralocorticoid and glucocorti- coid receptors and their differential effects on memory performance in people with Addison's disease. *Psychoneuroendocrinology* 29, 712–723.

Uno, H., Tarara, R., Else, J. G., Suleman, M. A., and Sapolsky, R. M. (1989). Hippocampal damage associated with prolonged and fatal stress in primates. *J. Neurosci.* 9, 1705–1711.

Vallee, M., Mayo, W., Darnaudery, M., Corpechot, C., Young, J., Koehl, M., Le Moal, M., Baulieu, E. E., Robel, P., and Simon, H. (1997). Neurosteroids: deficient cognitive performance in aged rats depends on low pregnenolone sulfate levels in the hippocampus. *Proc. Nat. Acad. Sci. U.S.A.* 94, 14865–14870.

Vallee, M., Mayo, W., and Le Moal, M. (2001). Role of pregnenolone, dehydroepiandrosterone and their sul- fate esters on learning and memory in cognitive aging. *Brain Res. Rev.* 37, 301–312.

Verbitsky, M., Yonan, A. L., Malleret, G., Kandel, E. R., Gilliam, T. C., and Pavlidis, P. (2004). Altered hip- pocampal transcript profile accom- panies an age-related spatial mem- ory deficit in mice. *Learn. Mem.* 11, 253–260.

Watanabe, Y., Gould, E., and McEwen, B. (1992). Stress induces atrophy of apical dendrites of hippocampal CA3 pyramidal neurons. *Brain Res.* 588, 341–346.

Webster, S. P., Ward, P., Binnie, M., Craigie, E., McConnell, K. M., Sooy, K., Vinter, A., Seckl, J. R., and Walker, B. R. (2007). Discovery and biological evaluation of adamantyl amide 11beta-HSD1 inhibitors. *Bioorg. Med. Chem. Lett.* 17, 2838–2843.

Wiegert, O., Joels, M., and Krugers, H. (2006). Timing is essential for rapid effects of corticosterone on synaptic potentiation in the mouse hippocampus. *Learn. Mem.* 13, 110–113.

Wilson, I. A., Ikonen, S., Gallagher, M., Eichenbaum, H., and Tanila, H. (2005). Age-associated alterations of hippocampal place cells are sub- region specific. *J. Neurosci.* 25, 6877–6886.

Wilson, I. A., Ikonen, S., Gureviciene, I., McMahan, R. W., Gallagher, M., Eichenbaum, H., and Tanila, H. (2004). Cognitive aging and the hippocampus: how old rats represent new environments. *J. Neurosci.* 24, 3870–3878.

Wolkowitz, O. M., Reus, V. I., Weingartner, H., Thompson, K., Breier, A., Doran, A., Rubinow, D., and Pickar, D. (1990). Cognitive effects of corticosteroids. *Am. J. Psychiatry* 147, 1297–1303.

Wong, E. Y., and Herbert, J. (2006). Raised circulating corticosterone inhibits neuronal differentiation of progenitor cells in the adult hippocampus. *Neuroscience* 137, 83–92.

Wright, R. L., and Conrad, C. D. (2005). Chronic stress leaves novelty-seeking behavior intact while impairing spatial recognition memory in the Y-maze. *Stress* 8, 151–154.

Wright, R. L., Lightner, E. N., Harman, J. S., Meijer, O. C., and Conrad, C. D. (2006). Attenuating corticos- terone levels on the day of mem- ory assessment prevents chronic stress-induced impairments in spa- tial memory. *Eur. J. Neurosci.* 24, 595–605.

Xiao, L., Feng, C., and Chen, Y. (2010). Glucocorticoid rapidly enhances NMDA-evoked neurotoxicity by attenuating the NR2A-containing NMDA receptor-mediated ERK1/2 activation. *Mol. Endocrinol.* 24, 497–510.

Yau, J., Noble, J., and Seckl, J. R. (1997). Site-specific regulation of corticosteroid and serotonin receptor subtype gene expression in the rat hippocampus following 3, 4- methylenedioxymetham- phetamine: role of corticosterone and serotonin. *Neuroscience* 78, 111–121.

Yau, J., Olsson, T., Morris, R., Noble, J., and Seckl, J. R. (1996). Decreased NGFI-A gene expression in the hip- pocampus of cognitively impaired aged rats. *Mol. Brain Res.* 42, 354–357.

Yau, J. L., McNair, K. M., Noble, J., Brownstein, D., Hibberd, C., Morton, N., Mullins, J. J., Morris, R. G., Cobb, S., and Seckl, J. R. (2007). Enhanced hippocam- pal long-term potentiation and spatial learning in aged 11beta-hydroxysteroid dehydrogenase type 1 knock-out mice. *J. Neurosci.* 27, 10487–10496.

Yau, J. L., Morris, R. G., and Seckl, J. R. (1994). Hippocampal corti- costeroid receptor mRNA expres- sion and spatial learning in the aged Wistar rat. *Brain Res.* 657, 59–64.

Yau, J. L., Noble, J., Graham, M., and Seckl, J. R. (2006). Central administration of a cytochrome P450-7B product 7 alpha- hydroxypregnenolone improves spatial memory retention in cog- nitively impaired aged rats. *J. Neurosci.* 26, 11034–11040.

Yau, J. L., Noble, J., and Seckl, J. R. (1999). Continuous blockade of brain mineralocorticoid recep- tors impairs spatial learning in rats. *Neurosci. Lett.* 277, 45–48.

Yau, J. L., Noble, J., and Seckl, J. R. (2011). 11beta-hydroxysteroid dehydrogenase type 1 defi- ciency prevents memory deficits with aging by switching from glucocorticoid receptor to min- eralocorticoid receptor-mediated cognitive control. *J. Neurosci.* 31, 4188–4193.

Yau, J. L., Noble, J., Kenyon, C. J., Hibberd, C., Kotelevtsev, Y., Mullins, J. J., and Seckl, J. R. (2001). Lack of tissue glucocorticoid reac- tivation in 11beta-hydroxysteroid dehydrogenase type 1 knockout mice ameliorates age-related learning impairments. *Proc. Natl. Acad. Sci. U.S.A.* 98, 4716–4721.

Yau, J. L., Noble, J., Hibberd, C., Rowe, W. B., Meaney, M. J., Morris, R. G., and Seckl, J. R. (2002). Chronic treatment with the antidepressant amitriptyline prevents impair- ments in water maze learning in aging rats. *J. Neurosci.* 22, 1436–1442.

Yau, J. L., Olsson, T., Morris, R. G., Meaney, M. J., and Seckl, J. R. (1995). Glucocorticoids, hip- pocampal corticosteroid receptor gene expression and antide- pressant treatment: relationship with spatial learning in young and aged rats. *Neuroscience* 66, 571–581.

# 25

# Route repetition and route retracing: effects of cognitive aging

***Jan M. Wiener*, Hana Kmecova and Olivier de Condappa***

*Psychology Research Centre, Bournemouth University, Poole, UK*

**Edited by:**
*Thomas Wolbers, University of Edinburgh, UK*

**Reviewed by:**
*Denise Head, Washington University in St. Louis, USA*
*John Philbeck, The George Washington University, USA*

***Correspondence:**
*Jan M. Wiener, Psychology Research Centre, Bournemouth University, Poole House, Talbot Campus, Fern Barrow, Poole, Dorset BH12 5BB, UK.*
*e-mail: jwiener@bournemouth.ac.uk*

Retracing a recently traveled route is a frequent navigation task when learning novel routes or exploring unfamiliar environments. In the present study we utilized virtual environments technology to investigate age-related differences in repeating and retracing a learned route. In the training phase of the experiment participants were guided along a route consisting of multiple intersections each featuring one unique landmark. In the subsequent test phase, they were guided along short sections of the route and asked to indicate overall travel direction (repetition or retracing), the direction required to continue along the route, and the next landmark they would encounter. Results demonstrate age-related deficits in all three tasks. More specifically, in contrast to younger participants, the older participants had greater problems during route retracing than during route repetition. While route repetition can be solved with egocentric response or route strategies, successfully retracing a route requires allocentric processing. The age-related deficits in route retracing are discussed in the context of impaired allocentric processing and shift from allocentric to egocentric navigation strategies as a consequence of age-related hippocampal degeneration.

**Keywords: route retracing, route learning, cognitive aging, spatial memory, wayfinding**

## INTRODUCTION

Age-related differences in navigation abilities are well established both in animal and human literature (Rosenzweig and Barnes, 2003; Moffat, 2009). While age-related performance declines have been reported for different navigation tasks, they seem to be particularly pronounced in unfamiliar environments (Devlin, 2001). One navigation ability crucial for navigating unfamiliar environments is retracing—navigating a recently traveled route from the end to the start—as it enables a navigator to return to a known part of the environment (Lorenz, 1952; Miller and Eilam, 2011). Specific age-related deficits in route retracing would increase the risk of getting lost when navigating novel environments and could thus explain why older adults often report avoiding unfamiliar places and routes (Burns, 1999). While route retracing is a common navigation task, especially when exploring unfamiliar environments, it has received surprisingly little attention in the literature and it is unclear how it is accomplished. In the current study we present a novel experimental paradigm to investigate the cognitive processes and strategies involved in route learning and route retracing in more detail. Moreover, by comparing route retracing performance between a younger and older age group we investigate the effects of cognitive aging on route retracing.

Route knowledge is typically conceptualized as a series of stimulus-response associations (Trullier et al., 1997). A single stimulus-response association consists of recognizing the current place (e.g., by recognizing a landmark associated with that place) and selecting the direction in which to proceed along the route Waller and Lippa, 2007). Learning a route with multiple decision points, therefore, requires knowledge of landmarks along the routes, associations of directional information with these landmarks, and knowledge about the order of landmarks.

Note that route knowledge that takes the form of stimulus-response pairs is inherently uni-directional, allowing a route to be repeated. The stimulus-response pairs are encoded in an egocentric reference frame during learning ("Turn left at X"). During route retracing, however, the decision points are approached from a viewpoint different to that experienced before. Accordingly, the egocentric stimulus-response pairs that were encoded during route learning do not support route retracing. Route retracing requires knowledge about the spatial relationship between the direction from which a decision point is approached and the direction in which the route proceeded. Such a representation is viewpoint independent—i.e., allocentric—and would support for route retracing.

Egocentric and allocentric navigation strategies are supported by different neuronal circuits: egocentric strategies involve the parietal cortex and the caudate nucleaus, while allocentric strategies are hippocampus dependent (McDonald and White, 1994; Wolbers et al., 2004; Burgess, 2008). While cognitive aging affects egocentric strategies (Barrash, 1994; Wilkniss et al., 1997; Moffat et al., 2001; Head and Isom, 2010), allocentric strategies seem to be more severely affected (Begega et al., 2001; Moffat and Resnick, 2002). As a result, a number of studies report shifts from allocentric to egocentric strategies with increasing age (Barnes et al., 1980; Nicolle et al., 2003; Rodgers et al., 2012; Wiener et al., under review). Age-related hippocampal degeneration offers an explanation for the impaired allocentric processing and according strategy shifts (Raz et al., 2010).

In the current study we used a novel experimental paradigm to investigate the cognitive processes and strategies involved in route retracing. Specifically, we tested the hypothesis that route retracing, in contrast to route repetition, relies on allocentric processing. In the experiment, participants were navigated along a complex route with multiple decision points each featuring a unique landmark. In the subsequent test phase they were guided along sections of the route either in the direction of original travel (route repetition) or in the opposite direction (route retracing). Their tasks were, first, to indicate travel direction (route repetition or route retracing), second to indicate the direction required to continue along the route to either reach the end or the start place (depending on travel direction), and third, to identify the next landmark encountered on route if the current travel direction was maintained. Comparisons of performance in these tasks between route repetition and route retracing trials allowed for first insights into the nature of route retracing. In order to test whether route retracing in fact involves allocentric processing, we compared performance between a younger and older participant group. In line with earlier research into the effects of cognitive aging on navigation abilities (Moffat et al., 2001; Head and Isom, 2010), we expected an overall effect of age on performance in all three tasks. If route retracing—as argued above—relied on allocentric processing, we expected additional age-related performance declines for route retracing trials as compared to route repetition trials reflecting the particularly adverse effects of cognitive aging on allocentric navigation strategies (Moffat and Resnick, 2002; Iaria et al., 2009).

## MATERIALS AND METHODS

### PARTICIPANTS

Forty participants [20 younger (eight females; mean age 20.53 ± 1.84 years, range 25–30); 20 older (11 females; mean age 69.45 ± 5.48 years, range 61–85)] took part in the experiment. The montreal cognitive assessment (MoCA; Nasreddine et al., 2005) was administered to all participants to screen for mild cognitive impairment (MCI). No participant had to be excluded based on the recently recommended MoCA cut-off score for the MCI of 23 (Luis et al., 2009). The average MoCA scores for the young and old age group were 27.56 (young) and 27.65 (old).

### THE VIRTUAL ENVIRONMENT

Using Vizard 3.0 (WorldViz) we created a virtual route consisting of 11 four-way intersections (see **Figure 1**). Each intersection could be identified by a unique single landmark—an image of an object—that was mapped onto a cube suspended from the wall. During the experiment, participants were passively transported along the entire route in the training phase and along parts of the route in the test phase.

### PROCEDURE

The experiment consisted of six experimental sessions. Each experimental session was composed of a training phase and a test phase. In the training phase, participants were transported along the entire route twice. Their task was to memorize the route. The test phase consisted of 18 trials, each of which was composed of three tasks:

- **Route Direction Task.** First, participants were transported along two intersections of the original route either in the same direction as during training (route repetition, nine trials) or in the opposite direction (route retracing, nine trials). For example, in a route repetition trial they would approach the intersection with the sofa, turn left and then approach the intersection with the football where movement stopped (see **Figure 1**). Participants were asked to indicate the direction of

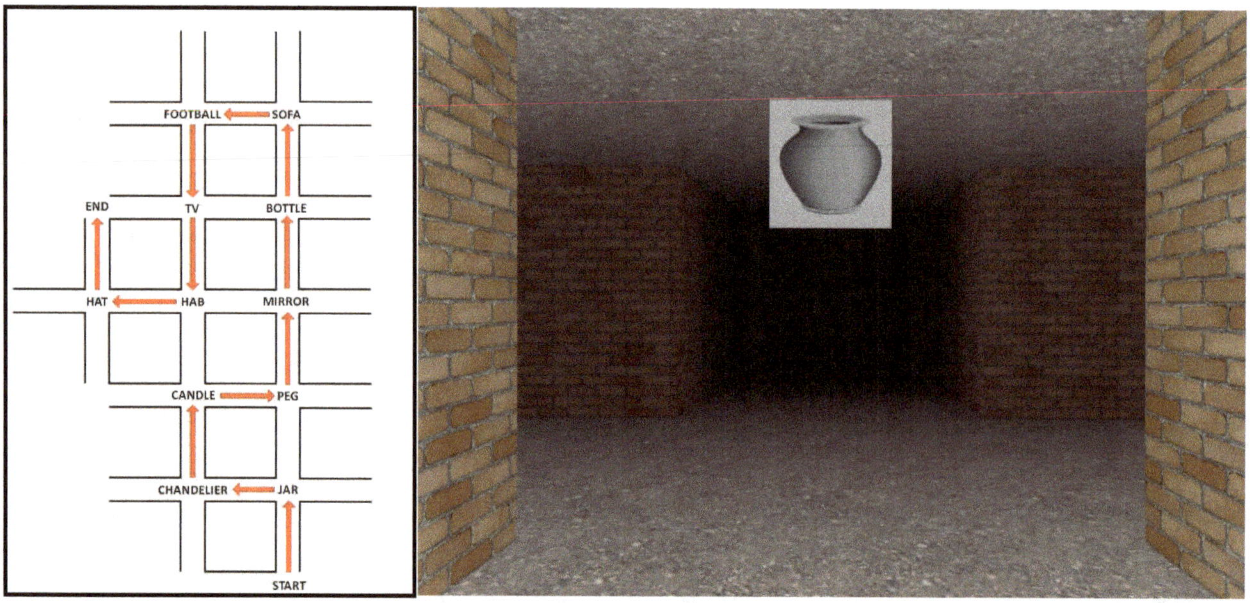


**FIGURE 1 | Left:** schematic drawing of the route consisting of 11 intersections; **right:** screen-shot of one of the intersections.

travel (repetition or retrace). Participants were instructed to respond as soon as they identified the travel direction, even if this occurred during the actual movement. Chance level for this task was 50%.

- **Intersection Direction Task.** Subsequent to the *Route Direction Task*, participants were asked to indicate the direction in which the route continued after movement stopped given the current travel direction. For route repetition trials, this involves indicating the direction required to follow the original route toward the end. In contrast, for route retracing trials this involves indicating the direction required to return to the start location while remaining on the route. With three possible movement directions and an equal amount of trials requiring a left, right, and straight responses, chance level for this task was 33.3%.
- **Landmark Sequence Task.** Finally, participants were presented with an image depicting three of the landmarks on the route. Their task was to indicate which of these landmarks would be encountered next, if the current travel direction was maintained. Chance level for this task was 33.3%.

Participants were instructed to respond as accurately and as quickly as possible by pressing the correspondingly labeled buttons on a response box (Cedrus RB-730).

The *Route Direction Task*, the *Intersection Direction Task*, and the *Landmark Sequence Task* were designed to test different aspects of route learning and route retracing. To solve the *Route Direction Task* participants needed to compare the sequence of landmarks and/or turns encountered during travel with their route memory. The *Intersection Direction Task* and the *Landmark Sequence Task* require participants to anticipate the upcoming movement direction or the next landmark, respectively. For repetition trials, these tasks are functionally equivalent to standard route learning tasks (Waller and Lippa, 2007; Head and Isom, 2010). Retracing trials, in contrast, require further processing: the *Landmark Sequence Task* requires manipulation of the temporal order of the landmarks; the *Intersection Direction Task* requires comprehending the spatial relationships between the direction from which an intersection is approached and the direction in which the route continues.

### ANALYSIS

We first analyzed performance for the *Route Direction Task*. Only trials in which participants correctly identified travel direction were included in the analyses of the *Intersection Direction* and the *Landmark Sequence Task*. As a result of removing incorrect *Travel Direction Task* trials, fewer data points were available for the remaining analyses. In order to analyze effects of learning on these two tasks we, therefore, pooled data from sessions 1–3 and 4–6.

## RESULTS

### ROUTE DIRECTION TASK

In order to enter the final data-set, participants' performance in repetition trials on the *Route Direction Task* had to exceed chance level (50%). This criterion was set to ensure that participants had acquired sufficient route knowledge during the training phases to investigate the effects of cognitive aging on route repetition. Performance for two older participants did not reach chance level. These participants were excluded from the final data-set.

To examine the impact of travel direction (route repetition and route retracing) on performance in the Route Direction Tasks between age groups, a repeated-measures ANOVA was conducted with the between-subject factors of age group (young, older) and sex and two within-subject factors of experimental session (1–6) and travel direction (repetition, retrace). We observed main effects of age [$F_{(1,\ 34)} = 9.74$, $p < 0.01$, $\eta^2 = 0.22$], session [$F_{(3.2,\ 111.17)} = 42.20, p < 0.001, \eta^2 = 0.55$], direction [$F_{(1,\ 34)} = 26.36$, $p < 0.001$, $\eta^2 = 0.44$], but not of sex [$F_{(1,\ 34)} = 0.16$, $p = 0.69$, $\eta^2 = 0.01$]. Specifically, younger participants performed better than older participants (86.19% vs. 74.97%), performance on repetition trials was better than on retracing trials (88.08% vs. 73.07%), and performance improved over experimental sessions (session 1: 60.96%, session 6: 89.94%).

The main effect of direction was primarily driven by the impaired performance of older participants on retracing trials (see **Figure 2**). This is reflected in the significant interaction of direction *x* age group [$F_{(1,\ 34)} = 10.31, p < 0.01, \eta^2 = 0.23$] and by *post-hoc* tests demonstrating that younger and older participants performed comparatively during route repetition trials [*t*-test (89.31% vs. 87.25%): $t_{(35.75)} = 0.73$; $p = 0.47$], but performed differently during route retracing trials [*t*-test (84.27% vs. 63.32%): $t_{(23.50)} = 3.59$; $p < 0.01$]. Only one other interaction, direction *x* session [$F_{(2.9,\ 100.7)} = 3.55, p = 0.02, \eta^2 = 0.10$] was significant.

Note that participants who entered this analysis were selected on basis of their performance on repetition trials. However, despite good performance on repetition trials, older adults showed impaired performance on retracing trials compared to young adults. In other words, the subsample of older adults that had no problems identifying travel direction during route repetition, exhibited a specific age-related impairment when traveling in the opposite direction along the route.

How did participants solve the *Route Direction Task*? In principle there are two ways: first, participants can compare the order in which the landmarks are encountered during training and test phase; second, for those test trials that feature a turn at the first intersection encountered, participants can compare the turning direction at this intersection between training and test. The analysis of response times for test trial with a turn at the first intersection allows us to distinguish between these two alternatives: Turning onset was 4.7 s after the test trial started. After 7.4 s the landmark of the second intersection was in sight. Response time for the relevant test trials was 10.25 s for young adults, 12.08 s for older adults, 11.06 s for repetition trials, and 11.26 s for retracing trials. There was a main effects of age [$F_{(1,\ 36)} = 8.33$, $p < 0.01$, $\eta^2 = 0.19$] but no main effect of direction [$F_{(1,\ 36)} = 1.91$, $p = 0.18$, $\eta^2 = 0.05$] and no significant interaction [$F_{(1,\ 36)} = 1.52$, $p = 0.23$, $\eta^2 = 0.04$] (see **Figure 2** right). Participants made their decision 3 s (younger) to 5 s (older) after the second landmark was in sight. This strongly suggests that participants analyzed the order in which landmarks were encountered during travel to inform their decision, rather than the turning direction at the first intersection encountered.

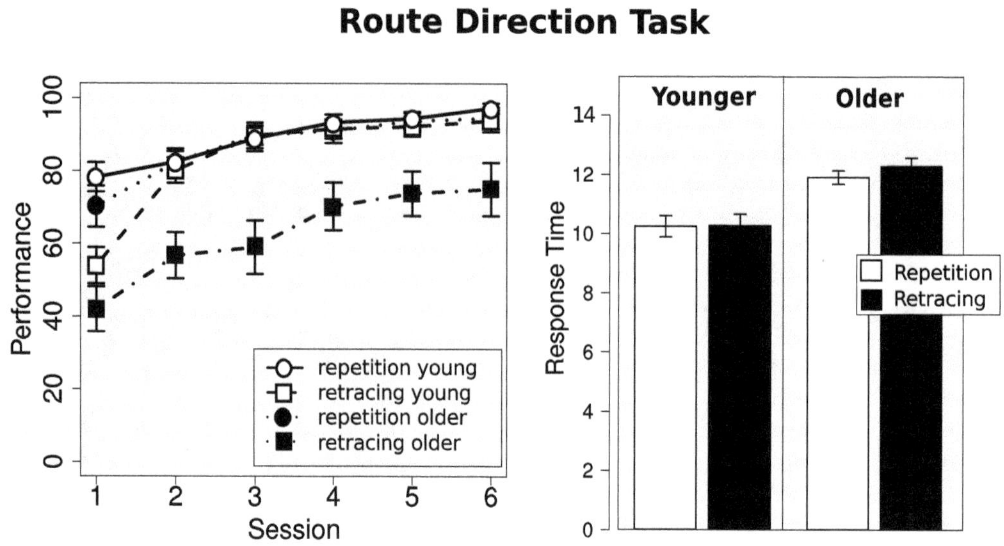


**FIGURE 2 | Left:** performance for the *Route Direction Task*; **right:** response time for test trials featuring a turn at the first intersection encountered.

## INTERSECTION DIRECTION TASK

As a result of removing two older participants from the final dataset and of excluding data from incorrect *Route Direction Task* trials from the further analysis, fewer trials from older participants (1446) than from younger participants (1720) entered the analysis of the *Intersection Direction Task* and the *Landmark Sequence Task*.

In order to examine performance differences between age groups in the *Intersection Direction Task*, a repeated-measures ANOVA was conducted with the between-subject factor of age (younger, older) and two within-subject factors of experimental session (first and second half of the experiment) and movement direction (repetition, retrace). We observed main effects of session [$F_{(1, 36)} = 29.76$, $p < 0.001$, $\eta^2 = 0.45$], direction [$F_{(1, 36)} = 29.51$, $p < 0.001$, $\eta^2 = 0.45$], and age [$F_{(1, 36)} = 17.39$, $p < 0.001$, $\eta^2 = 0.33$]. The main effect of age was driven both by repetition trials (*post-hoc*: $p < 0.001$) and by retracing trials (*post-hoc*: $p < 0.01$).

Of the interactions only direction *x* session [$F_{(1, 36)} = 9.07$, $p < 0.01$, $\eta^2 = 0.20$] and direction *x* session × age group [$F_{(1, 36)} = 4.12$, $p = 0.05$, $\eta^2 = 0.10$] were significant. These interactions were primarily driven by impaired learning in the older adults in the retracing trials: while young participants' performance improved over the course of the experiment for both repetition and retracing trials, the older adults' performance improved only on repetition trials, but not on retracing trials (see **Figure 3**). This is corroborated by additional separate repeated-measures ANOVAs for the young and the old age group: while main effects of direction and session were observed for both age groups (all $p < 0.05$), the interaction between direction and session was significant only in the older age group ($p = 0.02$), but not in the young age group ($p = 0.12$).

Note that performance for retracing trials in the older age group remained close to chance level performance (33%) for the entire experiment (see **Figure 3**).

## LANDMARK SEQUENCE TASK

In order to examine performance differences between age groups in the *Landmark Sequence Task*, a repeated-measures ANOVA was conducted with the between-subject factor of age (younger, older) and two within-subject factors of experimental session (first and second half of the experiment) and movement direction (repetition, retrace). We observed main effects of age [$F_{(1, 36)} = 11.54$, $p < 0.01$, $\eta^2 = 0.24$] and session [$F_{(1, 36)} = 95.07$, $p < 0.001$, $\eta^2 = 0.73$], but not of direction [$F_{(1, 36)} = 2.30$, $p = 0.14$, $\eta^2 = 0.04$]. Overall, performance was better for the young age group (young: 76.20%; old: 63.31%) and increased over the course of the experiment (first half: 62.22%; second half: 77.29%; see **Figure 3**). While none of the interactions was significant, the direction *x* age group interaction neared significance [$F_{(1, 36)} = 4.04$, $p = 0.052$, $\eta^2 = 0.10$].

## DISCUSSION

In this study we used a novel experimental paradigm to investigate the effects of cognitive aging on the ability to retrace a route—i.e., to navigate from the end of a route back to the start location. In the experiment, participants first viewed a visual presentation of a route and were then presented with short segments of the route either in the direction experienced during training (route repetition trials) or in the opposite direction (route retracing trials). For each of these presentations, participants were given three tasks: in the *Route Direction Task* they had to indicate the overall travel direction; in the *Intersection Direction Task*, they had to indicate the direction of movement required to remain on the route given the current travel direction; in the *Landmark Sequence Task* they had to indicate which landmark they would encounter next when proceeding in the current travel direction.

Consistent with earlier findings (Barrash, 1994; Wilkniss et al., 1997; Moffat et al., 2001; Head and Isom, 2010), the older age

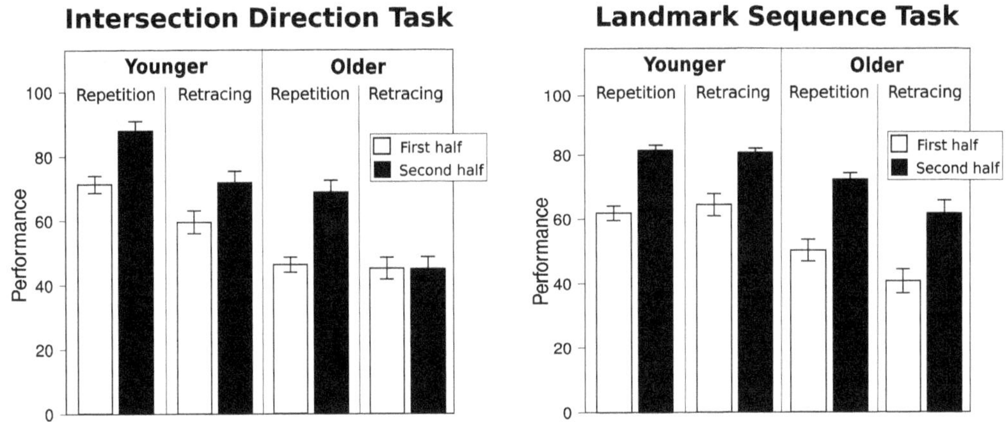


**FIGURE 3 | Left:** performance for the *Intersection Direction Task*; **right:** performancre in the *Landmark Sequence Task*.

group showed an overall performance deficit in route learning, even after removing two participants from the final data-set who did not reach chance level performance in route repetition trials in the *Route Direction Task*. In addition, older adults also showed specific deficits in retracing trials for both the *Route Direction Task* and the *Intersection Direction Task*. That is, older adults experienced difficulties when asked to identify the overall travel direction and to indicate the next movement direction when retracing the route, but not when repeating the route. Given the importance of successfully retracing a recently navigated route when exploring unfamiliar environments (Lorenz, 1952; Miller and Eilam, 2011), these effects offer an explanation for why age-related declines in navigation abilities are more striking in novel than in familiar environments (Devlin, 2001) and why older adults often report avoiding unfamiliar routes and places (Burns, 1999). In the following we consider results from the three tasks in the test phase in more detail.

### ROUTE DIRECTION TASK

The *Route Direction Task* assessed participants' ability to identify the current travel direction (route repetition or route retrace) while being passively transported along a short segment of the route. While this task can, in principle, be solved by comparing the turning direction at a single intersection during test with that experienced during training, participants of both age groups only responded after they encountered a second landmark. This suggests that they used the temporal ordering of landmarks to solve the task. Both younger and older adults performed well on route repetition trials. In contrast, for route retracing trials we found performance decrements in the older age group. In other words, while the older adults that entered the final data-set were perfectly able to recognize travel direction when it was identical to that during training, they had problems doing so when travel direction was reversed. This may be explained by the involvement of different cognitive processes during route repetition and route retracing: in the *Route Direction Task* participants are asked to identify travel direction by matching the order of landmarks experienced during the test phase to that experienced during training. Research in the area of sequence processing suggests that in repetition trials this task recruits a supervisory process that involves monitoring and selectively activating relevant items while suppressing irrelevant ones (Oberauer et al., 2000). For retracing trials, however, the sequence is reversed thus additionally requiring the coordination of the relative positions between the items. The efficiency of this coordination process has been found to be affected by cognitive aging (Bopp and Verhaeghen, 2007) which could explain the specific impairment for retracing trials in the older age group.

### LANDMARK SEQUENCE TASK

Older adults were also less accurate than young adults in the *Landmark Sequence Task* (see also Lipman and Caplan, 1992; Wilkniss et al., 1997; Head and Isom, 2010). However, the older adults reached performance levels clearly above chance level and performance increased over the course of the experiment. We did not observe a main effect of travel direction for the *Landmark Sequence Task*: both age groups performed at similar levels on repetition trials and on retrace trials. This seems surprising at first glance, but can be explained by (1) both the *Route Direction Task* and the *Landmark Sequence Task* requiring comparison between the temporal ordering of landmarks during the training phase with that experienced during the test phase; and (2) that only the data from correct *Route Direction Task* trials entered the *Landmark Sequence Task* analysis. In other words, as both tasks rely on similar processes and by pre-selecting trials on basis of performance in one task, potential effects of travel direction in the second task are reduced.

### INTERSECTION DIRECTION TASK

In line with earlier research (e.g., Head and Isom, 2010), older adults were less accurate in the *Intersection Direction Task* than young adults. This effect was observed both for route repetition trials as well as for route retracing trials. In addition, we found a specific learning deficit in retracing trials for the older age group: performance in retracing trials was close to chance level and, in contrast to repetition trials and the younger age group, did not improve over the course of the experiment. That is to say, not only did older adults perform weaker in indicating the correct direction when retracing a route, they were also unable learn the correct direction over the course of the experiment.

Egocentric route learning strategies (Trullier et al., 1997; Waller and Lippa, 2007) enable a navigator to solve the *Intersection Direction Task* in route repetition trials. Route retracing, in contrast, is not supported by egocentric strategies as intersections are approached from a different direction than during training. Route retracing, therefore, requires abstracting from the viewpoint-dependent memory encoded during the learning phase. This can be achieved by encoding the spatial relationship between the arm from which a particular intersection was approached and the arm in which the route proceeded. This form of representation is independent of the navigator's viewpoint and, therefore, allocentric. Recent research suggests that age-related deficits in allocentric processing (Moffat and Resnick, 2002; Moffat et al., 2007; Harris and Wolbers, in press) result from hippocampal degeneration during typical aging (Raz et al., 2010; Wiener et al., under review). This could also explain the age-related decline in performance on route retracing trials as these, in contrast to the route repetition trials, require allocentric processing.

In addition to the proposed deficits in allocentric processing resulting from age-related hippocampal degeneration, more general age-related declines in working memory and processing speed may contribute to the observed effects. The *Processing Speed Theory* states that declines in processing speed with increasing age can result in impairments in cognitive performance (Salthouse, 1996). This may be due to task-related time limitations or because results of earlier cognitive operations are no longer available when later operations are completed (simultaneity). While the current paradigm did not impose time limitations, allocentric processing is computationally more demanding than egocentric processes as it requires additional cognitive operations (Byrne et al., 2007). Any age-related processing speed effects are, therefore, more likely to affect retracing trials which rely on allocentric processing rather than repetition trials for which egocentric processes are sufficient.

We have argued that route retracing relies on allocentric processing. This is supported by a series of findings: route retracing provides a means to return to the start of a journey and has, therefore, been suggested to be crucial for exploring novel environments (Lorenz, 1952). Accordingly, in freely exploring rodents, route retracing is mainly observed during early stages of learning an environment (Miller and Eilam, 2011). Early stages of spatial learning primarily rely on allocentric place strategies, whereas egocentric response or route strategies only occur later (Tolman et al., 1946; Ritchie et al., 1950). Together with results from the current study this suggests that route retracing during the early stages of learning an environment relies on allocentric strategies.

Recent electrophysiological findings in rats suggest a neuronal mechanism that could support route retracing. Foster and Wilson (2006) recorded from hippocampal place cells and found that immediately after traversing a track, the hippocampal place cell activity observed during navigation was reactivated in reverse temporal order as if retracing the route. Importantly, these reverse replays were observed to a greater extent after navigating through a novel environment compared to a familiar environment, suggesting that such replays play an important role during spatial learning (see also Colgin and Moser, 2006).

To conclude, we have demonstrated age-related deficits in route retracing. Specifically, older participants showed impaired performance in both recognizing travel direction when navigating along the route in the reverse direction and in indicating the direction required to retrace the route. Given the importance of route retracing for learning novel environments these findings provide further insights into the effects of normal cognitive aging on wayfinding and orientation abilities.

## ACKNOWLEDGMENTS

Many thanks to Gemma Hanson for her help in collecting data.

## REFERENCES

Barnes, C. A., Nadel, L., and Honig, W. K. (1980). Spatial memory deficit in senescent rats. *Can. J. Psychol.* 34, 29–39.

Barrash, J. (1994). Age-related decline in route learning ability. *Dev. Neuropsychol.* 10,189–201.

Begega, A., Cienfuegos, S., Rubio, S., Santin, J. L., Miranda, R., and Arias, J. L. (2001). Effects of ageing on allocentric and egocentric spatial strategies in the wistar rat. *Behav. Processes* 53, 75–85.

Bopp, K. L., and Verhaeghen, P. (2007). Age-related differences in control processes in verbal and visuospatial working memory: storage, transformation, supervision, and coordina- tion. *J. Gerontol. B Psychol. Sci. Soc. Sci.* 62,239–246.

Burgess, N. (2008). Spatial cognition and the brain. *Ann. N.Y. Acad. Sci.* 1124, 77–97.

Burns, P. C. (1999). Navigation and the mobility of older drivers. *J. Gerontol. B Psychol. Sci. Soc. Sci.* 54,49–55.

Byrne, P., Becker, S., and Burgess, N. (2007). Remembering the past and imagining the future: a neural model of spatial memory and imagery. *Psychol. Rev.* 114, 340–375.

Colgin, L. L., and Moser, E. I. (2006). Neuroscience: rewinding the mem- ory record. *Nature* 440, 615–617.

Devlin, A. (2001). *Mind and Maze: Spatial Cognition and Environmental Behavior.* Westport, CT: Praeger.

Foster, D. J., and Wilson, M. A. (2006). Reverse replay of behavioural sequences in hippocampal place cells during the awake state. *Nature* 440, 680–683.

Harris, M., and Wolbers, T. (in press). Ageing effects on path integra- tion and landmark navigation. *Hippocampus.*

Head, D., and Isom, M. (2010). Age effects on wayfinding and route learning skills. *Behav. Brain Res.* 209, 49–58.

Iaria, G., Palermo, L., Committeri, G., and Barton, J. J. (2009). Age differences in the formation and use of cognitive maps. *Behav. Brain Res.* 196, 187–191.

Lipman, P. D., and Caplan, L. J. (1992). Adult age differences in memory for routes: effects of instruction and spatial diagram. *Psychol. Aging* 7, 435–442.

Lorenz, K. (1952). *King Solomon's Ring – New Light on Animal Ways.* New York, NY: Meridian Books (Penguin).

Luis, C. A., Keegan, A. P., and Mullan, M. (2009). Cross validation of the montreal cognitive assessment in community dwelling older adults residing in the southeastern US. *Int. J. Geriatr. Psychiatry* 24, 197–201.

McDonald, R. J., and White, N. M. (1994). Parallel information pro- cessing in the water maze: evidence for independent memory systems involving dorsal striatum and hip- pocampus. *Behav. Neural Biol.* 61, 260–270.

Miller, M., and Eilam, D. (2011). Decision making at a crossroad: why to go straight ahead, retrace a path, or turn sideways? *Anim. Cogn.* 14, 11–20.

Moffat, S. (2009). Aging and spatial navigation: what do we know and where do we go? *Neuropsychol. Rev.* 19,478–489.

Moffat, S., Kennedy, K., Rodrigue, K., and Raz, N. (2007). Extra- hippocampal contributions to age differences in human spatial naviga- tion. *Cereb. Cortex* 17, 1274–1282.

Moffat, S., and Resnick, S. (2002). Effects of age on virtual environ- ment place navigation and allo- centric cognitive mapping. *Behav. Neurosci.* 116, 851–859.

Moffat, S., Zondermann, A., and Resnick, S. (2001). Age differences in spatial memory in a virtual envi- ronment navigation task. *Neurobiol. Aging* 22, 787–796.

Nasreddine, Z. S., Phillips, N. A., Bedirian, V., Charbonneau, S., Whitehead, V., Collin, I., Cummings, J. L., and Chertkow, H. (2005). The Montreal cognitive assessment, MoCA: a brief screening tool for mild cognitive impairment. *J. Am. Geriatr. Soc.* 53, 695–699.

Nicolle, M. M., Prescott, S., and Bizon, J. L. (2003). Emergence of a cue strategy preference on the water maze task in aged C57B6 x SJL F1 hybrid mice. *Learn. Mem.* 10, 520–524.

Oberauer, K., Suss, H., Schulze, R., Wilhelm, O., and Wittmann, W. (2000). Working memory capac- ity facets of a cognitive ability construct. *Pers. Individ. Dif.* 29, 1017–1045.

Raz, N., Ghisletta, P., Rodrigue, K. M., Kennedy, K. M., and Lindenberger, U. (2010). Trajectories of brain aging in middle-aged and older adults: regional and individ- ual differences. *Neuroimage* 51, 501–511.

Ritchie, B., Aeschliman, B., and Pierce, P. (1950). Studies in spatial learn- ing. viii. Place performance and the acquisition of place dispositions. *J. Comp. Physiol. Psychol.* 43, 73–85. Rodgers, M. K., Sindone, J. A., and Moffat, S. D. (2012). Effects of age on navigation strategy. *Neurobiol. Aging* 33, 15–22.

Rosenzweig, E. S., and Barnes, C. A. (2003). Impact of aging on hippocampal function: plasticity, network dynamics, and cognition. *Prog. Neurobiol.* 69, 143–179.

Salthouse, T. A. (1996). The processing speed theory of adult age differ- ences in cognition. *Psychol. Rev.* 103, 403–428.

Tolman, E., Ritchie, B., and Kalish, D. (1946). Studies in spatial learning: place learning versus response learning. *J. Exp. Psychol.* 36, 221–229.

Trullier, O., Wiener, S. I., Berthoz, A., and Meyer, J. (1997). Biologically based artificial navigation sys- tems: review and prospects. *Prog. Neurobiol.* 51, 483–544.

Waller, D., and Lippa, Y. (2007). Landmarks as beacons and associative cues: their role in route learning. *Mem. Cognit.* 35, 910–924.

Wilkniss, S. M., Jones, M. G., Korol, D. L., Gold, P. E., and Manning, C. A. (1997). Age-related differences in an ecologically based study of route learning. *Psychol. Aging* 12, 372–375.

Wolbers, T., Weiller, C., and Buchel, C. (2004). Neural foundations of emerging route knowledge in complex spatial environments. *Brain Res. Cogn. Brain Res.* 21, 401–411.

# 26

# The relationship of topographical memory performance to regional neurodegeneration in Alzheimer's disease

**George Pengas[1†], Guy B. Williams[1], Julio Acosta-Cabronero[1], Tom W. J. Ash[1†], Young T. Hong[1], David Izquierdo-Garcia[1†], Tim D. Fryer[1], John R. Hodges[2] and Peter J. Nestor[1]***

[1] Department of Clinical Neurosciences, University of Cambridge, Cambridge, UK
[2] Neuroscience Research Australia, Sydney, NSW, Australia

**Edited by:**
Thomas Wolbers, University of Edinburgh, UK

**Reviewed by:**
Junming Wang, University of Mississippi Medical Center, USA
J. Arturo García-Horsman, University of Helsinki, Finland
Stefan Klöppel, University of Freiburg, Germany

***Correspondence:**
Peter J. Nestor, Department of Clinical Neurosciences, University of Cambridge, Herchel Smith Building for Brain and Mind Sciences, Robinson Way, CB2 0SZ, Cambridge, UK.
e-mail: pjn23@hermes.cam.ac.uk

The network activated during normal route learning shares considerable homology with the network of degeneration in the earliest symptomatic stages of Alzheimer's disease (AD). This inspired the virtual route learning test (VRLT) in which patients learn routes in a virtual reality environment. This study investigated the neural basis of VRLT performance in AD to test whether impairment was underpinned by a network or by the widely held explanation of hippocampal degeneration. VRLT score in a mild AD cohort was regressed against gray matter (GM) density and diffusion tensor metrics of white matter (WM) ($n = 30$), and, cerebral glucose metabolism ($n = 26$), using a mass univariate approach. GM density and cerebral metabolism were then submitted to a multivariate analysis [support vector regression (SVR)] to examine whether there was a network associated with task performance. Univariate analyses of GM density, metabolism and WM axial diffusion converged on the vicinity of the retrosplenial/posterior cingulate cortex, isthmus and, possibly, hippocampal tail. The multivariate analysis revealed a significant, right hemisphere-predominant, network level correlation with cerebral metabolism; this comprised areas common to both activation in normal route learning and early degeneration in AD (retrosplenial and lateral parietal cortices). It also identified right medio-dorsal thalamus (part of the limbic-diencephalic hypometabolic network of early AD) and right caudate nucleus (activated during normal route learning). These results offer strong evidence that topographical memory impairment in AD relates to damage across a network, in turn offering complimentary lesion evidence to previous studies in healthy volunteers for the neural basis of topographical memory. The results also emphasize that structures beyond the mesial temporal lobe (MTL) contribute to memory impairment in AD—it is too simplistic to view memory impairment in AD as a synonym for hippocampal degeneration.

**Keywords: topographical memory, Alzheimer's, MRI, PET, multivariate, support vector, retrosplenial cortex**

## INTRODUCTION

Memory impairment in Alzheimer's disease (AD) is often assumed to be a consequence of mesial temporal lobe (MTL) degeneration. The reasons for this are self-evident: neurofibrillary tangle (NFT) pathology in AD begins in the MTL (Braak and Braak, 1991); NFT load correlates with cognition in AD (Giannakopoulos et al., 2003); and the hippocampus is known to be atrophic in AD (Jack et al., 1997), including those at the mild cognitive impairment (MCI) stage whose deficit is restricted to memory (Pengas et al., 2010a). Such reasoning, however, might be an oversimplification. For instance, Braak and Braak (1991) used NFTs for their proposed staging protocol, precisely because they observed that NFT pathology followed a progressive pattern in AD; it is therefore expected that NFTs will correlate with other measures of disease severity. Furthermore, it is now well documented that prodromal AD is not simply a "hippocampal" disease: at a presymptomatic stage, carriers of familial, autosomal dominant AD mutations had both accelerated hippocampal and posterior cingulate volume loss (Scahill et al., 2002). This is also true of the MCI-stage of sporadic AD in which there is comparable atrophy of retrosplenial cortex, posterior cingulate cortex and hippocampus (Choo et al., 2010; Pengas et al., 2010a). Indeed, the earliest hypometabolic region identified in AD is the posterior cingulate/retrosplenial cortex (Minoshima et al., 1997; Nestor et al., 2003a) with posterior temporoparietal hypometabolism emerging as the next most affected isocortical region with disease progression (Nestor et al., 2003b; Chetelat et al., 2005).

This constellation of affected regions (MTL, posterior cingulate, retrosplenial cortex, posterior parietal lobe) is homologous with the network activated when healthy volunteers navigate in functional magnetic resonance imaging (MRI) paradigms (Ghaem et al., 1997; Maguire et al., 1998; Burgess et al., 2001; Ino et al., 2002; Shelton and Gabrieli, 2002; Rosenbaum et al., 2004; Wolbers et al., 2004; Wolbers and Buchel, 2005;

Ekstrom and Bookheimer, 2007; Iaria et al., 2007; Ino et al., 2007). It was therefore, previously, hypothesized that topographical memory impairment would be sensitive and specific for early AD. The virtual route learning test (VRLT), in which subjects have to learn routes in a virtual reality environment, was devised and found to be highly sensitive and specific in distinguishing patients with early AD from controls. Moreover, when compared to a range of other memory tests, the VRLT most strongly correlated with real world navigation problems (Pengas et al., 2010b).

To our knowledge, only one previous study has investigated the neural basis of route learning impairment in AD but it did so as a two population voxel-based morphometry (VBM) contrast of gray matter density (GM) in subjects who got lost ($n = 6$ AD plus $n = 5$ MCI) versus those that did not ($n = 4$ AD plus $n = 7$ MCI plus $n = 19$ controls) who did not (deIpolyi et al., 2007). It reported no significant regions in a whole brain analysis but focusing on regions of interest in inferior parietal lobule, parahippocampal gyri and hippocampi, the authors reported atrophy in inferior parietal regions with a rightward bias as well as a tiny area in the right hippocampal tail. The use of regions of interest, the two population design, and inclusion of controls mean that only limited conclusions can be drawn from this study.

The aim of the present study, therefore, was to map the neural substrate for impaired route learning in an unbiased manner with multimodal imaging, using scores from the VRLT, in a cohort of mild AD patients. These behavioral data were derived from the earlier neuropsychological study (Pengas et al., 2010b) and, because the aim of the present work was to understand the basis of route learning impairment in AD, only patients with this condition (i.e., no controls) were included. VRLT scores were regressed with GM density (as a measure of regional brain atrophy), normalized $^{18}$F-fluorodeoxyglucose (FDG) radioactivity concentration—used as a measure of resting cerebral glucose metabolism corrected for inter-subject variation in basal metabolism—and diffusion tensor imaging (DTI) parameters of white matter tracts (WM). GM density and FDG data were also examined using a multivariate approach to specifically look at overall network contributions to navigation performance.

## METHODS

### SUBJECTS

A cohort of $n = 30$ patients with mild AD was identified for the study that had undergone detailed clinical and neuropsychological assessments of whom $n = 16$ patients had MCI (Petersen et al., 2001), and $n = 14$ met National Institute of Neurological and Communicable Diseases and Alzheimer's Disease and Related Disorders Association (NINCDS-ADRDA) criteria for probable AD (McKhann et al., 1984) at the time of scanning. The MCI subjects were followed up longitudinally after scanning to confirm progressive decline in all subjects, therefore indicating that their MCI status was due to probable AD. All 30 underwent the MRI protocol and a subset ($n = 26$ of which 14 were designated MCI and 12 AD when scanned) also had FDG—positron emission tomography (PET) imaging (demographics summarized in **Table 1**). These patients were derived from the earlier neuropsychological study of topographical memory in AD (Pengas et al., 2010b). The study was approved by the Local Research Ethics Committee and the Administration of Radioactive Substances Advisory Committee, UK. Written informed consent was obtained from all subjects and care-givers.

**Table 1 | Demographics of the AD subjects that were included in the analyses (note: the PET subjects represent a subgroup of the MRI subjects; MMSE: Mini-mental state examination; ACE-r: Addenbrooke's Cognitive Examination-revised).**

| | MRI subjects Mean ± SD (range) | PET subjects Mean ± SD (range) |
|---|---|---|
| N (sex) | 30 (17*M*:13*F*) | 26 (15*M*:11) |
| Age, yrs | 69.2 ± 5.4 (59–78) | 68.8 ± 5.6 (59–78) |
| Education, yrs | 13.8 ± 3.0 (10–19) | 13.8 ± 3.1 (10–19) |
| MMSE | 24.6 ± 2.6 (18–28) | 24.5 ± 2.6 (18–28) |
| ACE-r | 74.2 ± 10.5 (55–88) | 74.3 ± 10.2 (55–88) |
| VRLT error score | 14.5 ± 5.3 (3–23) | 14.5 ± 5.1 (3–23) |

### TOPOGRAPHICAL MEMORY ASSESSMENT

Full details of the VRLT have been previously published (Pengas et al., 2010b). Briefly, the VRLT is s graded route learning task that employs four consecutively harder routes that subjects need to learn and reproduce by navigating with a joystick in a 3D first-person computer-generated virtual town. The task is scored in the number of errors a subject makes to complete all four routes, in a "learning-to-criterion" paradigm (Pengas et al., 2010b).

### IMAGING

#### *Image acquisition*

***MRI.*** Within days of the behavioral data collection, MR images were acquired on a Siemens Trio 3T system (Siemens Medical Systems, Erlangen, Germany) equipped with gradient coils capable of 45 mT/m and a slew rate of 200T/m/s, and a 12-channel phased-array total imaging matrix head-coil (Siemens Medical Systems, Erlangen, Germany). At acquisition, the field of view was aligned to stereotactic space: the anterior commissure—posterior commissure line was aligned with the axial plane and the inter-hemispheric fissure was aligned along the sagittal plane. In addition, the scanning bed was adjusted to place the scanner isocentre at the thalamus in the mid-sagittal plane. Volumetric T1-weighted images were obtained using 3D magnetisation-prepared radio-frequency pulses and rapid gradient-echo (MP-RAGE) sampling (relaxation time (TR)/ echo time (TE)/ inversion time (TI)/ number of excitations (NEX) = 2300 ms/ 2.86 ms/ 900 ms/ 1; flip angle 9; matrix 192 × 192; 144 slices; voxel size 1.25 × 1.25 × 1.25 mm$^3$ isotropic). Diffusion-weighted images (DWI) were acquired using a twice-refocused single-shot echo-planar imaging pulse sequence (Reese et al., 2003), with parameters TR/TE/NEX = 7800 ms/ 90 ms/ 1; matrix 96 × 96; 63 contiguous axial slices; isotropic voxel resolution of 2 × 2 × 2 mm$^3$; bandwidth of 1628 Hz/pixel and echo spacing of 0.72 ms). The diffusion tensor was acquired with diffusion-sensitising gradient orientations along 63 non-collinear directions ($b = 1000$ s/mm$^2$) that were maximally spread by considering the minimal energy arrangement of point charges on a sphere and one scan without diffusion weighting ($b = 0$ s/mm$^2$, b0). Parallel acquisition of independently reconstructed images was allowed for, using generalised autocalibrating partially parallel acquisitions or GRAPPA (Griswold et al., 2002), with acceleration factor of 2 and 39 reference lines.

***FDG-PET.*** FDG-PET scans were acquired within a few weeks of the MRI scans for all patients, using a GE Advance scanner (GE Medical Systems, Milwaukee, WI, USA) in 3D mode (voxel size $2.34 \times 2.34 \times 4.25\,mm^3$, field of view $30.0 \times 30.0 \times 15.3\,cm^3$). Subjects were scanned after a 6 h fast in a dimly lit, quiet room, without using ear-plugs or blindfolds. A 150MBq FDG intravenous bolus injection was given over 30 s. Prior to the acquisition of emission images 35–55 min after injection ($4 \times 5$ min), a 10 min geometrically windowed, coincidence mode transmission scan was performed using rotating germanium-68 rods for attenuation correction. PET emission images were reconstructed using the PROMIS 3D filtered back-projection algorithm (Kinnahan and Rogers, 1989) with corrections applied for dead time, randoms, normalisation, scatter, attenuation, sensitivity, and decay. Arterial sampling was not performed.

#### Data processing

***Voxel-based morphometry.*** Statistical parametric mapping 2005 (SPM5, http://fil.ion.ac.uk/spm) was employed to evaluate voxel-wise GM density using VBM (Ashburner and Friston, 2000). Recent studies have shown that skull-stripping and radio-frequency bias correcting MR images improve the performance of warping procedure so this was undertaken using a previously described algorithm (Acosta-Cabronero et al., 2008; Pereira et al., 2010). The resulting warped GM segments were modulated to compensate for volumetric differences introduced into the warped images, and smoothed using an 8 mm full-width half-maximum (FWHM) isotropic Gaussian kernel. Pre-processing and warping procedures need reasonable initial estimates; hence the origin of each structural volume was set manually to the anterior commissure prior to pre-processing. A relative masking threshold of 0.2 was applied for SPM5 analyses. The GM, WM and cerebrospinal fluid segments from SPM5 were summed together to calculate the total intracranial volume (Pengas et al., 2009), and entered as a nuisance covariate in the statistical regressions.

***FDG-PET.*** Mean FDG (35–55 min) radioactivity concentration maps were generated and their origins were also reset to the anterior commissure. The resulting volumes were skull-stripped using BET2 ($f = 0.7$, $g = 0$) (Smith, 2002), rigidly aligned to their corresponding pre-processed structural image and re-sliced (sinc interpolated) to the voxel size of the structural image using the VTK CISG registration toolkit v2.0.0 (Rueckert et al., 1999). Aligned mean FDG maps were then transformed into stereotactic space using the SPM5 warp transforms of pre-processed volumes and re-sampled to 2 mm isotropic using 7th degree b-spline interpolation. Finally, mean FDG maps were normalized by multiplying all voxels by the scaling factor required to equalize the mean cerebellar radioactivity concentration of each subject to the mean cerebellar radioactivity concentration of all subjects (Ichimiya et al., 1994), and smoothed with a 16 mm FWHM kernel. A relative masking threshold of 0.8 was applied for SPM5 analyses.

***Diffusion tensor imaging.*** The FSL package (http://www.fmrib.ox.ac.uk/fsl/) was employed to process and analyze the DWI data. First, each diffusion-weighted volume was affine-aligned to its corresponding b0 image using FMRIB's linear image registration tool v5.4.2 (Jenkinson and Smith, 2001) to correct for possible motion artefacts and eddy-current distortions. Prior to fitting the tensor, brain masks of each b0 image were generated using BET2 with $f = 0.1$ and $g = 0$. FMRIB's diffusion toolbox v2.0 was then used to fit the tensor and compute the orthogonal elements at each brain voxel, from which fractional anisotropy (FA), axial diffusivity ($\lambda_1$), radial diffusivity (RD) and mean diffusivity (MD) metrics were derived. Spatial normalization was performed to a target image; this was the map that required the least amount of non-linear warping to match all other images, which was then affine-aligned into MNI152 standard space. The combination of the two transformations was applied to each subject's FA image, and all warped FA maps were then averaged to create the mean FA template, from which the mean FA skeleton is derived (FA > 0.2). Finally, all subjects' normalized FA, $\lambda_1$, RD, and MD data were projected onto the skeleton for statistical analysis. The tract-based spatial statistics (TBSS) approach (Smith et al., 2006), whereby the nearest most relevant tract center in each subject's spatially normalized FA image is projected onto the mean FA skeleton containing the center of all tracts common to all subjects, was used to perform voxel-wise statistics at the tract centers only, thus minimizing the effect of residual misregistration.

#### Statistical analysis

***Univariate analyses.*** Whole brain analyses were carried out by regressing the VRLT error score with each of the three different imaging modalities: GM density, normalized FDG radioactivity concentration and diffusion metrics ($\lambda_1$, RD, MD, and FA). GM density and normalized FDG radioactivity concentration were analyzed using voxel-based multiple linear regressions in SPM5 and illustrated at a statistical threshold of $p$ (uncorrected) < 0.005 and with no voxel extent threshold ($k = 0$). Diffusion analyses employed permutation-based non-parametric inference on unsmoothed statistical maps in TBSS; 10,000 permutations of the data were generated to test against using "randomise v2.1," and cluster-like structures were enhanced using the threshold-free cluster enhancement algorithm (Smith and Nichols, 2009). Previous work has shown that $\lambda_1$, MD, and RD can be more sensitive to diffusivity changes in AD than FA (Acosta-Cabronero et al., 2010). Therefore $\lambda_1$, MD, RD (in addition to FA) were each assessed using multiple linear regression at $p$ (uncorrected) <0.05. It should be highlighted, however, that there is presently uncertainty as to how changes in these various diffusion metrics relate to neuronal loss in WM; as such, the diffusion analyses should only be considered as exploratory at this time (See "Discussion" also).

***Multivariate analyses.*** Support vector machines for use in regression contexts [support vector regression (SVR)], allow for cognitive scores to be predicted using independently acquired data such as imaging, and therefore to interrogate the algorithm as to which brain areas influenced the algorithm the most, i.e., which are most relevant to the predicted cognitive score.

The general method of use for statistical learning tools has two phases. The first is a "supervised learning" phase, where the model is "trained" on a subset of the data and is optimized over a cost function, such that it outputs optimal results for that training set. A separate test on the remaining subset of the data then validates the generalizability of the learned model. As the present dataset was relatively small, the data cannot reasonably be split into learning and testing subsets (as small subsets inevitably lead to overfitting), and so cross-validation utilized "leave-one-out" tests instead. In this strategy, one subject's image is removed and the algorithm learns over the rest of the dataset. Then a prediction is made, based on the learned model, for the left-out image. This is then repeated over all subjects, and the accuracy is computed over all tests. The correlation between predicted scores and actual scores for each image then gives a measure of how well the technique performed, and how reliable the model it outputs is. Importantly, if this correlation was not statistically significant, further analyses (to identify relevant brain regions) were not performed.

In the case of regression, optimization takes place by ensuring that predictions over the training set have minimal error, whilst maintaining as robust a predictive function as possible. There are two adjustable parameters, C, the regularisation parameter, which restricts how much influence a single training example can have on the learned model, and ε, an upper bound for the maximum acceptable error allowed without penalty. The predictive form is:

$$Prediction = \sum_{i}^{SVs} \alpha_i k(\boldsymbol{x}_i, \boldsymbol{z}) + b$$

where summation is over all training examples, α's are hyperparameters giving the influence each training example has on the final model, $b$ is a normalisation constant, and $k(\boldsymbol{x}_i, \boldsymbol{z})$ is a kernel function, which allows a model to take a non-linear form.

Visualization of the model is simple in the case of a linear kernel. The functional form of the classifier can be simplified by using the concept of the weight vector, $\boldsymbol{w}$:

$$\boldsymbol{w} = \sum_{i}^{SVs} \alpha_i \boldsymbol{x}_i$$

The predictive form of the SVR technique is then:

$$Prediction = \boldsymbol{w} \cdot \boldsymbol{z} + b$$

As the dot product of weight vector $\boldsymbol{w}$ with test vector $\boldsymbol{z}$ is taken, larger values of $\boldsymbol{w}$ represent regions of the trained model that are more sensitive to change in voxel intensity. In the present study, the SVR was implemented using SVM_light and employing default values from this algorithm for C and ε (Joachims, 1999). Displays of a thresholded version of the weight vector have been previously used in neuroscience work with support vector machines, e.g., Klöppel et al. (2008).

Interpretation of a weight vector is slightly different to interpretation of the more traditional mass univariate scheme. In a mass univariate scheme, an individual voxel is regressed to the score variable, and hence has an individual $p$-value associated with its correlation. In this multivariate case, a weighted version of the entire field of voxels is regressed to the score variable, and hence it is the overall pattern which has a $p$-value for correlation—the present technique cannot provide $p$-values for individual voxels, only for the entire pattern. Given that cognitive functions rely on distributed neural systems, this multivariate methodology is potentially very powerful as it offers the possibility to explain task performance at a network level.

## RESULTS

### UNIVARIATE ANALYSES

#### *Atrophy (GM density) correlations*

VRLT performance correlated bilaterally with GM density in the region of the isthmus/retrospenial junction and extreme tail of the hippocampus. Patchy correlations were also evident in parahippocampal gyrus (PHG), insula, parietal and frontal cortices that were bilateral but with greater right hemisphere involvement (**Figure 1**).

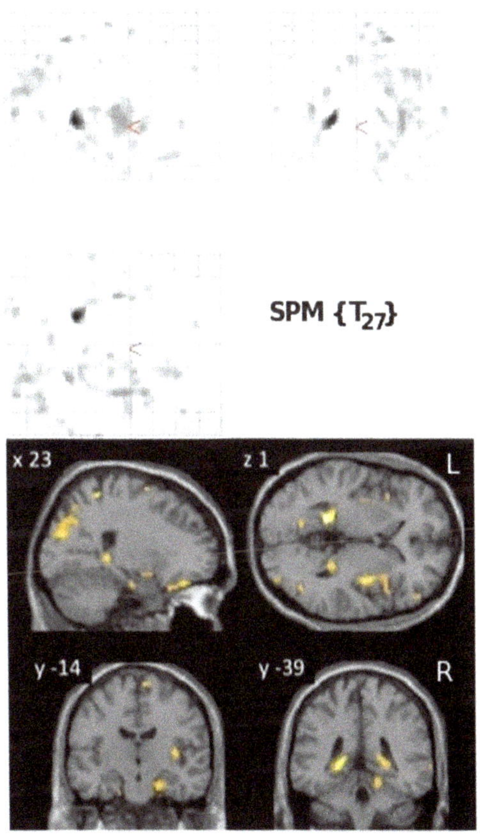


**FIGURE 1 | Results of the univariate linear regression of VRLT error score with GM density.** *Above panel*: glass brain; *below panel*: selected slices projected onto a single subject template. The slice labeled "$y = -39$" best illustrates the bilateral isthmus/retrosplenial lesion.

### *Metabolism (FDG) correlations*

Normalized FDG radioactivity concentration correlation with VRLT performance identified a confluent region spanning right posterior cingulate, retrosplenial cortex, precuneus, lateral posterior parietal cortex, and posterior PHG. A less extensive and less significant cluster was seen on the left side involving posterior parietal cortex (**Figure 2**).

### *Diffusion (WM) correlations*

VRLT performance correlated with $\lambda_1$ bilaterally in the WM of the cingulum bundle in the posterior cingulate/retrosplenial region. On the right side this was more extensive and confluently extended rostrally in the PHG to the level of the hippocampal head in the *y*-plane (**Figure 3**). RD, MD, and FA failed to produce confluent results in any tract.

## MULTIVARIATE ANALYSES

Using GM density within an SVR model to predict VRLT performance did not produce values that correlated significantly with the true values (2-tailed $p = 0.19$). There was a significant predictive correlation between actual and predicted VRLT performance using normalized FDG radioactivity concentration (2-tailed $p < 0.005$). This involved bilateral postero-lateral parietal and retrosplenial cortices as well as right caudate nucleus, right mediodorsal thalamus and a small area of right dorso-lateral prefrontal cortex. Overall, the regression was more extensive in the right hemisphere (**Figure 4**). Plotting the results of the SVR found that one data point was a potential outlier, re-running the correlation with this data point excluded diminished the significance of the correlation (1-tailed $p = 0.05$) (**Figure 5**).

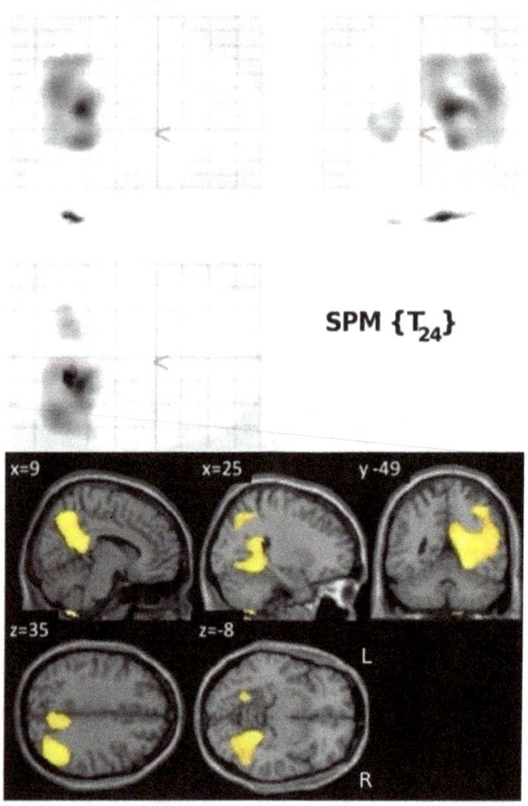


**FIGURE 2 | Results of the univariate linear regression of VRLT error score with FDG metabolism.** *Above panel*: glass brain; *below panel*: selected slices projected onto a single subject template.

## CONVERGENCE OF RESULTS ACROSS METHODS AND MODALITIES

The univariate analyses of GM and FDG and the multivariate FDG analysis identified a common area of correlation in the right retrospenial cortex/isthmus region extending to the region of the hippocampal tail. Axial diffusion ($\lambda_1$) in WM adjacent to this region was also significantly correlated (**Figure 6**).

# DISCUSSION

Performance on the VRLT, in which subjects attempt to learn routes in a virtual environment, was recently shown to have exquisite sensitivity for detecting impairment in very early AD; it also showed excellent ecological validity in that it correlated strongly with real world endorsements of route-finding difficulty (Pengas et al., 2010b). Univariate analyses of GM density, FDG (glucose metabolism) and WM axial diffusion found convergent correlations with the right retrosplenial/isthmus/posterior cingulate/hippocampal tail region. The multivariate analysis of FDG yielded a more distributed network of correlation that included this same region as well as lateral parietal association cortex, right caudate nucleus, and right dorso-medial thalamus. With the exception of the lateral parietal and retrosplenial regions, the network was exclusively right-sided. Though the present results offer considerably more detail, they are in general agreement with the GM density region of interest results of delpolyi et al. (2007) who reported greater right side atrophy in AD and MCI patients who got lost, and involvement of the extreme right hippocampal tail (n.b. their region of interest analysis included hippocampi, parahippocampal gyri, and inferior parietal lobules).

Correlation of topographical memory impairment with the retrosplenial region is in agreement with behavioral data from focal lesions to this region (Takahashi et al., 1997; Maeshima et al., 2001). Similarly, functional neuroimaging studies of healthy subjects navigating in virtual environments activate the retrosplenial region (Ghaem et al., 1997; Maguire et al., 1998; Maguire, 2001; Ino et al., 2002; Wolbers et al., 2004). It also resonates with the observation that this area is the earliest detectable hypometabolic region in the MCI-stage of AD (Nestor et al., 2003b). The present findings suggest that this lesion is a significant contributor to the emergence of memory impairment in AD. Furthermore, the observation that both metabolism and GM density in this region correlated with VRLT performance suggests that this is not just a functional lesion but, rather, a direct consequence of local neurodegeneration. The correlation with axial diffusion in the WM subtending this region would also be consistent with local degeneration causing disruption to axonal projections from this area. As already mentioned, however, the diffusion analysis should only be treated as exploratory at this time; none of the other diffusion metrics correlated with VRLT performance, and, at present, too little is known about the dynamics of change between specific diffusion metrics and axonal loss to have strong expectations for how these variables may relate to each other.

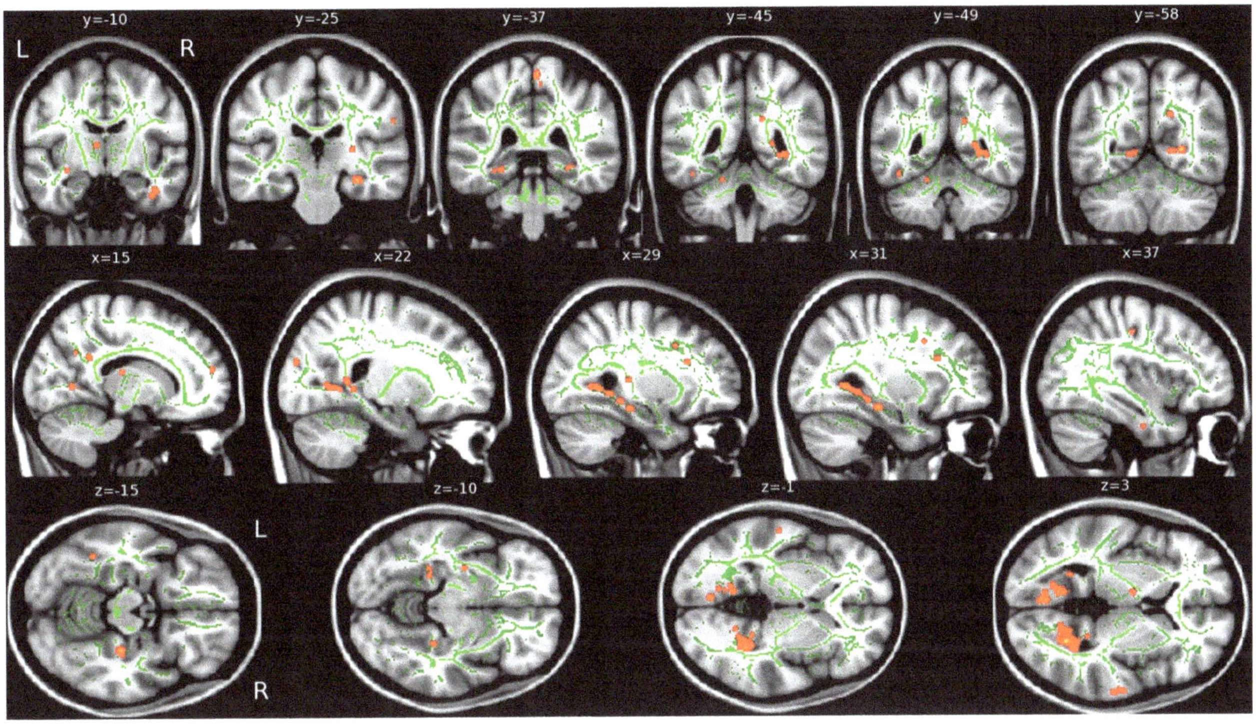


**FIGURE 3 | Areas of correlation between increased axial diffusion ($\lambda_1$, red) and VRLT error score.** The TBSS "skeleton" (i.e., the white matter tract centers on which the statistics are computed) is green.

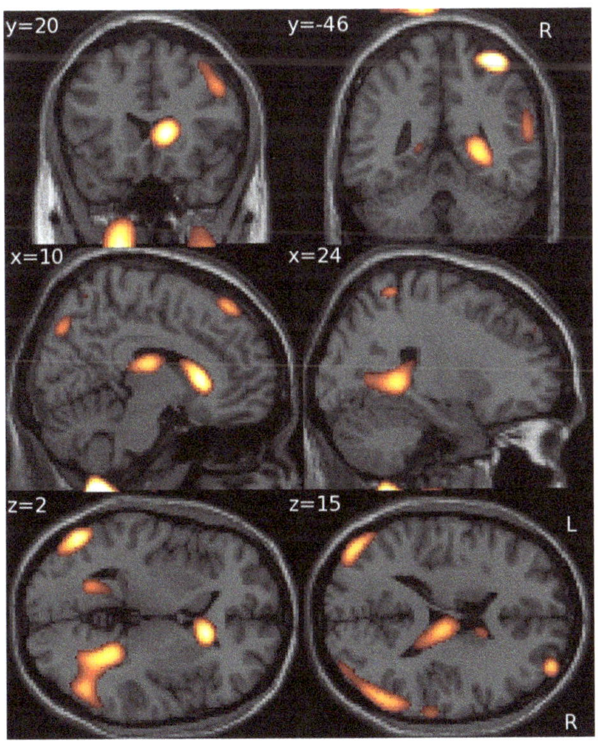


**FIGURE 4 | Multivariate support vector regression of VRLT performance with normalized FDG metabolism.**

The multivariate SVR analysis which estimates a significance level to the pattern of cerebral correlates as whole, and therefore could be viewed as giving a more informed picture of network level change, yielded a more complex picture than the mass univariate approach with respect to FDG. In addition to the retrosplenial lesion, this analysis revealed that lateral parietal regions—with a right-sided predominance—were also significantly related to VRLT performance. These findings highlight the homology between the fMRI pattern of activation during navigation (Ghaem et al., 1997; Maguire et al., 1998; Mellet et al., 2000; Burgess et al., 2001; Wolbers et al., 2004; Moffat et al., 2007) and the imaging profile in AD (Minoshima et al., 1997; Baron et al., 2001; Chetelat et al., 2002; Scahill et al., 2002; Nestor et al., 2003b; Acosta-Cabronero et al., 2010; Pengas et al., 2010a) that was the inspiration for developing this test. The analysis also highlighted right medio-dorsal thalamus in the correlation with VRLT performance. This location has not been a major feature of the spatial memory network in fMRI studies. Lesions to the thalamus are, however, an established cause of human amnesia (Stuss et al., 1988; Hodges and McCarthy, 1993) and, moreover, this area is part of the limbic-diencephalic network that is specifically hypometabolic in the amnesic prodrome of AD (Nestor et al., 2003a).

The failure to detect a significant network correlate with the multivariate GM SVR might suggest that the metabolic findings are predominantly physiological and separate from local degeneration (atrophy). It is important to emphasize, however, that this quite likely reflects the far greater sensitivity of FDG to detect local

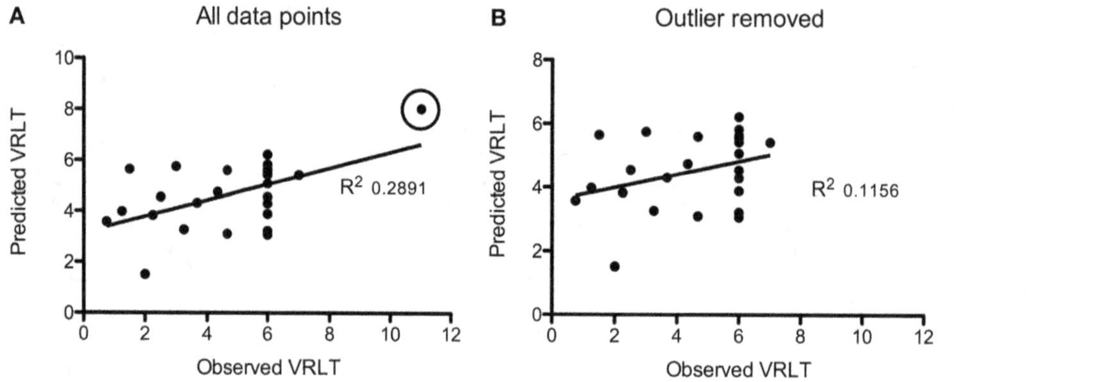


**FIGURE 5 | Plots of the Support Vector Regression (predicted versus observed VRLT score). (A)** Shows the full cohort: note that one data point (circled) appeared to be a potential outlier. Removing this data point **(B)** diminished the strength of the correlation though it remained significant ($p = 0.05$).

degeneration compared to GM density measurements. This phenomenon can be illustrated by contrasting the findings from two studies of the posterior cortical atrophy form of AD—one that examined glucose metabolism (Nestor et al., 2003c) and another that examined GM density (Whitwell et al., 2007). The lesion distribution in the two studies was identical suggesting a tight concordance between cerebral metabolism and atrophy; the key difference was that the FDG-PET result was generated from 16 subjects ($n = 6$ patients; $n = 10$ controls) whereas the GM density result came from 76 subjects ($n = 38$ in both patient and controls groups).

One finding in the multivariate FDG analysis probably does, however, represent a physiological network co-variance—this being the striking emergence that the right caudate nucleus was exerting an influence on performance. The right caudate nucleus is the one region identified to be part of the spatial memory network that is not a prominent component of the landscape of early degeneration in AD. It is, however, specifically activated during egocentric spatial memory tasks in healthy volunteers (Maguire et al., 1998; Doeller et al., 2008), and so would be expected to engage in a route learning test. Furthermore, there seems no reason to expect any disease-related caudate metabolism alterations in AD to be strongly right lateralized. We, therefore, propose that the unilateral right caudate finding in the current study offers direct evidence that this region is co-varying with posterior cortical regions involved in topographical memory performance. This observation reinforces the findings of previous fMRI studies in healthy volunteers that the right caudate nucleus is intimately involved in topographical memory processing using the complimentary model of a neurodegenerative disease that impairs this ability.

A very relevant negative in this study was the absence of prominent hippocampal correlation with task performance. Some analyses identified involvement of the extreme tail of the hippocampus, though, even then, it was never restricted to the hippocampus and could possibly have even been arising from correlation with neighbouring structures. Nevertheless, if real, it would be consistent with fMRI evidence that the tail may be the critical hippocampal component in spatial memory (Doeller et al., 2008). Arguably the more important point was that excluding the caudal couple of millimeters, no evidence was identified for hippocampal involvement in a topographical memory task that was previously shown to be highly sensitive to early AD. Without the current analyses, it is likely that many would assume topographical, indeed any kind of, memory test impairment in AD was a consequence of hippocampal damage. The present results challenge this view as an oversimplification. It would be overstating the case to suggest that the degree of hippocampal degeneration found in early AD is irrelevant to memory impairment—even in the present study it is possible that it exerted an influence that failed to reach statistical significance. It is, however, worth reflecting that the evidence that hippocampal degeneration causes memory impairment in AD is largely biased by the fact that studies finding correlation between these variables in the past have typically not examined regions beyond the MTL. Although many such studies found significant correlations (Kohler et al., 1998; de Toledo-Morrell et al., 2000a,b; Grundman et al., 2003; Reitz et al., 2009; Stoub et al., 2010), given that both MTL degeneration and memory impairment are a function of disease severity, one could ask, how could they fail to correlate? This risk of non-causal correlation is exemplified in studies in which non-mnemonic functions such as naming (Wilson et al., 1996) also correlated with MTL degeneration. The present results also offer explanation for the observation that patients with the non-Alzheimer disorder, semantic dementia, can perform the VRLT normally (Pengas et al., 2010b) yet have been previously shown to have greater MTL degeneration than is seen in AD (Chan et al., 2001; Galton et al., 2001; Nestor et al., 2006).

In conclusion, this study sought to investigate the neural basis of topographical memory impairment in AD. The traditional mass univariate regression approach employed with several different imaging modalities found correlations that particularly converged on a region encompassing retrosplenial/isthmus/posterior cingulate cortex and possibly hippocampal tail. A relatively novel multivariate approach, however, revealed that a, predominantly

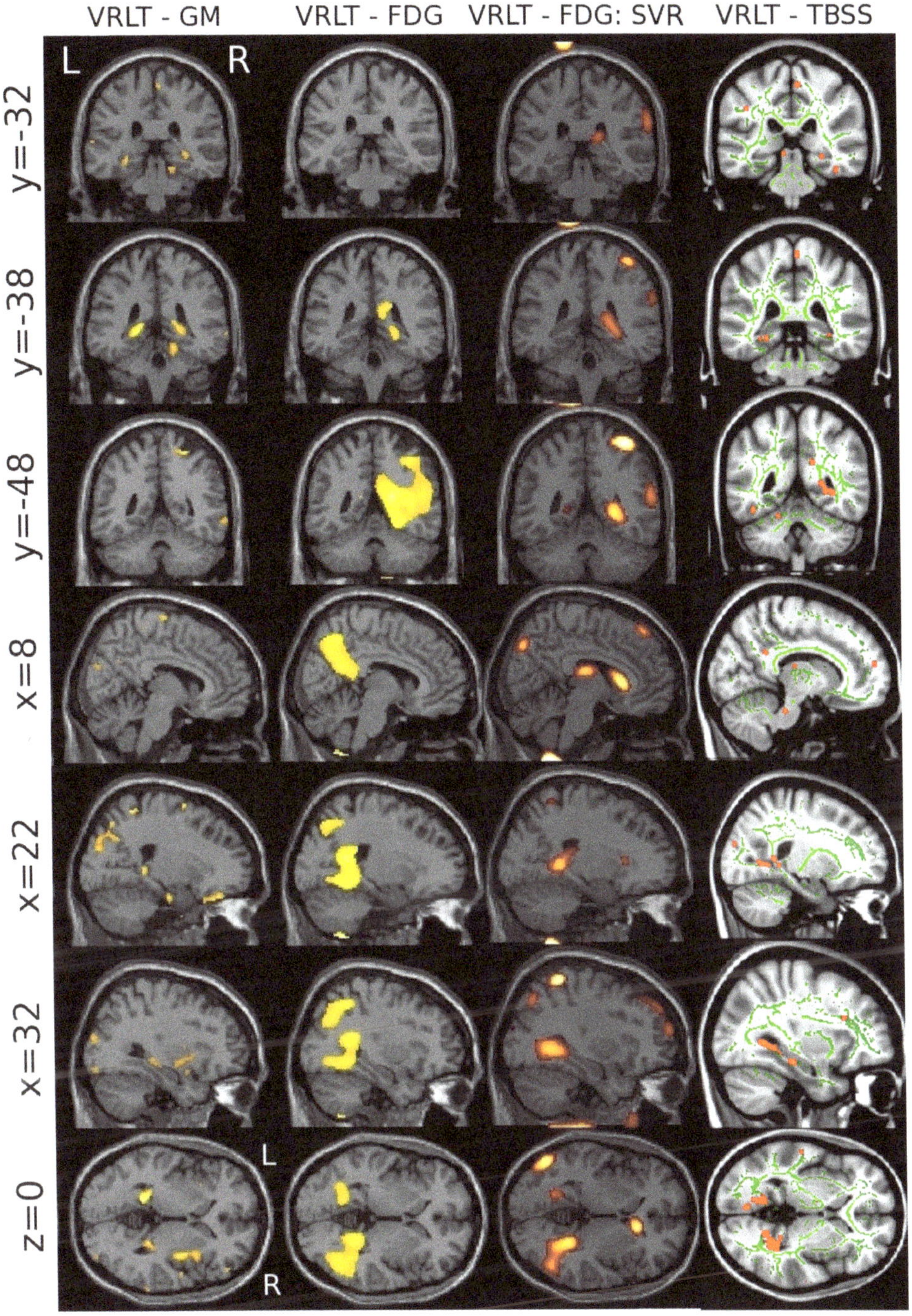


**FIGURE 6 | Convergence of results across different imaging modalities and analysis techniques.** Note that the retrosplenial/isthmus correlation is common to all analyses (see rows $y = -38$ and $z = 0$).

right hemispheric, network that reflected elements of (1) the limbic-diencephalic network known to be abnormal in incipient AD and (2) the topographical network highlighted in past fMRI studies of healthy volunteers, underpinned task performance in AD. These results, therefore, offer lesion evidence to corroborate observations made in healthy subjects regarding human route learning. Moreover, the findings highlight that memory impairment in AD is network-driven and unlikely to be simply a consequence of MTL damage.

## ACKNOWLEDGMENTS

This work was supported by funding from the Medical Research Council UK, Alzheimer's Research UK and the Cambridge Biomedical Research Centre.

## REFERENCES


Acosta-Cabronero, J., Williams, G. B., Pengas, G., and Nestor, P. J. (2010). Absolute diffusivities define the landscape of white matter degener- ation in Alzheimer's disease. *Brain* 133(Pt2), 529–539.

Acosta-Cabronero, J., Williams, G. B., Pereira, J. M., Pengas, G., and Nestor, P. J. (2008). The impact of skull-stripping and radio-frequency bias correction on grey-matter segmentation for voxel-based morphometry. *Neuroimage* 39, 1654–1665.

Ashburner, J., and Friston, K. J. (2000). Voxel-based morphometry-the methods. *Neuroimage* 11(6 Pt 1), 805–821.

Baron, J. C., Chetelat, G., Desgranges, B., Perchey, G., Landeau, B., de la Sayette, V., and Eustache, F. (2001). *In vivo* mapping of gray matter loss with voxel-based morphom- etry in mild Alzheimer's disease. *Neuroimage* 14, 298–309.

Braak, H., and Braak, E. (1991). Neuropathological stageing of Alzheimer-related changes. *Acta Neuropathol.* 82, 239–259.

Burgess, N., Maguire, E. A., Spiers, H. J., and O'Keefe, J. (2001). A tem- poroparietal and prefrontal network for retrieving the spatial context of lifelike events. *Neuroimage* 14, 439–453.

Chan, D., Fox, N. C., Scahill, R. I., Crum, W. R., Whitwell, J. L., Leschziner, G., Rossor, A. M., Stevens, J. M., Cipolotti, L., and Rossor, M. N. (2001). Patterns of temporal lobe atrophy in semantic dementia and Alzheimer's disease. *Ann. Neurol.* 49, 433–442.

Chetelat, G., Desgranges, B., De La Sayette, V., Viader, F., Eustache, F., and Baron, J. C. (2002). Mapping gray matter loss with voxel-based morphometry in mild cognitive impairment. *Neuroreport* 13, 1939–1943.

Chetelat, G., Eustache, F., Viader, F., De La Sayette, V., Pelerin, A., Mezenge, F., Hannequin, D., Dupuy, B., Baron, J. C., and Desgranges, B. (2005). FDG-PET measurement is more accurate than neuropsy- chological assessments to predict global cognitive deterioration in patients with mild cogni- tive impairment. *Neurocase* 11, 14–25.

Choo, I. H., Lee, D. Y., Oh, J. S., Lee, J. S., Lee, D. S., Song, I. C., Youn, J. C., Kim, S. G., Kim, K. W., Jhoo, J. H., and Woo, J. I. (2010). Posterior cin- gulate cortex atrophy and regional cingulum disruption in mild cog- nitive impairment and Alzheimer's disease. *Neurobiol. Aging* 31, 772–779.

delpolyi, A. R., Rankin, K. P., Mucke, L., Miller, B. L., and Gorno-Tempini, L. (2007). Spatial cognition and the human navigation network in AD and MCI. *Neurology* 69, 986–997.

de Toledo-Morrell, L., Dickerson, B., Sullivan, M. P., Spanovic, C., Wilson, R., and Bennett, D. A. (2000a). Hemispheric differences in hippocampal volume predict verbal and spatial memory performance in patients with Alzheimer's disease. *Hippocampus* 10, 136–142.

de Toledo-Morrell, L., Goncharova, I., Dickerson, B., Wilson, R. S., and Bennett, D. A. (2000b). From healthy aging to early Alzheimer's disease: *in vivo* detection of entorhi- nal cortex atrophy. *Ann. N.Y. Acad. Sci.* 911, 240–253.

Doeller, C. F., King, J. A., and Burgess, (2008). Parallel striatal and hip- pocampal systems for landmarks and boundaries in spatial memory. *Proc. Natl. Acad. Sci. U.S.A.* 105, 5915–5920.

Ekstrom, A. D., and Bookheimer, S. Y. (2007). Spatial and temporal episodic memory retrieval recruit dissociable functional networks in the human brain. *Learn. Mem.* 14, 645–654.

Galton, C. J., Patterson, K., Graham, K., Lambon-Ralph, M. A., Williams, G., Antoun, N., Sahakian, B. J., and Hodges, J. R. (2001). Differing patterns of temporal atrophy in Alzheimer's disease and semantic dementia. *Neurology* 57, 216–225.

Ghaem, O., Mellet, E., Crivello, F., Tzourio, N., Mazoyer, B., Berthoz, A., and Denis, M. (1997). Mental navigation along memorized routes activates the hippocampus, pre- cuneus, and insula. *Neuroreport* 8, 739–744.

Giannakopoulos, P., Herrmann, F. R., Bussiere, T., Bouras, C., Kovari, E., Perl, D. P., Morrison, J. H., Gold, G., and Hof, P. R. (2003). Tangle and neuron numbers, but not amy- loid load, predict cognitive status in Alzheimer's disease. *Neurology* 60, 1495–1500.

Griswold, M. A., Jakob, P. M., Heidemann, R. M., Nittka, M., Jellus, V., Wang, J., Kiefer, B., and Haase, A. (2002). Generalized autocalibrating partially parallel acquisitions (GRAPPA). *Magn. Reson. Med.* 47, 1202–1210.

Grundman, M., Jack, C. R. Jr., Petersen, R. C., Kim, H. T., Taylor, C., Datvian, M., Weiner, M. F., DeCarli, C., DeKosky, S. T., van Dyck, C., Darvesh, S., Yaffe, K., Kaye, J., Ferris, S. H., Thomas, R. G., and Thal, L. J. (2003). Hippocampal vol- ume is associated with memory but not monmemory cognitive perfor- mance in patients with mild cog- nitive impairment. *J. Mol. Neurosci.* 20, 241–248.

Hodges, J. R., and McCarthy, R. A. (1993). Autobiographical amnesia resulting from bilateral paramedian thalamic infarction. A case study in cognitive neurobiology. *Brain* 116(Pt4), 921–940.

Iaria, G., Chen, J. K., Guariglia, C., Ptito, A., and Petrides, M. (2007). Retrosplenial and hippocampal brain regions in human navigation: complementary functional contri- butions to the formation and use of cognitive maps. *Eur. J. Neurosci.* 25, 890–899.

Ichimiya, A., Herholz, K., Mielke, R., Kessler, J., Slansky, I., and Heiss, W. D. (1994). Difference of regional cerebral metabolic pattern between presenile and senile dementia of the Alzheimer type: a factor analytic study. *J. Neurol. Sci.* 123, 11–17.

Ino, T., Doi, T., Hirose, S., Kimura, T., Ito, J., and Fukuyama, H. (2007). Directional disorientation following left retrosplenial hemorrhage: a case report with fMRI studies. *Cortex* 43, 248–254.

Ino, T., Inoue, Y., Kage, M., Hirose, S., Kimura, T., and Fukuyama, H. (2002). Mental navigation in humans is processed in the anterior bank of the parieto-occipital sulcus. *Neurosci. Lett.* 322, 182–186.

Jack, C. R. Jr., Petersen, R. C., Xu, Y. C., Waring, S. C., O'Brien, P. C., Tangalos, E. G., Smith, G. E., Ivnik, R. J., and Kokmen, E. (1997). Medial temporal atrophy on MRI in nor- mal aging and very mild Alzheimer's disease. *Neurology* 49, 786–794.

Jenkinson, M., and Smith, S. (2001). A global optimisation method for robust affine registration of brain images. *Med. Image Anal.* 5, 143–156.

Joachims, T. (1999). "Making large scale SVM learning practical," in *Advances in kernel methods - Support vector learning,* eds B. Schollkopf, C. Burges, and A. Smola (Cambridge, MA: MIT press), 169–184.

Kinnahan, P. E., and Rogers, J. G. (1989). Analytic 3D image recon- struction using all detected events. *IEEE Trans. Nucl. Sci.* 36, 964–968.

Klöppel, S., Stonnington, C. M., Chu, C., Draganski, B., Scahill, R. I., Rohrer, J. D., Fox, N. C., Jack, C. R. Jr., Ashburner, J., and Frackowiak, R. S. (2008). Automatic classifica- tion of MR scans in Alzheimer's disease. *Brain* 131(Pt 3), 681–689.

Kohler, S., Black, S. E., Sinden, M., Szekely, C., Kidron, D., Parker, J. L., Foster, J. K., Moscovitch, M., Winocour, G., Szalai, J. P., and Bronskill, M. J. (1998). Memory impairments associated with hip- pocampal versus parahippocampal-gyrus atrophy: an MR volume- try study in Alzheimer's disease. *Neuropsychologia* 36, 901–914.

Maeshima, S., Ozaki, F., Masuo, O., Yamaga, H., Okita, R., and Moriwaki, H. (2001). Memory impairment and spatial disorien- tation following a left retrosplenial lesion. *J. Clin. Neurosci.* 8, 450–451. Maguire, E. A. (2001). The retrosplenial contribution to human navigation: a review of lesion and neuroimag- ing findings. *Scand. J. Psychol.* 42, 225–238.

Maguire, E. A., Burgess, N., Donnett, J. G., Frackowiak, R. S., Frith, C. D., and O'Keefe, J. (1998). Knowing where and getting there: a human navigation network. *Science* 280, 921–924.

McKhann, G., Drachman, D., Folstein, M., Katzman, R., Price, D., and Stadlan, E. M. (1984). Clinical diagnosis of Alzheimer's disease: report of the NINCDS-ADRDA Work Group under the auspices of Department of Health and Human Services Task Force on Alzheimer's disease. *Neurology* 34, 939–944.

Mellet, E., Briscogne, S., Tzourio Mazoyer, N., Ghaem, O., Petit, L., Zago, L., Etard, O., Berthoz, A., Mazoyer, B., and Denis, M. (2000). Neural correlates of topo- graphic mental exploration: the impact of route versus survey per- spective learning. *Neuroimage* 12, 588–600.

Minoshima, S., Giordani, B., Berent, S., Frey, K. A., Foster, N. L., and Kuhl, D. E. (1997). Metabolic reduction in the posterior cingulate cortex in very early Alzheimer's disease. *Ann. Neurol.* 42, 85–94.

Moffat, S. D., Kennedy, K. M., Rodrigue, K. M., and Raz, N. (2007). Extrahippocampal contri- butions to age differences in human spatial navigation. *Cereb. Cortex* 17, 1274–1282.

Nestor, P. J., Fryer, T. D., Smielewski, P., and Hodges, J. R. (2003a). Limbic hypometabolism in Alzheimer's disease and mild cognitive impairment. *Ann. Neurol.* 54, 343–351.

Nestor, P. J., Fryer, T. D., Ikeda, M., and Hodges, J. R. (2003b). Retrosplenial cortex (BA 29/30) hypometabolism in mild cognitive impairment (pro- dromal Alzheimer's disease). *Eur. J. Neurosci.* 18, 2663–2667.

Nestor, P. J., Caine, D., Fryer, T. D., Clarke, J., and Hodges, J. R. (2003c). The topography of metabolic deficits in posterior cortical atrophy (the visual vari- ant of Alzheimer's disease) with FDG-PET. *J. Neurol. Neurosurg. Psychiatry* 74, 1521–1529.

Nestor, P. J., Fryer, T. D., and Hodges, J. R. (2006). Declarative memory impairments in Alzheimer's disease and semantic dementia. *Neuroimage* 30, 1010–1020.

Pengas, G., Hodges, J. R., Watson, P., and Nestor, P. J. (2010a). Focal pos- terior cingulate atrophy in incipi- ent Alzheimer's disease. *Neurobiol. Aging* 31, 25–33.

Pengas, G., Patterson, K., Arnold, R. J., Bird, C. M., Burgess, N., and Nestor, P. J. (2010b). Lost and found: bespoke memory testing for Alzheimer's disease and semantic dementia. *J. Alzheimers Dis.* 21, 1347–1365.

Pengas, G., Pereira, J. M., Williams, G. B., and Nestor, P. J. (2009). Comparative reliability of total intracranial volume estimation methods and the influence of atrophy in a longitudinal semantic dementia cohort. *J. Neuroimaging* 19, 37–46.

Pereira, J. M., Xiong, L., Acosta Cabronero, J., Pengas, G., Williams, G. B., and Nestor, P. J. (2010). Registration accuracy for VBM studies varies according to region and degenerative dis- ease grouping. *Neuroimage* 49, 2205–2215.

Petersen, R. C., Stevens, J. C., Ganguli, M., Tangalos, E. G., Cummings, J. L., and DeKosky, S. T. (2001). Practice parameter: early detec- tion of dementia: mild cognitive impairment (an evidence-based review). Report of the quality standards subcommittee of the American academy of neurology. *Neurology* 56, 1133–1142.

Reese, T. G., Heid, O., Weisskoff, R. M., and Wedeen, V. J. (2003). Reduction of eddy-current- induced distortion in diffusion MRI using a twice-refocused spin echo. *Magn. Reson. Med.* 49, 177–182.

Reitz, C., Honig, L., Vonsattel, J. P., Tang, M. X., and Mayeux, R. (2009). Memory performance is related to amyloid and tau pathology in the hippocampus. *J. Neurol. Neurosurg. Psychiatry* 80, 715–721.

Rosenbaum, R. S., Ziegler, M., Winocur, G., Grady, C. L., and Moscovitch, M. (2004). "I have often walked down this street before": fMRI studies on the hip- pocampus and other structures during mental navigation of an old environment. *Hippocampus* 14, 826–835.

Rueckert, D., Sonoda, L. I., Hayes, C., Hill, D. L., Leach, M. O., and Hawkes, D. J. (1999). Nonrigid reg- istration using free-form deforma- tions: application to breast MR images. *IEEE Trans. Med. Imaging* 18, 712–721.

Scahill, R. I., Schott, J. M., Stevens, J. M., Rossor, M. N., and Fox, N. C. (2002). Mapping the evo- lution of regional atrophy in Alzheimer'sdisease:unbiased anal- ysis of fluid-registered serial MRI. *Proc. Natl. Acad. Sci. U.S.A.* 99, 4703–4707.

Shelton, A. L., and Gabrieli, J. D. (2002). Neural correlates of encod- ing space from route and sur- vey perspectives. *J. Neurosci.* 22, 2711–2717.

Smith, S. M. (2002). Fast robust auto- mated brain extraction. *Hum. Brain Mapp.* 17, 143–155.

Smith, S. M., and Nichols, T. E. (2009). Threshold-free cluster enhance- ment: addressing problems of smoothing, threshold dependence and localisation in cluster inference. *Neuroimage* 44, 83–98.

Smith, S. M., Jenkinson, M., Johansen- Berg, H., Rueckert, D., Nichols, T. E., Mackay, C. E., Watkins, K. E., Ciccarelli, O., Cader, M. Z., Matthews, P. M., and Behrens, T. E. (2006). Tract-based spatial statis- tics: voxelwise analysis of multi- subject diffusion data. *Neuroimage* 31, 1487–1505.

Stoub, T. R., Rogalski, E. J., Leurgans, S., Bennett, D. A., and deToledo-Morrell, L. (2010). Rate of entorhi- nal and hippocampal atrophy in incipient and mild AD: relation to memory function. *Neurobiol. Aging* 31, 1089–1098.

Stuss, D. T., Guberman, A., Nelson, R., and Larochelle, S. (1988). The neu- ropsychology of paramedian tha- lamic infarction. *Brain Cogn.* 8, 348–378.

Takahashi, N., Kawamura, M., Shiota, J., Kasahata, N., and Hirayama, K. (1997). Pure topographic disorien- tation due to right retrosplenial lesion. *Neurology* 49, 464–469.

Whitwell, J. L., Jack, C. R. Jr., Kantarci, K., Weigand, S. D., Boeve, B. F., Knopman, D. S., Drubach, D. A., Tang-Wai, D. F., Petersen, R. C., and Josephs, K. A. (2007). Imaging correlates of posterior cortical atrophy. *Neurobiol. Aging* 28, 1051–1061.

Wilson, R. S., Sullivan, M., deToledo- Morrell, L., Stebbins, G. T., and Bennett, D. A. (1996). Association of memory and cognition in Alzheimer's disease with volu- metric estimates of temporal lobe structures. *Neuropsychology* 10, 459–463.

Wolbers, T., and Buchel, C. (2005). Dissociable retrosplenial and hippocampal contributions to successful formation of survey representations. *J. Neurosci.* 25, 3333–3340.

Wolbers, T., Weiller, C., and Buchel, C. (2004). Neural foundations of emerging route knowledge in com- plex spatial environments. *Brain Res. Cogn. Brain Res.* 21, 401–411.

# 27

# Differential effects of aging on spatial learning through exploratory navigation and map reading

***Naohide Yamamoto* and Gregory J. DeGirolamo***

*Department of Psychology, Cleveland State University, Cleveland, OH, USA*

**Edited by:**
*Thomas Wolbers, University of Edinburgh, UK*

**Reviewed by:**
*Scott Moffat, Wayne State University, USA*
*Jon Kelly, Iowa State University, USA*

***Correspondence:**
*Naohide Yamamoto, Department of Psychology, Cleveland State University, 2121 Euclid Avenue, Cleveland, OH 44115, USA.*
*e-mail: n.yamamoto@csuohio.edu*

It has been shown that abilities in spatial learning and memory are adversely affected by aging. The present study was conducted to investigate whether increasing age has equal consequences for all types of spatial learning or impacts certain types of spatial learning selectively. Specifically, two major types of spatial learning, exploratory navigation and map reading, were contrasted. By combining a neuroimaging finding that the medial temporal lobe (MTL) is especially important for exploratory navigation and a neurological finding that the MTL is susceptible to age-related atrophy, it was hypothesized that spatial learning through exploratory navigation would exhibit a greater decline in later life than spatial learning through map reading. In an experiment, young and senior participants learned locations of landmarks in virtual environments either by navigating in them in the first-person perspective or by seeing aerial views of the environments. Results showed that senior participants acquired less accurate memories of the layouts of landmarks than young participants when they navigated in the environments, but the two groups did not differ in spatial learning performance when they viewed the environments from the aerial perspective. These results suggest that spatial learning through exploratory navigation is particularly vulnerable to adverse effects of aging, whereas elderly adults may be able to maintain their map reading skills relatively well.

**Keywords: aging, spatial learning, navigation, map, ground-level, aerial, route, survey**

## 1. INTRODUCTION

Abilities in spatial learning and memory are adversely affected by both normal and pathological aging. Many senior citizens experience great difficulty in navigation in unfamiliar environments (Burns, 1999), and it is often the case that topographical disorientation is among the earliest symptoms displayed by patients with Alzheimer's disease (Pai and Jacobs, 2004). Results from experimental studies have been consistent with these epidemiological observations, showing that elderly participants (either healthy or demented) performed worse than young participants in a variety of spatial learning and memory tasks (for review, see Iachini et al., 2009; Moffat, 2009; Vlček, 2011). In spite of these converging and accumulating findings in the literature, psychological mechanisms of this age-related decline are poorly understood. For example, it is largely unknown whether aging has equal consequences for all types of spatial learning or impacts certain types of spatial learning selectively. The objective of the present study was to address this issue by contrasting the effects of normal aging on spatial memories acquired through two major methods of spatial learning: exploratory navigation in a ground-level (also called *route*) perspective and map reading in an aerial (also called *survey*) perspective (Siegel and White, 1975; Thorndyke and Hayes-Roth, 1982).

Previous studies demonstrated age-related decrements of spatial learning both in exploratory navigation and in map reading. Extensive research has been carried out by having participants learn environments through exploratory navigation in the first-person (i.e., ground-level) perspective. Some studies involved real navigation in physical environments (e.g., Kirasic, 1991; Barrash, 1994; Wilkniss et al., 1997; Newman and Kaszniak, 2000; Iachini et al., 2005), and others utilized simulated navigation in virtual environments (e.g., Moffat et al., 2001; Moffat and Resnick, 2002; Lövdén et al., 2005; Iaria et al., 2009; Zakzanis et al., 2009; Liu et al., 2011). These studies commonly found that young participants acquired knowledge of the environments more accurately or quickly than senior participants (see also Cushman et al., 2008). Similarly, when participants learned specific routes on maps first and attempted to trace them in actual environments later, older adults were slower and less accurate (Wilkniss et al., 1997; Carelli et al., 2011). In addition, young adults tended to use maps more effectively for spatial learning than elderly adults: young adults recalled more landmark locations than elderly adults after studying street maps (Thomas, 1985; De Beni et al., 2006; Meneghetti et al., 2011), and having a map of an environment during exploratory navigation did not enhance elderly adults' learning of object locations (Sjölinder et al., 2005). All of these findings indicates that certain degrees of decline in spatial learning abilities take place in later life regardless of the ways in which an environment is learned. However, because spatial learning by exploratory navigation and spatial learning by map reading were examined separately in the previous studies, it remains unclear whether these two kinds of spatial learning show the same level of decline or one goes down more significantly than the other. Thus, the present study was designed to make a direct comparison between exploratory navigation and map reading to investigate possible differential effects of aging on these two types of spatial learning.

Neuroimaging and neurological studies have provided important clues for addressing this issue. On one hand, neuroimaging studies have suggested that activation in the medial temporal lobe (MTL), hippocampus and parahippocampal cortex in particular, is a key to distinguishing spatial learning through exploratory navigation and spatial learning through map reading. For example, Shelton and colleagues found that encoding of spatial information through exploratory navigation and map reading elicited activations in overlapping areas of the young adult brain, but the MTL was activated more strongly by exploratory navigation than map reading (Shelton and Gabrieli, 2002; Shelton and Pippitt, 2007). When Borghesani et al. (2008) applied the same paradigm to healthy elderly adults who did not carry the apolipoprotein E ε4 allele, a known genetic risk factor for Alzheimer's disease (Strittmatter et al., 1993), they found that MTL activity during spatial learning through exploratory navigation but not through map reading was correlated with subsequent performance on a spatial memory test. Furthermore, when similar activations in the MTL were observed while participants learned environmental layouts in other studies, they typically learned environments through exploratory navigation (e.g., Aguirre et al., 1996; Grön et al., 2000; Moffat et al., 2006; Antonova et al., 2009; Iglói et al., 2010; Marchette et al., 2011; but see also Blanch et al., 2004). On the other hand, cross-sectional and longitudinal studies of age-related brain volume changes have revealed significant atrophy of the MTL in healthy elderly populations (Golomb et al., 1993; Jack et al., 1997, 1998; Šimić et al., 1997; Insausti et al., 1998; Jernigan et al., 2001; Scahill et al., 2003; Raz et al., 2004; but see also Sullivan et al., 1995, 2005). Importantly, this shrinkage of the MTL has actual behavioral consequences on spatial learning: Nedelska et al. (2012) demonstrated that smaller volume of the right hippocampus corresponds to larger impairment of spatial learning in the first-person perspective. Similarly, impaired performance of elderly adults in spatial learning through exploratory navigation correlated with reduced activation of the MTL, which might result from the atrophy of this brain region (Meulenbroek et al., 2004; Moffat et al., 2006; Antonova et al., 2009). Together, these neuroimaging and neurological findings lead to a hypothesis that vulnerability of the MTL to age-related atrophy makes spatial learning through exploratory navigation more susceptible to detrimental effects of increasing age. By contrast, because the MTL is engaged to a lesser extent while encoding spatial information from maps, it is also predicted that spatial learning through map reading would be affected by aging less significantly.

These hypotheses were tested in an experiment reported below. Young and senior participants learned locations of landmarks in virtual environments by viewing them either from a perspective of an observer walking through the environments (i.e., exploratory navigation) or from an aerial perspective that had a constant orientation relative to the environments (i.e., map reading). After learning each environment, they attempted to reproduce the layout of landmarks in a smaller scale. It was predicted that senior participants would reconstruct the layouts less accurately than young participants. More specifically, a greater difference between young and senior groups would be observed following spatial learning through exploratory navigation than that through map reading.

## 2. MATERIALS AND METHODS

### 2.1. PARTICIPANTS

Forty-eight participants gave their informed consent to participate in the experiment. They included 24 young participants (9 males and 15 females, 18–33 years old) and 24 senior participants (13 males and 11 females, 60–80 years old). Means ($M$) and standard deviations ($SD$) of their ages were as follows: $M = 21$, $SD = 4.76$ (young); and $M = 68.5$, $SD = 5.19$ (senior). The exact age of one young participant was not available. These two groups differed significantly in mean ages but not in ratios of males and females, $t_{(45)} = -31.95, p < 0.001$ and $\chi^2_{(1)} = 1.34$, $p = 0.25$, respectively. They received either monetary compensation or partial credit in a psychology course in return for their participation. They were native or fluent speakers of English and reported normal or corrected-to-normal vision.

All but one senior participant were enrolled in courses at Cleveland State University at the time of the experiment. Thus, although no formal screening was conducted, it was reasonable to assume that they were cognitively healthy individuals.

### 2.2. DESIGN AND PROCEDURE

The experimental protocol described below was approved by the institutional review board of Cleveland State University. Four virtual environments of the same size (110 × 130 ft in virtual space) were presented on the display of a desktop computer by using the PsyScope program (Cohen et al., 1993). They were visually distinct from each other (see **Figure 1** for examples), and each environment contained 10 large landmarks and seven small objects in a unique configuration. They were the same environments as those used in previous studies by Shelton and colleagues (e.g., Shelton and Gabrieli, 2002; Shelton and McNamara, 2004; Shelton and Pippitt, 2007). Each participant viewed all four environments, two from the perspective of a six-foot-tall observer walking through the environments (navigation condition; **Figure 1A**) and the other two from the perspective of an observer who was 70 ft above the ground and looking straight down (map condition; **Figure 1B**). In both conditions, approximately 2–3 landmarks were visible in their entirety at any given time (see **Figures 1A** and **B**). The walk-through of an environment in the navigation condition always began at the southwest corner and proceeded clockwise along the perimeter of the environment (**Figure 1C**). At each corner, the observer made a 90°-turn to face the new direction of travel. Viewing of an environment in the map condition was carried out in a similar manner. The observer was initially at the southwest corner and moved along four legs of the environment in the same direction. An important difference is that in the map condition the observer maintained the initial orientation (indicated by the arrow labeled as Leg 1 in **Figure 1C**) within each environment. Variable orientations and the fixed orientation were utilized in navigation and map conditions, respectively,

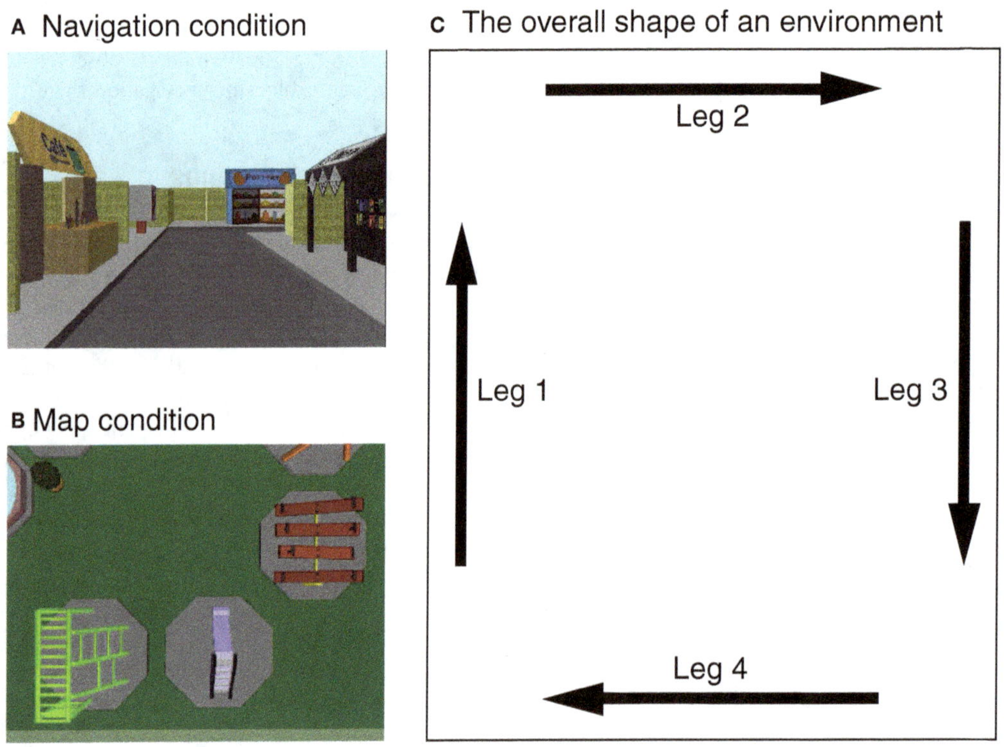


**FIGURE 1 | Examples of virtual environments learned by participants in the experiment.** They were presented either from a ground-level perspective in varying orientations **(A)** or from an aerial perspective in a fixed orientation **(B)**. The presentation of each environment began at its southwest corner (lower left corner in the figure) and proceeded clockwise along the four legs **(C)**. These virtual environments were originally created and used by Shelton and colleagues (Shelton and Gabrieli, 2002; Shelton and McNamara, 2004).

in order to capture essential aspects of corresponding types of spatial learning: exploratory navigation is conducted in the first-person perspective that varies with an observer, whereas maps are typically read in a single orientation (Shelton and Pippitt, 2007).

Participants were instructed to learn the locations of the 10 landmarks for a later memory test. They were given a diagram similar to **Figure 1C** and informed that they would view environments along the four legs in clockwise direction. They were also told that environments would be presented from either a ground-level or an aerial perspective. During the first run of each environment, an experimenter named 10 landmarks that were to be learned. Subsequently, participants viewed six additional runs of the environment by themselves. They were encouraged to pay close attention to all of the subsequent showings of the environment by naming the landmarks every time they appeared on the screen. To clearly indicate which leg they were in at any given moment, a label specifying a leg number was presented for 4 s right before each leg was shown. Each run of an environment took 56 s including the leg labels.

After learning each environment, participants were presented with a dry-erase board on which a rectangle representing the perimeter of the environment was drawn in scale ($17.92 \times 21.18$ cm). It also specified the southwest corner (i.e., the starting point) of the environment and the direction of the first leg, which was aligned with participants' egocentric orientation at the time of initial presentation of the board. Participants were free to turn the board, if they so chose. They were given 10 identical magnet disks (2 cm diameter), which were to be placed at the locations of landmarks within the rectangle. They were also given names of the 10 landmarks and used them to indicate which disk represented which landmark. They were allowed to place the landmarks in any order and spend unlimited time to complete this task. No error feedback was given to participants.

Following completion of the memory test, participants were presented with a new environment in the same procedure. This study-test sequence was repeated until all four environments were learned and tested. The order of two perspectives was counterbalanced over participants. Four environments were randomly assigned to each perspective with the constraint that each environment appeared in each position of the sequence with equal frequency.

### 2.3. DATA ANALYSIS

The dependent measure was accuracy of the reconstructed layouts of landmarks. It was obtained through extension of bidimensional regression (Tobler, 1994). In this technique, a reconstructed layout first undergoes translation, rotation, and linear scaling so that it is transformed into the correct layout as much as possible. The best-fit layout can be uniquely determined by the least square method, and the regression coefficients associated with this transformation are converted into a distortion index (DI), which reflects the overall accuracy of the reconstructed layout independent of translation, rotation, and scaling factors. The DI is a dimensionless value ranging from 0 to 100, with 0 indicating accurate reconstruction of the layout and 100 corresponding to the case in which all landmarks are placed in a single point. Details of the computational procedure are described by Waterman and Gordon (1984).

Although primary independent variables in this experiment were participant groups (young vs. senior) and types of spatial learning (navigation vs. map), it included an additional variable that was not relevant to the present study: once within each type of learning, the four legs of an environment were presented in random order. However, other than increasing the overall distortion of reconstructed layouts of landmarks, this variable showed virtually no interactions with group or learning type. Thus, this additional variable was not included in the analysis. Dropping this variable did not introduce any bias in results reported below because its effect was equally distributed across all conditions (i.e., the three variables were factorially combined).

## 3. RESULTS

DIs from the two environments learned in the same type of learning were averaged within each participant, and then their means and standard deviations were calculated for each age group and for each learning type. They were as follows (see also **Figure 2**): $M = 47.07$, $SD = 19.63$ (young, navigation); $M = 34.27$, $SD = 13.66$ (young, map); $M = 65.51$, $SD = 22.02$ (senior, navigation); and $M = 35.46$, $SD = 14.27$ (senior, map).

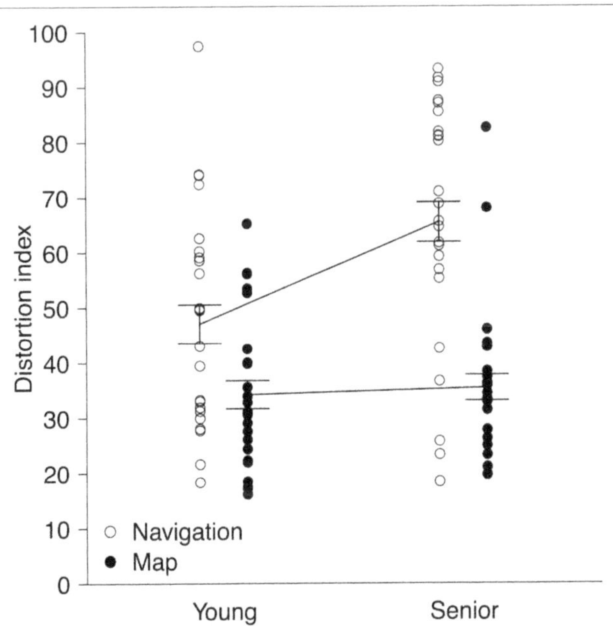


**FIGURE 2 | Distortion indices (DIs) as a function of group (young vs. senior) and type of learning (navigation vs. map).** Each dot shows a DI of one participant. For each type of learning, a solid line connects the means of the age groups. Error bars represent ±1 standard error of the mean.

Data were checked for outliers, but only one data point of a senior participant in the map condition fell outside the range of $M \pm 3$ $SD$, and excluding this participant did not alter the results at all. Thus, all data points were included in the analysis. DIs were subjected to a split-plot analysis of variance with group (young vs. senior) as a between-subject factor and type of learning (navigation vs. map) as a within-subject factor. Generalized eta squared ($\eta^2_G$) values are reported below as effect size statistics (Olejnik and Algina, 2003; Bakeman, 2005).

**Figure 2** shows DIs as a function of group and learning type, revealing two major findings. First, following spatial learning through exploratory navigation senior participants created more distorted layouts of landmarks than young participants, but following spatial learning through map reading these two groups performed equivalently. Consistent with these observations, the interaction between group and learning type was significant, $F_{(1, 46)} = 7.54$, $p = 0.0086$, $\eta^2_G = 0.056$. Simple main-effect tests comparing the two age groups yielded a significant result within the navigation condition but not within the map condition, $F_{(1, 46)} = 12.40$, $p < 0.001$, $\eta^2_G = 0.21$, and $F_{(1, 46)} = 0.052$, $p = 0.82$, $\eta^2_G = 0.0011$, respectively. Additionally, this substantial worsening of senior participants' performance in the navigation condition made the main effect of group significant, $F_{(1, 46)} = 5.49$, $p = 0.024$, $\eta^2_G = 0.071$. Second, there was an overall difference in the quality of reconstructed layouts between navigation and map conditions: participants reproduced the layouts more accurately after spatial learning through map reading than that through exploratory navigation. This was indicated by the significant main effect of learning type, $F_{(1, 46)} = 46.56$, $p < 0.001$, $\eta^2_G = 0.27$. Furthermore, a simple main-effect test comparing the two conditions in the young group was also significant, $F_{(1, 46)} = 8.31$, $p = 0.0060$, $\eta^2_G = 0.15$, showing that accuracy of reproduced layouts was reliably different between navigation and map conditions even among young participants.

## 4. DISCUSSION

The present study was conducted to investigate whether increasing age has differential impacts on spatial learning through exploratory navigation in the first-person (i.e., ground-level) perspective and map reading in an aerial perspective. On the basis of previous findings that encoding of spatial information from the first-person perspective strongly engages the MTL and that this brain region is susceptible to age-related atrophy, it was hypothesized that elderly adults would be especially impaired at learning an environmental layout by navigating in the environment. Results from the experiment supported this hypothesis, showing that (1) senior participants constructed the layouts of landmarks less accurately than young participants after learning them through exploratory navigation; and (2) young and senior participants reproduced the layouts with equivalent accuracy after learning them through map reading. These data suggest that not all types of spatial learning are affected equally by aging. Rather, it is suggested that seniors' ability in learning environments from maps is better maintained through normal aging processes than their ability to acquire spatial knowledge from actual navigational experiences.

It is noteworthy that in the experiment young and senior participants performed equivalently after learning environments through maps. This suggests that the observed difference between the two age groups in the navigation condition cannot be explained entirely by general age-related factors such as slower speed of information processing and less familiarity with computers. In navigation and map conditions, the environments were presented at comparable rates (i.e., approximately the same number of landmarks were visible at any given time in both conditions), and identical learning and test procedures were employed. Furthermore, the competent performance of senior participants in the map condition supports the observation that they were cognitively healthy individuals. Thus, it is reasonable to conclude that the decreased accuracy of spatial memories in the navigation condition was indicative of specific effects of normal aging on spatial learning through exploratory navigation.

It is also important to note that although the present study found little difference between young and senior participants in the map condition, it does not necessarily indicate that there would be no age-related decline in map reading abilities. As discussed in the introduction, previous studies showed that elderly adults had a tendency to acquire spatial knowledge from maps less proficiently than young adults (Thomas, 1985; De Beni et al., 2006; Meneghetti et al., 2011). A notable difference from the present study is that in these studies participants were asked to recall both landmark identities and their locations. On the other hand, in the present study, participants were given names of to-be-remembered landmarks in the beginning of a test phase. This most likely reduced the burden on their spatial memories, helping senior participants perform competently in the map condition. Nevertheless, in the navigation condition, this advantage did not eliminate the age difference in spatial learning and memory.

Previous studies on age-related changes in spatial learning suggested that among various processes of spatial learning elderly adults have trouble in cognitive mapping in particular, a process with which observers build the mental representation of a configuration of object locations that are experienced separately (e.g., Iaria et al., 2009; Liu et al., 2011). In these studies, participants learned large-scale environments through exploratory navigation in the first-person perspective and subsequently attempted to create layouts of landmarks from an aerial perspective. Consistent with the navigation condition of the present study, senior participants in the previous studies were impaired at this task compared to young participants. By contrast, although the same cognitive mapping process was involved in the map condition of the present study, senior participants reconstructed the layouts as accurately as young participants. This suggests that the integration process itself with which landmark locations are combined into the entire layout remains intact in elderly adults. Instead, impaired performance observed in the previous studies and in the navigation condition likely stemmed from declines in the ability of (1) encoding spatial information from the ground-level perspective, (2) transforming spatial information from ground-level into aerial perspectives, or (3) aligning landmarks learned from multiple orientations with each other, as none of these was necessary in the map condition.

Related to the above, it should be explicitly pointed out that in the present study the memory test was conducted in an aerial perspective that was also used for encoding spatial information in the map condition. As a consequence, participants had to transform spatial information from ground-level to aerial perspectives only in the navigation condition. This transformation was expected to have minimal influence (at least in young participants) because when a similar task was performed by young adults in previous studies, layouts of equivalent accuracy were constructed after learning environments from ground-level and aerial perspectives (Shelton and Gabrieli, 2002; Shelton and McNamara, 2004; Shelton and Pippitt, 2007). However, in the present study, even young participants created more accurate layouts of landmarks in the map condition than in the navigation condition. Although it is not readily clear why there was this discrepancy in findings, the present result does indicate that effects of perspective transformation were not negligible in the navigation condition. This is potentially important for explaining the observed age-related difference in this condition, given that the MTL has been shown to be involved in manipulation of viewpoints in spatial memory (King et al., 2002; Lee et al., 2005); that is, the ability to mentally transform perspectives can decline in aging, possibly causing selective impairment in the navigation condition (Inagaki et al., 2002; Joanisse et al., 2008; Devlin and Wilson, 2010). Thus, in future studies it would be informative to include tasks that do not require transforming perspectives between learning and test in both navigation and map conditions (e.g., a scene recognition task; Shelton and McNamara, 2004). Such tasks would help clarify whether it was types of spatial learning *per se* or mental transformation of spatial information that impacted performance of senior participants in the present study.

Spatial learning through exploratory navigation and spatial learning through map reading are different in a number of respects. The present study focused on two most notable differences between them: perspectives and orientations. Exploratory navigation is carried out in a ground-level perspective with variable orientations, whereas maps are read from an aerial perspective in a stable orientation. In the present study, they were varied simultaneously between navigation and map conditions for achieving naturalistic simulation of exploratory navigation and map reading. Although this approach was effective in revealing the selective effect of aging on spatial learning through exploratory navigation, the present data alone cannot determine whether it originated from viewing environments from the ground-level perspective or learning environmental layouts with varying orientations. Similarly, for the purpose of making strict comparisons between the two conditions, some characteristics of each type of spatial learning were not captured in the present study. For example, one typical advantage of map reading over exploratory navigation is that observers can learn a greater portion of an environment from a single point of view. However, this advantage was not available in the present experiment because approximately the same number of landmarks were made visible at any given time in both conditions in order to avoid a potential confound of general age difference in information processing speed. It is important for future studies to examine possible roles of these unexplored factors in age-related changes in spatial learning abilities. Such investigations should bring about a clearer understanding of elderly adults' challenges in spatial learning and memory, and eventually a solution for easing their difficulties.

## ACKNOWLEDGMENTS

The authors thank Amy Shelton for providing materials used in the experiment, and Albert Smith, Jesse Sargent, and Lucinda Rohde for comments on drafts of this article.

## REFERENCES

Aguirre, G. K., Detre, J. A., Alsop, D. C., and D'Esposito, M. (1996). The parahippocampus subserves topo- graphical learning in man. *Cereb. Cortex* 6,823–829.

Antonova, E., Parslow, D., Brammer, M., Dawson, G. R., Jackson, S. H. D., and Morris, R. G. (2009). Age- related neural activity during allo- centric spatial memory. *Memory* 17, 125–143.

Bakeman, R. (2005). Recommended effect size statistics for repeated measures designs. *Behav. Res. Methods* 37,379–384.

Barrash, J. (1994). Age-related decline in route learning ability. *Dev. Neuropsychol.* 10,189–201.

Blanch, R. J., Brennan, D., Condon, B., Santosh, C., and Hadley, D. (2004). Are there gender-specific neural substrates of route learning from different perspectives? *Cereb. Cortex* 14,1207–1213.

Borghesani, P. R., Johnson, L. C., Shelton, A. L., Peskind, E. R., Aylward, E. H., Schellenberg, G. D., and Cherrier, M. M. (2008). Altered medial temporal lobe responses during visuospatial encoding in healthy APOE*4 carriers. *Neurobiol. Aging* 29,981–991.

Burns, P. C. (1999). Navigation and the mobility of older drivers. *J. Gerontol. B Psychol. Sci. Soc. Sci.* 54B, S49–S55.

Carelli, L., Rusconi, M. L., Scarabelli, C., Stampatori, C., Mattioli, F., and Riva, G. (2011). The transfer from survey (map-like) to route repre- sentations into virtual reality mazes: effect of age and cerebral lesion. *J. Neuroeng. Rehabil.* 8,6.

Cohen, J., MacWhinney, B., Flatt, M., and Provost, J. (1993). PsyScope: an interactive graphic system for designing and controlling experi- ments in the psychology laboratory using Macintosh computers. *Behav. Res. Methods Instrum. Comput.* 25, 257–271.

Cushman, L. A., Stein, K., and Duffy, C. J. (2008). Detecting naviga- tional deficits in cognitive aging and Alzheimer disease using virtual reality. *Neurology* 71, 888–895.

De Beni, R., Pazzaglia, F., and Gardini, S. (2006). The role of men- tal rotation and age in spatial perspective-taking tasks: when age does not impair perspective-taking performance. *Appl. Cogn. Psychol.* 20,807–821.

Devlin, A. L., and Wilson, P. H. (2010). Adult age differences in the ability to mentally transform object and body stimuli. *Aging Neuropsychol. Cogn.* 17, 709–729.

Golomb, J., de Leon, M. J., Kluger, A., George, A. E., Tarshish, C., and Ferris, S. H. (1993). Hippocampal atrophy in normal aging. *Arch. Neurol.* 50,967–973.

Grön, G., Wunderlich, A. P., Spitzer, M., Tomczak, R., and Riepe, M. W. (2000). Brain activation during human navigation: gender-different neural networks as substrate of performance. *Nat. Neurosci.* 3, 404–408.

Iachini, T., Iavarone, A., Senese, V. P., Ruotolo, F., and Ruggiero, G. (2009). Visuospatial memory in healthy elderly, AD and MCI: a review. *Curr. Aging Sci.* 2,43–59.

Iachini, T., Poderico, C., Ruggiero, G., and Iavarone, A. (2005). Age differ- ences in mental scanning of loco- motor maps. *Disabil. Rehabil.* 27, 741–752.

Iaria, G., Palermo, L., Committeri, G., and Barton, J. J. S. (2009). Age differences in the formation and use of cognitive maps. *Behav. Brain Res.* 196, 187–191.

Iglói, K., Doeller, C. F., Berthoz, A., Rondi-Reig, L., and Burgess, N. (2010). Lateralized human hippocampal activity predicts navigation based on sequence or place memory. *Proc. Natl. Acad. Sci. U.S.A.* 107,14466–14471.

Inagaki, H., Meguro, K., Shimada, M., Ishizaki, J., Okuzumi, H., and Yamadori, A. (2002). Discrepancy between mental rotation and perspective-taking abilities in normal aging assessed by Piaget's three-mountain task. *J. Clin. Exp. Neuropsychol.* 24,18–25.

Insausti, R., Insausti, A. M., Sobreviela, M. T., Salinas, A., and Martínez-Peñuela, J. M. (1998). Human medial temporal lobe in aging: anatomical basis of memory preser- vation. *Microsc. Res. Tech.* 43, 8–15.

Jack, C. R., Petersen, R. C., Xu, Y., O'Brien, P. C., Smith, G. E., Ivnik, R. J., Tangalos, E. G., and Kokmen, E. (1998). The rate of medial tem- poral lobe atrophy in typical aging and Alzheimer's disease. *Neurology* 51,993–999.

Jack, C. R., Petersen, R. C., Xu, Y. C., Waring, S. C., O'Brien, P. C., Tangalos, E. G., Smith, G. E., Ivnik, R. J., and Kokmen, E. (1997). Medial temporal atrophy on MRI in nor- malagingandverymildAlzheimer's disease. *Neurology* 49, 786–794.

Jernigan, T. L., Archibald, S. L., Fennema-Notestine, C., Gamst, A. C., Stout, J. C., Bonner, J., and Hesselink, J. R. (2001). Effects of age on tissues and regions of the cere- brum and cerebellum. *Neurobiol. Aging* 22,581–594.

Joanisse, M., Gagnon, S., Kreller, J., and Charbonneau, M.-C. (2008). Age-related differences in viewer-rotation tasks: is men- tal manipulation the key factor? *J. Gerontol. B Psychol. Sci. Soc. Sci.* 63B, P193–P200.

King, J. A., Burgess, N., Hartley, T., Vargha-Khadem, F., and O'Keefe, (2002). Human hippocampus and viewpoint dependence in spatial memory. *Hippocampus* 12, 811–820.

Kirasic, K. C. (1991). Spatial cognition and behavior in young and elderly adults: implications for learning newenvironments. *Psychol. Aging* 6, 10–18.

Lee, A. C. H., Buckley, M. J., Pegman, S. J., Spiers, H., Scahill, V. L., Gaffan, D., Bussey, T. J., Davies, R. R., Kapur, N., Hodges, J. R., and Graham, S. (2005). Specialization in the medial temporal lobe for processing of objects and scenes. *Hippocampus* 15,782–797.

Liu, I., Levy, R. M., Barton, J. J. S., and Iaria, G. (2011). Age and gender differences in various topographi- cal orientation strategies. *Brain Res.* 1410, 112–119.

Lövdén, M., Schellenbach, M., Grossman-Hutter, B., Krüger, A., and Lindenberger, U. (2005). Environmental topography and postural control demands shape aging-associated decrements in spatial navigation performance. *Psychol. Aging* 20,683–694.

Marchette, S. A., Bakker, A., and Shelton, A. L. (2011). Cognitive mappers to creatures of habit: dif- ferential engagement of place and response learning mechanisms pre- dicts human navigational behavior. *J. Neurosci.* 31, 15264–15268.

Meneghetti, C., Fiore, F., Borella, E., and De Beni, R. (2011). Learning a map of environment: the role of visuo-spatial abilities in young and older adults. *Appl. Cogn. Psychol.* 25, 952–959.

Meulenbroek, O., Petersson, K. M., Voermans, N., Weber, B., and Fernández, G. (2004). Age differ- ences in neural correlates of route encoding and route recognition. *Neuroimage* 22, 1503–1514.

Moffat, S. D. (2009). Aging and spatial navigation: what do we know and where do we go? *Neuropsychol. Rev.* 19,478–489.

Moffat, S. D., Elkins, W., and Resnick, S. M. (2006). Age differences in the neural systems supporting human allocentric spatial navigation. *Neurobiol. Aging* 27,965–972.

Moffat, S. D., and Resnick, S. M. (2002). Effects of age on virtual environ- ment place navigation and allo- centric cognitive mapping. *Behav. Neurosci.* 116, 851–859.

Moffat, S. D., Zonderman, A. B., and Resnick, S. M. (2001). Age differences in spatial memory in a virtual environment naviga- tion task. *Neurobiol. Aging* 22, 787–796.

Nedelska, Z., Andel, R., Laczó, J., Vlcek, K., Horinek, D., Lisy, J., Sheardova, K., Bureš, J., and Hort, J. (2012). Spatial navigation impairment is proportional to right hippocampal volume. *Proc. Natl. Acad. Sci. U.S.A.* 109, 2590–2594.

Newman, M. C., and Kaszniak, A. W. (2000). Spatial memory and aging: performance on a human analog of the Morris water maze. *Aging Neuropsychol. Cogn.* 7,86–93.

Olejnik, S., and Algina, J. (2003). Generalized eta and omega squared statistics: measures of effect size for some common research designs. *Psychol. Methods* 8, 434–447.

Pai, M.-C., and Jacobs, W. J. (2004). Topographical disori- entation in community-residing patients with Alzheimer's dis- ease. *Int. J. Geriatr. Psychiatry* 19, 250–255.

Raz, N., Gunning-Dixon, F., Head, D., Rodrigue, K. M., Williamson, A., and Acker, J. D. (2004). Aging, sex- ual dimorphism, and hemispheric asymmetry of the cerebral cortex: replicability of regional differences in volume. *Neurobiol. Aging* 25, 377–396.

Scahill, R. I., Frost, C., Jenkins, R., Whitwell, J. L., Rossor, M. N., and Fox, N. C. (2003). A longitudinal study of brain volume changes in normal aging using serial registered magnetic resonance imaging. *Arch. Neurol.* 60,989–994.

Shelton, A. L., and Gabrieli, J. D. E. (2002). Neural correlates of encod- ing space from route and sur- vey perspectives. *J. Neurosci.* 22, 2711–2717.

Shelton, A. L., and McNamara, T. P. (2004). Orientation and perspec- tive dependence in route and sur- vey learning. *J. Exp. Psychol. Learn. Mem. Cogn.* 30, 158–170.

Shelton, A. L., and Pippitt, H. A. (2007). Fixed versus dynamic ori- entations in environmental learning from ground-level and aerial per- spectives. *Psychol. Res.* 71, 333–346. Siegel, A. W., and White, S. H. (1975). "The development of spatial representations of large-scale envi- ronments," in *Advances in Child Development and Behavior,* ed H. W. Reese (New York, NY: Academic Press), 9–55.

Šimić, G., Kostović, I., Winblad, B., and Bogdanović, N. (1997). Volume and number of neurons of the human hippocampal formation in normal aging and Alzheimer's disease. *J. Comp. Neurol.* 379, 482–494.

Sjölinder, M., Höök, K., Nilsson, L.-G., and Andersson, G. (2005). Age differences and the acqui- sition of spatial knowledge in a three-dimensional environ- ment: evaluating the use of an overview map as a navigation aid. *Int. J. Hum. Comput. Stud.* 63, 537–564.

Strittmatter, W. J., Saunders, A. M., Schmechel, D., Pericak-Vance, M., Enghild, J., Salvesen, G. S., and Roses, A. D. (1993). Apolipoprotein E: High-avidity binding to β- amyloid and increased frequency of type 4 allele in late-onset familial Alzheimer disease. *Proc. Natl. Acad. Sci. U.S.A.* 90, 1977–1981.

Sullivan, E. V., March, L., Mathalon, D. H., Lim, K. O., and Pfefferbaum, A. (1995). Age-related decline in MRI volumes of temporal lobe gray matter but not hip- pocampus. *Neurobiol. Aging* 16, 591–606.

Sullivan, E. V., Marsh, L., and Pfefferbaum, A. (2005). Pre- servation of hippocampal volume throughout adulthood in healthy men and women. *Neurobiol. Aging* 26, 1093–1098.

Thomas, J. L. (1985). Visual memory: adult age differences in map recall and learning strategies. *Exp. Aging Res.* 11, 93–95.

Thorndyke, P. W., and Hayes-Roth, B. (1982). Differences in spatial knowl- edge acquired from maps and navi- gation. *Cogn. Psychol.* 14, 560–589.

Tobler, W. R. (1994). Bidimensional regression. *Geogr. Anal.* 26, 187–212. Vlček, K. (2011). "Spatial naviga- tion impairment in healthy aging and Alzheimer's disease," in *The Clinical Spectrum of Alzheimer's Disease: The Charge Toward Comprehensive Diagnostic and Therapeutic Strategies,* ed S. M. de la Monte (Rijeka, Croatia: InTech), 75–100.

Waterman, S., and Gordon, D. (1984). A quantitative-comparative app- roach to analysis of distortion in mental maps. *Prof. Geogr.* 36, 326–337.

Wilkniss, S. M., Jones, M. G., Korol, D. L., Gold, P. E., and Manning, C. A. (1997). Age-related differences in an ecologically based study of route learning. *Psychol. Aging* 12, 372–375.

Zakzanis, K. K., Quintin, G., Graham, S. J., and Mraz, R. (2009). Age and dementia related differences in spatial navigation within an immersive virtual environment. *Med. Sci. Monit.* 15, CR140–CR150.

# Permissions

All chapters in this book were first published in EAREBB & SMAUWHPA, by Frontiers; hereby published with permission under the Creative Commons Attribution License or equivalent. Every chapter published in this book has been scrutinized by our experts. Their significance has been extensively debated. The topics covered herein carry significant findings which will fuel the growth of the discipline. They may even be implemented as practical applications or may be referred to as a beginning point for another development.

The contributors of this book come from diverse backgrounds, making this book a truly international effort. This book will bring forth new frontiers with its revolutionizing research information and detailed analysis of the nascent developments around the world.

We would like to thank all the contributing authors for lending their expertise to make the book truly unique.

They have played a crucial role in the development of this book. Without their invaluable contributions this book wouldn't have been possible. They have made vital efforts to compile up to date information on the varied aspects of this subject to make this book a valuable addition to the collection of many professionals and students.

This book was conceptualized with the vision of imparting up-to-date information and advanced data in this field. To ensure the same, a matchless editorial board was set up. Every individual on the board went through rigorous rounds of assessment to prove their worth. After which they invested a large part of their time researching and compiling the most relevant data for our readers.

The editorial board has been involved in producing this book since its inception. They have spent rigorous hours researching and exploring the diverse topics which have resulted in the successful publishing of this book. They have passed on their knowledge of decades through this book. To expedite this challenging task, the publisher supported the team at every step. A small team of assistant editors was also appointed to further simplify the editing procedure and attain best results for the readers.

Apart from the editorial board, the designing team has also invested a significant amount of their time in understanding the subject and creating the most relevant covers. They scrutinized every image to scout for the most suitable representation of the subject and create an appropriate cover for the book.

The publishing team has been an ardent support to the editorial, designing and production team. Their endless efforts to recruit the best for this project, has resulted in the accomplishment of this book. They are a veteran in the field of academics and their pool of knowledge is as vast as their experience in printing. Their expertise and guidance has proved useful at every step. Their uncompromising quality standards have made this book an exceptional effort. Their encouragement from time to time has been an inspiration for everyone.

The publisher and the editorial board hope that this book will prove to be a valuable piece of knowledge for researchers, students, practitioners and scholars across the globe.

# List of Contributors

**Eric S. Allard and Elizabeth A. Kensinger**
Cognitive and Affective Neuroscience Laboratory, Department of Psychology, Boston College, Chestnut Hill, MA, USA

**Manuel C. Voelkle, Ulman Lindenberger and Michaela Riediger**
Center for Lifespan Psychology, Max Planck Institute for Human Development, Berlin, Germany

**Natalie C. Ebner**
Department of Psychology, University of Florida, Gainesville, FL, USA

**Natalie C. Ebner**
Psychology, Social Cognitive and Affective Development Lab, Department of Psychology, University of Florida, Gainesville, FL, USA

**Håkan Fischer**
Department of Psychology, Stockholm University, Stockholm, Sweden

**Michaela Riediger, Markus Studtmann, Andrea Westphal and Antje Rauers**
Max Planck Research Group "Affect Across the Lifespan, "Max Planck Institute for Human Development, Berlin, Germany

**Hannelore Weber**
Institute for Psychology, University of Greifswald, Greifswald, Germany

**Raluca Petrican, Morris Moscovitch and Cheryl Grady**
Departmen of Psychology and Psychiatry, Rotman Research Institute, University of Toronto, Toronto, ON, Canada

**Tammy English**
Department of Psychology, Washington University in St. Louis, St. Louis, MO, USA

**Laura L. Carstensen**
Department of Psychology, Stanford University, Stanford, CA, USA

**Sanda Dolcos and Yuta Katsumi**
Department of Psychology, University of Illinoisat Urbana-Champaign, Champaign, IL, USA

**Roger A. Dixon**
Department of Psychology, University of Alberta, Edmonton, AB, Canada

**Philipp C. Opitz and Heather L. Urry**
Department of Psychology, Tufts University, Medford, MA, USA

**Ihno A. Lee and James J. Gross**
Department of Psychology, Stanford University, Stanford, CA, USA

**Didem Pehlivanoglu, Shivangi Jain and Robert Arie land Paul Verhaeghen**
School of Psychology, Georgia Institute of Technology, Atlanta, GA, USA

**Ute Kunzmann and Cathleen Kappes**
Institute of Psychology, University of Leipzig, Leipzig, Germany

**Carsten Wrosch**
Department of Psychology, Concordia University, Montreal, QC, Canada

**Joakim Svärd**
Aging Research Center, Karolins ka Institutet and Stockholm University, Stockholm, Sweden

**Håkan Fischer**
Aging Research Center, Karolins ka Institutet and Stockholm University, Stockholm, Sweden
Department of Psychology, Stockholm University, Stockholm, Sweden

**Daniel Lundqvist**
Department of Clinical Neuroscience, Karolinska Institutet, Stockholm, Sweden

**Kyoko Konishi and Véronique D. Bohbot**
Department of Psychiatry, Douglas Institute, McGill University, Verdun, QC, Canada

**Linda Truong and Lixia Yang**
Department of Psychology, Ryerson University, Toronto, ON, Canada

**Veronique D. Bohbot, Sam Mc Kenzie, Kyoko Konishi, Celine Fouquet and Vanessa Kurdi**
Department of Psychiatry, Douglas Institute, McGill University, Verdun, QC, Canada

**Russel Schachar**
Hospital for Sick Children, Toronto, ON, Canada

**Michel Boivin**
Deptartment of Psychology, Université de Laval, Quebec, QC, Canada

**Philippe Robaey**
Department of Psychiatry, Ste-Justine Research Center, Montreal, QC, Canada

**Brittany S. Cassidy and Angela H. Gutchess**
Department of Psychology, Brandeis University, Waltham, MA, USA

**Trey Hedden**
Athinoula A. Martinos Center for BiomedicalI maging, Massachusetts General Hospital, Boston, MA, USA

**Carolyn Yoon**
University of Michigan, Ann Arbor, MI, USA

**Mara Fölster and Katja Werheid**
Clinical Gerontopsychology, Department of Psychology, Humboldt-Universität zu Berlin, Berlin, Germany

**Ursula Hess**
Social and Organizational Psychology, Department of Psychology, Humboldt-Universität zuBerlin, Berlin, Germany

**R. Shayna Rosenbaum**
Neuroscience Graduate Diploma Program, Department of Psychology, York University, Toronto, ON, Canada
Rotman Research Institute, Baycrest, Toronto, ON, Canada

**Gordon Winocur**
Rotman Research Institute, Baycrest, Toronto, ON, Canada
Department of Psychology, University of Toronto, Toronto, ON, Canada
Department of Psychiatry, University of Toronto, Toronto, ON, Canada
Department of Psychology, Trent University, Peterborough, ON, Canada

**Malcolm A. Binns**
Dalla Lana School of Public Health, University of Toronto, Toronto, ON, Canada
Rotman Research Institute, Baycrest, Toronto, ON, Canada

**Morris Moscovitch**
Rotman Research Institute, Baycrest, Toronto, ON, Canada
Department of Psychology, University of Toronto, Toronto, ON, Canada
Department of Psychology, Baycrest, Toronto, ON, Canada

**Marsha R. Penner and Sheri J .Y. Mizumori**
Laboratory of Neural Systems, Decision Science, Learning and Memory, Department of Psychology, University of Washington, Seattle, WA, USA

**Mathew A. Harris**
Centre for Cognitive and Neural Systems, University of Edinburgh, Edinburgh, UK
Centre for Cognitive Ageing and Cognitive Epidemiology, University of Edinburgh, Edinburgh, UK

**Jan M. Wiener**
Psychology Research Centre, Bournemouth University, Poole, UK

**Thomas Wolbers**
Centre for Cognitive and Neural Systems, University of Edinburgh, Edinburgh, UK
Centre for Cognitive Ageing and Cognitive Epidemiology, University of Edinburgh, Edinburgh, UK
German Center for Neurodegenerative Diseases, Otto-von-Guericke University, Magdeburg, Germany

**Ivana Gazova, Zuzana Nedelska, Jan Laczó and Jakub Hort**
Department of Neurology, Memory Disorders Clinic, 2nd Faculty of Medicine, Charles Universityin Pragueand University Hospital Motol, Prague 5, Czech Republic
International Clinical Research Center and St. Anne's University Hospital Brno, Brno, Czech Republic

**Kamil Vlcek**
International Clinical Research Center and St. Anne's University Hospital Brno, Brno, Czech Republic
Department of Neurophysiology of Memory, Institute of Physiology Academy of Sciences of the Czech Republic v.v.i., Prague, Czech Republic

**Eva Hyncicova and Ivana Mokrisova**
Department of Neurology, Memory Disorders Clinic, 2nd Faculty of Medicine, Charles Universityin Pragueand University Hospital Motol, Prague 5, Czech Republic

**Katerina Sheardova**
International Clinical Research Center and St. Anne's University Hospital Brno, Brno, Czech Republic

**Diane E. Adamo**
Eugene Applebaum College of Pharmacy and Health Sciences, Wayne State University, Detroit, MI, USA
Institute of Gerontology, Wayne State University, Detroit, MI, USA

**Emily M. Briceño**
Department of Psychology, Wayne State University, Detroit, MI, USA

**Joseph A. Sindone**
Department of Linguistics, University of Michigan, AnnArbor, MI, USA

**Neil B. Alexander**
Mobility Research Center, Geriatrics Centerand Division of Geriatric Medicine, University of Michigan Hospitals and Veterans Affairs Ann Arbor Health Care System Geriatric Research Education and Clinical Center, Ann Arbor, MI, USA

**Scott D. Moffat**
School of Psychology, Georgia Institute of Technology, Atlanta, GA, USA

**Heikki Tanila**
A. I. Virtanen Institute, University of Eastern Finland, Kuopio, Finland

**Heather M. Holden**
Department of Psychology, San Diego State University, San Diego, CA, USA

**Paul E. Gilbert**
Department of Psychology, San Diego State University, San Diego, CA, USA
San Diego State University, University of California San Diego Joint Doctoral Programin Clinical Psychology, San Diego, CA, USA

**Joyce L. W. Yau and Jonathan R. Seckl**
Centre for Cognitive Ageingand Cognitive Epidemiology and Endocrinology Unit,Centre for Cardiovascular Science, The Queen's Medical Research Institute, University of Edinburgh, Edinburgh, UK

**Jan M. Wiener, Hana Kmecova and Olivier de Condappa**
Psychology Research Centre, Bournemouth University, Poole, UK

**George Pengas, Guy B. Williams, Julio Acosta-Cabronero, Tom W. J. Ash, Young T. Hong, David Izquierdo-Garcia, Tim D. Fryer and Peter J. Nestor**
Department of Clinical Neurosciences, University of Cambridge, Cambridge, UK

**John R. Hodges**
Neuroscience Research Australia, Sydney, NSW, Australia

**Naohide Yamamoto and Gregory J. DeGirolamo**
Department of Psychology, Cleveland State University, Cleveland, OH, USA

# Index

www.ingramcontent.com/pod-product-compliance
Lightning Source LLC
LaVergne TN
LVHW080925210926
848485LV00004B/730